Housing and Home Services for the Disabled

Guidelines and Experiences in Independent Living

GINI LAURIE
Editor/Publisher and Founder,
Rehabilitation Gazette,
St. Louis, Missouri

With contributions by Donna McGwinn and Joseph Scott Laurie

Cartoons by Robert E. Tanton, Jr.

WITHDRAWN

Medical Department
Harper & Row, Publishers
Hagerstown, Maryland
New York, San Francisco, London

77–78–79–80–81–82–10–9–8–7–6–5–4–3–2–1

HD
7293.
L38

Text and cover designed by Alice J. Sellers

HOUSING AND HOME SERVICES FOR THE DISABLED: Guidelines and Experiences in Independent Living. Copyright © 1977 by Harper & Row, Publishers, Inc. All rights reserved. No part of this book may be used or reproduced in any manner whatsoever without written permission except in the case of brief quotations embodied in critical articles and reviews. Printed in the United States of America. For information address Medical Department, Harper & Row, Publishers, Inc., 2350 Virginia Avenue, Hagerstown, Maryland 21740

Library of Congress Cataloging in Publication Data

Laurie, Gini, 1913–
  Housing and home services for the disabled.

  Includes bibliographies and index.
  1. Housing for physically handicapped. 2. Architecture and the physically handicapped. 3. Home care services. I. McGwinn, Donna, 1936– joint author.
II. Laurie, Joseph Scott, 1908– joint author.
III. Title.
HD7293.L38   362.4   76–19924
ISBN 0–06–141518–9

Vivamus atque amemus

Contents

Contributors ix
Foreword I xi
Foreword II xiii
Preface xv
Acknowledgments xvii

1 Signposts to Barrier Free Living 1
2 Adaptations to Housing 11
3 Kitchen Adaptations 32
4 Bathroom Adaptations 56
5 Independent Living Experiences 64
   Donna McGwinn
6 Attendant Care 84
   Donna McGwinn
7 Organized Home Services 100
8 California Attendant Programs 119
9 Transitional Projects 139
10 Apartment Living Arrangements 162
11 Long-Term Residential Facilities 186
12 Mobile Homes 204
13 HUD-Assisted Housing Projects 212
14 Projects in the United States That Faded or Failed 247
15 Alternatives for the Developmentally Disabled 256
16 Statistics, Legislation, Standards, Codes, and Studies 286
17 Canada 306
18 International Experiences 334

APPENDICES

Appendix A—International Symbol of Access   389

Appendix B—Accessibility for Disabled Persons—   390
Norms in Different Countries

Appendix C—Michigan State Housing Development   392
Authority Mentally Retarded Housing Program—
Guidelines—February, 1974

Appendix D—The Swedish Fokus Society   396

Appendix E—Rehabilitation Gazette Available   401
Back Issues

Appendix F—Resources for Architects and Planners   403

INDEX   417

Contributors

Marji Cappel
Chapter 18
Germany section
Elmstein/Pfalz, West Germany

D. J. Forward
Chapter 18
South Australia section
Member, International Association of Mouth and Foot Painting Artists, Blackwood, South Australia

Erich Krell
Chapter 18
South Australia section
Member, International Association of Mouth and Foot Painting Artists, Blackwood, South Australia

Joseph Scott Laurie
Foreword II
Co-Editor, Rehabilitation Gazette, St. Louis, Missouri

Donna McGwinn
Chapters 5, 6
Book Editor, Rehabilitation Gazette, Grand River, Ohio

Adolf Ratzka, M.A.
Chapter 18
Sweden section
Doctoral Candidate, University of California, Los Angeles; Stockholm, Sweden

Isabel P. Robinault, Ph.D.
Foreword
Supervisor, Research Utilization Laboratory, ICD Rehabilitation and Research Center, New York, New York

Foreword I

This book is written by the right people at the right time. Few workers in the field of rehabilitation have the contacts with recipients of the helping services that Gini Laurie and her husband, Joe, have as volunteers. Most professionals know *about* disabled people whom we see more or less periodically during established appointments. The Lauries have known them as colleagues and friends since 1949 and as reader contributors since their first journal *Toomey j Gazette* was launched in 1958 for and by the disabled. It is the disabled who turned *Toomey j* into an international journal, now called *Rehabilitation Gazette,* by using it as an around-the-world forum for their opinions, their goals, and their experiences. As a result, every concept and project mentioned within this book is people-generated and people-tested. All over the world, creative disabled people have found some living arrangement, some housing format, or some environmental adjustment suitable to their needs and to their tastes, and they have shared these in this book. Indeed, this book is written with the right people—Donna McGwinn and dozens of others who are severely disabled.

To say that it is written at the right time may seem overoptimistic during the present lull in funding for more functional construction, barrier-free environments, and varied patterns of community living. Moreover, there are about 300 million people in the world with highly visible deformities, and in 1973 the disabled population of the United States was estimated to be 20,608,900. These people are still waiting for action. How can this be the right time?

Until recently, the disabled had been lumped into one amorphous mass—they were *different.* As long as that attitude persisted, housing and living solutions were simplistic in concept and delayed because they were considered a minority need. However, modern research has shown that the disabled are not a homogeneous entity—physically, mentally, or emotionally. The pilot projects discussed in this book demonstrate a wide variety of solutions for some people with a wide variety of disabilities. What's more, the general population can take advantage of many of these solutions. Many of these pilot projects for the disabled can also be seen as more thoughtful prototypes of better living for the able-bodied, including our senior citizens. The authors of this book have taken the information explosion on this subject and have translated it into ways-of-living prototypes, useful to both the able and the disabled. Now is the right time for all of us to reap from this harvest of ingenuity. What are we waiting for?

Isabel P. Robinault, Ph.D.
Research Utilization Laboratory,
ICD Rehabilitation and Research Center,
New York, New York

Foreword II

HOUSING AND HOME SERVICES FOR THE DISABLED is being published at a time when the problems of the disabled are finally being recognized universally. It is a time when many of the previous efforts to effect legislation have become reality. Now, attempts to further this legislation so that it will encompass services, health care, integrated housing, and the abolition of environmental barriers are the goal of concerned groups and individuals. Coalitions of the disabled are coming together to weld their separate efforts into a task force with the power of concerted action.

Architectural barriers are being slowly supplanted through education and enactment of building codes which recognize the monstrosity of what has been built in the past and how cheaply modifications can be incorporated. New standards of accessibilities help to lessen the problems of the disabled and elderly and add safety and a new convenience to the general environment for all persons. However, elimination of architectural barriers involves the efforts of relatively few individuals influencing relatively few members of the government and governmental agencies. Sadly, it is the attitudinal barriers which will more slowly be eliminated—the barriers of prejudice founded on fear . . . fear of the palsied, fear of the physically impaired, and fear of the retarded . . . almost as if these disabled might be contagious. Too many people look on the disabled with pity, not with understanding; with revulsion, not with sympathy. Would that there were methods and means to provide and encourage more personal relationships between these faint-hearted and their less fortunate fellows, then the future might see a rebirth of care for one's neighbor, for the aged next door, and for the disadvantaged. These selfsame skeptics might realize that *all* are capable of enjoying fulfilling love, as basic human beings, without corresponding to Madison Avenue's projected image of the perpetually youthful idol. It will come, but it will come slowly.

Joseph Scott Laurie
Co-Editor, Rehabilitation Gazette,
St. Louis, Missouri

Preface

Society has a new complex of housing problems because the elderly live longer and many people survive catastrophic accidents and diseases that in the past were usually fatal. Although many of these healthy elderly and healthy but disabled persons could live independently with supportive services, they are kept in hospitals, shunted into nursing homes, or suppressed at home because society is not prepared to cope with them. To liberate themselves from these circumstances, some disabled individuals and voluntary groups have developed innovative experiments in humane living. Many efforts failed, but much more importantly, many succeeded.

The primary purpose of this book is to present information on a worldwide assortment of housing experiments in order to enable government agencies, voluntary organizations, groups of disabled persons, and individuals to find either specific solutions to problems or pertinent examples to use as models. Although the information here is specific and useful, I have sought also to provide a unique insight into the subjective reactions of severely disabled individuals to their environment and to demonstrate that even the most severely disabled individuals can be self-supporting. Thus, this book should not only provide facts but also should be of creative assistance to architects, occupational and physical therapists, social workers, rehabilitation counselors, and government housing, rehabilitation, and veterans agencies as well as volunteer organizations in the United States, Canada, England, and many other countries.

HOUSING AND HOME SERVICES FOR THE DISABLED includes summaries of legislation and of principal professional surveys and studies, lists of equipment sources and literature related to housing around the world, and the experiences and criticisms of a great many disabled persons. I have presented the material in this way to demonstrate the ingenuity and adaptability of severely disabled individuals in coping with independent living situations and to stress that the problems of housing, employment, supportive services, and transportation are inextricably intertwined with successful rehabilitation.

This smorgasbord of examples of housing arrangements and services emphasizes that there is no universal solution to the housing problem and that each individual, each group, and each community not only can learn from the experiences of others but must also create its own special solution. Further, these examples trace the development of housing from segregation in large facilities toward integration within the community in a variety of barrier free housing at all economic levels.

Costs of care of the elderly, retarded, and disabled can be substantially reduced by alternatives to institutionalization. Several studies have estimated that when the costs of home services are balanced against nursing home costs, four severely disabled individuals can live at home for the cost of maintaining one in a nursing home. For both economic and humane reasons, the rules of government must be amended to make independent living as feasible as nursing home subsistence.

This book includes references to legislation and housing projects designed for the elderly and developmentally disabled because they are also significant to the physically disabled. It includes their common problems of rigid licensing procedures and zoning that inhibit group living arrangements and covers their common needs for central information services, ombudsmen, adaptations to existing housing, equipment, respite care, transitional facilities, involvement in planning and management, modifications of building codes, and ongoing support from rehabilitation centers. Many of these adaptations and modifications will benefit also the general public; though the problems of the wheelchaired are the most obvious, one in ten persons has trouble negotiating steps, going through revolving doors, getting up curbs, finding accessible housing, and using public transportation.

Through sharing the actual experiences of thousands of groups and individuals with housing and home services in many countries, readers who are disabled will learn ways of adapting existing housing, of handling attendants, of acquiring the techniques which make living with a disability less handicapping, and of working together to create integrated housing in a more hospitable total environment. I hope that professional personnel will also find these experiences, resources, and information useful in understanding and solving the problems of persons who are disabled, retarded, and elderly.

G.L.

Acknowledgments

The acknowledgments for this book could cover many pages because so many generous people, both disabled and nondisabled, have given their time to help create it. Among the nondisabled, I am most grateful to my husband Joe and to Eleanor Bjorkman for their extraordinary helpfulness. I wish to express my warm appreciation to Nancy Cole, Dorothy Davis, Frances Payne, Judy Raymond, Kathy Sheehan, and Richard Ward who helped with the proofing, typing, and preparation of the manuscript. I am deeply grateful to all who supplied data and who corrected the chapters relating to their fields of expertise.

My bounteous thanks to our many friends who are severely disabled for their invaluable assistance in gathering facts about housing projects and services in this country and abroad and in sharing their own experiences in homemaking, in achieving independent living, and in adapting their homes. I am particularly indebted to Donna McGwinn who contributed the chapters on attendants and independent living experiences, to Bob Tanton who created the cartoons, to Adolf Ratzka for his section on Sweden, and to Marji Cappel for her section on Germany.

Disability has been a part of my life since the year before I was born when an epidemic of poliomyelitis caused the deaths of two sisters and left an older brother severely disabled. Until his death, 15 years later, I acted as his auxiliary arms and legs. My concern for the problems of the disabled was rekindled during the epidemic of 1949 when I started working as a volunteer with "iron lung polios." During the ensuing 27 years of volunteering, my husband and I through our *Rehabilitation Gazette* have made thousands of severely disabled friends in every state and in 83 countries. Indirectly, they have all contributed to this book.

Without such treasured help, this book could not have been written.

G.L.

Housing and Home Services for the Disabled

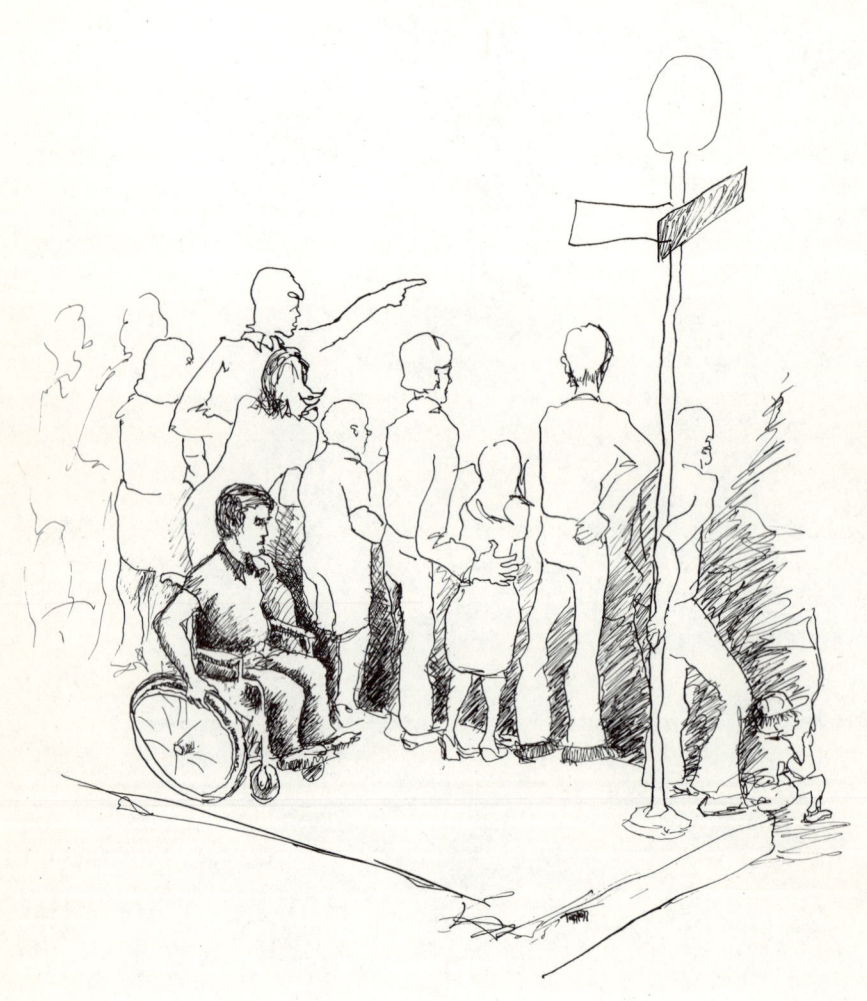

"A person who is severely impaired never knows his hidden sources of strength until he is treated like a normal human being and encouraged to shape his own life."

Helen Keller

1
Signposts to Barrier Free Living

The starting point for solving the housing problems of the disabled and the elderly is to treat them like normal human beings; to see them as people with disabilities, not as disabled people; to see them as people who are aging, not as aged people; to see them as people who are mentally retarded, not as mentally retarded people; to see their essential humanity, their need to love and to be loved, their vitality, their potential for growth and accomplishment. It is essential to realize that their housing problems are inextricably intertwined with the housing problems of the entire population and can be solved only as the problems of all others are solved, not separately, but through integration within normal housing.

Housing for most severely disabled and many elderly persons must include services to replace the helping hands of the old days. Services are even more important than housing. Accessible housing without services is useless to the severely disabled and fully liberating to those less severely disabled only if solutions to the other problems of income, employment, and transportation are also available. No one knows how many disabled persons are unemployed because of a lack of accessible public transportation and accessible housing. It is certain that many more would be employed if these two problems were solved.

The most basic service needed is a source of information with individualized attention. National, regional, and local independent living information centers should be established. These information centers, largely staffed by disabled individuals and working with existing voluntary and government agencies, should provide information on a face-to-face basis, or by telephone, or letter. They should maintain lists of accessible housing, attendants, and respite and holiday facilities. They should furnish information on employment, transportation, welfare programs and legislation as well as provide peer counseling and act as ombudsmen.

Housing is not a farm house or a townhouse or an apartment or a flat. Housing is the total environment—the people who share the housing, the neighbors, the neighborhood, the shops, the recreation, the employment, and the transportation. Housing is the focus of the human need for security and shelter, for privacy and independence, for the approval of family, friends, and neighbors.

Eventually, the total environment—physical and psychological—must be made hospitable to those with problems of mobility, of sight, of hearing, of retardation, or of aging. Public transportation, public buildings, public schools, public sidewalks, and all facilities used and financed by the public must be made accessible. Awareness of the problems of accessibility must be made an integral part of the education and training of architects, urban planners, real estate personnel, builders, and contractors. Accessibility specifications must be built into local building codes as well as national standards.

Percentages of residential units must be made accessible and adaptable. A choice of housing in a range of prices, areas, and types must be made available so that disabled and elderly individuals have the same freedom to move as nondisabled and younger persons. They have this freedom of choice only if they have a selection of accommodations and the income or its equivalent in subsidies and services to afford a choice.

POST-WAR CHANGES IN HOUSING PATTERNS

World War II triggered a massive change in the housing patterns of most of the civilized world. Movements from farms and small communities to cities, from large households of many generations to small families and apartments, caused far-reaching upheavals in lifestyles. The more recent scarcities of reasonably priced houses, of public transportation, and of gasoline complicate the lives of those on both sides of the Atlantic and Pacific. Unemployment and inadequate educational facilities are common problems. Inflation and recession stalk the world.

INCREASING NUMBERS OF DISABLED AND ELDERLY

World War II also spurred changes in medical management and technologic advances that resulted in a large increase in the number of disabled and older persons. In the United States, for instance, there are now more than 20 million people who are 65 years of age or older, representing nearly 10% of the population. These numbers have increased dramatically since 1900, when the average life span was 47 years and only 4% were 65 and older. The percentage will increase further in response to the declining birthrate and improved health care services. Medical discoveries, particularly the antibiotics that conquer pneumonia and infections, are adding years to the lives of the elderly and the disabled. The problem now is to discover ways and means to add life to those years.

HOUSING IN THE 1950s AND EARLY 1960s

These were the years when "iron lung polios" demonstrated that even the most severely disabled individuals can live fulfilling lives in their own homes if they have comprehensive rehabilitation, a resource center, and financial support for equipment, home adaptations, and attendant care. These vital supporting factors were made possible through the generosity of the public to their polio societies. People in Great Britain, Europe, Canada, South America, Australia, New Zealand, and the United States opened their purses to help polio disabled and kept them open until their fears were removed by the vaccine.

Economy was behind the exodus from custodial care in hospitals to home care. The March of Dimes in the United States began in 1950 to put an end to the tremendous cost of maintaining respiratory poliomyelitis patients on custodial care in hospitals and nursing homes. It initiated a superb system of 17 respiratory and rehabilitation centers at teaching hospitals of medical schools throughout the country, totaling over 500 treatment and rehabilitation beds. These centers demonstrated the tremendous value of the team approach; of quickly available money at the local chapter level for equipment, home adaptations, and attendant care; of a center of information and support; and of a one-to-one relationship with the local chapters of the March of Dimes.

The team approach included the hospital staff as well as the patient, his family, his physician, and his community. The key to rehabilitation was the weekly staff–patient conference and the cooperative relationship that developed, plus the carefully orchestrated trial home visits. The flow of monies covered everything from remodeling kitchens and bathrooms to hydraulic lifts, every conceivable type of respiratory equipment, including duplicates of equipment for emergencies, generators, and free maintenance of all equipment.

It was the payment for attendant care, however, that was the magic ingredient that made it possible for families to take care of their disabled husband, wife, or child. The payments averaged $100–$300/month, varying widely around the country.

Specific figures attesting to the value of the system were reported by Dr. Kenneth S. Landauer at the Fourth International Poliomyelitis Conference in Geneva, Switzerland, in 1957. Because of improvements in medical management, the case fatality rate fell from 6.5 in 1949 to 3.6 in 1956. From the opening of the first center in 1950 to September, 1956, 4196 severely paralyzed poliomyelitis patients had been admitted to the centers, and 3802 had been discharged. Most significant, of the 918 who were permanently dependent upon artificial respiratory equipment, 845 (92%) were released from hospitals to return to their homes.

Dr. Landauer estimated that the costs of caring for patients at home were one-tenth to one-fourth of what hospital costs would have been. He pointed out another fact of economic significance that is important in all types of chronic illness, "The later in the disease the patient is admitted for rehabilitation, the harder the job, the longer the period needed, the less the benefits, and the greater the cost."

After Salk and Sabin vanquished poliomyelitis, the funds no longer poured into the March of Dimes, and the organization eventually turned its energies to birth defects. It was forced to curtail support of individuals, except for equipment maintenance, and to close the respiratory centers. The sudden cessation of attendant care funds caused waves of fright. Fortunately, the disabled had had enough years of experience at home to toughen them, and they managed to muddle through. Several of these "old polios" were the leaders of the many unsuccessful efforts during these years to establish housing facilities for the disabled in the United States.

With the exception of the special attention given to those disabled by poliomyelitis, the 1950s and early 1960s were the years of various forms of institutionalization as solutions to the lack of housing and home service arrangements for the growing numbers of disabled and elderly. They ranged from England's geriatric hospitals and altruistic segregated residences to the United States' nursing home "industry." Denmark alone pioneered an apartment building with a mix of disabled and nondisabled persons, including special provisions for a few disabled by poliomyelitis who required respiratory aids.

HOUSING IN THE LATE 1960s AND EARLY 1970s

Shortly after the regional respiratory centers were closed in the early 1960s, the number of spinal cord injured and other disabled individuals began to rise. The timing was tragic, for the expertise of the team approach and the comprehensive resource functions acquired in dealing with poliomyelitis quadriplegics could have been transferred to those who are quadriplegic because of disease or injury. Currently, the rehabilitation and needs for housing and home service programs of the spinal cord injured are the most obvious around the world, and it is for them that most of the present housing for the physically disabled is being planned. Though England pioneered the treatment and set up centers around the country, only the principal center has a small hostel for those who need a further adjustment period and those who are unable to return home. Canada's nationwide system, directed by spinal cord injured persons, most nearly approaches the regional respiratory center system of following through and dealing directly with each individual's problem.

In the United States, there is no comprehensive nationwide system that approaches that of the poliomyelitis regional centers. Though there are a few regional spinal cord injury centers for civilians and VA spinal cord injury centers for the large number of injured Vietnam veterans, there are not enough centers. There are no comparable programs of payments for attendant care, equipment, home adaptations, or after-care. There are no accurate counts of spinal cord injured individuals, or of those with any disability, and realistic plans cannot be made until realistic numbers are available.

Planning should be based on market studies and an accurate count of the disabled and elderly population that would include information on the type of housing needed, functional ability, and requirements in the areas of services, adaptations, and equipment. A mere listing of disabilities or a census count of wheelchair users is not enough because individuals vary so widely in the way they are affected or how they cope with disability. They vary widely not only in relation to others with the same disability but in their own developing or regressing ability to deal with disability.

Based on the respiratory center experiences, the sums being wasted on custodial care might well pay for enough additional centers to orchestrate home adaptations, attendant care, and other services so that disabled individuals could be assisted to work out their solutions, singly or in groups, to fit their particular choices of lifestyles. When the costs of home services are balanced against nursing home costs, four severely disabled individuals could live at home for the cost of one in a nursing home.

The early 1970s are the years of the beginning of deinstitutionalization. The tide around the world is starting to turn from the large specialized housing projects that separated those who are disabled from the community to housing integrated within the community. The disabled are becoming involved in planning their own integrated facilities and attendant services. The mentally retarded are being represented by well-organized advocates.

NEW POSSIBILITIES IN THE 1970s

In the United States, new possibilities for services, housing, and the removal of attitudinal and architectural barriers are opening through legislation such as the Rehabilitation Act of 1973, the Housing and Community Development Act of 1974, the Developmental Disabilities Acts, the Rehabilitation Act Amendments of 1974, and the Social Services Amendments of 1974 and through an increased consciousness of human rights and needs.

NATIONAL CENTER FOR A BARRIER FREE ENVIRONMENT

Convened by Goodwill Industries of America in Houston and sponsored by HUD and HEW, a national conference on housing in September, 1974, brought together individuals and representatives of the voluntary and governmental agencies concerned with housing for the disabled. One of the most active participants was the National Center for a Barrier Free Environment, 8401 Connecticut Avenue, Washington, D.C. 20015, which had been established in January, 1974.

Membership in the nonprofit organization is open to professional as well as disabled persons. It publishes a newsletter, REPORT, and is developing an information exchange and referral system related to barrier free design, to serve as a clearinghouse of information on such topics as legal and court action, legislation, building and zoning codes, housing, affirmative action plans for employers, transportation and travel, community surveys, and school accessibility. Meanwhile, it responds to inquiries on barrier free design or refers them to experts among its membership.

One of its major projects is the administration of a national design competition for adaptable housing with funding of $100,000 from HUD and the sanction of the American Institute of Architects. The winning design may be built as a prototype for adaptable housing and as a testing mechanism for the new American National Standards Institute (ANSI) criteria developed by Syracuse University School of Architecture.

WHITE HOUSE CONFERENCE ON HANDICAPPED INDIVIDUALS

Legislated by the Rehabilitation Act Amendments of 1974, the White House Conference on Handicapped Individuals should prove as effective for the disabled as a similar conference did for the elderly, delineating their problems and pointing the way toward solutions. The executive director of the Conference, scheduled for the spring of 1977, is Jack F. Smith, who is wheelchaired as the result of poliomyelitis. The Conference is concerned with attitudes of the general public, civil rights, the elimination of environmental barriers, residential and community based programs, and educational and recreational opportunities. The Conference is designed to provide an opportunity for disabled persons to make their concerns known and to take a major leadership role. Headquarters for the Conference is 1832 M Street, N.W., Suite 801, Washington, D.C. 20036.

STATE REPORTS ON NEEDS OF THE DISABLED

An outstanding example of involvement on the state level is documented in the *Final Report of Wisconsin's Task Force on Problems of People with Physical Handicaps. July 19, 1974.* This 416-page report reflects 18 months of work directed by Representative James W. Wahner, 201 East Washington Avenue, Room 269, Madison, Wisconsin 53702. It is the product of eight regional public hearings that totaled 135 hours of testimony by 400 witnesses and extensive committee meetings. The report considers each phase of the environment as it affects the disabled—civil rights, architecture, transportation and streets, education, rehabilitation, employment, recreation, taxation, and Medicare—and makes specific recommendations to the governor, the legislature, and various state departments, agencies, and bureaus.

A similar statewide summary of needs was prepared in Minnesota and presented in a 21-page statement at the 1974 Minnesota Governor's Conference on Handicapped Persons. The statement, developed by a coalition of over 80 committees, consumer groups, public agencies, and private organizations, discussed early and periodic screening, education, health, environmental barriers, community alternatives and institution reform, rehabilitation and employment, human and legal rights, consumer concerns. Copies are available from Minnesota Commission for the Handicapped, 492 Metro Square, St. Paul, Minnesota 55101.

BARRIER FREE DESIGN CONSULTING FIRM

INTERFACE, Box 5688, Raleigh, North Carolina 27607, is organized by a firm of human factors design consultants specializing in barrier free design. It offers complete consulting services for new and remodelled buildings and residential and recreation facilities. The firm is compiling a research and information clearinghouse and it will assist organizations to develop workshops on architectural barriers.

LIBERATION MOVEMENTS OF THE ELDERLY

Following the White House Conference on Aging in 1961 the organized groups of older persons have been increasingly successful in accomplishing their objectives through legislation. Gale's *Encyclopedia of Associations* lists about 15 organizations concerned with aging. Among those listed are The American Association of Retired Persons, the National Council on the Aging, the National Retired Teachers Association, the National Council of Senior Citizens, the Golden Ring

Council of Senior Citizens, the League of Elderly Gentlemen in Reduced Circumstances, the Gray Panthers, and Flying Senior Citizens of the U.S. They have influenced legislation such as the Older Americans Act and have effected tax relief, low cost housing, day care centers, reduced fares on mass transportation, and regional centers to promote their needs. Some of the groups offer housing directories, travel tours, insurance, counseling, purchase of drugs at reduced rates, and information services.

In England, Age Concern (National Old People's Welfare Council) is a national center for information and advice on all aspects of care of the elderly. It advises the government on legislation affecting the elderly, represents their needs to the public, operates a comprehensive information service, and supports local groups.

LIBERATION MOVEMENTS OF THE DISABLED

One of the earliest and most successful of the liberation movements was England's Disablement Income Group (DIG). As part of the organization's efforts to prod the government into action, a protest parade to 10 Downing Street in September, 1969, by some of the 70 surviving respiratory polios dramatized the need of all disabled for an allowance to enable them to live at home instead of in hospitals. About 20 men and women, in iron lungs on truck beds or using respirators in wheelchairs, led the parade.

In October, 1974, about 1000 disabled members of DIG Scotland marched in wheelchairs in the pouring rain to the music of the pipers to publicize the plight of the Scottish disabled. Union of the Physically Impaired Against Segregation (UPIAS) presents the view of actual or potential recipients of institutional care in England. In Canada, Action League for Physically Handicapped Advancement (ALPHA) has devoted its efforts to legislation for a guaranteed income and transportation for the disabled.

In the United States there are over 1000 clubs and local chapters of organizations of the disabled. A few of the older organizations are still primarily social clubs, but the majority of the clubs now reflect the growing mood of activism and self-determination that is emerging as disabled individuals discover in themselves a new source of strength.

One of the most colorfully titled organizations, World Association to Remove Prejudice Against the Handicapped (WARPATH) is headquartered in Florida. The disabled students organizations on the university campuses of New York City have named themselves Student Organization For Every Disability United for Progress (SO FED UP). One of the members of the group says that it is easy for people who are disabled to be sympathetic with the Black movement, "Blacks were relegated to the back of the bus; we can't even get on the bus." Physically Impaired Association of Michigan (PAM) is working to establish a communication network among consumers and advocate organizations. California Association of The Physically Handicapped, Inc. (CAPH) is "dedicated to helping the physically handicapped become self-dependent." Committee for the Rights of the Disabled (CRD) represents the concerns of the disabled of the Los Angeles area, including those who are Spanish-speaking. Disabled in Action (DIA) made a dramatic demonstration during the gasoline shortage when its wheelchaired members blocked city streets to protest gasoline allocations.

A significant trend has been developing in the last few years. Individuals and organizations representing persons who are blind, developmentally disabled, physically disabled, and elderly are beginning to work together to effect legislation to solve their common problems. In California, for instance, when the attendant care program was threatened by cutbacks in December, 1974, several hundred persons met to protest. Joining the disabled and blind protestors were elderly persons wearing large buttons proclaiming "Senior Power."

AMERICAN COALITION OF CITIZENS WITH DISABILITIES

Though a national coalition has been needed for years, it was not formed until the 1974 annual meeting of the President's Committee on Employment of the Handicapped (PCEH) when 150 individuals affiliated with or representing 52 disability groups met to discuss coalition and elect a steering committee to structure the organization.

After a year of consolidation, the organization met at the 1975 annual meeting of PCEH and elected officers and board members. The new president, Eunice Fiorito, is director of the Mayor's Office for the Handicapped in New York City and vice-president of the American Council of the Blind of New York State. With one exception, all the officers and board members are wheelchaired, blind, or deaf. Member organizations include the Paralyzed Veterans of America, National Association of the Deaf, American Council of the Blind, New York's Congress of People with Disabilities, Berkeley's Center for Independent Living, Massachusetts Council of Organizations of the Handicapped, and the Florida Council of Organizations of the Handicapped. Local chapters of the National Paraplegia Foundation and the National Association of the Physically Handicapped are represented. Among the nonvoting member organizations are the National Association for Retarded Citizens and the National Rehabilitation Association. Write to American Coalition of Citizens with Disabilities, Inc. 1346 Connecticut Avenue, N.W., Room 308, Washington, D.C. 20036.

The Coalition is concentrating its energies on two of the areas that are of vital concern to the disabled population: 1) an amendment to the federal Civil Rights Act of 1964 to bar discrimination against disabled persons in housing, employment, and public accommodations (such an amendment would allow the disabled access to the Act's complaint mechanisms and to the expertise of its enforcement offices) and 2) a national health security system as advocated by the Health Security Action Council, which would include prostheses and mechanical, electronic, and technologic aids, appliances, and devices.

The Coalition is wise to start its activities by working toward an amendment of the Civil Rights Act of 1964. Attitudinal barriers are more inhibiting and impeding than architectural barriers. The most direct and effective way to improve attitudes toward the disabled is to legislate and enforce behavior change. Attitudes will be changed when people who are disabled are treated as equals and when the environment is modified so that they can function as equals. Increased exposure to the normality of the disabled and the elderly will bring about a lasting understanding.

THE DISABLED ARE THEIR OWN BEST ADVOCATES

Since the 1950s, a few concerned voluntary organizations have been effective leaders in accomplishing legislation, facilities, and services for the disabled. Recently, throughout the world, the disabled themselves are beginning to assume the responsibility of advocacy in their own behalf. Collectively and individually, they are making themselves heard in the voluntary organizations and in government; they are making their needs known.

Organizations of the elderly and disabled are demonstrating innumerable possibilities for cohesive action: group insurance programs; a nationwide chain of transitional, retirement, recreational, and permanent living accommodations; a cooperative "seal of approval" on equipment; pharmacy services; travel tours; employment; equipment manufacturing; equipment information; ombudsmen; counseling; group therapy; accessibility information; equipment exchange; vacation and home exchanges; attendant registers; accessible housing registers; legislation information; and wheelchair maintenance and repair.

The feelings of disabled individuals worldwide echo those of the English Union of the Physically Impaired Against Segregation: "We reject the whole idea of 'experts' and professionals holding forth on how we should accept our disabilities, or giving learned lectures about the 'psychology' of disablement. We already know what it feels like to be poor, isolated, segregated, done good to, stared at, and talked down to—far better than any able-bodied expert. We as a Union are not interested in descriptions of how awful it is to be disabled. What we are interested in are ways of changing our conditions of life, and thus overcoming the handicaps which are imposed on top of our physical disabilities by the way society is organized to exclude us."

Bibliography

Abroad in the Land: Legal Strategies to Effectuate the Rights of the Physically Disabled. By Ann Gailis and Keith M. Susman. THE GEORGETOWN LAW JOURNAL, Vol. 61, No. 6, pages 1501–1523, July, 1973.

AGE AND VITALITY. Commonsense Ways of Adding Life to Your Years. By Irene Gore. London, published for Age Concern by George Allen & Unwin Ltd., 1973.

THE AMERICAN PEOPLE. By E.J. Kahn, Jr., Baltimore, Penguin Books Inc., 1975.

Barrier Free Design, Report of a United Nations Expert Group Meeting. Special Issue, INTERNATIONAL REHABILITATION REVIEW, Vol. XXVI, No. 1, pages 1–36 First Quarter, 1975.

Changes in Attitudes Toward People With Handicaps. By Beatrice A. Wright, PhD. REHABILITATION LITERATURE, Vol. XXXIV, No. 12, 354–357 December, 1973.

THE CITY IS THE FRONTIER. By Charles Abrams. New York, Harper & Row, 1965.

"Crip Lib:" The Disabled Fight For Their Own Cause. By Gregg W. Downey. MODERN HEALTHCARE, pages 21–26, February, 1975.

"Crips" Unite to Enforce Symbolic Laws: Legal Aid for the Disabled: An Overview. By Jack Achtenberg. UNIVERSITY OF SAN FERNANDO VALLEY LAW REVIEW, Vol. 4, No. 2, pages 161–213, Fall, 1975.

From Problem to Solution: The New Focus in Fighting Environmental Barriers For the Handicapped. By Rita McGaughey. REHABILITATION LITERATURE, Vol. 37, No. 1, pages 10–12, January, 1976.

The Handicapped Majority. INDUSTRIAL DESIGN, Vol. 21, No. 4, pages 22–41, May, 1974.

Helping the Disabled to Live to Capacity. By Dr. Margaret Agerholm, MA. Address delivered at the Annual Conference of the Cheshire Foundation Homes, July 11, 1964. Printed in REHABILITATION, journal of the British Council for Rehabilitation of the Disabled.

The Minority That Has It Harder Than Anybody. By Bert Shanas. NEW YORK SUNDAY NEWS, pages 8–9, 20, April 20, 1975.

A National Program of Respiratory and Rehabilitation Centers. By Dr. Kenneth S. Landauer. In POLIOMYELITIS: PAPERS AND DISCUSSIONS PRESENTED AT THE FOURTH INTERNATIONAL POLIOMYELITIS CONFERENCE. Philadelphia. J. B. Lippincott Company, 1958.

OLD AGE. THE LAST SEGREGATION. Ralph Nader's Study Group Report on Nursing Homes. By Claire Townsend. Baltimore, Bantam Books, Inc. 1971.

PHYSICAL DISABILITY—A PSYCHOLOGICAL APPROACH. By Beatrice A. Wright. New York, Harper & Brothers, 1960.

THE PHYSICALLY HANDICAPPED AND THE COMMUNITY. Some Challenging Breakthroughs. By Louis Arthur Michaux. Springfield, Charles C. Thomas, 1970.

Three Little Stairs. By Ronald J. Dickson. THE ROTARIAN, pages 28–31, October, 1968.

What Kind of Public Building Access Do the Handicapped Need? By William B. Hopkins. THE BUILDING OFFICIAL AND CODE ADMINISTRATOR, pages 14–17, October, 1974.

A WORLD TO CARE FOR. The Autobiography of Howard A. Rusk, MD. By Howard A. Rusk, MD. New York, Random House, Inc., and The Reader's Digest Association, Inc., 1972.

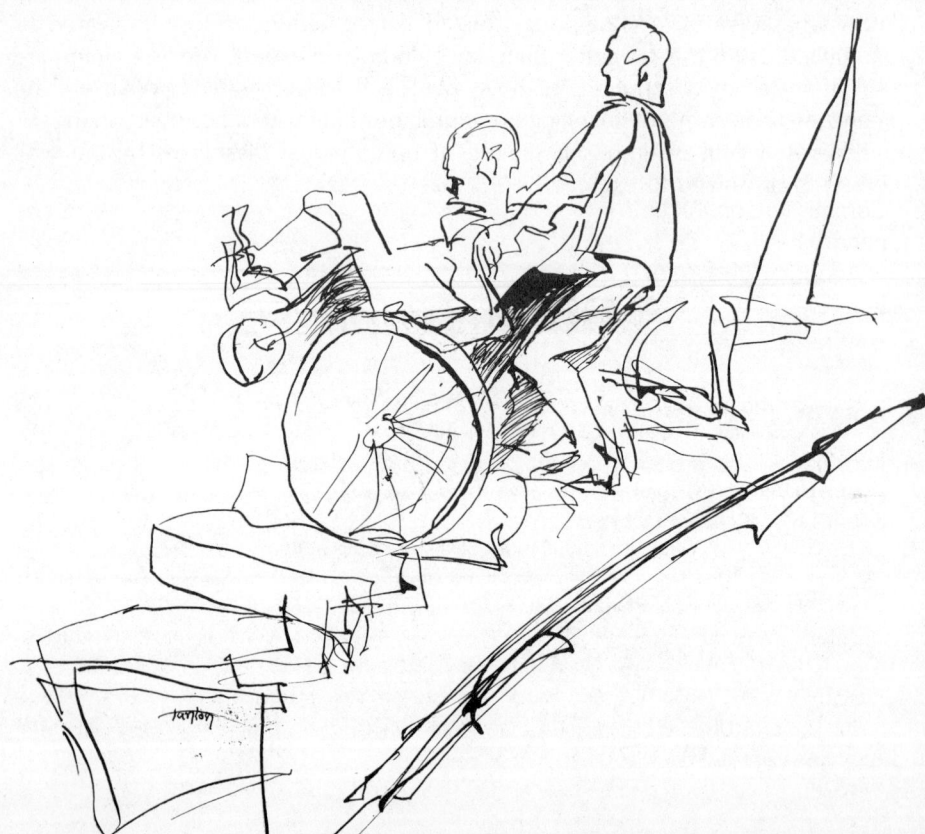

"Now that I have been cooking and keeping house for over a year I realize that there are no easy solutions for the quad housewife. At this point I think motivation and experience are the most important factors."

—Barbara Cory Good

2
Adaptations to Housing

Adapting to disability is a two-way street; the individual must adapt to the environment, and the environment must be adapted to the individual. For those who are severely disabled, of course, the most important element of a living arrangement is the accompanying service from other people, and the primary aim of adapting housing is to reduce the need for service.

Whatever the disability, there are common elements in adapting. The most important are motivation and information. Though the capacity to adapt depends on an individual's overall pattern of adjusting, the degree of success can be augmented by support and information from family, friends, therapists and doctors, and the experiences of others with similar disabilities.

This chapter, a potpourri of ideas on adaptations, is a mixture of all these sources—the experiences of disabled persons, books by therapists, and sources of supply. Some of it will be familiar to long-time readers of *Rehabilitation Gazette* because parts of it are an updating of material written by its severely disabled readers over the years. Though the sources of supply given are all in the United States, the ideas are universal. Similar sources in England and Europe can be found through the Disabled Living Foundation in England and International Commission on Technical Aids (ICTA) in Sweden (see Information Centers, Appendix B).

Adapting a house or apartment to fit the needs and quirks of an individual who is severely disabled involves three Ms—motivation, methods, and money—mixed with creativity and knowledge of what has been done and is available.

A BASIC LIBRARY

Information about existing adaptations, techniques, remodeling plans, and specifications is vital, the starting point for individual creativity. Ten books have been selected as being economical and basic. For $12.50, you can purchase this treasure collection of information, most of it compiled by occupational therapists who are experts in the field of living with disabilities.

ADAPTATIONS AND TECHNIQUES FOR THE DISABLED HOMEMAKER. By K. Hodgeman, OTR, and E. Warpeha, OTR. Publications Department, Sister Kenny Institute, 1800 Chicago Avenue, Minneapolis, Minnesota 55404. $1.75.

PLANNING KITCHENS FOR HANDICAPPED HOMEMAKERS. By V. H. Wheeler. Publications Unit, Institute of Rehabilitation Medicine, New York University Medical Center, 400 East 34th Street, New York, New York 10016. Rehabilitation Monograph XXVII. $2.

SOURCES OF INFORMATION ON SELF-HELP DEVICES FOR THE HANDICAPPED. Annotated bibliography. The National Easter Seal Society for Crippled Children and Adults, 2023 West Ogden Avenue, Chicago, Illinois 60612. Free.

SELF AIDS. By Wendy M. Davis, SROT, MAOT. The Thistle Foundation, 22 Charlotte Square, Edinburgh, EH2 4DF, Scotland. 37 pence ($1).

EASY-TO-USE KITCHENS and EASY TO USE SINK CENTER. Cooperative Extension Service, University of Nebraska-Lincoln, East Campus, Lincoln, Nebraska 68503. Free.

WHEELCHAIR BATHROOMS. By Harry A. Schweikert, Jr. Paralyzed Veterans of America, Inc., 7315 Wisconsin Avenue, Suite 301-W, Bethesda, Maryland 20014. $1.

MEALTIME MANUAL FOR THE AGED AND HANDICAPPED. By J. L. Klinger, OTR, MA. Simon & Schuster. Paperback available from FashionABLE, Rocky Hill, New Jersey 08553. $2.98 including postage.

ON YOUR OWN NEWSLETTER. Office of Independent Study, Division of Continuing Education, Box 2967, University of Alabama, University, Alabama 35486. Free.

SELF-HELP MANUAL FOR ARTHRITIS PATIENTS. By J. L. Klinger, OTR, MA. The Arthritis Foundation, 1212 Avenue of the Americas, New York, New York 10036. $1.25.

THE WHEELCHAIR IN THE KITCHEN. By J. Chasin and J. Saltman. Paralyzed Veterans of America, Inc. 7315 Wisconsin Avenue, Suite 301-W, Bethesda, Maryland 20014. $2.50.

OUTDOORS AND ENTRANCES

WALKS

Though adult wheelchairs average about 2 ft. 1 in. wide, some motorized chairs may be 2 ft. 5 in. wide, so the walks should be about 3 ft. wide for a casual leeway. Existing paths and walks may be widened by the addition of rows of cement blocks, bricks, or railroad ties.

GARAGES

At least 12 ft. in width should be allowed for transfer and maneuvering of a wheelchair or hydraulic lift. Ideally, the door should be opened remotely by radio beam from within the car or electric switch reachable from it.

RAMPS

Individualized ramps need not conform to the more rigid standards of public ramps, which must cover a wide variety of disabilities, but they must follow certain general rules of safety. The gentlest slope for self-propelling is a 1-ft. rise in 20 ft. (5%); the most often recommended slope is a 1-ft. rise in 12 ft. (8.3%). (Those figures mean that for every 1-ft. rise, there should be 12 ft. in length; thus, 3 ft. high steps require a 36 ft. long ramp.) With an electric wheelchair, strong arms, or a good "pusher," steeper slopes can be used. In Canada, even public ramps can be as steep as a 1-ft. rise in 7 ft. if they have two handrails and are for wheelchairs only.

The ramp need not protrude from the house but can be wrapped around its walls, perhaps starting at the side driveway, making a 90° turn at a platform, and ending in front at the entrance door. It can be decorative and imaginative, concealed with a lattice, vines, or shrubs. If a wrapped around ramp would interfere with a basement door, it can be hinged to open as if it were a moat gate. Since an extremely long ramp is tiring, it should be no more than 30 ft. long in a section, with the sections separated by a level platform at least 5 ft. long.

A low guardrail at the edge of the ramp is essential to prevent rolling off. There should be a minimum of 2 ft. 8 in. and, preferably 3 ft. between these rails. Descent can be braked by turning against the guardrails. Ascent can be assisted with an electric tow (Power Pull, 820 Griffs Avenue, Fort Worth, Texas 76103). The ramp should have handrails on at least one side, 2 ft. 8 in. high. If there are two rails, people with strong arms and hands can use them to brake or to give an extra heave upwards. Handrails should be easy-to-grip wood or "slip-covered" metal.

The surface of the ramp should be fireproof and nonslip. It can be made slip-proof by sprinkling sand on the wet paint, using cleats, covering it with a rough-surfaced roofing paper, or painting it with a skid-resistant paint. Safety-Walk, used on the stairs of 727s and DC-9s, resists icing and skidding. If snow and ice are a problem, the ramp should be enclosed, roofed, made with built-in electric heating cables, or covered with electric carpet strips.

The platform at the door should be at least 3 ft. deep if the door swings in and 5 ft. deep if it swings out; the open area at the bottom of the ramp should be at least 6 ft. deep.

Most important: always go up forward and down backward, whether self-propelled or pushed. Leaning slightly forward will make the trip a bit easier and safer.

If the house or apartment is only a step or two off the ground a portable ramp can be used. Here are a number of commercial ramps that are portable, as well as one that could be made by a local machine shop.

Handi-Ramp, Inc., 1414 Armour Boulevard, Mundelein, Illinois 60060, pioneered the manufacturing of folding ramps. The company's products are now available from leading automobile dealers in the United States, and there are export offices for the Far East and dealers in Canada and Europe. Handi-Ramp has developed two folding ramps, one for buses and vans and the other for steps

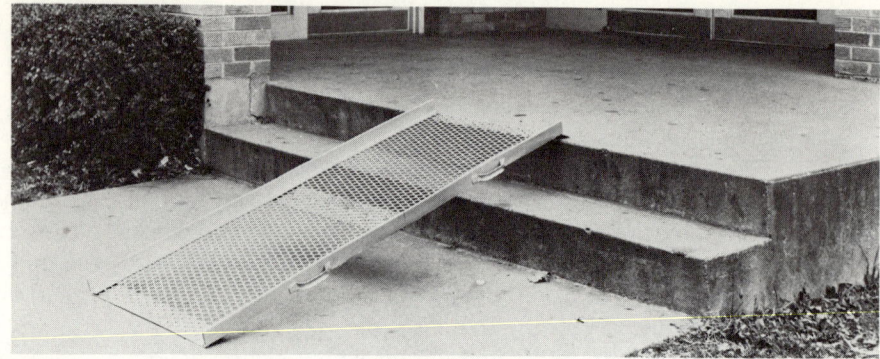

Fig. 2–1. Folding ramp of expanded metal made by Handi-Ramp.

Fig. 2–2. The Handi-Ramp folds in half.

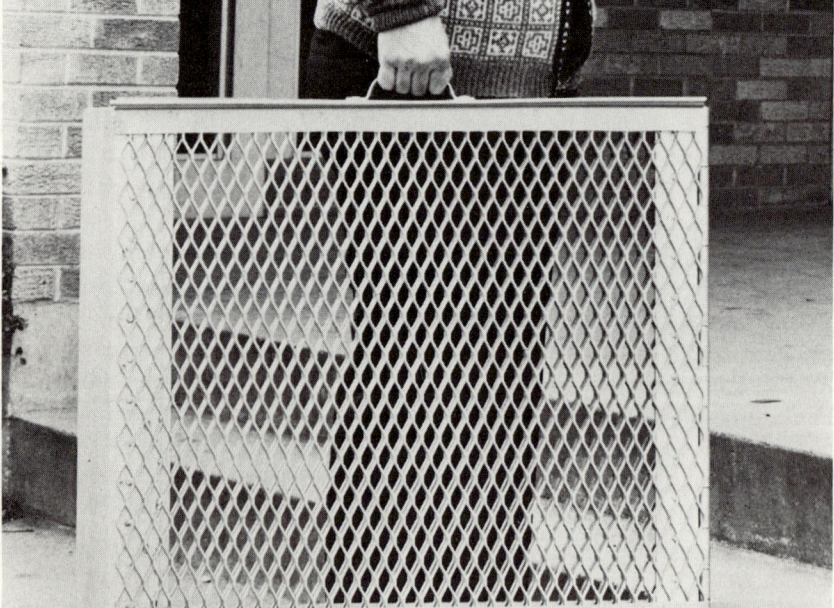

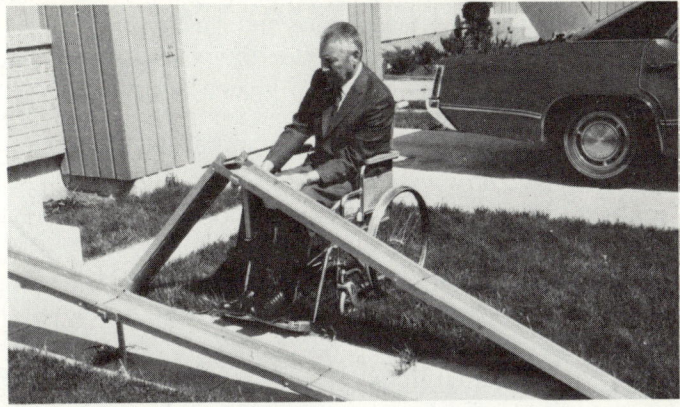

Fig. 2-3. Canadian folding ramp. The middle section has an adjustable leg to support weight and prevent damage to the hinge joint.

(Fig. 2-1). The latter, which folds in half (Fig. 2-2), opens to 2 ft. 2 in. wide × 5 ft. (44 lb.) or 2 ft. 2 in. × 7 ft. (54 lb.). Its rough surface provides good traction.

A fiberglass ramp, which adjusts to steps 4–8 in. high, weighs 18 lb, is 2 ft 5 in. wide and 2 ft 8 in. long, and has a skid-resistant surface is made by Port-A-Ramp, Inc., 4019 S.W. 12th Street, Plantation, Florida 33314.

A portable ramp was developed for the Canadian Paraplegic Association's loan service for use at summer cottages. It is 13 ft long, made of four sections of 3 ft 4 in. each (Fig. 2-3). Weighing about 14 lb per section, the ramp may be easily loaded into a car and used for visiting friends' houses or traveling. Spacers can adjust for any width wheelchair. The edges of the runners are made of rectangular steel tubing approximately ¾ in. × 1-⅜ in. The deck is a lightweight metal, welded to the tubing. The non-slip surface was obtained by sprinkling sand onto the paint while wet. (More information from Canadian Paraplegic Association, Central Western Division, 825 Sherbrook Street, Winnipeg, Manitoba R3A 1M5).

Commercially made models of the folding metal channel ramps are available from Donald S. Crawford, 5948 East 129th Street, Grandview, Missouri 64030 and Fred Scott & Sons, 70 Scott Street, Elk Grove, Illinois 60007.

A pair of motorcycle ramps, casually available from many local sources, may be an inexpensive solution to some ramping needs.

ELEVATORS

WHEELCHAIR ELEVATORS

Most of the elevators on the market have been developed by disabled persons who wanted to be elevated in their wheelchairs without the strain of transferring to a fixed seat. Some were developed primarily for outdoor use; others have models for both indoor and outdoor use. Tony Mathews of Savannah, Georgia, designed an inexpensive and simple porch lift for himself and his wheelchair (Fig. 2–4). He had it made by welding supporting rods on the forks of a worm type bumper jack and bolting a platform of ½-in. plywood onto this frame.

Another inexpensive solution is a lift of the type used in warehouses to handle heavy materials. Mounted on a concrete slab, it can be left safely in place in all weathers. An on-off switch which has a lock or is mounted in the house prevents neighborhood children from playing with the controls.

All of the following manufacturers of outdoor elevators should be contacted for their latest brochures and prices. All these elevators use 110 volts and have weatherproofed controls.

Wheelchair Elevators, Inc., Box 489, Broussard, Louisiana 70518. Measuring 4 ft × 4 ft 6 in., the elevator will take all sizes of wheelchairs and will raise loads

Fig. 2–4. Tony Mathews and his porch lift made with a worm type bumper jack.

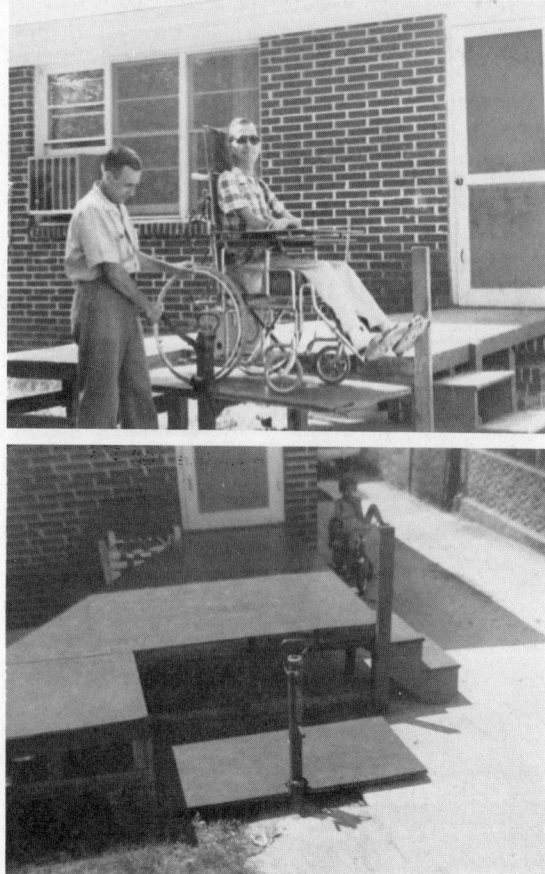

of 350 lb to heights of up to 6 ft. Approved for veterans, it may be rented from some hospital supply companies.

R. J. Chair Lift Company, 7228½ West Madison Street, Forest Park, Illinois 60130. Available in stock sizes up to 12 ft high, it has folding gates mounted on the unit or at top and bottom stations and is large enough for a wheelchair and an attendant. A key-operated switch prevents unauthorized use. Models are available for indoor and outdoor use.

American Stair-Glide Corporation, 4001 East 138th Street, Grandview, Missouri 64030. The new Porch-Lift can be placed at the porch or at the side of an interior stairway; key-operated, it elevates to a maximum of 4 ft 5 in.

Earl's Stairway Lift Corporation, Highway 218 North, Cedar Falls, Iowa 50613. With a capacity of 250 lb, the lift will carry a wheelchair up any size straight stairsteps, inside or outside, including hillsides (Fig. 2–5).

The Cheney Company, 7611 North 73rd Street, Milwaukee, Wisconsin 53223. The company, which has been building the Wecolator Stairway Elevator for 40 years, has added wheelchair lifts for indoors, porches, and vans. The porch lift will carry up to 350 lb vertically. The stairway lift will carry 250 lb along a straight stairway; the platform stores on the bottom floor to allow normal use of the stairway.

Fig. 2–5. Earl's stairway lift operates both indoors and outdoors.

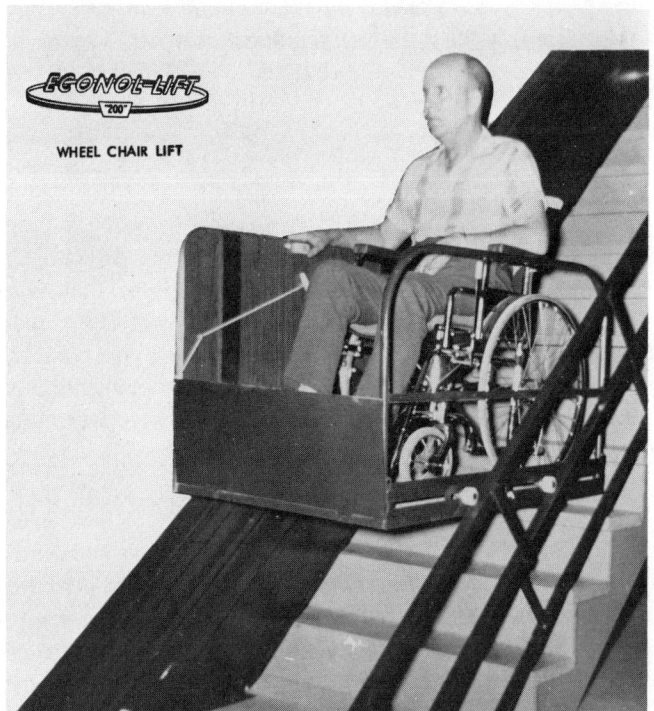

Fred Scott & Sons, 70 Scott Street, Elk Grove, Illinois 60007. The hydraulic InvaLift is engineered for interior or exterior use; it may be portable or stationary, semi- or fully automatic. With a deck size of 2 ft 8 in. $\times$ 5 ft, it is adjustable to any style entrance and stores flush with the surface when not in use. The maximum load is 2000 lb.

STAND-UP OR SIT-DOWN ELEVATORS

For those who are not wheelchaired, but who cannot climb stairs, there are a number of compact units for use indoors, as well as outdoor models for lakefront homes and houses on steep hills. Check with the American Stair-Glide Corporation, the Cheney Company, and Earl's Stairway Lift Corporation, whose addresses have been given. In addition, brochures may be obtained from Dover Corporation/Elevator Division, Box 2177, Memphis, Tennessee 38102 and Inclinator Company of America, 220 Paxton Street, Harrisburg, Pennsylvania 17105.

REHABILITATION ELIGIBILITY

Both the portable ramps and the elevators are removable, so they qualify as a medical expense for income tax purposes. Also, before making a purchase, the local vocational rehabilitation office should be contacted. Since an elevator or a ramp may be essential to getting out of the house to work or school or managing the household, the cost has frequently been assumed by this office as a rehabilitation expense, especially since the Rehabilitation Act of 1973 made it mandatory to rehabilitate those who are severely disabled.

DOORS

WIDENING A DOORWAY

If the doorway is just a little too narrow for a wheelchair, an inch or so may be gained by replacing the door hinges with a "step-back" hinge that swings the door free of the frame and allows it to lie flat against the wall. If the hinges are not available at a local hardware store, they can be ordered from MED, Inc. 1215 South Harlem Avenue, Forest Park, Illinois 60130. Alternatively, the door may be removed and replaced with a heavy curtain, such as a shower curtain.

NARROWING A WHEELCHAIR

A chair-narrowing device may be installed on either side of a standard wheelchair that will reduce its width by as much as 4 in. while the user is in the chair. The narrower, which is operated by rotating a lever located at the armrest, may be detached when it is not in use. This device is also available from MED, Inc. Another narrower is manufactured by Narro-Matic, Inc., 1 Pennsylvania Plaza, New York 10001. A folding wheelchair may be narrowed by hooking a coat hanger over the pushing handles or by tightening a heavy belt across the frame at the back or under the knees.

Another method of getting through narrow doors is to transfer to a kitchen type chair to which castors have been attached. A transfer board, one that has been beveled at both ends, helps bridge the gap from wheelchair to chair or car or bed or wherever. A lightweight one of white plastic is made by G. E. Miller, Inc., 484 South Broadway, Yonkers, New York 10705.

DOOR KEYS

The difficulties of managing a key with minimal hand function may be overcome by attaching a short length of dowel to the key or by screwing a wood handle to it. A commercially made model is available from VABCO Products, 160 North Gilbert Street, Fullerton, California 92633.

DOOR HANDLES

It is unfortunate for the disabled that the United States became the land of the round doorknob rather than of the lever knob used in most of the rest of the world. However, round knobs can be less troublesome and frustrating if heavy rubber bands, 2-in. diameter hose clamps, or bathtub nonslip strips are put around the knobs and if the hand is placed behind the knob, with the knob between the index and middle fingers and the palm outward. A "doorknob helper" is available from FashionABLE, Rocky Hill, New Jersey 08553. This heavy rubber bulb stretches over the round knob and extends to a 4-in. leverlike device. A hole in the bulb makes the keyhole accessible. The lever may be pushed with the arm, elbow, or hip to open or close a door. An aid to closing a door may be made by attaching a cord or strap with a loop wide enough to insert a wrist or foot.

TELEPHONES AND ALARM SYSTEMS

SPECIAL TELEPHONE SERVICES

The Bell System publishes an informative and free booklet, *Services for Special Needs,* that includes the various services available to compensate for different disabilities. In addition to these services, local phone companies can arrange special combinations of services to meet individual needs, including calls for assistance to neighbors or emergency community agencies. Special services and equipment listed in the booklet include

For hearing and speech impairment: column control handset, amplifier for coin phones, adjustments for hearing aids, bone conduction receiver, headset amplifier, an instrument to convert sound into sight or touch signals, an aid for lipreaders, and dataphone service linking the telephone to telewriting devices. Signals to indicate a phone's ring include tone ringer, loud bell, gongs, sounds in different frequencies, lights or electric fans that are activated by a ring.

For impaired vision: illuminated key set, seeing aid switchboard

For speech loss: electric larynx

For motion impairments: card dialer, one-number dialer, touchtone service, trimline phones, speakerphones (hands free operation), single-button phone, on/off switches, and a variety of lightweight headsets

For education by telephone: connections between school or college and home or hospital

The telephone company can also turn a home's extension phones into an intercom system. By switching one of the phones to intercom one can broadcast his voice throughout the house from speakers mounted near each extension phone. Anyone can answer without picking up the phone because a tiny microphone in the base of each phone picks up the replies from anywhere in the room. The front door, too, can have a microphone and a speaker so that the door can be answered from any phone in the house.

In addition to these services, still more can be created by studying two comprehensive books on telephones. *Telephone Services for the Handicapped* is an invaluable handbook that shows an amazing variety of attachments that can be affixed to a telephone to make it more usable by even the most severely disabled person. With the cooperation of the American Telephone and Telegraph Company, it was published by the Institute of Rehabilitation Medicine, New York University (Publications Office, 400 East 34th Street, New York, New York 10016. $2.50). The telephone company translated these services into its manual, *Telephone Services for the Motion Handicapped*. It is not usually given to customers, but a copy should be available for reference in most telephone offices.

PERSONAL ALARM SYSTEMS

Most of the specialized equipment catalogs have signal buzzers, ranging from the very simple to electronic genii, operated by minimum touch and used to call for assistance. Security and Fire Enterprises, 443 Elm Street, Stamford, Connecticut 06902, manufactures a wireless panic button device, the size of a pack of cigarettes, that can be used to call a doctor, an ambulance, the police or fire department, family, or neighbors. By a slight pressure on the device a prerecorded series of different telephone messages are sent to preselected agencies or persons. Its applications are almost unlimited, including the device's ability to detect smoke, fire, or gases and to call the fire department.

Hammacher Schlemmer, 147 East 57th Street, New York, New York 10022, sells an Electronic Caretaker that plugs into any phone jack or phone line junction and dials any number, local or long distance, when it is triggered by fire, heating system failure, or intrusion. It includes step-on mat and 50 ft of cord; it may be shut off with a special whistle.

REMOTE CONTROLS

Though many of the remote control systems are still in the experimental stage or in very limited production, it is tantalizing to dream of the optimum independence through environmental control that bioengineering can give to severely disabled individuals through these systems.

BRITISH REMOTE CONTROL SYSTEMS

The earliest and most widely used remote controls are in Great Britain, where the National Health Service issues the Possum Selector Unit to individuals with severe motion impairment of arms and hands. Possum enables them to exercise remote on/off control over as many as 11 electrical devices, such as bell and buzzer alarm systems, light, heat, TV, radio, intercom to front door, electric door lock, and a specially adapted loudspeaking telephone with self-dialing facilities. The unit is operated by a flicker of movement on a microswitch or by breath (pneumatic control). Other Possum systems operate electric typewriters by pneumatic controls. Information on all Possum equipment is available from POSM Research Project, 63 Mandeville Road, Aylesbury, Buckinghamshire, England. Another system, PILOT, is operated by a light directed onto photoelectric cells. Information on this system may be obtained from Hugh Steeper, Ltd., Queen Mary's Hospital, Roehampton, London S.W.15, England.

Other systems used in Great Britain are the Corseford Selector, Medical Aids Electronic Development Company, 19 Cochrane Street, Glasgow C.1, Scotland; System Seven, Zambette Electronics, Ltd., 17 High Street, Southen-on-Sea, Essex, England; and Electraid, J.W.F. Electraid Systems, 8 Bramcote Close, Aylesbury, Buckinghamshire, England. For details on the systems, contact the consultant on electronic equipment of the Disabled Living Foundation, Roger M. Jefcoate, Willowbrook Swanbourne Road, Mursley, Buckinghamshire, England.

NASA'S SIGHT SWITCH AND OTHER CONTROLS

In the United States, the most dramatic device is the sight switch (Fig. 2–6), originally developed by the National Aeronautics and Space Administration (NASA) to solve the problems of the astronaut whose arms would be pinned by gravity force. The device consists of a cylinder mounted on the earpiece of eyeglass frames. The tiny cylinder contains an infrared light source, amplifier, sensitivity control, and infrared sensor. It is operated simply by looking at it and controlled by moving the eyes to the left or right. More information is available in NASA Tech Brief #SSB65–10079, which can be obtained from the Clearinghouse for Federal Scientific and Technical Information, 5285 Port Royal Road, Springfield, Virginia 22151.

The Veterans Administration (VA) has developed an environmental control system called VAPC Environmental Controllers which employs pneumatic switches and an operational logic which is different from the Possum type. It requires sequential sucking on an air tube to actuate the selected channels. The

VA is using the system for some of its spinal cord injured. The controls enable the operator to turn the TV on and off and select channels, turn lights and radio on and off, operate a motorized bed, and work a call buzzer. It is available from R. & D. Engineering, P.O. Box 3584, Los Amigos Station, Downey, California 90242.

In the last 10 years, numerous sophisticated electronic control systems have been developed by hospital research departments with HEW funding, by individual engineers, and by commercial firms. Among the firms and individuals are 1) Adaptive Therapeutic Systems, Inc., 36 Howe Street, New Haven, Connecticut 06511; 2) Bio-Med Technology, Inc., 1081 Clinton Avenue North, Rochester, New York 14621; 3) Cyber Systems, Inc., P.O. Box 2354, Fullerton, California 92633; 4) Cybernetics Research Institute, 2233 Wisconsin Avenue, N.W., Washington, D.C. 20007; 5) NIRE., Pompton Lakes, New Jersey 07442; 6) Scientific Systems International, 2024 Wooddale Drive, Huntsville, Alabama 35801; 7) Scope Electronics, Inc., 1860 Michael Faraday Drive, Reston, Virginia 22090; 8) Southwest Research Institute, 8500 Culebra Road, P.O. Drawer 28510, San Antonio, Texas 78284; 9) Dean Tougas, 923-23rd Street East, Seattle, Washington 98112.

Some of these firms make one particular device, such as a remote controlled wheelchair; others design equipment for a particular individual's special needs. Most of the equipment is expensive and should be prescribed only by experts. Two other firms have presented a few electronic items in nontechnical language in illustrated brochures: MED, 1215 South Harlem Avenue, Forest Park, Illinois 60130 and Prentke Romich Company, 2111 Acacia Park Drive, #106, Cleveland, Ohio 44124. MED lists a Med-i-lectric zero-pressure remote power control for one or more electrical units. The controls may be operated by a light touch or by breath. Another remote control unit by MED turns a television set on and

Fig. 2–6. The sight switch is operated simply by looking at it; it has been used experimentally to operate a wheelchair.

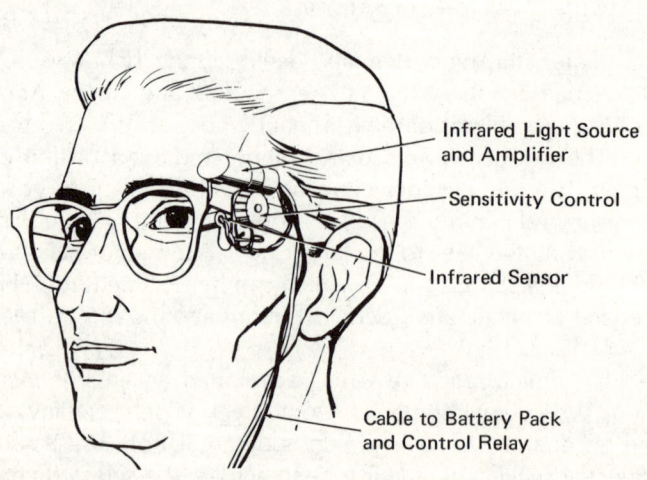

off when someone breathes on the receptor. MED also has Sip 'N' Puff systems for controlling wheelchairs and dialing telephones. Prentke Romich makes automatic dialing telephones and other electronic devices to control alarm systems, wheelchairs, or radios.

Edited by Keith Copeland, *Aids for the Severely Handicapped* is a comprehensive 152-page book in which remote control devices used in England, Canada, and Finland are described in detail by 29 authors. Also included is a list of the organizations involved in research on remote controls in Australia, Austria, Canada, Denmark, Finland, Germany, Italy, The Netherlands, Sweden, United Kingdom, and the United States. Published in 1974, it is available from Grune & Stratton, Inc., 111 Fifth Avenue, New York, New York for $12.50.

The remote control devices included are: POSSUM, PILOT, LOT, VOTEM, Typewriter control by dental plate key, Systems 7 and 8, GMMI, TARC, COMHANDI, Talking Brooch, Lightwriter, Communication display/print out with memory, and Interlock. The modes of operation include: pneumatic mouth-operated, head-mounted light source, light source attached to spectacles, voice-operated using Morse code, key-mounted dental plate using Morse code, movement of lips, and push button or toggle switches.

SIMPLE SOUND SWITCHES

Several catalogs list switches that turn on or off lamps, electrical appliances, TVs, or Christmas tree lights when triggered by a whistle, a shout, a handclap, or a key chain rattle. Two of the companies that list them in their catalogs are Joan Cook, 853 Eiler Drive, Ft. Lauderdale, Florida 33316 and Suburbia, Inc., 366 Wacouta, St. Paul, Minnesota 55101. Signal Science, 140 Lowland Street, Holliston, Massachusetts 01746 sells a whistle switch. The uses of whistle switches are limited, however, because they are triggered by all sorts of extraneous noises such as barking dogs or clanking pots or pans. Another disadvantage is that there is no selection; if two or more appliances or lights are plugged in, they are all either on or off. Nevertheless, they are relatively inexpensive, and they have an aura of magic and fun as well as some possibilities for usefulness.

USE YOUR HEAD

ROBERT B. MCCOWN

Dr. McCown, a physicist, has been quadriplegic because of poliomyelitis since age 15. He received a BA from Hastings College in Nebraska and his MS and PhD in physics from Stanford University in California.

When you cannot use your hands, it is all the more important to use your head. Use it to make appliances and doors and telephones work for you (Fig. 2–7). Try these simple modifications of existing equipment and soon you will be happily thinking up others for yourself.

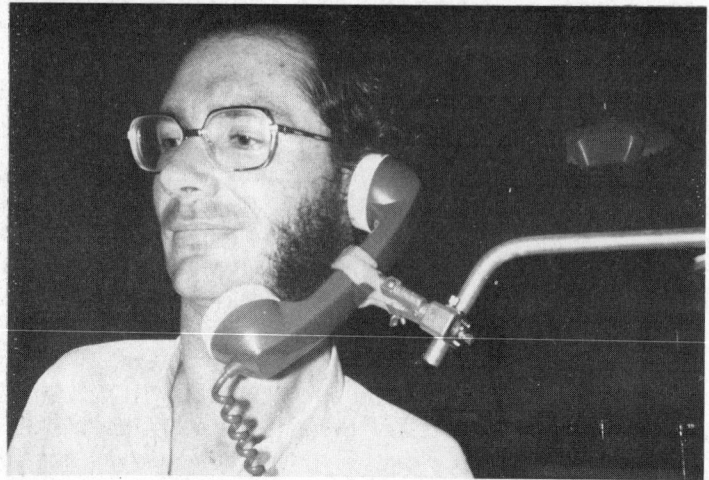

Fig. 2–7. Fisher brand flask holder supports a telephone handset for Dr. McCown. The flask holder can be attached to any rod by a thumbscrew.

WALL SWITCHES

If you are in a wheelchair, the usual wall switch is too high for you. You can, of course, have it relocated lower down on the wall, but this is expensive and unnecessary. Instead, you can replace the conventional switch with one of the push on-push off type, which you can operate by pushing it with your head or whatever.

This solution illustrates a basic principle that you should follow whenever you approach a problem: choose the least complicated solution that produces the end result desired. Try to think of many different ways to accomplish your goal without regard at first to their apparent feasibility. Include the fantastic and far-out ideas as well as the obvious possibilities. Do not insist on doing everything the same way in which it has always been done. Examine each idea carefully and make sure that it is impossible before you discard it.

APPLIANCES

You can turn lights and electric appliances off and on by adding an extension cord which has its own special switch. Buy toggle switches at your electronic supply shop, and if necessary, lengthen the toggle lever by slipping any desired length of plastic drinking straw over it and filling the straw with epoxy glue. Remember to wire the switch to an extension rather than to the appliance cord itself; in that way you can add it quickly to any appliance—including borrowed items. The kind of plastic box that is supposed to hold 3 × 5 file cards is ideal for holding the switch. Drill a hole in the box, feed the cord through the hole, and tie a knot in it; this will prevent a wire from being pulled loose and causing an electrical hazard.

You can modify some appliances, such as radios and TV sets, by gluing levers

Adaptations to Housing   25

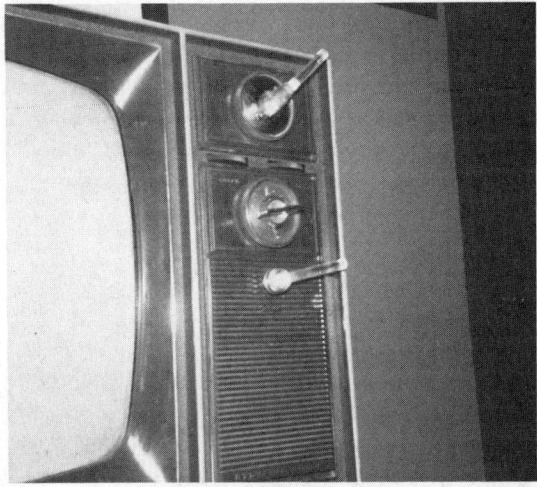

Fig. 2–8. Small rods have been glued to the knobs on this TV set to reduce the force necessary to turn them.

Fig. 2–9. Electric door opener. The rectangular box contains control relays and the radio control receiver. The wire projecting from the bottom of the box is the antenna for the receiver. The small black thing at the upper right corner of the doorway is a switch that senses when the door is closed.

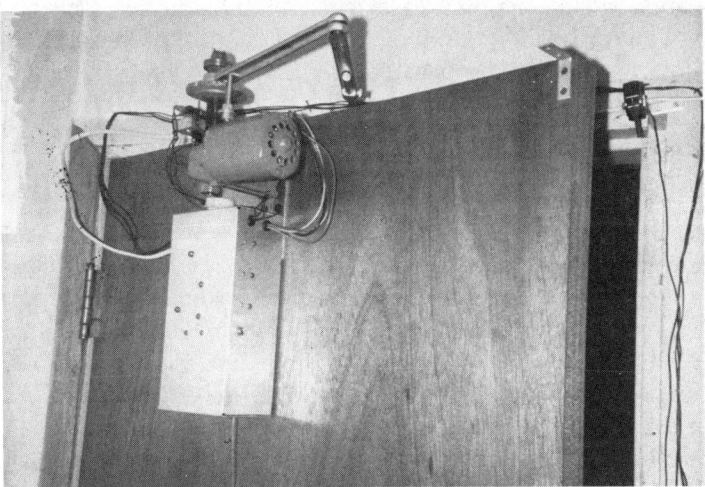

or extensions onto the control knobs. It is wise to obtain replacement knobs from a repair shop before you begin, so that the appliance will not be temporarily out of order if the experiment fails. Some of the plastics used to make these knobs seem to repel any adhesive you use. In this case, fasten the extension to the knob with a small piece of tape and liberally coat the entire knob and the extension with epoxy glue (Fig. 2–8). Some may think this looks messy, but it works.

DOORS

Radio-controlled garage door openers were originally intended for use by able-bodied persons who, for whatever reason, did not wish to get out of their car to open the garage door. You can adapt these gadgets for your use in opening and closing any door (Fig. 2–9). When the door so equipped is closed, it is locked. When it is locked, the only way you or anyone can open it from the outside is with a radio transmitter that is operating at the correct frequency. You can further equip the door with doorbell buttons, one on the outside and another on the inside, so that anyone can open or close it without using the transmitter when it is not locked from the inside.

A transmitter is about the size of a pack of cigarettes and can be clipped to your belt, sun visor, or wheelchair.

These door openers are most easily adapted to the heavy, sliding, glass type. However, you can adapt yours to operate any standard hinged door, although it may not look as neat. If the appearance is important to you, you can buy just the transmitter and the receiver (about $65) and build the mechanical part from scratch. This approach requires more work and costs almost as much, but it does look better.

You may also want to build a door check, which is the mechanism that keeps the door from closing too fast and thereby injuring someone. You can buy the linkage arms separately from an industrial supply firm and connect them to an electric motor (of about 3–5 rpm) by means of a work arbor with a standard ½–20 thread and castle nut. Cut two washers from cork at least ½ in. thick and place them on the arbor on each side of the linkage arm. Tighten the castle nut just enough to allow the motor to operate the door—never any tighter. A cotter pin will keep the nut from turning.

You can also add an electric lock to your existing door latch. Place it in the jamb on the frame, and you will not have to change your present lock and bolt. This lock can be activated by your transmitter or used manually.

SIGNALS FOR HELP

The applications of garage door openers are limited only by your imagination. The receiver is a remote-controlled switch which is turned on as long as the button on the transmitter is pushed. While the receiver cannot switch on high currents, it can switch on an electric relay which in turn *can* switch on high currents. It can therefore be used as a personal alarm or call for help. For this purpose, you would want to wear your transmitter on your belt and have the receiver connected to an alarm bell. The receiver can be located as much as 150 ft away from the transmitter, and the alarm can be even farther away as long as it is connected to the receiver by a wire.

TELEPHONES

You should begin by buying your own telephone. When you own it, you are free to modify it as you wish, which you cannot do to one owned by the telephone company. Do *not* buy telephone equipment from the local electronic discount shop—it is often neither dependable nor durable. Buy only from telecommunications supply companies, such as Graybar Electric, because they sell only top quality equipment and they can supply whatever you need: speakers, headsets, long cords, extension ringers, plugs, jacks. The prices are surprisingly low (about $16 for a standard phone). If your supply company refuses to sell to an individual, have a church or local business buy it for you. You may have to obtain special permission from the local telephone company to connect your phone to their lines.

You can add a toggle switch to turn the phone on or off, and the handset can be off the hook all the time. Buy a test tube holder at a chemical supply company; it can hold the handset in a position that allows you to talk and listen. You will not have to move the handset to answer or to hang up. Instead, the phone is electrically connected to the line and disconnected from it. If you attach a large pulley to the dial, you can rotate the dial by pulling the string. You can glue a peg into the "O" hole which will prevent the dial from rotating too far and will make it easy for you to dial the operator. Then, of course, once you have explained your disability, the operator can dial the number for you.

Using electronic computer logic circuits, I have built a telephone dialer that is easy to operate. A single push-button switch controls the phone in a manner similar to a push-operated electric wall switch. Push the switch to answer the phone and push again to hang up. To dial the operator, push the button as if you were answering the phone and hold it down for 3 sec. This is the same, electrically speaking, as dialing "O."

The dialer is not wired directly into a phone but instead has a phone plug and jack so that any unmodified phone can be plugged into it, and the dialer can be plugged into any phone jack. Because the phone is disconnected from the line when it is "hung up," its bell will not signal an incoming call. You can install an extension ringer in the dialer or at the jack.

You should have a battery-powered telephone. True, telephones usually continue to operate even when an entire city loses its electric power, and that is just when you are most likely to need to telephone for help. However, the card dialers and other automatic equipment obtained from the telephone company use electricity to operate.

LOCATING EQUIPMENT

Many excellent ideas have been abandoned because the necessary parts could not be found. Look in the yellow pages of your phone book, and do not hesitate to ask questions. Sometimes the people you have called do not have what you want but can direct you to someone else who does carry it.

For toggle switches, look under Electronic Equipment and Supplies or Switches—Electric. For test tube holders, try Laboratory Equipment and Supplies or Chemicals. For garage door openers and transmitters and receivers, look under Doors; you can also obtain them from Heath-Kit, Benton Harbor, Michigan 49022. One of the largest suppliers of phones is Graybar Electric Company, which is often listed under Electric Equipment and Supplies—Wholesale. Keep trying, and good luck!

If you want to design your own telephone equipment, a large amount of technical information is available. Write to Western Electric, Commercial Relations, P.O. Box 1579, Newark, New Jersey 07102, and ask for *Technical Reference Catalog Index and Price List, Publication 40000.*

Bibliography

ADAPTATIONS AND TECHNIQUES FOR THE DISABLED HOMEMAKER. By Karen Hodgeman, OTR, and Eleanor Warpeha, OTR. 32 pages. Illustrated. 8½ × 11. 1973. Order from Publications Department, Sister Kenny Institute, 1800 Chicago Avenue, Minneapolis, Minnesota 55404. $1.75.

This manual, designed for disabled homemakers, occupational therapists, and nurses, replaces the earlier Kenny publication, *Homemaking Aid for the Disabled*. With more than 60 photographs and drawings, it clearly illustrates both equipment and techniques. The adaptive devices described are simple and inexpensive; explicit directions are given for constructing as well as purchasing equipment.

Of value not only to those who work from a wheelchair or crutches but also to those who have the use of only one hand or who have arthritic or weak hands, it covers the whole range of household work. Most importantly, the techniques and the equipment are not designed for the dream kitchen, but any kitchen, any range, any refrigerator. Nothing special is needed except know-how, inexpensive devices, and a good lapboard for a working area.

For instance, if it is impossible to remove doors and make an opening under the sink, it suggests approaching the sink sideways with the stronger or good arm next to the sink. It shows a wooden spoon being used to set range dials that are out of reach; it shows how to make a Velcro strap for opening oven doors, a wooden bowl holder, a one-handed rolling pin, and enlarged faucet handles. Bedmaking, one of the most difficult tasks from a wheelchair, is made easier by using specially folded bed linens and doing all the work for one side at one time.

AIDS TO INDEPENDENT LIVING. Self-help for the Handicapped. By Edward W. Lowman, MD, and Judith Lannefeld Klinger, OTR, MA. 796 pages. 8½ × 11¼. 1969. Order from McGraw–Hill Book Company, Inc., 1221 Avenue of the Americas, New York, New York 10020. $41.

This encyclopedia of aids, gadgets, and techniques, represents two decades of creative rehabilitation and research at the Institute of Rehabilitation Medicine, New York University School of Medicine.

It classifies the tasks and jobs of daily living into 65 categories for easy reference. Following each category are lists of relevant books, periodicals, and agencies; at the end of the book is a list of equipment sources. Emphasis is placed on devices and gadgets that are commercially available through mail order catalogs.

Following are the general topics included: basic tasks of daily living, ambulation, housing, furniture and posturpedic equipment, homemaking, communications and vocations, recreational and avocational interests, transportation and travel, education, speech, and organizations designed to help the disabled.

COPING WITH DISABLEMENT. Edited by Edith Rudinger. 230 pages. Illustrated. 6 × 8. 1974. Order from Consumers' Association, 14 Buckingham Street, London WC2N 6DS, England. £1.25. (About $2.50)

A good source of practical advice and information about ways of overcoming difficulties in everyday living, the book has detailed explanations of the services for disabled and elderly people that are provided by local authorities through social services departments and by the national health services through area health authorities. In addition, it includes sources of information on special aids. Topics covered include wheelchairs, housework, cooking and eating, pastimes, travel, clothes, bathrooms, cars, and voluntary organizations.

INDEPENDENT LIVING FOR THE HANDICAPPED AND THE ELDERLY. By Elizabeth Eckhardt May, Neva R. Waggoner, and Eleanor Boettke Hotte. 271 pages. Illustrated. 7 × 10. 1974. Order from Houghton Mifflin Company, 110 Tremont Street, Boston, Massachusetts 02107. $9.95.

This is not a how-to-do book, but a you-can-do book. Its impact is in the photographs of disabled people around the world maintaining their homes and caring for their families. The emphasis is on Lillian M. Gilbreth's techniques of applying work simplification principles to enable those who are elderly or disabled to live more independently. The chapters on clothing, for both adults and children, and caring for children are especially helpful. A sit-to-work chair is of interest to the elderly and those with limited energy; it is made by cutting off the legs of a comfortable old chair and fastening it to a castered platform built of plywood and bumpered with rubber tubing.

MEALTIME MANUAL FOR THE AGED AND HANDICAPPED. By Judith Lannefeld Klinger, OTR, MA, Fred H. Frieden, MD, and Richard A. Sullivan, MD. 242 pages. Spiral bound. Illustrated. 5½ ×

8½. 1970. Order B461 from FashionABLE, Rocky Hill, New Jersey 08553. $2.98 (including postage).

This treasure, with a foreword by Howard A. Rusk, MD, was compiled by the Institute of Rehabilitation Medicine, New York University Medical Center. Financed with a $200,000 grant from the Campbell Soup Fund, it is the culmination of 2 years of research by a team composed of medical advisors, two occupational therapists, a home economist, a bioengineer, an electrical engineer, and a graduate engineering student. All this professional talent is well blended. The book, though extraordinarily helpful and factual, has a feeling of joyousness.

It is universally useful, whether the individual is just learning to slow down with age or a new quadriplegic who is trying to cook again. Specifically, it includes hints for homemakers who are elderly, who work with one hand, who have weakness in their upper extremities, who have arthritis, or who use wheelchairs. In addition, it includes hints for the upper-extremity amputee and demonstrates how to do housework and cook with loss of sensation, with limited vision, or with incoordination.

A very important point is made about the possibilities of qualifying for assistance under the vocational rehabilitation program which considers homemaking a remunerative occupation. "Retraining can include counseling, diagnostic and physical restorative services, and tools or equipment. . . . Equipment includes kitchen changes—both material and labor costs."

The chapter on small electrical appliances is particularly useful for those who cannot do any major remodeling. Such appliances can be placed on a low table or wheel-around cart at any convenient height. Included is good general advice on planning the purchases. Among the appliances brand-named, photographed, and priced are: can openers, five electric and two manual, that can be used with one hand or weak hands; table ranges; electric skillets, with ideas for replacing a cover knob with a large wooden handle and attaching a metal-spoked or dowel handle to the temperature control; broilers and broiler–ovens; mixers; blenders; electric knives; toasters; hot pots; and grinders.

Sinks and dishwashing are covered in detail in another helpful chapter which suggests a way of determining the comfortable depth of a sink for a seated or wheelchaired cook. Stretch the palms of the hands as far as possible toward the bottom of the sink without leaning forward; if the bottom cannot be reached, a rack can be placed on the bottom of the sink to bring the dishpan up to a pleasant working height. For an average sized seated cook, the counter should be 31 in. high, and the sink 5½ in. deep; a long-legged person might like a 4 in. deep sink. To reach faucets, use an ordinary S-shaped closet hook screwed into the end of a dowel. Rubbermaid, 1205 East Bowman, Wooster, Ohio 44692, manufactures lazy Susans, drawer dividers, rubber mats, and rubber sink dividers.

The 82-page section on menus is full of sensible, inexpensive ideas, many of them using canned soups as a short cut. Quite practically, the section starts off with descriptions of a gadget and knives to open cartons that seem ironclad. The gadget is the Zip-Cut Box Opener by Ekco Housewares Company, 9234 West Belmont Avenue, Franklin Park, Illinois 60131; the knives, a linoleum knife or a steel utility knife also made by Ekco. A safety spoon that clips to the side of the pan so that it does not fall into the pan but stays relatively cool to the touch is made by the American Foundation for the Blind, 15 West 16th Street, New York, New York 10011. A Rubbermaid waffled pattern mat prevents slithering of hot pans.

THE ONE HANDER'S BOOK. A Basic Guide to Activities of Daily Living. By Veronica Washam. 126 pages. Illustrated. 8×10. 1973. Order from The John Day Company, 257 Park Avenue South, New York, New York 10010. $10.

A handsome book with large photographs, it was written for those who are able-bodied except for the full or partial loss of one arm. Subjects include dressing and grooming, hair styling and care, fashion, housework, cooking, sewing, baby and children care, dining out, traveling, at work, at school, social occasions, and recreation and sports.

SELF AIDS. Compiled by Wendy M. Davis, SROT, MAOT. 83 pages. Illustrated. 6×9½. 1970. Order from Thistle Foundation, 22 Charlotte Square, Edinburgh, EH2 4DF, Scotland. 37 pence (From U.S. send $1.)

This is a delightful booklet of inexpensive, do-it-yourself aids and appliances that covers every area of daily living. Among the homemade items illustrated are a tipping stand for teapots, a buttering board, a bathtub seat, key grips, shoe remover, and a long shoehorn.

SELF-HELP MANUAL FOR ARTHRITIS PATIENTS. By Judith Lannefeld Klinger, OTR, MA. 124

pages. Illustrated. 6×9. 1974. Order from The Arthritis Foundation, 1212 Avenue of the Americas, New York, New York 10036. $1.25.

This paperback "Bible" of rehabilitation equipment, gadgets, techniques, and sources is a people's version of the gold-plated *Aids to Independent Living,* which Mrs. Klinger created with Dr. Lowman. Its title is misleading, however, since it is not for arthritics alone, but for all elderly and disabled people who want to "open new areas of excitement and life or bring back ones they have enjoyed in the past."

An ingenious method of keying products to their sources is used. Emphasis is placed on aids that are commercially available through mail catalogs intended for the general public.

The table of contents lists the following headings: managing your time, protecting your joints, ambulation, bed transfer, posture, accessories, toilet aids, bathing and showering aids, grooming, dressing, housing and furnishings, aids around the house, kitchen planning and meal preparation aids, eating, sewing and needlework, communication and vocational aids, travel and shopping, recreation and leisure time, sources for equipment, and bibliography.

The positive spirit of the book is set in the introduction, "Delve into the bibliography. Check out the catalogues of suppliers. The world is your oyster, and you might just find the pearl that will allow you to do something you thought impossible."

WHAT YOU CAN DO FOR YOURSELF. By Patricia Galbreaith. 272 pages. Illustrated. 6×9½. 1974. Order from Drake Publishers, Inc., 381 Park Avenue South, New York, New York 10016. $12.

Mrs. Galbreaith is known to many disabled individuals through her nationally syndicated newspaper column on hints for the handicapped. She has put together a comprehensive collection of ideas gathered from her columns and her own 15 years in a wheelchair.

WHEELCHAIR INTERIORS. By Sharon C. Olson and Diane K. Meredith. 46 pages. Illustrated. 8½ × 11. 1973. Order from National Easter Seal Society for Crippled Children and Adults, 2023 West Ogden Avenue, Chicago, Illinois 60612. $1.50.

This booklet was derived from the authors' research projects toward degrees in interior design from the University of Wisconsin. The specifications and suggestions were obtained from a local organization of disabled individuals. Included are wheelchair dimensions, average reach from a wheelchair, and suggestions for kitchens, bathrooms, laundry, bedrooms, and working and storage areas.

YOU CAN DO IT FROM A WHEELCHAIR. By Arlene E. Gilbert. 144 pages. Illustrated. 6¼ × 9¼. 1973. Order from Arlington House Publishers, 81 Centre Avenue, New Rochelle, New York 10801. $6.95.

The author, wheelchaired by multiple sclerosis, shares her experiences in child care, homemaking, and general living problems.

"The disabled must take the responsibility for their own lives."

—Jan Posker, Chairman of the Disabled Persons' Housing Cooperative, Czechoslovakia

3
Kitchen Adaptations

Kitchen adaptations are the prime target of every specialist in housing for the disabled and elderly, of every therapist preparing hospitalized patients for a return to normal living, of every housewife who becomes disabled, and of every disabled bride or bachelor. In this chapter, the disabled themselves describe their kitchens, methods, equipment, and gadgets. Their adaptations, lifestyles, and attitudes are strongly individual. They are not stereotyped drawing-board disabled. They are homemakers who are homemaking from a wheelchair. These wide variations indicate that kitchens for the disabled can be adjustable and adaptable to each individual and that disabled individuals are adaptable.

FIVE WHEELCHAIR KITCHENS

Following are descriptions of five kitchens designed by five wheelchaired individuals. The kitchens range from superspecial to quite normal. All have single lever tap handles, countertop range burners, and wall ovens—features of many new homes. One of the designers has upper cupboards that can be raised and lowered mechanically. Another uses six pull-out breadboards as work areas. Another uses her lapboard exclusively as a work area. One has open space under the sink and range. One has 33 in. high counters; one has 32 in. high counters. Another prides herself on being able to work at standard height counters.

WHERE DID THE KITCHEN GO?

JERRY WINTER

Jerry Winter of Denver, Colorado, is quadriplegic at C-5 level because of idiopathic transverse myelitis. She and her husband, Dick, have four children 14–20 years of age. She has acted as a consultant for Kitchen Distributors, Inc. and has demonstrated her kitchen to therapists and the disabled in the Denver area. (Photographs are by Paul Currier.)

In 1965, I came home from the hospital in a wheelchair with good use of only one hand. Home was a two story house with a basement and no bath on the main floor. Four small children were scattered among a few antiques and some classy junk. I practiced being a lady in a wheelchair while my husband, Dick, sold the house out from under me and started building a new one with the help of an architectural designer and a builder.

Dick didn't do any actual building but kept everyone thinking from a sitting position. His words, "Let's sit down and discuss it," were more than a courtesy. We had an old decrepit wheelchair at the building site. Plumbers, electricians, and carpenters sat in the chair to discuss with Dick ways of installing drains under sinks to prevent hot water burns to legs with no sensation, placing light switches 42 in. from the floor and electric outlets 20 in. high to allow an easy reach from a sitting position, and building 33 in. high countertops everywhere to be used as functional work levels. Considering how many craftsmen sat in that chair, we must have seemed like a delegation for a hire the handicapped committee. Ed Warner, our designer, was the most experienced. He has one useless arm as a result of Chinese polio, which is the same as ours except he got it in China. Ed measured the turning radius of my wheelchair and drew the plans that were right for us.

Building the new house took longer than we expected. Working from a sitting position in a standard kitchen while waiting for our new home required the creative imagination of the cook. The higher countertops with built-in cupboards underneath meant all food preparation had to be done from a side position. Since I couldn't get my knees under the counter, additional work space was added with a fold-down extension the same depth as the counter but at a height more functional. The extension was fastened to the counter with two card table hinges. The sink was not usable for me. I did all clean up work with a plastic bowl on my lap. The bowl was filled and emptied with a small pitcher. Later I discovered the value of a plastic turkey baster, good for filling a steam iron or removing hot liquid from a container with less danger of spills. Reachable storage space was added with boxlike units mounted under top cabinets. Similar plastic units are now available at most department stores in addition to plug-in fluorescent lighting if back lighting presents a visual problem. Pegboard attached to the outside door of a low cabinet was used for hanging heavier tools such as a frying pan and other often used pans and cooking utensils.

In the years we have lived in our new house I have received a number of questions about my wheelchair kitchen. The design of the kitchen stumped both Dick and Ed, so I designed my own. I hate to cook but realized this kitchen was a bonus for my grandmother, who is 4 ft 10-½ in. tall. A sensible kitchen doesn't have to be designed specifically for wheels.

Built-in appliances are no more expensive than individual pieces if starting from scratch. The most dangerous appliance in the kitchen is the standard stove. The burners are too high for the sitting cook to use safely, and the hot oven door must be hinged to pull toward the individual. Bending from the side of the chair and forward into the hot oven is a most dangerous experience and impossible with a heavy, large roaster. I found sturdy countertop burners and had them mounted into one corner. Since they come in sets of two, it wasn't difficult to have one set follow the counter one way and the other placed at an angle to the first (Fig. 3–1), allowing the cook to rest both arms on the counter for balance when stirring.

The ovens are built into the wall with the bottom rack 31 in. from the floor and close enough to the counter or bread board to slide a heavy roaster (Fig. 3–2). The doors of the ovens are hinged to raise toward the ceiling rather than pull

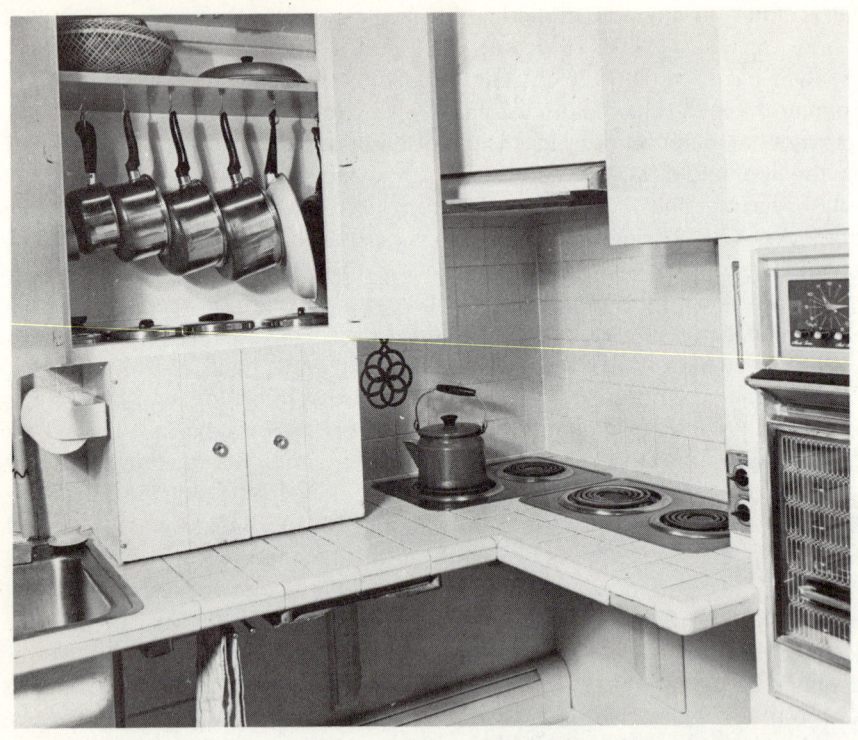
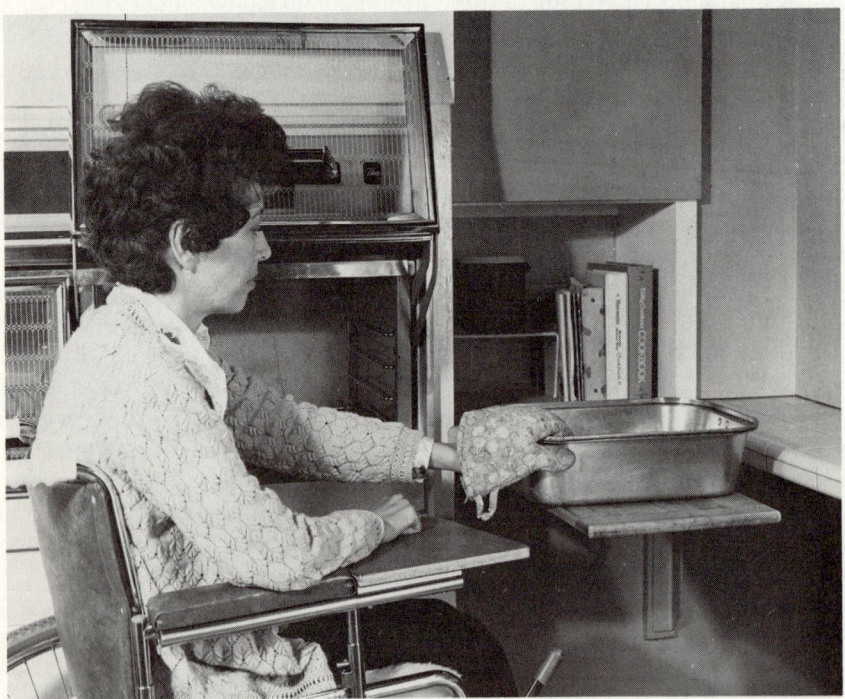

Kitchen Adaptations 35

Fig. 3–1. Built-in burners are installed flush with counter surface for ease in sliding pots and pans instead of lifting. Controls are mounted on wall to the immediate right. Pots and pans are not stacked and can be removed and replaced individually. (Kitchen display from Kitchen Distributors, Inc.)

Fig. 3–2. Undercounter bread boards in strategic locations limit handling of heavier utensils. Countertops are made on 1-1/8 in. subflooring covered with ceramic tile and are supported by ½ × 2 × 2 in. fabricated steel brackets mounted on back walls. (Kitchen display from Kitchen Distributors, Inc.)

Fig. 3–3. Double oven with doors opening upward. Drawers are used for hot pads, baster, mixing spoons, spatula, etc. Bottom drawer and top cabinets have vertical dividers for roasters, cookie sheets, carving boards, etc. (Kitchen display from Kitchen Distributors, Inc.)

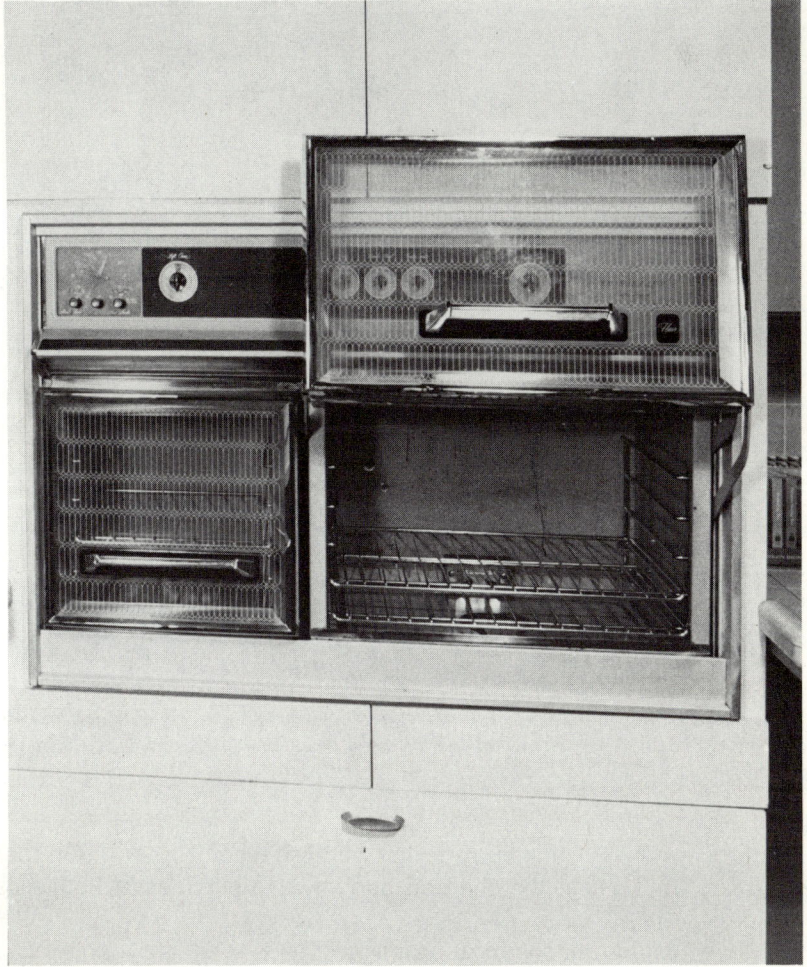

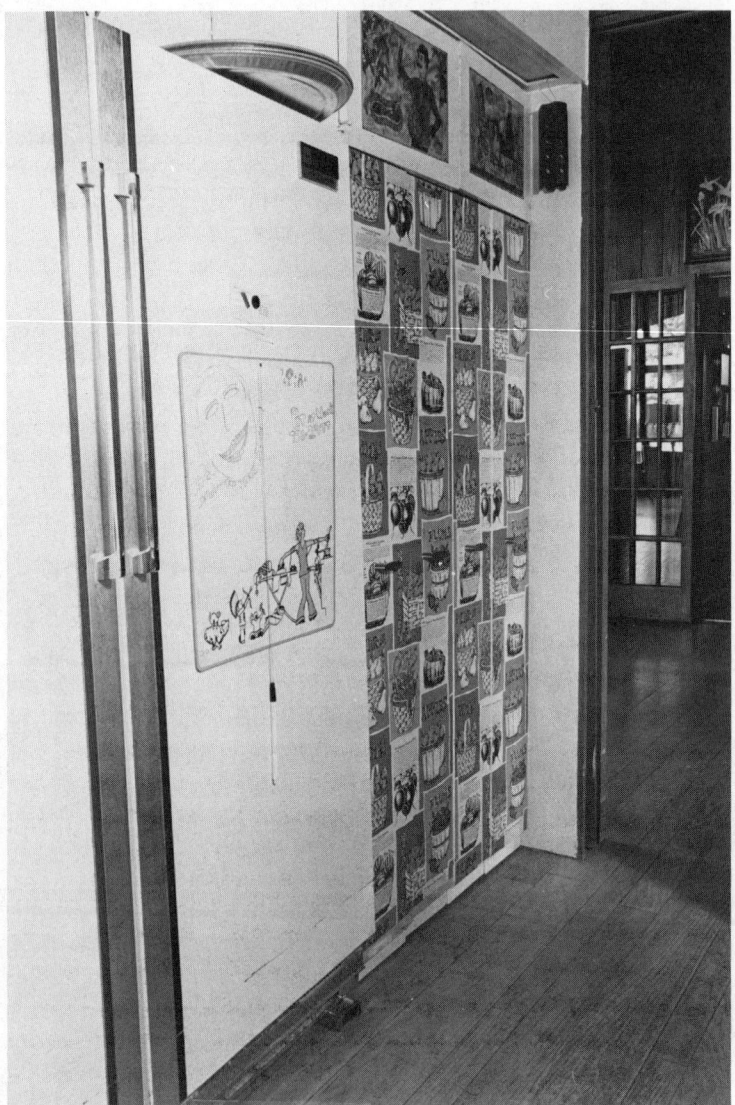

Fig. 3–4. Position of the side-by-side refrigerator–freezer allows 180° opening of doors. The entry to the kitchen is closed off by a folding wood door recessed in wall return. (Kitchen display from Kitchen Distributors, Inc.)

toward the cook, eliminating burns for all who use them (Fig. 3–3). On today's market ovens can be hinged at the side, and it is possible to have the hinges on either side.

The refrigerator–freezer combination is large (Fig. 3–4). All shelves pull out, and it is positioned to extend an inch or two from the cupboards and counter on either side. This allows the doors to swing open as wide as possible, and I can make

Fig. 3–5. Vertical upended drawers serve as the pantry. Cabinets, pantry, and counters were built on the job by carpenters. Free use was made of particle board and plywood. (Kitchen display from Kitchen Distributors, Inc.)

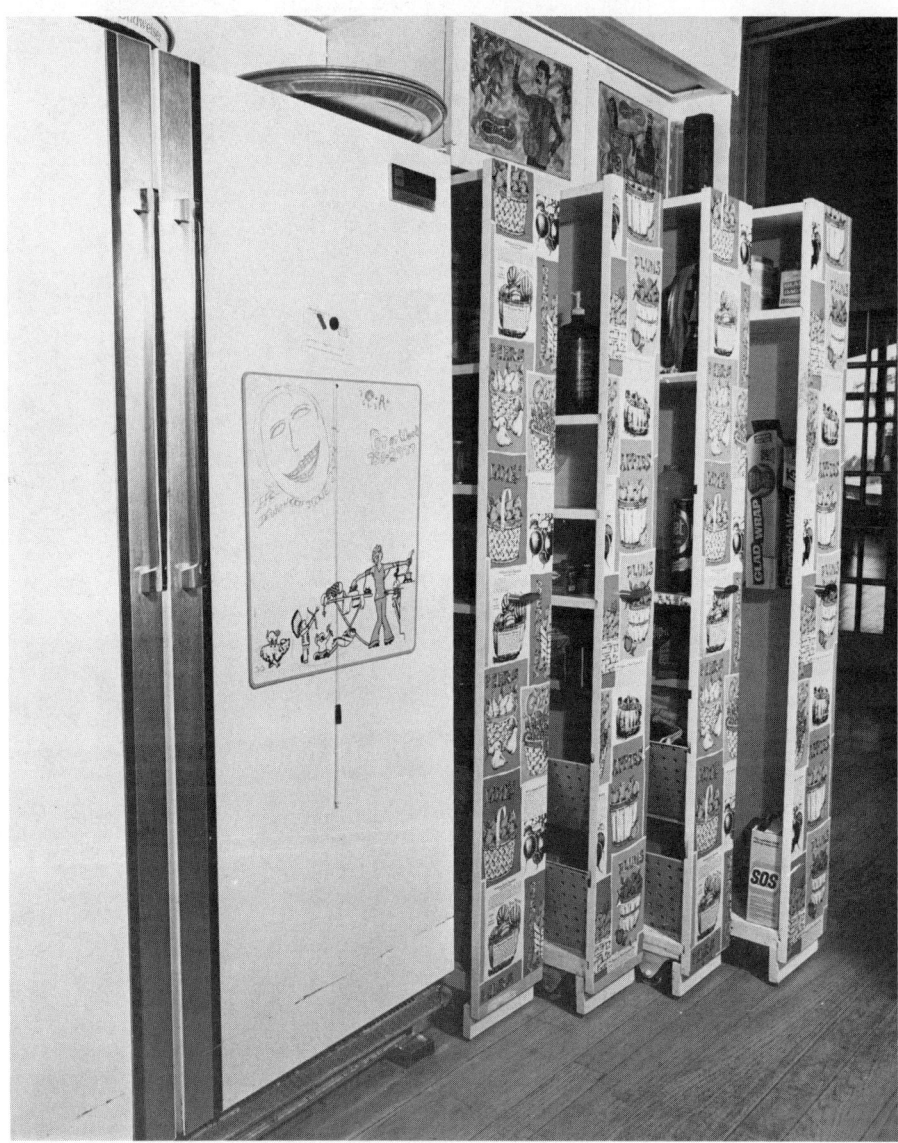

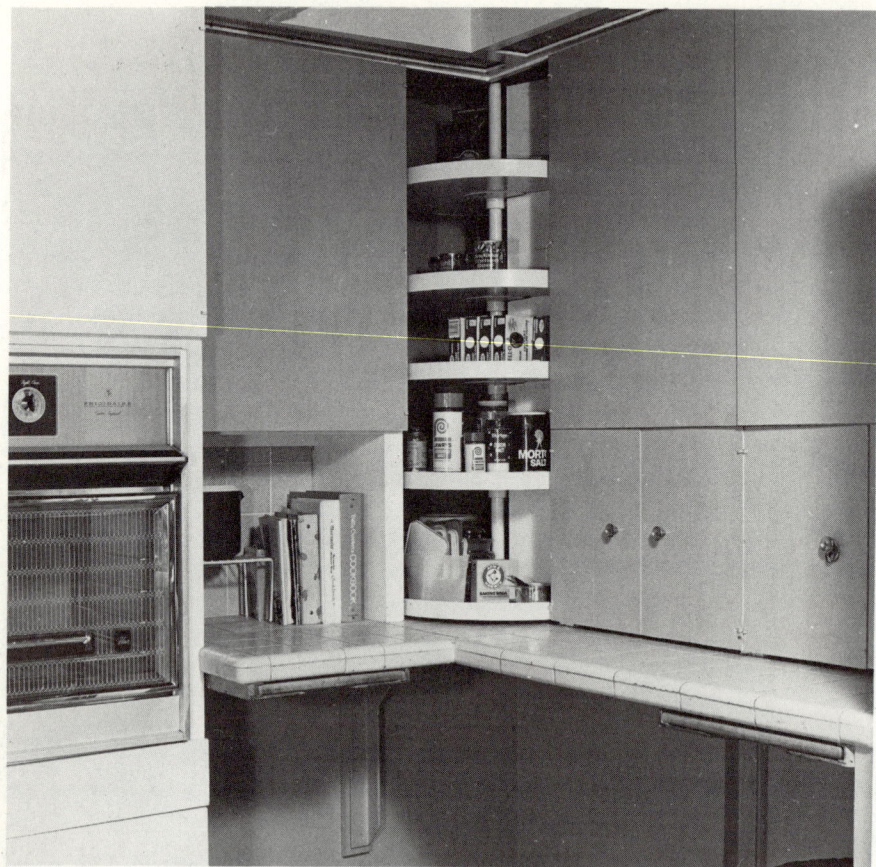

Fig. 3–6. Smaller lazy Susan with baking needs. Mixer and bowls are stored behind countertop doors to the right. Tiled countertop is open underneath; access for chair under counter allows easy reach to low shelves. (Kitchen display from Kitchen Distributors, Inc.)

a side approach rather than leaning forward. Stocking a standard size refrigerator requires thinking ahead, since the top shelf is not conveniently reachable and heavier items, such as a gallon of milk, usually end up on that shelf.

The pantries to the side of the refrigerator are built like upended 9 in. deep drawers (Fig. 3–5). They pull out individually, gliding on 6 in. rubber rollers and guided by a track at top. They are only deep enough for one or two cans of whatever and are, perhaps, the handiest things in the kitchen. In opposite corners are two lazy Susans that revolve in complete circles. The smaller of the two holds spices, flour, and other baking needs (Fig. 3–6) and is located between the ovens and the electric mixer and mixing bowls. The larger lazy Susan houses dishes, glasses, and glass cookware and is between the dishwasher and a section of drawers where I keep flatware, placemats, napkins and other table needs (Fig. 3–7). On top of the drawers is a microwave oven with a side hinged door, a useful new addition to the kitchen. The table where we share our meals, snacks, conversation and do homework is just beyond the drawers. Lighting directed onto working areas is fluorescent, mounted inside soffits above cabinets. The double sink has single lever control. The left sink is 4 in. deep with the drain at the rear. The drain pipe is quick turned and plumbed to wall. The right sink is deeper and has a disposer. The cutting board on the left sink slides over the sink. The low window allows a view from a sitting position.

For me there is one complete advantage of an accessible kitchen: the ability to entertain instead of the dread of isolation. To live in a wheelchair is to face a world of steps, curbs, and narrow doorways. These barriers are difficult in public places but can be impossible in the homes of friends and acquaintances. The ability to prepare a meal or a simple snack means a party, a meeting, any gathering in my own home.

Fig. 3–7. Dishes are rinsed at the sink, then loaded into the dishwasher. The dishwasher is unloaded into the lazy Susan, and the silverware is put into the drawers at left. The dishwasher countertop is at the conventional height; other counters are approximately 4 in. lower. (Kitchen display from Kitchen Distributors, Inc.)

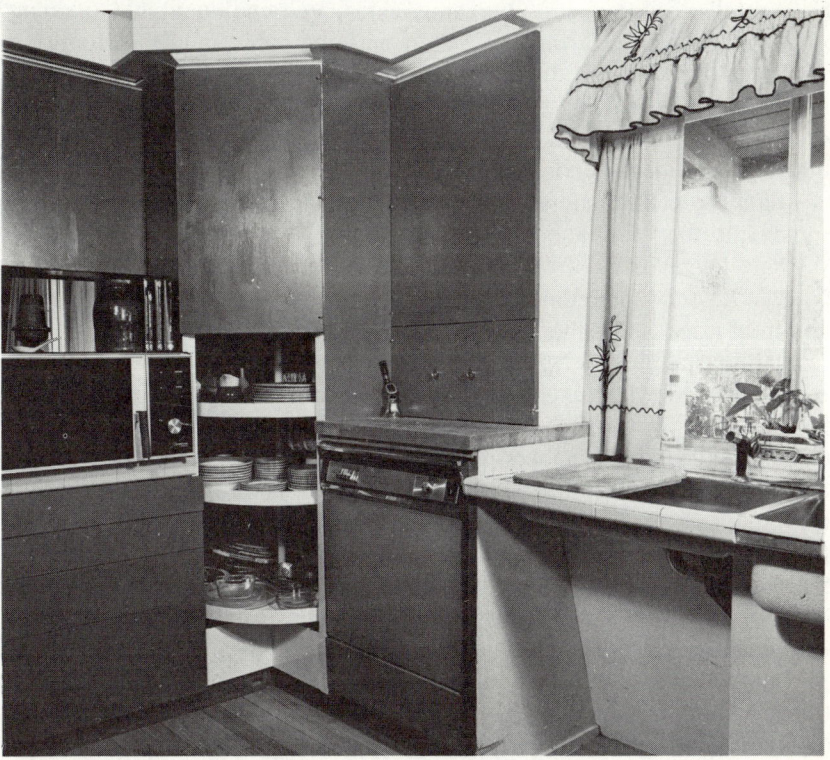

A REDESIGNED HOUSE

MARENE AULGER

Marene Aulger and her husband, Aulton, are wheelchaired. She was disabled by polio in 1937; he was injured while a flyer in the Navy Air Corps during World War II. Both went back to college after an interim of about 30 years. They teach wheelchair dancing—square dancing and other forms of dancing on rear wheels. They have made a sound and color movie of their dancing groups which they rent for a nominal amount.

After 21 years of living with the veteran's paraplegic house that we had designed and built, we did extensive redesigning to correct some of the mistakes and to add some things we discovered we needed.

Everything is planned so I can work with a good left hand and a not so good right one; I do all my own cooking, dishwashing, laundry, and house cleaning. Aulton works three mornings a week at Manufacturing Production Services, a firm of which he is part owner, that makes hand controls and car ramps. We both have hand-controlled automobiles. Our garage doors are radio-controlled, opening or closing at the touch of a button. Aulton built the cabinets in the laundry and service area and panelled the lower half of his den.

We expanded our living room to enclose a front porch and added parquet floors. We now have a total of about 2000 sq ft, with three bedrooms and two bathrooms. Our master bedroom is 16 ft square. We have an extra large curving sofa which has built-in end tables to make it easier to clean and to prevent our bumping into them and knocking them over.

We have telephones in the bedroom, kitchen, and den, plus a number of phone jacks. We have an intercom system throughout the house, including the bathroom, front door, and patio.

Our bathrooms are extra wide. The shower has a swing-away seat which locks into position while you are getting onto it, then it can be unlocked and swiveled around in place. In the bathtub we have an hydraulic lift.

I am delighted with the pantry which I designed. In a space 4 ft wide, 2 ft deep, and 7 ft high I have more than two dozen shelves, and I can keep everything I need within easy reach. The inner sides of the two doors are filled with shelves; a full-length shelved panel pulls out to the left, behind this are more shelves that are staggered so that I can see what is on them without sliding out the panel.

Most of our changes were made in the kitchen to take advantage of new developments such as the speed-cooking electronic oven and the Corning range, the "counter that cooks." We installed a luminous ceiling and a new kitchen door with top-to-bottom louvered glass panels. In addition, we replaced all the old cabinets. We have a low dishwasher now at the end of the cabinets (Fig. 3–8). The counters and the sink are all 32 in. high, and we had our "toe-kick" area under the cabinets made 9 in. high and 6 in. deep so it is easy to get our chairs close to the counters. Our wall oven is 32 in. high at the base. There are drawers for a blender and a mixer. Lazy Susan shelves spin around in the corners, and we had six pull-out bread boards put in because I find them so helpful that I want them in every working area. A set of plans showing all the details of our kitchen

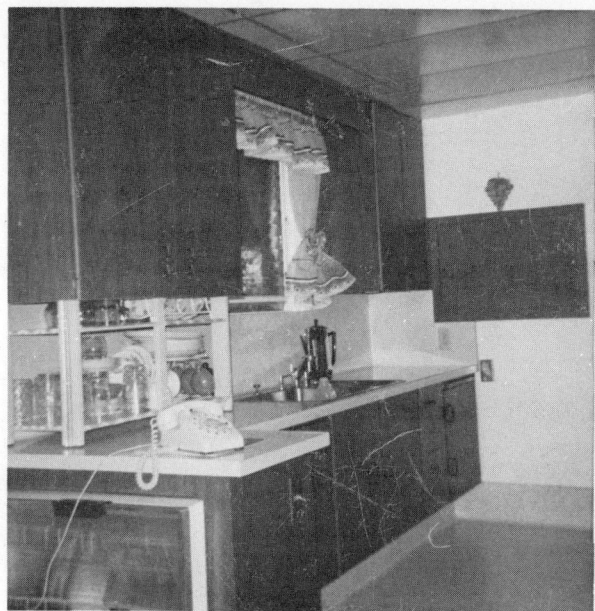

Fig. 3–8. The new dishwasher is at the end of the counter. The press of a button brings the upper cabinet shelves down a full 17 in.

is available for $20. Our address is Mr. and Mrs. Aulton A. Aulger, 4275 View Place, San Diego, California 92115.

MY KITCHEN IS BUILT FOR ME

MONALEE CHAMBERS

Monalee Chambers of Unionville, Michigan, was working as a nurse when she became quadriplegic because of poliomyelitis in 1959. She and her husband, Jack, and their 18-year-old son, Jeff, live in a ranch house which they had specially designed so she could do as much as possible by herself.

In the beginning my vital capacity was a little more than 400 cc, and I could only wiggle the toes on my left foot and move my arms slightly. As the years have passed I've grown stronger and needed less and less help. Now I just have a cleaning lady twice a month.

My kitchen is built for me so I can do everything myself. I have an automatic dishwasher, and my utility room, where I have an upright freezer and my washer and dryer, is near the kitchen. I find carpeting so much easier to care for than tile floors that I have my kitchen carpeted also. The once in 2 months or so shampooing is easier than daily mopping. I have an electric rug shampooer and can run it myself.

My countertops are higher than most, but I sit on 4 in. of foam rubber in my chair so I don't get so tired of sitting. There is enough room under my oven so

42   Housing and Home Services for the Disabled

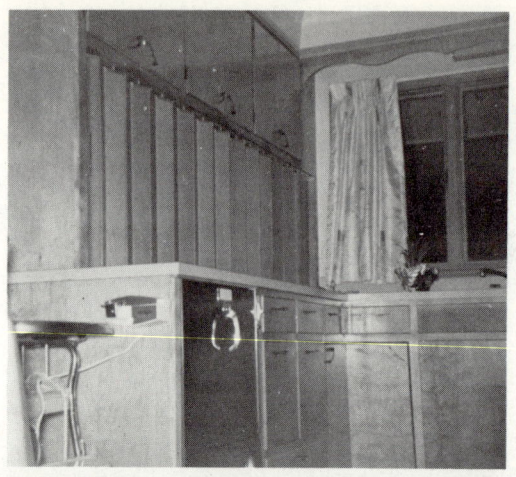

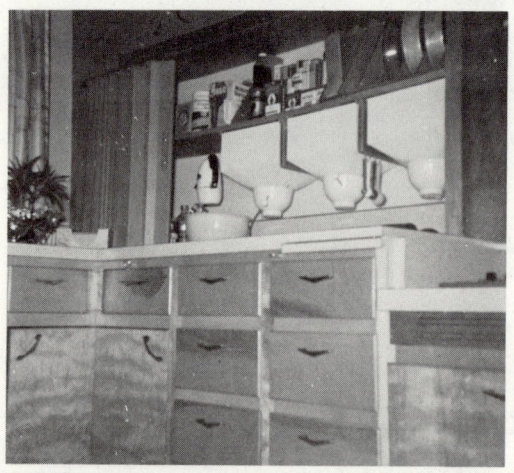

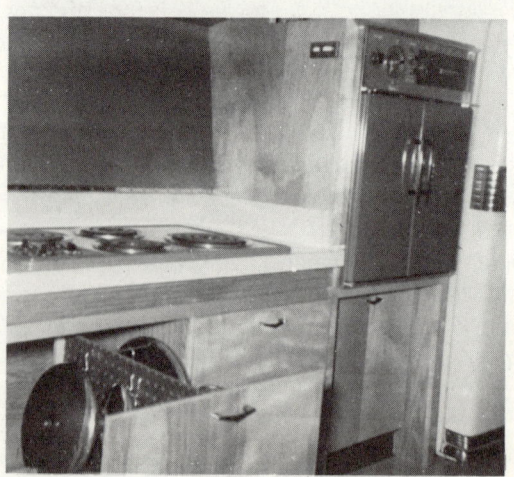

Fig. 3–9. All table dishes, toaster, etc. are on shelves behind the folding wooden curtain. There is a lazy Susan in each corner. Drawers hold bread, cereal, and silverware.

Fig. 3–10. The baking area has flour and sugar bins, little steps for spices, and a shelf divided vertically for cake and pie pans.

Fig. 3–11. The oven doors are French—no reaching over a hot oven door. A cover drops down over the burners.

I can face it, and the door under my sink opens back so I can roll under. My refrigerator is a Frigidaire. It is frost-proof, and I like the slide-out shelves. Unfortunately, the top freezer door opens from the top down so I must reach over the door.

All of my bottom cupboards are drawers and lazy Susans. The space between my top and bottom cupboards is closed by an accordion type wooden door (Fig. 3–9). One side of my kitchen has two shelves for storage of table dishes; the other side is a baking area (Fig. 3–10). My cooking pans and utensils hang from a hook on pegboard in the center of a big drawer just below my burners (Fig. 3–11).

The only real barrier for me to function quickly in my kitchen is that I must use my hands to move. For me the most unpleasant task is washing dishes; I am so thankful for my dishwasher. My most difficult kitchen task is cleaning my oven —in fact I just can't do it, or I'm not able to use my arms the rest of the day.

I am happy and thankful to be able to do my own housework. I love to cook and wash and iron. It just is a thrill for me knowing I've done it myself, to see my clothes sparkling white and ironed smoothly, to see my family nicely dressed, and to see my husband's and son's eyes and hear their comments of pleasure as they enjoy their food. The old saying about not missing the water until the well is dry is so true.

I'M A REAL LAPBOARD FREAK

JAN SERVICE

Jan Service, an artist at stitchery and entertaining, attributes her ability to adjust to existing houses to her constant use of a lapboard. Jan and her husband, Dean, live in a condominium in Phoenix.

Since becoming a paraplegic 22 years ago, I've lived in four different homes. Two of them we had custom-built, and two of them were existing homes. I feel that a house does not have to be drastically changed to meet my needs as a homemaker. Many friends have asked why my kitchen looks just like their own, why I haven't eliminated cabinets under the sink and range so that I could wheel under.

From the beginning, I've just naturally wheeled along side and worked easily when doing dishes, cooking, or cleaning. Perhaps it's because I'm a real lapboard freak. I'm seldom without my small lapboard, which fits easily over the desk arms of my chair. I've always worn the arms reversed; rolling is much easier this way, as there is room for my arms to wheel more freely.

Using a lapboard I can easily carry things back and forth from stove to sink without spilling or burning. I cut and chop food on the lapboard. I find it easy to carry everything for setting a table on it and to use it again for clearing the table. Getting things from the refrigerator is simple when you can pile it all on a lapboard.

I even iron on the board after placing a folded towel on it. I write on it; I wrap on it; I lean on it when doing stitchery; I always have an ash tray, cigarettes, lighter, and glasses on it. So you can see why I'm a lapboard freak and couldn't keep house without it. The lapboard is the reason we haven't drastically changed the basic parts of the kitchen. Perhaps I didn't want to sacrifice any cupboard space. Perhaps I was thinking of resale of the houses; it certainly could change a prospective buyer's mind if he thought he had to spend a large amount of money to make a kitchen normal again.

I have always been happy that I started right out using things as they were, adjusting myself to the current situation. Sometimes I found it terribly difficult and had to make some minor changes. With very few exceptions, I really don't think a kitchen must be structurally changed. Instead of wheeling underneath for a straight shot at whatever you're doing, roll along side and work easily from either side.

I ENJOY DOING IT MYSELF

DIANE SMITH

Diane Smith and her late husband, Bob, were both disabled by poliomyelitis in the 1940s and 1950s. Diane is ambulatory with one long leg brace and two long hand–wrist splints. When they built their house in Carmi, Illinois, they included some unusual features to fit their particular needs.

I have no upper arm muscles, a pretty fair left hand, and a poor right hand. I keep the buckle straps of my long hand splints extra long. I can raise my arm by grasping my upper forearm strap in my teeth. I can carry nearly anything I need up to about 4 lb. For closer reaching or lifting, I use the wrist strap. I discovered this method myself and have found it extremely functional for me. It has made me much more independent.

I do not use a regular wheelchair but an office type chair with casters which I find very useful. It eliminates much getting up and down, and still I am not stationary as I would be in a regular chair. I use this at my desk and to watch TV. I stand when I am cooking.

Prior to living in our adapted home my biggest problem was not having a work area my special height; I had a wheelchair then. Now my work space is a large pull-out board, 24-½ in. from the floor, which fits in the cabinets like a drawer. When not in use it is pushed back out of the way. The height of my work board is very basic to my being functional (Fig. 3–12).

I find the single lever faucet most convenient. I can reach the lever by holding the hand splint in my teeth. To fill a large pan or kettle, I relay the water from sink to stove with a measuring cup. If the pan is small, I hold it in my hand under the faucet and the hand splint strap in my teeth until it is full, then transfer it.

Our GE refrigerator has a left hand door, as my left is my "good" hand. It has the advantages of swing-out shelves, foot pedal to open, door storage, and an ice bucket for cube storage in freezer above. An ice-maker type would be much better as it is very difficult to empty ice trays, however, and I would prefer the freezer below. The push buttons on the built-in GE table top range are low and

Fig. 3–12. The kitchen is split-level, with some of the counters low and some at normal level for nondisabled helpers.

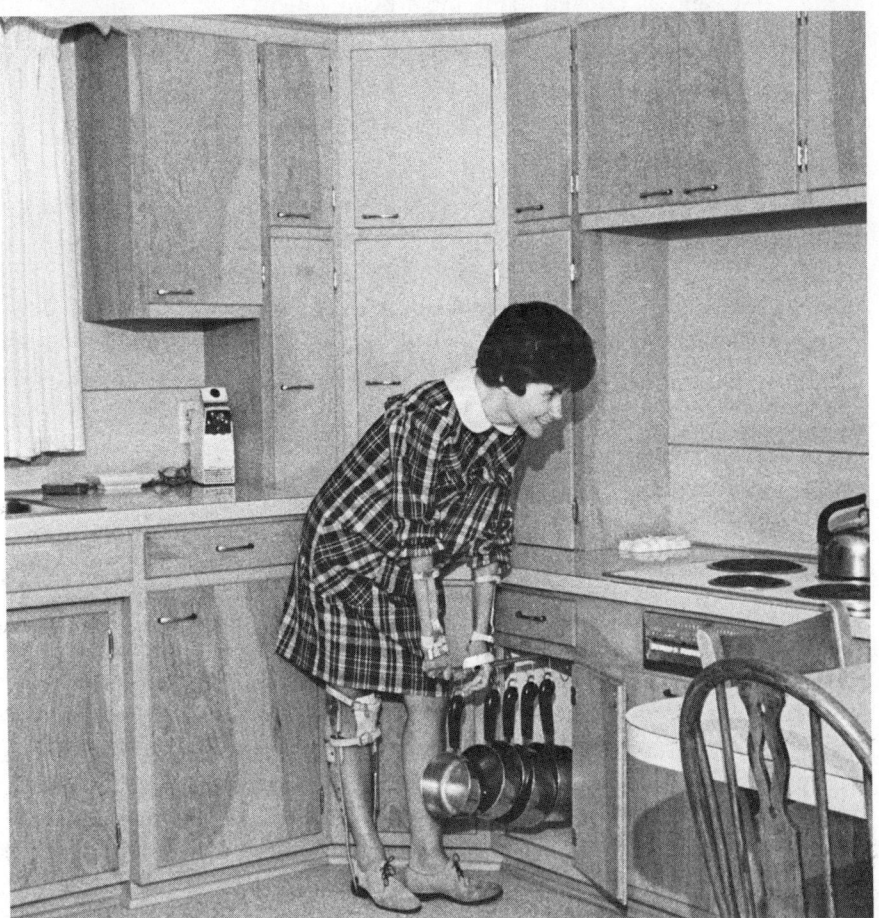

easy to push. The built-in GE oven is low so I don't have to reach up, but I would prefer a side-hinged oven door.

FORTY QUADRIPLEGIC COOKS

Forty quadriplegic cooks, 39 ladies and 1 gentleman, filled out extensive questionnaires for *Rehabilitation Gazette* on how they adapted their kitchens and their methods to cooking from a wheelchair with limited arm use. Following are the gleanings from these questionnaires. Only five of the cooking quads reported that they have specially built kitchens; the rest manage with modifications and ingenuity. The numbers of meals they cook per week range from 50 to 21, averaging 14. They are disabled by poliomyelitis quadriplegia (21), respiratory poliomyelitis quadriplegia (9), traumatic quadriplegia (5), muscular dystrophy (2), multiple sclerosis (1), muscle atrophy (1), and dystonia (1). They live in 19 different states and in Alberta and Ontario, Canada.

The following are mentioned as sources of gadgets and equipment. Most catalogs are free, and all contain many more helpful items.

Aristera Organization, 9 Rice's Lane, Westport, Connecticut 06880

Be O.K. Sales Co., P.O. Box 32, Brookfield, Illinois 60513

Breck's of Boston, 100 Breck Building, Boston, Massachusetts 02210

Cleo Living Aids, 3957 Mayfield Road, Cleveland, Ohio 44121

Colonial Garden Kitchens, 270 West Merrick Road, Valley Stream, New York 11582.

FashionABLE, Rocky Hill, New Jersey 08553. (25¢ for catalog)

MED, 1215 South Harlem Avenue, Forest Park, Illinois 60130.

Miles Kimball, 41 East Eighth Avenue, Oshkosh, Wisconsin 54901.

Rubbermaid, Inc., Wooster, Ohio 44691.

APRONS AND CARRY-ALLS

"A pocket on the side of my wheelchair holds things I like to have with me."

"Most notion counters have a plastic apron held on by a plastic clip. You can make your own by buying the clip from Cleo."

BAKING

"Be O.K. has a one-handed rolling pin."

"An easy-to-grip biscuit and cookie cutter can be made by removing both ends from a used soup can."

"I can't put puddings or liquid pies in the oven without spilling, so I set the pie shell on the oven rack, the liquid in a container on the oven door, and ladle the liquid into the shell with a soup dipper."

CUTTING AND CHOPPING

"Use paper towels to secure foods such as boiled eggs, pickles, and onions when cutting. A board gets slick after cutting a few of these things."

"Partially cooked potatoes are easier to slice."

"Scissors chop and slice many vegetables more easily than a paring knife."

"Thin knives cut through anything with little pressure. They cannot be bought. Find great grandma's or one in a second-hand store and have someone grind it down."

"I have a suction cup cutting board with nails to hold vegetables."

"Vegetables are easier to slice if cut in two first and the flat side placed against the board."

"I found left-handed scissors and peelers at Aristera."

ELECTRICAL OUTLETS AND EXTENSIONS

"If you can't reach the over-counter outlets, use short extension cords with outlets on the end."

"Put little off-on snap switches on such things as coffee pots that you can't plug in. Use the type that can be placed anywhere on the cord."

"Get an extension cord with a plug-in strip and have it put under the overhang of the countertop."

FAUCETS

"I turn on the water by hitting the faucet handles with the end of my extension brake."

"I walk my fingers around the sink to the water faucets."

"I tap faucets on and off with a small hammer with a long handle."

"I use a long wooden spoon with four nails in the bowl section that have been wrapped with electrician's friction tape."

"I have had the plumber replace the old ones with long-handled faucets."

FILLING PANS WITH WATER

"I put the pan on the stove and fill it, a cup at a time, with lots of patience."

"I fill a pan on my lap and take it to the stove."

"I fill a pan partly, place it on the stove, and finish filling it with a pan of water kept there."

"Sometimes I carry water to the kettle in two or three trips; sometimes I carry a sloshing kettle; sometimes I take the coward's way and ask my son or my husband to carry it."

"I use a hair shampoo spray with the head removed to fill pans and rinse dishes."

GRIPPING AND LIFTING

"I wrap handles of heavier saucepans with rubber-foam strips."

"We buy milk in plastic cartons as they are so much easier to handle than glass bottles."

"A gallon jug with a spigot to hold milk, juice, or water saves lifting the bottle out of the refrigerator and pouring."

"Rivet a large handle on lids to make them easier to handle."

"It is amazing what can be moved with small lifting power by using a propped elbow as a pivot."

HANDLING HOT STUFF

"I keep a magnetic potholder on the oven door."

"I have a pull-out board even with the opened door of the oven for sliding hot pans from the oven."

"I tried barbecue mitts but they were too unwieldy. I sewed three big potholders together and slip my hand between."

"Miles Kimball has a giant spatula, the Oven Hand, for putting things in and getting them out of the oven."

MIXING

"Before buying a mixer, check blade insertion and removal; make sure it has a bowl resting place and that you can operate the switch."

"I prefer the larger mixer to a junior because I get tired holding bowl and mixer."

"Instead of using regular mixing bowls I use 1- and 2-quart pitchers. They have nice handles I can hold whereas the bowl gets away from me."

"Use pans instead of mixing bowls. Tuck handle of pan under useless arm for security."

"A damp dish towel or cloth may be used to keep a pot or bowl in place while stirring."

"I've discovered Dycem is as stubborn as a Missouri mule; it anchors mixing bowls, telephones, dishes on lapboards, feet for transfers, and the pieces make grips for jar lids and door knobs. MED has it."

"I bought dog-feeding bowls at a pet shop; they're tipproof and have rubber suction bases."

"I emptied a drawer and put a board with a cut-out hole on top to hold the mixing bowl."

OPENING CANS AND JARS

"Before they leave the house in the morning, I have my family open all the jars and cans I will need for the day's meals and put them in the refrigerator."

"I use a nut cracker to grip bottle caps."

"Colonial Gardens has a jar and bottle opener with gear driven jaws and a large wooden handle that can be operated easily."

"The electric can openers vary so much that it is best to go to the store and find the one that will fit you. Check them with several different sizes of cans."

OPENING DOORS AND DRAWERS

"I have touch latches on cabinet doors. They can be opened with an elbow or head. I have drawer pulls that can be hooked into with toes, thumbs, or coat hangers."

"Rubber bands on small knobs give a good grip."

"If you are unable to use the hardware on drawers and cabinets, just skip it and fasten on inexpensive towel racks for easy pulling."

"If opening drawers is too much of an energy hassle, keep all your favorite utensils in heavy jars on top of the counter, the way artists keep their brushes."

PEELING

"The easiest way to peel vegetables is to anchor the peeler and move the vegetable against the peeler. This takes less strength and frees both hands to hold the vegetable."

"Colonial Gardens has a peeler that can be adjusted to right or left hand use."

"Be O.K. has a maple paring board with suction feet."

REACHING AND PICKING UP

"I have two magnetic hooks on the side of my chair from which I hang a pair of tongs and a 29 in. long ½ in. wood dowel with a hook on the end. With the latter I snag the refrigerator door open."

"I use a magnet on a string for picking up small steel things (including my tongs)."

"I have a 12 in. long dowel with a magnet on the end."

"I have an old fashioned grocery store reacher to grab things far away from me."

"I keep reachers all over the house."

"I use utility tongs of several sizes to reach things on the second shelf of the cupboard. Also, I have a heavy yardstick with an L-shaped hook fastened to the end."

"A child's rake can be used to retrieve things and to straighten curtains."

"I use barbecue utensils for a longer reach."

"I have a pulled-out wire coat hanger to hook towels from shelves."

REMOVING FOODS FROM COOKING WATER

"I don't attempt the impossible or take chances of getting burned or scalded just to prove how independent I can be."

"I use a straining spoon for removing vegetables. For spaghetti, I use a very small saucepan to ladle out the water first."

"Colonial Gardens has a colander–scoop with an easy-to-hold handle so you can take the vegetables or rice right from the boiling water."

"I learned to cook vegetables and spaghetti in a fry basket and remove them from the water easily."

"Frozen vegetables can be cooked in a casserole with a little water and butter added and a slow oven."

SERVING CARTS

"We converted a metal laundry cart into a utility cart by replacing the wire basket with a rimmed Formica tray. It has four swivel casters, and a mere nudge sends it sailing across the room. Since it is so easy to push from my chair, I use it for everything that has to be transported from one room to another and from icebox to sink or stove."

"We bought a used pill-dispensing cart from a hospital supply store. I take all the serving dishes from the kitchen to the dining room by pushing it ahead of me."

STORAGE

"Revolving shelves are the quad's answer to accessible storage in any cabinet in any room."

"Clear plastic containers make it possible to check on quantity of contents without opening them."

"We solved all our storage problems with Rubbermaid's slide-out drawers, racks, and turntables. You can find them at most dime stores or hardware stores or get a catalog from Rubbermaid."

"Kimball has magnetic steel cup hooks."

"We put pegboard on the back of our counters and hang our pots and utensils on hooks."

STOVE AND STOVELESS COOKING

"I can't reach the stove top so I have a two-burner electric burner on a low table."

"The electric skillet on my work table saves reaching. The glass top lets me see what's cooking."

"My stove is too high so I have a low table for all my electrical appliances: hand mixer, fry pan with a broiler in the lid, cooker, knife sharpener, can opener, coffee pot, and blender."

"An angled mirror over my stove shows what's going on in the pans on my back burners."

"I can cook simple things right on the table by using a heating coil hooked into an extension cord with an on-off switch."

THINKING AHEAD

"A lot of short cuts can be made by thinking ahead, doing things in order, doing them ahead of time, and allowing extra time for yourself in doing them."

"Fatigue is my problem if I attempt what I think I ought to accomplish in 1 day."

"When making something that can be frozen, I usually make enough for 2–3 times, then I have half the cooking to do."

"I keep a small grocery store in the basement so that my family only has to shop every 2 or 3 weeks."

USING HELPING HANDS

"I plan ahead and every night have the boys get down any seldom used supplies from the upper cupboards."

"When I have able-bodied help, I have them peel potatoes and chop onions and freeze them for later use."

"Several ladies from my church have volunteered their services to do many of the sticky jobs for me such as cleaning the stove, defrosting the refrigerator, cleaning and relining drawers and cupboards."

WASHING DISHES

"Don't waste energy putting dishes and glasses away after every meal. Stack them in a drainer for air drying, cover with a towel, and then set the table from the drainer."

"Washing dishes at the sink was a problem until I had the doors underneath removed. Now I swing my chair pedals backward, roll forward to the sink, and set my feet on the lower shelf of the cabinet. This way I am able to rest my arms on the edge of the sink. It is easier than trying to reach over. We had the pipes insulated so I don't burn my knees."

WELL, THE NEED AROSE

CASEY JONES

Casey Jones of Eugene, Oregon, the lone gentleman who responded to the questionnaire, elaborated on his thoughts about being a cooking quad. Jones, a C5-6 quadriplegic, is a fifth-grade teacher.

I have felt for a long time that disabled people in general have not done what they could along the lines of housework, child care, and such chores so I'd like to get in my two cents worth. Maybe the reason they haven't is because it is tedious, rather unglamorous, and without much recognition. Quite often handicapped people are seeking something more spectacular which will have greater compensatory value. Seeking recognition, they often overlook the obvious and tend to forget that little things are important, too. Of course, it often takes us a lot longer and requires a lot more effort from us to perform these little tasks than it does for the nondisabled around us, so we tend to shrug our shoulders and let them do it while we dream of more exciting ventures. However, if we enjoy our work, it really shouldn't matter if it takes us longer.

I was guilty of the same sin of omission for 6 years as a C5-6 quad. With dear old mother around to do the housework, I never lifted a hand toward those chores. In fact, it never really dawned on me that perhaps I could. Then, with mother gone, my wife away at college except on weekends, and housework piling up, I found that I could do all kinds of things that I had heretofore considered outside my realm of activity. I guess it was partly a labor of love; the thought of pleasing my new bride as she came home on weekends inspired me to greater efforts.

I learned to wash dishes by holding the dishes between my two hands. (We soon bought unbreakable dishes.) I found that, with a hose, I could fill the laundry tubs and washing machine; with a hooked stick I could put the clothes in the machine, fish them out, put them through the wringer, rinse them and even hang them on the line. Luckily we had a huge laundry room with a cement floor and a drain so I could spill and splash all I wanted to. I soon had indoor lines strung up at my level and could hang clothes up to dry inside. I threw the clothespins away and just draped the clothes over the lines. I never tried ironing; with no feeling in my hands I was chicken about getting singed. Sweeping wasn't hard at all with the broom cradled between my two hands. I never did learn to use the dustpan though; it was much more convenient to sweep the dust into a pile under the bed or behind the garbage can. Then I could ask my wife to sweep it up, and that meant that I'd be sure to get recognition for sweeping it all into the neat pile.

Mopping was the next step, and with a sponge mop equipped with a squeeze lever this proved no problem except once or twice when I tipped the mop pail over.

With a tray on my lap, and spoons, forks, spatulas, knives, and peelers with special handles, I soon found to my amazement that I could peel potatoes, open cans, mix bread (I learned to make 25-loaf batches in two big dishpans and then freeze them after they were baked; that way I only had to bake bread about once a month), make cakes, fry hamburger, and cook steaks. I got some great padded mitts for taking hot things out of the oven. Long tongs work beautifully to reach things up in the cupboards. I use hooked sticks to pick things up from the floor after I drop them. I soon trained the dog to lick up any spills and destroy the evidence.

Stew, baked beans, and meat loaves were my specialties. I soon learned to make huge batches at one time and then freeze the rest. I was so lazy that I was an efficiency expert. For instance, I would make a large stew and keep it going, that is, reheat it at least once a day and add to it occasionally for a week or two. A good stew should never die.

I don't do housework, or cooking, or cleaning very often anymore, but it sure is nice to know that I can when and if I want to or need to. I do think that severely disabled people need to specialize somewhat and capitalize on their greatest talents. For some, it might be a waste of time to knock themselves out trying to be a housekeeper or cook all their lives when they could earn a good income using some specialized skill. However, housework can be fun, and it's something that must be done in all homes. It's mighty handy sometimes to be able to pitch in and help. Also, for those who are not gainfully employed, it certainly is a chance to help out in some way. It's a thousand times better than doing nothing, even if you can't perform efficiently at the tasks. It can be a challenge, a hobby, a change from your regular job.

Bibliography

"EASY-TO-USE KITCHENS." "EASY TO USE SINK CENTER." Order from Cooperative Extension Service, University of Nebraska-Lincoln, East Campus, Lincoln, Nebraska 68503. Free.
These two leaflets are concise and helpful.

KITCHENS FOR WOMEN IN WHEELCHAIRS. By Helen E. McCullough and Mary B. Farnham. 31 pages. Illustrated. 8½ × 11. 1961. Order Circular #841 from Information Office, College of Agriculture, Mumford Hall, University of Illinois, Urbana, Illinois 61803. 50¢
One of the first guides to designing special kitchens, it is based on an earlier study of 26 wheelchaired homemakers. The authors emphasize the importance of the three major work centers in the kitchen—sink, range, and food preparation. Counters 30–32 in. high and work spaces 27 in. high for mixing and beating are recommended. Open space for knees under counters is of primary importance: knee space should be a minimum of 24 in. high and 24 in. wide. Suggestions for adapting commercial cabinets are included. The suggestions for storage in drawers are particularly helpful. The mix center, with cupboards concealed by a bamboo curtain, vertical files, and a pegboard backing of the counter area, is attractive and functional.

KITCHEN SENSE FOR DISABLED PEOPLE OF ALL AGES. By Sydney Foott, Marian Lane, and Jill Mara. 218 pages Illustrated. 7 × 8. Order from Disabled Living Foundation, 346 Kensington High Street, London W14 8NS, England. 1.25. (about $2.50)
Based on the work of a housewife who is disabled by arthritis, a home economist, and an occupational therapist, the book covers all aspects of the use of a kitchen. It includes plans, choice of equipment, diet and menus, aids and short cuts in preparing and cooking, shopping, sources of advice, and manufacturers.

A PILOT STUDY OF DISABLED HOUSEWIVES IN THEIR KITCHENS. By Phyllis M. Howie. 104 pages. Illustrated. 8¼ × 12. 1967. Order from Disabled Living Foundation, 346 Kensington High Street, London W14 8NS, England. Price: 25s. (about 50¢
The study examined the work patterns and movements of 30 disabled housewives with an assortment of disabilities and 30 nondisabled housewives—all in existing kitchens. It concluded that, in planning a kitchen, the size and shape are of less importance than the layout and the inclusion of work centers with appropriate storage nearby. These work centers include storage (refrigerator), sink, cooking, and serving. A clear pathway from range to sink is important. A low preparation center is essential for disabled housewives; they need home visits and follow-ups. A cart is a vital piece of equipment; "it can make the difference between managing and not managing at home." A design for a kitchen cart with a sliding tray is included; the average dimensions are 18 × 20 in. with a height of 30 in. It has two shelves, the bottom one level with the most used shelf in a low oven.

PLANNING KITCHENS FOR HANDICAPPED HOMEMAKERS. By Virginia Hart Wheeler. 83 pages. Illustrated. 8½ × 11. 1965. Order Rehabilitation Monograph XXVII from Publications, Institute of Rehabilitation Medicine, New York University Medical Center, 400 East 34th Street, New York, New York 10016. $2.50
The Institute's kitchen planning consultant has created a fascinating and basic handbook for the planning of new kitchens as well as modifying and learning how to make the most of existing kitchens. It is a useful guide for rehabilitation counselors, architects, and disabled individuals.
The focus of the book is on the ideal kitchen for the disabled cook. According to the author, the ideal kitchen is U-shaped (L-shaped also has potential); on the left leg of the U, there is a lazy Susan in the corner, next to it a 36 in. high dishwasher, then the L-shaped 31 in. high work counter with open space below. The bottom of the U contains a built-in range top and a built-in oven (31 in. from the floor), which has a side-opening door. The sink in the countertop on the right leg is 6 in. deep, and next to it is a pull-out board. Across the backs of the lowered counters are 8 in. deep storage cabinets with sliding doors and pull-out drawer containers for staples.
An interesting chapter, titled "Practical Compromises," includes ways of making the most of limited space and money. According to the author, the starting point in adapting a kitchen is the sink; first, try to open it up underneath, then see if it can be lowered. If neither can be done, some kind of work top at a good wheelchair working height of 25–29 in. must be created from a shelf, drop-leaf shelf, pull-out board, or a table. Before and after examples clearly illustrate the changes made to kitchens

in a low-rent housing project, an old country house, and to one that seemed "impossible." A source list of equipment and appliances is included.

THE WHEELCHAIR IN THE KITCHEN. A Guide to Easier Living for the Handicapped Homemaker. By Joseph Chasin and Jules Saltman. 32 pages. Illustrated. 8½ × 11. 1973. Order from Paralyzed Veterans of America, Inc., 7315 Wisconsin Avenue, Suite 301-W, Bethesda, Maryland 20014. $2.50.

An attractive and informative presentation of basic ideas on kitchen construction, renovation, and layout, the booklet is useful both for those considering an apartment or for those planning the perfect wheelchair house. It includes clear diagrams and explanations of how much space a wheelchair needs (27 in. clear for head-on approach to doors and 30 in. for an oblique approach); the dimensions of a wheelchair (width of adult chairs from 22-½ in. to 26-½ in.); and ways of narrowing, heightening, and shortening chairs. It covers the cooking center, refrigerator, sink, storage, and designs for wheelchair trays and reachers.

The five-page section on how to make do with existing facilities in a rented house or apartment is especially creative. The suggestions include removing the doors of the cabinets to make them more reachable; using lazy Susans on the shelves; converting a broom closet into a pantry; hanging a shallow closet on the back of a door; installing a heavy duty outlet control center with an on-off switch, safety light, and its own fuse box to handle the array of tabletop cookers and electrical appliances it suggests using; and keeping a party-sized coffee maker with a spigot filled with water for a supply away from the sink.

"Even the most severely disabled people retain an ineradicable conviction that they are still fully human in all that is ultimately necessary."

—Paul Hunt, editor of Stigma, The Experience of Disability

4
Bathroom Adaptations

The bathroom is the most frequently inaccessible room because of a damnable door that is only 2 ft. wide. If the door is wide enough for a wheelchair, then the open space within most bathrooms is too small to allow for transfer, turning, or even closing the door for privacy.

The designers of bathrooms for the disabled are not in agreement as to the best height of a toilet or a sink. Recommended toilet heights range 15–23 in., and the sink heights range 21–36 in. In a private home, one can make the choice that is best suited to one's particular dimensions. In public housing, whichever height is chosen will be a help for some and a hindrance for others, and individual adaptations will be necessary.

Theoretically, the wheelchair bathroom would have a door with a minimum width of 32 in. that would swing out or slide. The clear floor space would be at least 5 × 5 ft. Handrails would be placed as needed near the toilet. The lavatory would be high enough to clear wheelchair arms and would have single lever controls and insulated water pipes. The toilet would be at a height for convenient transfer. A tub would have a built-in transfer area and handrails or a lift. A shower would be free of curbs and have at least 3 ft. 6 in. × 4 ft 6 in. clear space inside with a folding seat at wheelchair height and reachable single lever controls. Medicine cabinets and mirrors would be reachable and usable. Wall outlets would be no less than 16 in. from the floor. Floors would be slipproof, and there would be an alarm system for calling for assistance.

Actually, few existing bathrooms are utopian, and most disabled individuals have had to work out their own adaptations. Most of the devices, aids, and equipment mentioned in this chapter are available from local hospital supply and rental agencies. They are also available from many specialized mail order houses, including the following:

SOURCES OF EQUIPMENT

Abbey Rents Medical Catalog Sales Department, 13500 South Figueroa, Los Angeles, California 90061 or nearest Abbey Rents

American Standard, 40 West 40th Street, New York, New York 10018

E. F. Brewer Co., 13901 Main Street, Menomonee Falls, Wisconsin 53051

Edco Surgical Supply Company, Inc., 43 West 61st Street, New York, New York 10023

FashionABLE, Rocky Hill, New Jersey 08553. Send 25¢ for catalog.

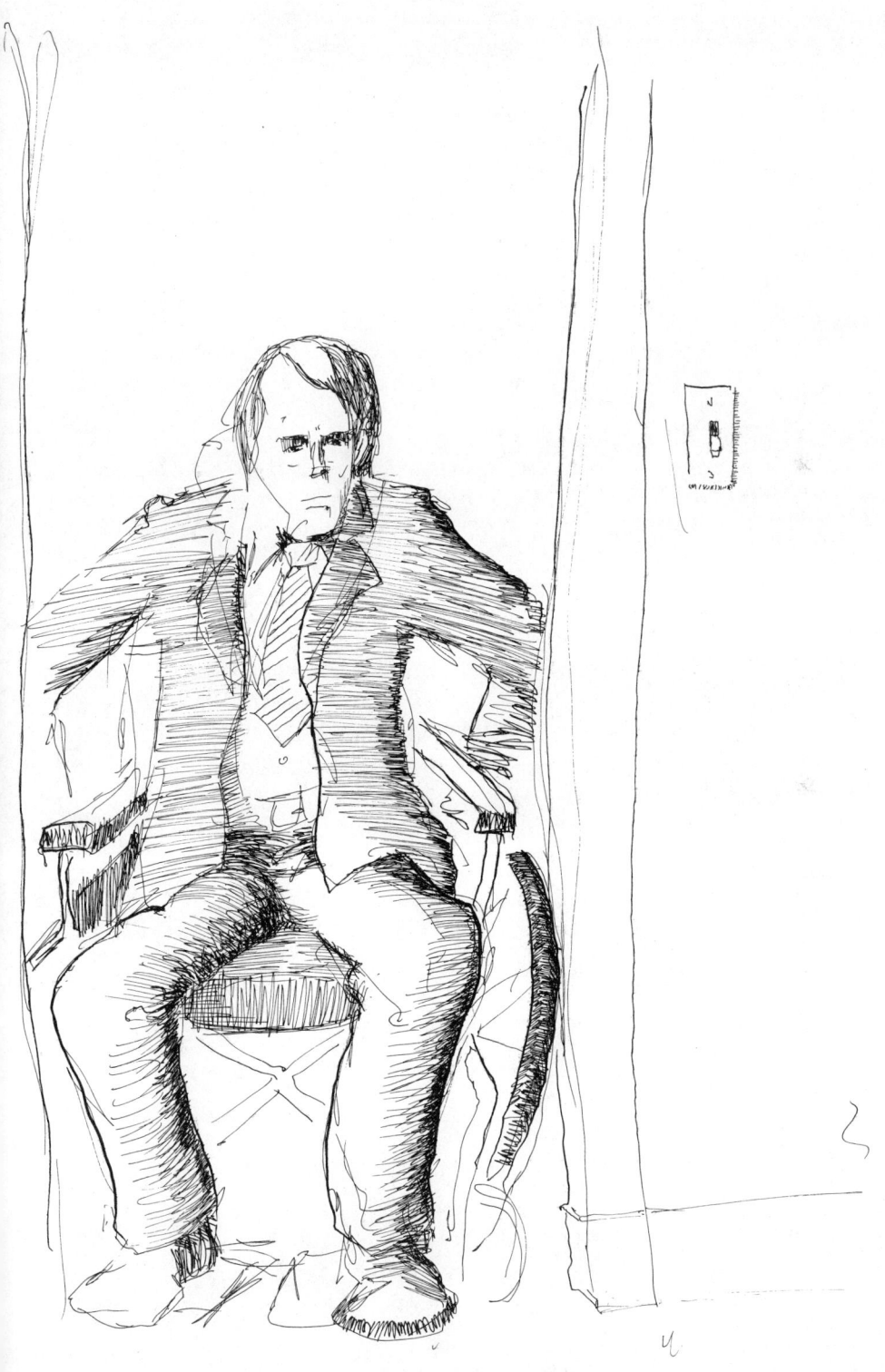

Lumex, Inc., 100 Spence Street, Bay Shore, New York 11706

MED, 1215 South Harlem Street, Forest Park, Illinois 60130

Nelson Medical Products, 3112 Wilder Avenue, Sarasota, Florida 33580

Rehabilitation Products, 2020 Ridge Road, Evanston, Illinois 60201

Sears, Roebuck and Company, Department 141, 925 South Homan Avenue, Chicago, Illinois 60607. Request *Catalog of Home Care and Convalescent Needs.*

Trujillo Industries, 5726 West Washington Boulevard, Los Angeles, California 90016

VABCO Products, 160 North Gilbert, Fullerton, California 92633

TOILETS

If the toilet is too low, it can be raised to a more comfortable height of 1 ft 6 in. or 1 ft 8 in. by relocating it on a wood block or platform or by using a raised toilet seat. Most of the self-help catalogs have portable models with raised padded seats to prevent decubiti, similar to the one illustrated by VABCO Products (Fig. 4–1) which can be ordered in a choice of full circle, open front, or open front and rear. If transfer is difficult, the toilet may be turned. Armrests may be easily attached to the seat bolts, or a toilet chair can be used. Most of the catalogs have a wide selection of safety bars that will fit any special need for support or transfer. The photograph of the Scandinavian supports that fold up against the wall should be studied carefully. Perhaps a plumber could copy them (see Fig. 18–15.)

American Standard, manufactures a toilet especially for the wheelchaired that is 4 in. higher than normal, has a slotted bedpan holder rim, and may be had with tank or flush valve operation. MED manufactures gadgets which give independence to those with paralyzed or flail hands, such as devices for inserting rectal suppositories and for replacing manual stimulation.

REMOTE CONTROL CLEANSING

A number of toilet seat attachments and a special water closet direct a gentle flow of warm water to the perineal area, eliminating the use of toilet paper and the need for hands. Sani-Seat, Inc., 5835 North Tripp Street, Chicago, Illinois 60646 makes the Sanitet. Clos o Mat Samoa (Hans Maurer, 8125 Zollikerberg/Zurich, Switzerland and Spies Trading Company, 75 Valentine Road, Bloomfield, New Jersey 07003) automatically supplies a warm water douche for hygienic personal cleansing (Fig. 4–2).

EXTRACURRICULAR TOILETING

Urinals can be a boon to women as well as men, saving many wrestles with clothes and trips to the bathroom. Those for women are contoured anatomically for proper fit and can be used either sitting or lying down. If women wear pants,

58 Housing and Home Services for the Disabled

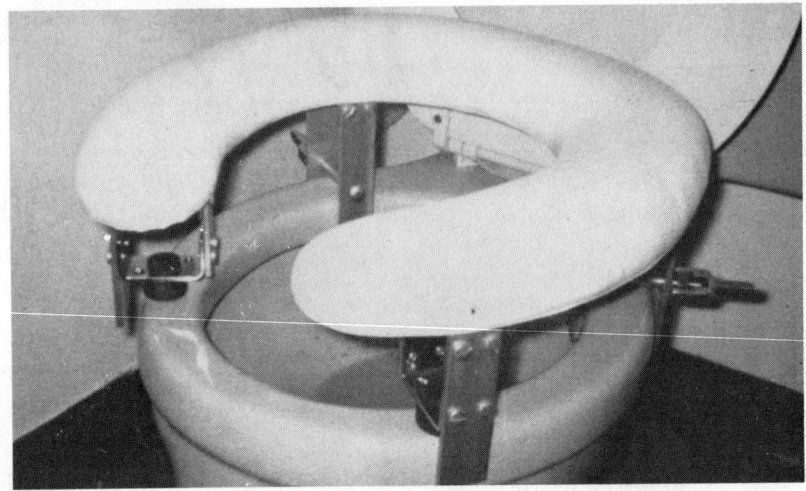

Fig. 4–1. Raised, padded, and portable seat by VABCO.

Fig. 4–2. Clos-o-Mat supplies warm water and air for cleansing and drying.

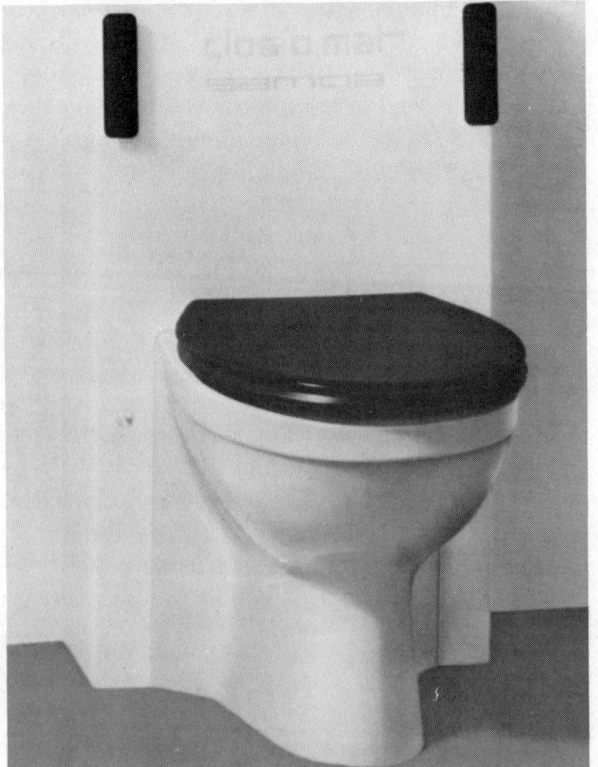

ripping 6 in. or so down each inner side seam at the crotch and reclosing the seams with easy-to-undo Velcro (at notion counters or from FashionABLE) avoids the need to lower them.

Jones-Zylon, Inc., P.O. Box 158, West Lafayette, Ohio 43845, which manufactures the Combo—a male or female urinal—is working on a special seated or wheelchair model for those unable to change their positions. Using a female urinal is easier if one slides far forward when sitting in a chair and if one almost assumes the Pap test position when horizontal. A funnel attached to a rubber tube can be used with a jug or near a toilet. A wide-mouthed jar or ice bag can be almost as effective as a urinal. The latter is handy for traveling, since its innocent appearance can hide the fact that it has not yet been convenient to empty it.

Throw-away plastic bleach jugs are useful for disposable bedside drainage, but they are light and tip over easily. Nelson Medical Products sells a jug holder that is held to a solid base by a stainless steel band.

At night incontinent ladies can sleep on a shower cap stuffed with cellucotton. A built-in bedpan can be made by cutting out a piece larger than the pan at the bedpan location on a foam rubber mattress. Bind the edges with tape and cover the cut-out foam rubber with a pillow case to be replaced at nonpanning times. Cut and bind corresponding holes in bottom sheets. For extra comfort, have pillows at the hips when using the pan. No lifting is necessary; just roll on and off. To skidproof an ordinary bedpan, put it on a bathmat with suction feet.

Hospital supply companies, MED, Sears, and most of the specialized mail order firms make commode chairs that roll over a toilet or commodes that conceal their purpose. Sears' catalog, *Home Health Care and Convalescent Needs,* describes portable commodes; some flush, and some look like modern armchairs or walnut cabinets with adjustable armrests.

The manufacturers that supply trailers, vans, and motor homes have developed inexpensive and functional chemical toilets and other bathroom fixtures that could be used to make a bathroom in a corner of a bedroom or in a closet. For information, check the yellow pages of the phone book for recreational vehicle suppliers, or send for the various free catalogs listed in *Trailer Travel* or *Camping and Trailering Guide.* Several firms specialize in designing trailers and motor homes that are accessible to the disabled and should be particularly helpful: 1) Skyhawk Industries, Inc., Route 2, Box 129, Marcellus, Michigan 49067; 2) McHenry Trailer & Lift Sales, Pilot Knob, Missouri 63663; and 3) Harvest Recreational Vehicles, Inc., Handicapped Division, Box 3206, El Monte, California 91733.

Another type of portable toilet, the Destroilet, is a combination toilet and incinerator that can be used anywhere with 115-volt electricity and a supply of either bottled or natural gas. It is self-contained and does not require a septic system, plumbing, holding tanks, or any water. Manufactured by La Mere Industries, Inc., 227 North Main Street, Walworth, Wisconsin 53184, it is available through local LP gas dealers. Incidentally, it must be vented through a chimney or a separate flue.

BATHTUBS

Most catalogs of specialized equipment have illustrations of shower and bathtub seats and benches, safety rails, grab bars, hand-held shower heads, slipproofing tapes and tub pads, as well as various hydraulic and water-powered lifts that can be used for raising and lowering someone onto the toilet or into the tub.

Safe-T-Bath, 2837 West 21st Street, Tulsa, Oklahoma 74107 makes a fiberglass tub that is raised 18 in. off the floor and has a side door that opens to let the bather sit down easily and swing around. An inflatable on-the-bed tub (Bob Whalen, P.O. Box 7141, Stanford, California 94305) is made of plastic and nylon cloth. It can be rolled under a person, then inflated with a small blower and filled with water from a special faucet connection, which also empties the tub (Fig. 4–3).

Bed-Bath (Hoffman Manufacturing Co., 22346 Hesperian Boulevard, Hayward, California 94541), another on-the-bed tub, is put together by snapping plastic sheeting onto a collapsible tubular framework. Filler hose connects to standard plumbing fixtures, and a venturi tube drains the water quickly.

A Swedish Tub-on-Tub distributed by MED is mounted on top of an existing tub. It consists of a wood base that rests on top of the bathtub, a padded bottom cushion, and a vinyl tub with a metal frame. The side of the tub lowers for entering. The bather uses a hand-held shower head mounted on a flexible hose and drains the water into the tub below through a drain hole.

Fig. 4–3. Inflatable on-the-bed tub. As a variation, a child's swimming pool can be used.

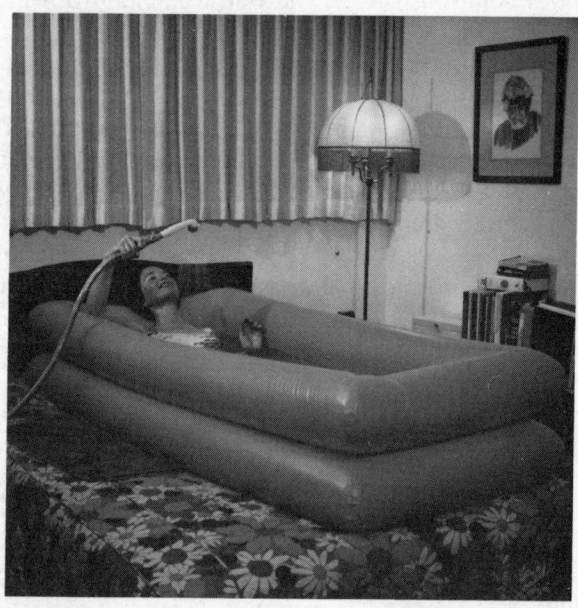

LAVATORIES

If the existing lavatory is hung too low on the wall, it might be raised so a wheelchair can roll under it. Most importantly, the pipes should be insulated to prevent accidental burning. A special wheelchair lavatory is available from American Standard. It has a concave front, a shallow bowl, faucets with 4-in. lever handles, a goose neck spout, and a height of 34 in. from the floor. If the faucet handles on the existing sink cannot be replaced with lever type handles, tap turners can be made by removing the present handle, flattening one side of a 4-in. length of dowel or broomstick, and wingnutting it in place.

GADGETS

If an electric shaver cannot be grasped with the fingers, it can be held on the back of the hand with a Velcro strap. Electric toothbrushes are useful not only for those with weak hands but for those who must have someone else do the brushing. A tooth paste dispenser, Dent-A-Matic, sold by Miles Kimball Company, Oshkosh, Wisconsin 54901 delivers tooth paste with just the push of a lever. It is well worth the time to comb through the trivia of the mail order catalogs to find devices that can be adapted for the disabled, since they are cheaper than when labeled for the disabled and sold by medical supply houses.

ELECTRIFIED PLUMBING

Temperature and flow are controlled by a hand-or foot-operated switch (Tempflow Manufacturing Co., P.O. Box 187, Prairie Grove, Arkansas 72753).

LIFTS

The specialized mail order houses and the local branches of medical supply houses carry an assortment of hydraulic lifts to be used in transferring from wheelchair to car or to bed, as well as to tub or to toilet. A free 16-page booklet describing a full line of lifters for home or travel is available from Ted Hoyer & Company, Inc., 2222 Minnesota Street, Oshkosh, Wisconsin 54901.

The Ted Hoyer Company has a new hydraulic bathlift with a safety stop. The Eaton-E-Z-Bath (P.O. Box 712, Garden City, Kansas 67846) is VA tested and approved as a lift. Made of welded aluminum, it is completely portable and fits all standard tubs and most old style ones. Mecanaids, Inc., 540 Hollywood Way, Burbank, California 91505 has developed a new bath lift, called the Autolift, whose main column is bolted to the floor and holds a plastic bathing seat. The user transfers to the seat, swings it over the tub, and lowers it. J. E. Nolan & Son, Inc., P.O. Box 22181, Louisville, Kentucky 40222 manufactures a bath chair which is water powered, using an ordinary shower or tub faucet. Requiring no installation, the lift is self- or attendant-operated, lifts 300 lb, and weighs 21 lb. (Fig. 4–4).

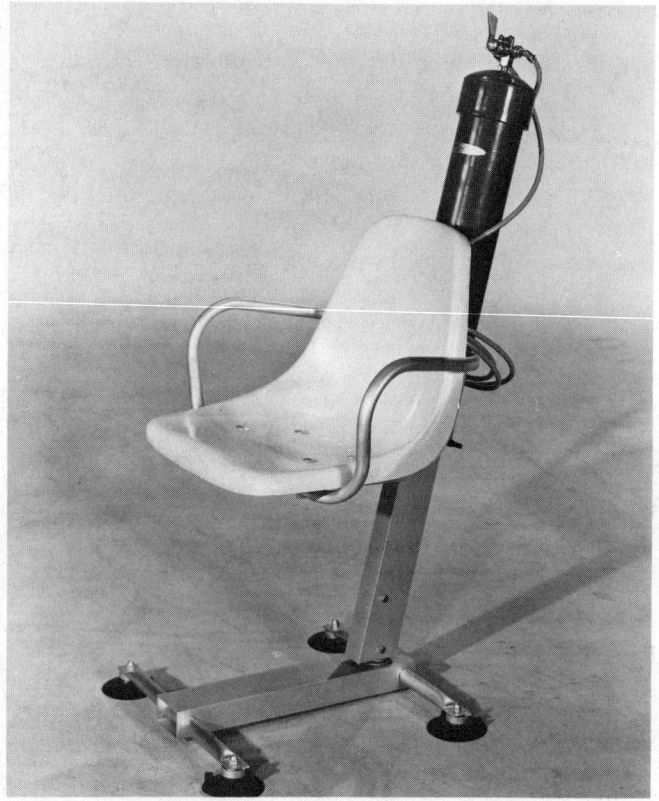

Fig. 4–4. Nolan's water-powered bath chair.

Other lifts are manufactured by Holeck Engineering Co., 9255 Clancey Avenue, Downey, California 90240 and Porto-Lift Manufacturing Co., Higgins Lake, Michigan 48627.

Bibliography

THE BATHROOM. By Alexandra Kira. 272 pages. Illustrated. 8 × 10. 1976. The Viking Press, Inc., 625 Madison Avenue, New York, New York 10022. $7.95 paper.

A witty and serious study of the bathroom by a professor of architecture at Cornell University, this new and revised edition is a critical reexamination of the changes in design and attitudes that have taken place in the last 10 years. In addition to developing the designs that were included in the first study, this edition includes the problems of public facilities and the diversity of special problems of the aged and the disabled.

Professor Kira suggests the height of the lavatory be in the 34- to 36-inch range, the depth be 4 inches, and the front-to-back dimension be in the 18- to 22-inch range. In addition to lever handle controls, he suggests the wrist-operated controls used with surgical basins or "perhaps ideally the controls should be of the electronic push-button variety for maximum ease of use" with a button that can be activated by the fist or ball of the hand rather than by a finger.

The toilet should be located so as to effect a direct horizontal transfer from a wheelchair and the seat should be at the same height as the wheelchair. The door should be a minimum of 36 inches wide; a sliding or bifold door is easier to manage. The minimum space for a wheelchair user should be approximately twice the space allotted in the standard minimum bathroom. The minor variations in facilities must be determined on the basis of the unique requirements and capabilities of the user. Other planning criteria include the careful location of luminous light switches and space-heating elements, a fountain type of water supply, and door locks that can be opened in an emergency from the outside.

The book concludes, "The ultimate irony is that most of the 'special' requirements necessary for aged and disabled persons are really not that special. Basically they represent careful attention to human needs and in many cases would be equally as suitable and useful for the normal population."

WHEELCHAIR BATHROOMS. By Harry A. Schweikert, Jr. 20 pages. Illustrated. 8½ × 11. 1971. Order from Paralyzed Veterans of America, Inc., 7315 Wisconsin Avenue, Suite 301-W, Bethesda, Maryland 20014. $1.

Schweikert, a paraplegic, considers the bathroom the most important room in the house for the spinal cord injured. He is deeply impressed by Professor Alexander Kira's first book, *The Bathroom: Criteria for Design*. He quotes from it at length, "It is important that we master these devices rather than be victimized by them." We must design "our physical environment and the objects in it so that they accommodate us rather than our having to accommodate ourselves to them."

Included are addresses of commercial sources for the equipment illustrated. According to Schweikert, a normal bathroom is 8 ft × 5 ft 6 in. A paraplegic can maneuver tightly in this space, but any size larger would be a comfort.

"Above all, they would retain their right to choose their own risks, and, within their new limits, they would continue to live their lives to capacity."

—*Dr. Margaret Agerholm, England*

5
Independent Living Experiences
DONNA McGWINN

Every person sculpts his life in his own style. The styles of those in unusual circumstances tend to be unusual, often revealing imagination and resourcefulness if not downright recklessness. How some of the disabled, with little or no mobility and few funds, have managed to set up independent lives is something most able-bodied social workers could not have planned. Necessity and desire make innovators of us. Frequently in retrospect we are amazed at the chances we took and the mad schemes we concocted for survival and freedom. None of us regretted them, even if they had their harrowing moments, and we encouraged each other to make similar moves. We exchanged and elaborated upon ideas and exulted or lamented at the results.

The following examples of how some of us coped with life are shared to continue this exchange of information and inspiration. It should be remembered that these short summaries of thoughts and experiences do not convey the frustrations, fears, disappointments, and joys that were their substance. Most successful lifestyles came after many trials and errors. No one learns quickly how to live fully and happily as a disabled individual in an able-bodied society.

STUDENT LIVE-IN ATTENDANTS

James Graaskamp is a quadriplegic as a result of having polio in 1951. He has no breathing problems, but requires help with his personal care and transportation. At 42, he is an Associate Professor and Chairman of the Real Estate and Urban Land Economics Department at the University of Wisconsin. His university salary is about $20,000/year, augmented by an equal amount of revenue from his real estate consulting firm and investments.

Before the reader is overwhelmed with envy, he should be advised that Jim works very hard to perform the duties that reward him so well monetarily. He rises at 5 or 6 A.M. and is in his wheelchair 15–18 hours/day. He reports, "I have tremendous stamina, and since my initial bout with polio, my only medical needs have been for an appendix and a broken leg. I use no therapy or tilt boards. As a result I do not require professional medical care."

Jim owns a home at the edge of the university campus. He employs three male students who live with him and provide his morning and night personal care, get him up and put him to bed, cook, and do certain household chores, such as emptying wastebaskets and changing light bulbs. The students receive room and

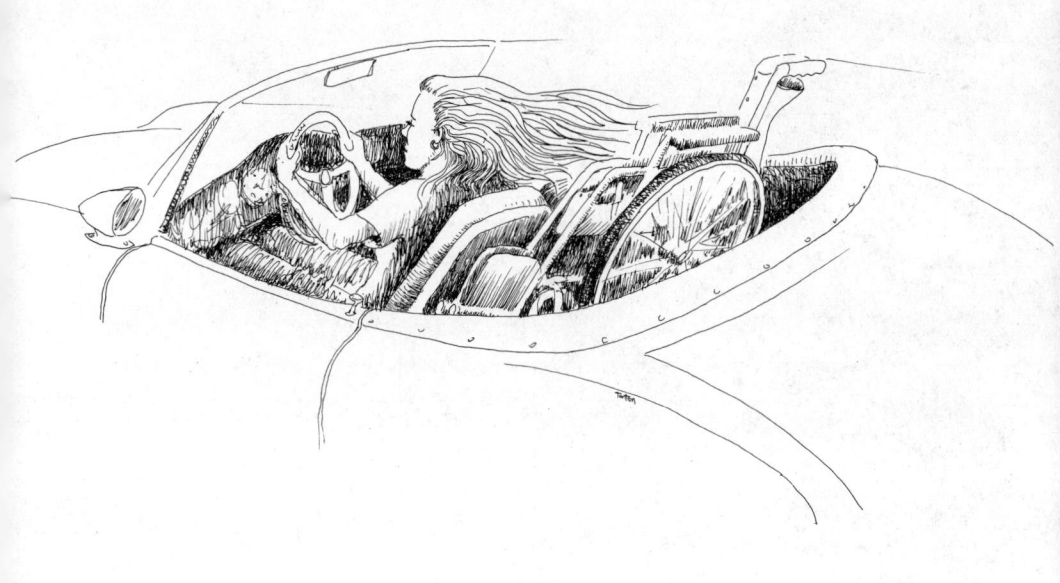

board and $10/week. Jim also employs two students as drivers who receive $2/hour and $2.50/hour for yard work, snow shoveling, etc. In addition he employs a regular secretary, whom he describes as "the rock on which everything rests," and two part-time secretaries.

On his home care routine, Jim says,

Each student works every third day. In the morning I leave a note as to the dinner menu, and the duty trick begins with the man of the day coming in at 4:30 P.M. to prepare dinner for the four of us, unless he has started a baked dinner on our oven timer (which is often). Dinner is always at 5:30 P.M., so everyone including me plans accordingly. If I don't warn the crew that I will be late, my share is 'et' by the rest of those at the trough. While I have an option on the duty man's evening if I want to go to bed early, I almost never do. The man on duty is due back then at 9:30 or 10 P.M. to put me down for the night. The alarm is set in my room for 5 or 6 in the morning when I give the duty man a ring on the buzzer system. Once he has me up and has given me breakfast, his duty tour is over.

During the summer when the boys are not in school and work solely for me, the duty man is on call to 5 in the afternoon for driving, shopping, yard work, etc., on an hourly basis. I try to anticipate needs so he can plan his day, but when there are surprises his schedule must yield on the assumption that the fringe benefits generally outweigh the irritations. Over the years, the pattern has evolved that on Friday and Saturday nights the man with the duty will be driving me out to dinner or a movie, etc., if I plan to go, but otherwise any driving is at the hourly rate.

While we have a cleaning lady for most household chores, the man on duty does the dishes (with a dishwasher), empties wastebaskets, and sorts the solid waste between paper salvage, incinerator, and garbage cans. The Friday night duty includes doing my socks and T shirts, etc.; the Saturday night chore includes a Sunday morning spruce-up of hair wash, fingernails, etc.; and the Sunday night chore includes grocery lists and burnt-out light bulbs or whatever. The inside crew has first chance at any travel opportunity on the basis of seniority. For the boys who drive, we try to balance the income earned to approximate the targets which the students have set at the outset of the semester.

The system works reasonably well and has minimum rules aside from fair play. I have been working at this since 1952 and have had only a couple of personality conflicts of any significance and only one theft in all that time. Most of the boys who work for me are friends of those who worked for me earlier and graduated or were married. I probably don't have to find more than one person who wasn't referred to me each year so far as the inside crew is concerned. The overwhelming majority of students are considerate, responsible, and flexible in adapting to a unique situation. My association with them is probably the only reason that I remain young and progressive for a man of my advanced years.

When asked if there were any problems involved in living with three attendants and how they were solved, Jim answered,

It is difficult to explain, but the personnel management requires an acute sense of when a sin of omission is simply attributable to youth and college pressures and when, rarely, it is a direct confrontation with my wishes and objectives. The former requires a gentle and oblique reminder so that instructions never appear as command, which in turn requires a constant appreciation on my part that management of the logistics is peripheral to my prime objectives in living my own life just as the chores involved for the students are and should be peripheral to the living of their own lives. Such a perspective, plus my natural self-confidence, means that there are very few oversights, mistakes, or whatever by the students that really threaten me or the subconscious me, an anxiety which would lead to overresponse and excessive supervision on my part. As a result, things run along without too much input on my part.

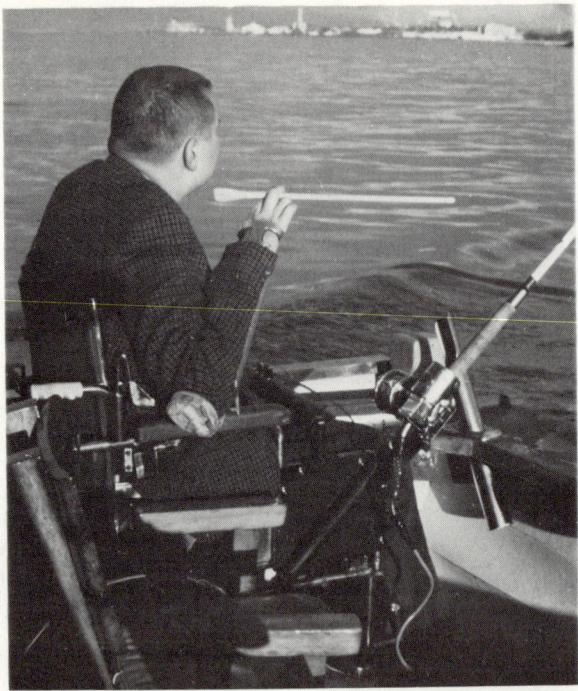

Fig. 5–1. Professor Graaskamp is an avid fisherman. He operates an electric reel with a mouthstick.

Fig. 5–2. Ruby Heine has learned to live independently with the help of her mother and daily live-in attendants.

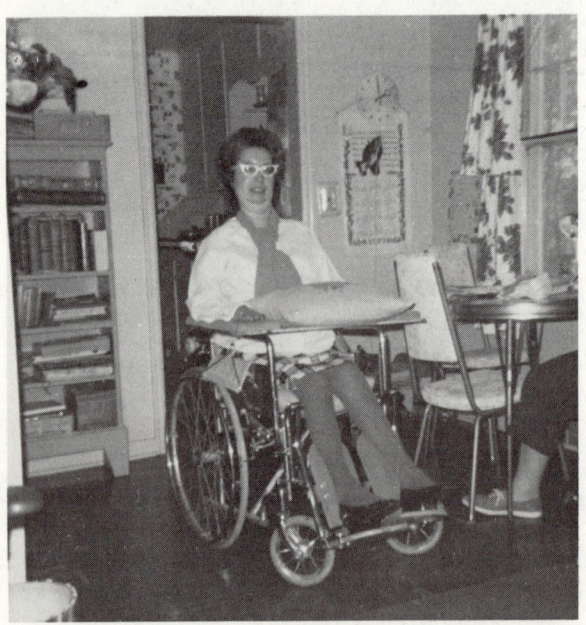

Jim has a Chevrolet Suburban van with a Hoyer Kar-Top lift. He likes to travel, one year going to the Bahamas on a chartered boat and another time to the northern edge of Great Slave Lake in the Yukon by float plane (Fig. 5–1).

Commenting on his social life, Jim says,

Teaching requires constant extroverted interaction with large and small groups of students, together with constant personal contact in performing administrative duties and in consulting so that my recreational social needs tend to be more private, such as fishing, travel, and reading. My unique circumstances leave me relatively isolated from my peer group of faculty families and married contemporaries. While business meetings and visits with friends on travels keep me out many evenings, I dislike social pastimes such as card playing and cocktail parties and do almost no entertaining at home, partly because it interferes with the normal pattern of attendant duties. Expensive recreational tastes and staff require some devotion to work and to making money. This desire to play hard is probably the reason I was able to become independent before obtaining my PhD."

DAILY LIVE-IN ATTENDANTS

Disabled by polio in 1949, Ruby Heine shares her home, which is rented through the Omaha Housing Authority, with her mother (Fig. 5–2). The monthly rent as of mid-1974 was $42. Ordinarily the house would rent for $125 month.

Ruby uses full-time respiratory assistance. She has very little movement in her arms and types and operates the adding machine with her mouthstick. She works from her rocking bed, selling Avon cosmetics, Amway household products, and wedding supplies. Most of her work is done by telephone, using an operator's headset clipped onto her glasses and operator dialing service. When Ruby completes one call, the operator asks her if she wants another number. Her income from these endeavors is about $250/month.

Most of Ruby's expenses, like those of most other severely disabled people, are for attendant care. Her income is not sufficient to meet these costs, and she is assisted by the county in which she lives in Omaha, Nebraska. She hires attendants on a 24-hour basis, from 4 P.M. one day to 4 P.M. the next. The payment for a 24-hour period is $21, for a total of $147/week. One of her attendants comes three times a week and high school students work on weekends. If one of the students cannot come, she has a sister or friend substitute for her. Ruby prefers having many different attendants because she thinks it best if two people are not confined together all the time. "People are more refreshed if they go home, resulting in fewer personality conflicts between attendant and employer."

Ruby explains her schedule:

Every day a housekeeping task is done in addition to my personal care. Dusting and ironing are done one day, vacuuming the next, cleaning cupboards another day, washing and other necessary tasks are all spaced out over the remaining days so that each attendant has an equal amount of work. I try not to be too much of a perfectionist because it makes both of us, the attendant and myself, uncomfortable if I am too demanding. There are also volunteers who help with bookkeeping, washing, and ironing.

There has to be a lot of give and take in an attendant–employer relationship. It's like a marriage. There are differences in likes and dislikes in food, television shows, and manner of living. The disabled individual should also remember that attendants have families, boyfriends, and projects of their own and when it comes to personal concerns, their interests come ahead of his. For instance, if I needed an attendant to work, would she give up a date? Usually, no. Thus, I have learned not to be tied to one person for my physical well-being, which means my emotional and psychologic well-being as well.

Ruby continues, "Everyone is not emotionally or psychologically equipped to live in a house or apartment alone with an attendant. He should be mature in both these areas for success in independent living."

Ruby's attendants are paid by the county under the Direct Vendor Service. With this system the attendants are paid directly. Unfortunately, there is an initial 3-week delay before payment, so Ruby pays her attendants at the end of each week and is reimbursed when they receive their checks and sign them over to her. When an attendant works hourly, payment is $2.10/hour.

A typical day in Ruby's life begins at 6 or 7 A.M. when she gets up in the wheelchair, where she stays until lunch time. She returns to bed via the hydraulic lift and eats lunch while rocking. After lunch she gets up again until dinner, for which she returns to bed unless she is going out.

Ruby is transportation chairman for the local chapter of the National Association for the Physically Handicapped, which meets monthly. She likes to go to the Omaha Symphony series of concerts, is active in church, and plays bridge. One of her more unusual activities is to bowl with a mouthstick.

Transportation is a problem, as Ruby needs strong people to get her and her respirators in and out of a car. Taxis are expensive and there is no handicapped bus service in her city. Because of these obstacles, Ruby has to turn down many invitations. This is especially true during the day, when most people are at work. On several occasions, local firemen helped get her in or out of the car.

To the newly disabled, Ruby says,

Don't get discouraged when you see other quads living full lives and think that their success came about in the short time of a year or two. You have to learn step by step, taking each day at a time. Enjoy the people you're with. New devices are always being invented that may help you. The rocking bed wasn't invented until 5 years after I got polio. There was no center at that time where I could learn to use one. It is important to associate with other disabled people to share common problems, frustrations, and goals. In this way you keep up with new ideas and medical and social advancements.

DISABLED COUPLE WITH LIVE-IN ATTENDANTS

Bill Clark was introduced to Connie Kowalski on the telephone by a friend. They became friends and then, as often happens with friends, fell in love. In October, 1973, they were married (Fig. 5-3). There was much publicity attending the wedding because both the bride and groom were in wheelchairs. Since then, they have been living with two attendants in an apartment house designed to accommodate the disabled.

Bill and Connie both come from Edmonton, Alberta, Canada. Connie was a victim of polio in 1953 when she was 15 years old. She uses full-time respiratory assistance—the rocking bed at night and part of the day, and the pneumobelt when sitting up. Her attendant handles all her personal care. Bill has multiple

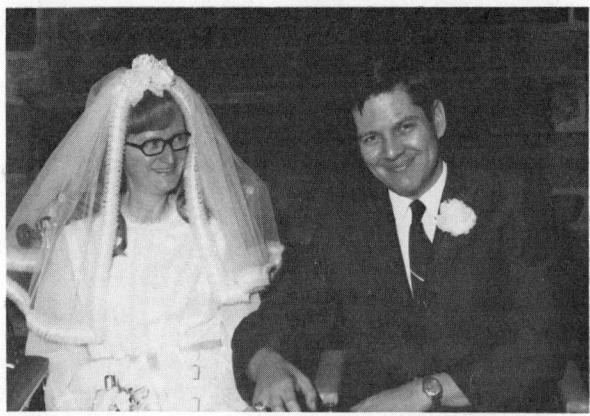

Fig. 5–3. Bill and Connie Clark, who are both in wheelchairs, share an apartment with two attendants.

sclerosis, first detected when he was studying to become a chiropractor. His eyesight was failing, his handwriting becoming shaky, and his sense of balance deteriorating. He continued his studies despite his physical problems, graduated, and set up a practice in 1960. It lasted only 6 months, for one day he could no longer walk up the stairs to his office. He can still use his hands and arms, although they are weak and spastic. Both attendants are required to lift him in and out of bed and help him to the bathroom. He has partial eyesight, but has been declared legally blind.

It was not a simple matter for Bill and Connie to get married and live independently. Bill had to present a passionate, 4-hour argument to the officials of the Alberta Social Services Department convincing them that marrying Connie and living outside the hospital would be cheaper for the government. He won his point. The Clarks receive $1116.75/month in aid from the province. Of this, $200–$250/month goes to each attendant. Bill and Connie describe their income as "just barely sufficient." They are now trying to get raises for their attendants.

The Clarks have a two-bedroom apartment. Connie has her rocking bed in the living room, leaving one bedroom for her attendant and the other for her husband and his attendant. She says, "We always treat our attendants like one of the family, as the feeling is much nicer that way. Also, I think they appreciate it." Finding attendants is difficult because, in Connie's view, "Most people don't want this type of work anymore. Our help often get bored as there isn't a great amount of work to do, especially if you're an organized person."

Bill and Connie have never had any serious problems with their attendants. Only one has been fired and the cause was alcoholism. Despite the fact that four people live close together, they usually get along well with each other. Their main problem is a lack of privacy.

The Clarks' apartment is in the center of town and convenient to everything. Connie's mother does their shopping. One of Bill's activities is answering the telephone for the Kinsmen Club paper bingo games. He also likes talking books, and one of his greatest pleasures is having his wife read to him. Connie can paint with an arm splint and a brush taped to her index finger. She designs and sells note paper. They do not try to earn too much extra income because earning more than $35/month would jeopardize their social assistance checks.

RENTING A HOUSE WITH STUDENT ATTENDANT AND FRIENDS

Dottie SantaPaul (Fig. 5–4) is disabled by amyotonia congenita, a progressive disease that has been stable since she was 12 years old. For most of her life she lived with her family and then stayed in a nursing home for 26 months. She says of this experience,

It felt like 26 years. I found it very depressing to live with 99 old people, ¾ of whom were senile. The rational ones were often the sickest physically and sometimes didn't get out of bed at all. I found the rules there very oppressing and I was discouraged from taking any responsibility in the decisions in my life at all. The atmosphere was one of death and awaiting death. The employees at this particular place were constantly at each other's throats and that—even apart from the institutional atmosphere—was hard to stand constantly.

Her dissatisfaction moved her to attempt independent living. She found the arrangements difficult and frustrating to work out.

I had tried nearly full time to coordinate housing, financial security, and some sort of attendant set-up for 6 months. Nothing ever lined up. As one thing got straightened out, another fell through. I finally gave up to God out of total frustration and extreme depression. Within 1 week, everything fell together in perfection.

Fig. 5–4. Dottie SantaPaul lives in a rented house with students and friends.

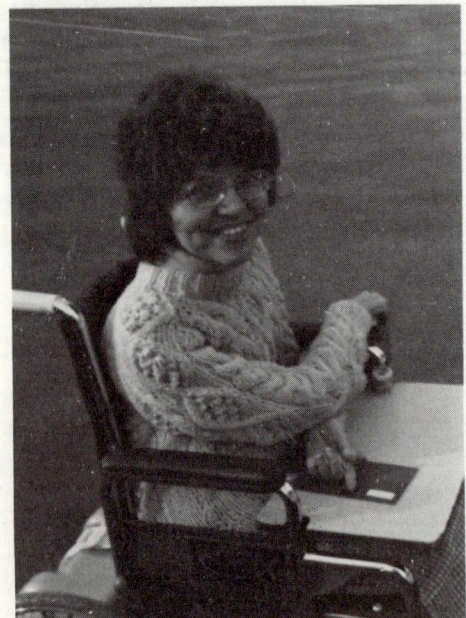

I had set a deadline of 8:30 on a certain night to decide whether to keep an apartment I had secured. If I hadn't found an attendant by then, I would give up the apartment. At 8:13 a girl called and said she'd heard I was looking for an attendant. I told her the situation and she agreed to live with me. She was a seminary student and one of her friends, also a student, decided to come with her.

Instead of taking the apartment, Dottie and her two new friends rented a 12-room, fully furnished house for $100/month. It had five acres of land, six fireplaces, a two-car garage, a view of a golf course, a glade of pines, and the ocean on three sides. Dottie's comment: "I thought I'd died and gone to heaven!"

The living arrangement worked well, and eventually Dottie moved to a house closer to town and church. The rent is $225/month. Three girls live with her and receive for their attendant help an equal portion of the $200/month Dottie receives from Supplemental Security Income. They help with her morning and night personal care, cooking, cleaning, laundry, and grocery shopping. Dottie says,

Schedules are flexible. I usually get up somewhere between 6 and 7:30 A.M. and go to bed between 11 and 12 P.M. We agree on who does what on which days, and if someone is going to be away for a weekend or even a week, we rearrange the schedule. If two or more are to be away at the same time, I have friends come in.

Financially, I make out pretty well, but have learned to live without luxuries. I get $200/month Supplemental Security Income and $90/month in a rental assistance grant. We share expenses. Independent living is about $150–$200/month cheaper than nursing home living.

Dottie finds most of her attendants through bulletin board notices at a nearby seminary and Christian college. She refers to them as roommates, even though they are paid.

We don't have an employer/employee relationship. We are friends and more of a family.

I'd say the biggest problem involved in needing attendants is that the structure of our 'family' changes frequently. Because we have a common bond in Christ, we have good groundwork on which to build relationships, but building good relationships takes work. It is my hope that someday there would be established a more permanent Christian community with sisters and brothers in Christ who are able to make long-term commitments. Even so, most of my roommates have stayed at least 1 or 2 years.

For transportation, Dottie has a Volkswagen van that is driven by a retired lady volunteer or young friends. She suggests that persons who need drivers contact local senior citizens groups.

Two of the devices that increase Dottie's independence are a long, wooden, scissorslike gadget she uses to pick up things and a brake left over from an old wheelchair. With the brake, "I pull things, open things, pry things, bang things. It's got 1001 uses. To push the toaster lever down, I put one end of the brake on the lever and the other against my head, and push down with my head."

Dottie has a degree in social work, but at the time of this writing was not employed. She is a volunteer receptionist at a treatment center for emotionally disturbed adolescents and enjoys many activities, such as bowling and crafts.

SPECIAL ALTERATIONS AND EQUIPMENT FOR SOLO LIVING

If a disabled individual were asked where in the world he would find life easiest, one of his first choices would certainly be Berkeley, California. By means of hard work the disabled there have attained improvements in attendant care, convenient and fast wheelchair repair, architectural accessibility, curb ramping, and other concerns.

One of the persons who worked hardest for these improvements is John Hessler, a 33-year-old C5–6 quadriplegic. John serves as director of the Physically Disabled Students Program (PDSP), a group he helped to organize at the University of California at Berkeley. John's salary as director comfortably covers his living expenses, including the extra expenses associated with a disability. Without the job, he could still manage on Supplemental Security Income and the monies provided by the state for attendant care.

After John broke his neck in a diving accident in 1957 when he was 16 years old, he spent 6 years in the rehabilitation ward of a county hospital. The main rehabilitative focus was on exercise and equipment which left much of John's potential untouched. The frustration and anger from his hospital experience shaped his belief that institutions, no matter how benevolent, create problems while attempting to cure others.

While in the hospital, John finished high school and then commuted to a junior college. The 2-year program there took him 4 years to complete because of illness and poor preparation for college. From junior college John went to the University of California at Berkeley for 6 years, majoring in German and French. There he received his BA and MA. During that time he lived at Cowell Hospital on the University campus. He was hesitant about moving into an apartment at that time because of a lack of supportive services in the community.

John spent a year in France as part of his study, sharing housing with several able-bodied people. His transportation was a Volkswagen van with a bed in the back. After he returned he decided to move out of Cowell Hospital into an apartment with two able-bodied roommates. A few months later another disabled student moved in with them, a situation that lasted until 1972, when John moved into an apartment where he lives by himself.

John's apartment was chosen because it is easily rampable and is large enough so he can move freely from room to room in his motorized chair. The kitchen is set up so that he can cook. He does most of his cooking in an electric frying pan that sits on a table high enough for him to put his legs under. Cooking utensils with adaptive devices, regularly used staples and spices, and an electric can opener sit on countertops that can be easily reached. A small refrigerator is raised on blocks so that all parts of it are accessible. The sink and faucets are within easy reach.

The bedroom is large enough for John to go completely around the bed. One side is kept clear for transferring in and out of the wheelchair. The other side is against a bookshelf that holds the telephone, water pitcher, and controls for the lights and stereo record player. All these things can be reached from the bed or chair. Any other electrical things that John wants to use can be plugged into a control box that contains four to six openings and switches for each plug. His telephone has a direct connection to the operator that is activated by lifting the receiver.

The Balkan frame on John's bed allows him to move around on and get in and out of bed. It is a structure built with metal posts on each corner of the bed supporting four parallel bars over the bed that have loops made of safety belt material hanging down in strategic spots. While hanging on to the loops, John is able to maneuver in bed.

John can undress himself in bed and hook up to his night drainage system. Velcro strips have been sewn into all his shirts and pants, replacing buttons. His sandals were especially made, have Velcro on the straps, and are bolted to the foot pedals of his wheelchair. This makes it possible for him to take his feet out of the sandals and put his legs on the bed without worrying about getting his shoes off after he gets in bed. The leg on which he wears the urine drainage bag has a Velcro seam on the inside seam of the pants so that he can empty his own drainage bag.

In the mornings John has an attendant come in for 2 hours. He also has an arrangement with someone who lives nearby to come in for emergency situations, such as unscheduled bowel movements. Two attendant pools are maintained in Berkeley, making attendants readily available to students and people in the community. Most attendants are students. They are chosen for the pool by counselors who have had experience as attendants or who use attendants. But the disabled individual hires, trains, and pays his own attendant, thereby controlling the quality of care he receives. John teaches his attendants what his body is supposed to look like, feel like, and how to recognize pressure sores.

John's typical day begins at 8 A.M. His attendant arrives and assists him by irrigating his catheter, bathing and dressing him, and helping him get into his wheelchair. Once up, John does his shaving, tooth brushing, and other grooming while his attendant straightens things up and sets out the necessary articles for meal preparation. John then leaves the apartment, gets into his specially equipped van, and drives to work. His work entails dictating letters, using a push-button phone to make calls, attending meetings on campus and in the community, supervising the office staff, and handling any large problems that may arise.

At the end of the workday and on weekends, John engages in several activities. He goes out on dates to accessible restaurants and theaters, visits friends, or goes to meetings. He may spend an evening at home, cook dinner, read, or entertain. John likes to travel, by van or plane. He is a member of the Board of Directors of the Center for Independent Living, a consumer-run organization for the disabled in Berkeley, and a trainer in a rehabilitation counselor training program.

LIVE-IN FRIEND AND HOURLY ATTENDANT

Nell Blaine is a well-known painter who lives with another artist friend in New York City (Fig. 5-5). Her paintings have been bought by over 300 collectors and for over 30 permanent public collections, including those of the Whitney Museum of American Art, The Brooklyn Museum, and the Virginia Museum of Fine Arts.

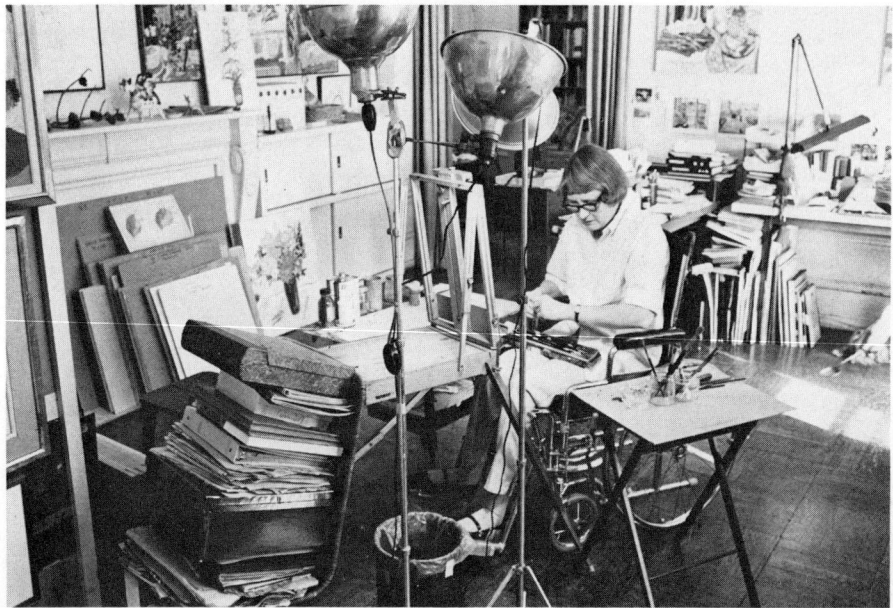

Fig. 5–5. Nell Blaine, the painter, in her New York studio. She lives with a friend and hires hourly attendants. (Photograph by Carol Crawford, Creative Artists Service Program)

She has been described as "an outstanding American painter, who may claim the unusual distinction of being a leader in the abstract movement in the 1940s, and in the forefront of the figurative movement in the 1950s."

This success is especially impressive when one is informed of the fact that most of this work was done by the left hand of a normally right-handed artist.

Nell Blaine contracted bulbar-spinal polio in 1959 while painting on the island of Mykonos, Greece. She was flown to Mount Sinai Respirator Center in New York, where she remained for nearly 8 months. When she left the hospital, she was confined to a wheelchair with paralysis in her back, stomach, right shoulder, diaphragm, and legs. As she could not lift her right arm, she slowly taught herself to paint in oils mainly with her left.

Nell's friend assists with her personal care evenings, which includes painting set-ups. Her daytime care is done by an attendant who comes for 8 hours each weekday. Still another attendant helps 1 or 2 days each weekend and one evening during the week. Nell pays her weekday attendant $135/week and her friend and her other helpers $135 and over weekly. Her own income is dependent on the number of paintings she sells and occasional grants she receives. In 1972 she received a CAPS grant and in 1974–1975 a Guggenheim. She estimates, "I sell roughly 25 pictures a year, oils for several thousand dollars depending on size and period; watercolors vary from $375 for the smallest to $1125 for an 18 × 25 in., which I consider large. Drawings range from $290 to approximately $950 (prices as of 1975). Except for my disability, I would be earning an excellent wage."

Nell has found that live-in help does not work well, except for one or two cases. To the question of whether she could live alone or not, she responds,

No, if my friend left I'd need to find another person to fill her place somehow. I need a number of helpers. My solutions are not wonderful, and I always think they should be improved upon. Sometimes it goes very poorly. People who work for me get sick or are unreliable and the burden falls on my friend. She is already overburdened and thus, guiltily, I impose dreadfully on her and on others. Naturally I long for greater independence.

She continues,

When getting an attendant I advertise in the *New York Times* (Sunday) and I've gotten several from reading their ads. I don't hire nurses or attendants always. I've tried housekeepers and cleaning people, offering them more than their usual wages. However, those who have stayed up to and over 2 years have always had at least nurses' aide experience previously. The worst part for me is interviewing and training. I find it takes months to break one in completely and often we hire three or four before one sticks, as it's a demanding job requiring lots of patience.

By the way, I've had some lulu experiences interviewing potential attendants. Once a very friendly voice on the telephone materialized with her arm in a splint up over her head and massive bandages; she was about half my size, a heavy smoker, and as lonely as they come. I felt a tower of strength by comparison!

To get a really first-rate attendant, one often needs a lot of money. One still needs to have a friend or relative about unless one can do certain basic things—get up and dress and go to the john.

TWO STUDENT LIVE-IN ATTENDANTS

This disabled individual receives welfare assistance as well as undeclared monthly income from her parents. Anonymity is advisable because disclosure of this latter fact would topple the financial structure of her independence, but knowing the amounts will help the reader understand how Jane manages to live on her own.

Disabled since birth, Jane decided in her early 30s to try living apart from her parents. She enrolled in a state university about 40 miles from her home and rented an apartment near the campus. Physically dependent on others, she offered free room and board to two students in return for attendant care. Despite the high turnover in attendants and the necessary personality adjustments with each change, Jane earned her BA and went on to graduate study in sociology.

Jane receives monthly $127 welfare assistance, $100 from her parents, approximately $40 in typing earnings which she reports as $30, and $118 in food stamps for which she pays $24. Her monthly expenses are $170 for rent, $15 for electricity, $18 for phone but averages $20 with toll calls, $110 for food, and $30 for cleaning fees. She keeps a van for transportation, and her father pays maintenance costs.

Most of Jane's problems center around attendant care. Finding two personalities that get along with each other as well as with her is one problem. Another is learning how to apportion duties. For a long time, Jane let her attendants work out duty arrangements, but she found this system usually resulted in many resentments and much work left undone. She gradually realized that she would have to allot housekeeping and attendant tasks herself. This eliminated much of the discord.

Commenting on the effects of living with many different attendants, she says

My statistics are 46 attendants in 6 years, or an average of 7.66/year. The advantages are obvious. It keeps a person from settling into a comfortable rut and there is the constant stimulation of new ideas. The disadvantages are more subtle—the difficulty of maintaining a sense of continuity, the anxiety, the constant struggle to preserve one's self-image in the face of continual change.

One thing that bothers me about this way of living is that I view my surroundings as an extension of myself, while to somebody who just comes in for a brief stay the apartment is merely a place to sleep and store junk—like a dorm room. They couldn't care less about cigarette burns in the couch, scratches in the furniture, etc. I am continually frustrated in my desire to have a nice apartment. There's no point in buying anything really nice because the others won't treasure it and take care of it.

Another major problem is boyfriends staying over. It makes me uncomfortable, and I feel as long as I'm paying the rent I have some say about what goes on. The attendants feel that they have earned their room and should be able to do what they want in it.

When asked what type of person makes the best attendant, Jane replied,

All kinds of people are attracted to the free room and board involved. What I look for now is just the right blend of toughness and sensitivity. I'd rather have an attendant who is slightly compulsive than a free spirit, because I can only be free within a well-structured framework. I have to know that someone will be here at a given time to perform a given task. Otherwise all my attention is directed toward worrying about basic necessities, and I can't function on any other level.

Generally, people attracted to the attendant role are the independent type. I wouldn't expect a sorority chick type to apply. (It's interesting to note that response to my ad has been better since I call myself a 'disabled Ms.') They are usually girls who are working their way through college, so I guess I could generalize and call them 'highly motivated.' Some might be hypochondriacs who are curious about the physical aspects of being disabled. Of course, there are the neurotics who are looking for somebody to relate to. They can be good attendants if the neurosis is complementary to yours.

A few things I've learned through the years are, it's best not to get too emotionally attached to your attendant. It may sound cold, but it's best to keep in mind the purpose the attendant was hired for, and the fact that attendants are interchangeable. It's possible to do this and yet relate on a human level. Some attendants will remain friends after they leave; others won't. This depends on mutual interests and is on another level than the attendant–attendee relationship. Also, it's absolutely necessary to remain in control of the situation. You have to learn to be firm and insist on having your needs taken care of without seeming like an ogre. The best way to do this is to make a schedule and stick to it rigidly. If it's bath day, take a bath—whether you feel like it or not. If the attendant knows what's expected, things work a lot more smoothly and everybody has more freedom.

One further note; some of my best attendants have been those who had the ability to project into my situation. One attendant had been in a car accident and had needed to be taken care of, another's brother was a paraplegic, one was an actress and could assume different roles, and one had suffered from severe asthma as a child.

I've learned that the success or failure of this arrangement largely depends on me. I believe I've become an easier person to live with, more assured, and more aware of myself.

EXCHANGING LODGING FOR SERVICES

Bernard Brett has cerebral palsy and describes himself as "about 96% disabled." He has the use of only one hand and cannot communicate effectively verbally.

After living for 7 years in a home for the disabled, he bought a large house near the center of town. Over the years he had learned the importance of being within walking or pushing distance of shops, restaurants, and theaters.

Five bed-sitting rooms are rented out in Bernard's house. Many of his lodgers are young couples who have had trouble finding a place that would accept children. They are grateful to have a home and are usually willing to help Bernard. Some of them trade attendant services in the evenings or on weekends for free accommodations. During the day Bernard employs attendants.

Most of my lodgers stay until they can get public housing, which often takes several years. The lodgers who pay rent cover the cost of running the house, rates, heating, and cooking. I am fortunate in receiving an allowance from my family. For transportation I have a van which has a ramp.

Sometimes there are as many as three children living here, which is fun but noisy. It is fortunate that I tend to be very tolerant (many of my helpers say much too tolerant of rows, mess, squabbles, and stealing). Still, if it provides help and support, this is what matters, particularly if it provides a second or third line of defense in case of illness or household upset. The greatest drawbacks in this system are a dire lack of privacy and being involved with people with many more problems and hang-ups than in the average population.

Bernard lives an active and useful life. Much of his time is occupied in taking an MA course in Social Policy Administration at Essex University. He likes to travel. One year he went to Northern Ireland and later to Montreal, Canada for 5 weeks. He also visited New York City and discovered a city "with a very special magic." Organizations that receive his help are Christian Action Housing, Adventure Playground Association, and the Disablement Income Group. With Bernard's help and that of many others, the Disablement Income Group won the Constant Attendant Allowance for the disabled in England.

Bernard feels,

The most challenging problem for any disabled person living on his or her own is loneliness, especially in times of difficulty or stress, when the burdens of depression can bring one very close to disaster. I also find many medics do not provide much support or treatment if they encounter disabled persons who are very depressed, because they regard this as natural. They are quite wrong in my view because often these times of depression are caused through factors of health, circumstances, and the time of year. Of course, financial worries are an important reason and this is why we in Britain are fighting for a National Disability Income as a right.

COOPERATIVE COMMUNAL LIVING

Mickie McGraw is an art therapist at Highland View Hospital (Fig. 5–6). She is a quadriplegic, but can use her hands and arms for her work and activities such as eating, combing her hair, washing her face, etc. A motorized wheelchair makes her mobile. For most of her personal care, transferring and transporting, she needs assistance.

Mickie had lived with her parents during the time she was an art student and for the first few years of her employment. To develop her independence further, she decided to try communal living. She rented a large house for $300/month and shared it with four friends. Their part of the rent was determined by their

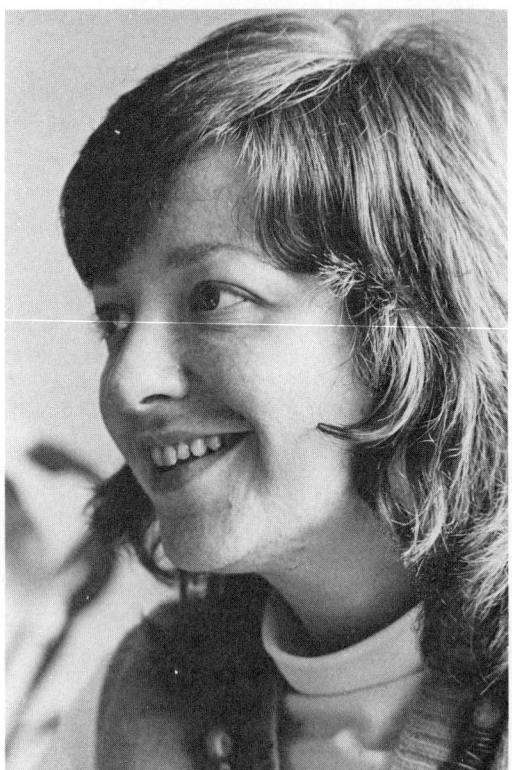

Fig. 5-6. Mickie McGraw is an art therapist in a rehabilitation hospital.

services. For instance, if one of the residents painted a room or acted as Mickie's driver, he paid less rent. The amount was agreed upon between Mickie and the other resident. Each person was responsible for providing his own food.

Each member of the group had a room of his own, and everyone shared the kitchen and dining room. Mickie's room was on the second floor and was made accessible by a stair lift. Unfortunately, it was the type of lift which she could not use without assistance. This limited her independence if she was alone in the house.

During the 18 months that Mickie lived with her friends, various attendant care arrangements were tried. The way that worked best was having one friend help her in the morning and another at night. This put less pressure and responsibility on one person. "Mixing the responsibility of attendant care and friendship is oftentimes difficult because the responsibility of attendant care is always difficult. It is often better to hire an attendant than burden a friendship with physical dependency."

Mickie suggests that anyone considering communal living first decide whether he has the right type of personality for it.

I discovered I was a private person. I needed more time to myself than was possible given my personality and a communal living situation. The more people there are, the more stimulation and intensities, and I found myself responding to every problem or need. My work involves contact on an intense level with many people, and I need a time for resting when I come home. Perhaps there are some people who can live and work as I do, but limit their receptivity enough to live successfully in a communal lifestyle.

She considers communal living a good transitional experience between a hospital or family situation and independent living. There is more than one person for the disabled individual to rely on to answer his needs. It is a stimulating way of living for a person who stays at home and does not go out to work because there is exposure to people and activities. Communal living is economically easier than independent living.

Mickie advises that a definite structure of responsibility, such as who does what when, be set up for successful cooperative communal living. "A clearly defined housekeeping schedule is necessary to eliminate a person's feeling resentful that he is doing more work than anyone else."

"It helps to have someone else of a peer age in the house," concludes Mickie. "You need someone of a proximal age and life understanding to share thoughts and interests with. It should be noted, too, that communal living has built-in limitations. Our experience was that most people involved in it felt a need to leave it after a year or a year and a half. But it can be good and useful experience for its duration."

LIVE-IN STUDENT AND HOURLY ATTENDANT

Caryl Smith is an assistant professor of psychology at a midwestern university and plans to develop a private clinical practice. She is married to a psychiatrist and at the time of this writing, they were expecting a baby. A quadriplegic, she requires help with her personal and home care. This is provided by an 8 hour/day, 5 days/week attendant, a weekend attendant, and a live-in student who gives week-night assistance.

The Smiths have a four-bedroom, four-bath "rambling old roomy place" that rents for $435/month. They looked for a year before finding it, having to pass up many others where the elevator was too small, too low in power to lift Caryl's motorized wheelchair and her in it, or where there was no elevator. Architectural problems also limit the social gatherings that Caryl can attend.

As are most of the disabled who live independently, Caryl accepts the inherent difficulties in finding attendants.

Living in an urban setting, I have found that newspaper advertising is the most effective way of securing attendants. Of course, advertising is not an easy way. You must answer numerous calls, many from people clearly unsuitable. Then you must interview promising callers in person. Anywhere from 25%–50% fail to show up for the interview. Of those who come, however, I have always found at least one whose references were good. Unfortunately, I have learned that attendants rarely stay 6 months, if that long. We have just come to accept this fact and are ready to place our ad whenever necessary. For interim fill-ins and emergencies we also rely on a local nurses' registry. Our salary range falls between that paid by nursing homes and that charged by nurses' registries. This is $2.50–$2.60/hour. The student who helps me to bed during the week receives free room and board.

Caryl comments further,

> The major problem with attendants is that at the salary level we can afford, one attracts people who are generally not part of the full-time permanent work force. Their lives are often not geared toward working consistently (they have all kinds of family problems requiring that they take time off from work), and many times jobs such as ours are accepted because they need to get out of debt, are separated from their spouse, etc. Any change in their personal situation is often reflected by a change in their job.
>
> My solution to transportation problems has been to have my own. I presently own a Checker Marathon Medic (high roof to accommodate my wheelchair and extra large rear door with which I use a plywood ramp for the wheelchair). When I hire a full-time attendant, she must have a current driver's license, express no fear of highway driving, and agree to drive as part of the job. I then assess their handling of the car once they begin the job (or, if time permits, *prior* to their first day).

When asked whether her husband helped with her personal care and what effect this had on their marital relationship, Caryl responded,

> My husband does assist in my personal care, but only on a part-time or pinch-hit basis. We just accept it in stride (it neither adds to nor detracts from 'romance' in our marriage). However, I would counsel couples in doubt on this point to go the 'live together for a while' route before signing the marriage license to see how it will work in practice. It is probably best to have an attendant do most of the personal care because 1) you can be more exacting if you're paying for the service and 2) your mate will feel less tied down, a feeling which invariably leads to anger, a definite detriment to romance.

LIVE-IN ATTENDANT SUPPLEMENTED BY FRIENDS AND NEIGHBORS

Having been a respiratory polio quadriplegic for 23 years, I have experienced several ways of living. I am totally dependent on respirators and cannot use my hands or arms, resulting in a 24-hour/day need for attendant care. For the first 5 years after I left the hospital, I lived with my mother and a live-in attendant. Weekends I spent with my father and a cousin who helped him with my personal care and cooking. The next 7 years I lived full-time with my father and a live-in attendant. In 1967 my father died and I have lived since then with various live-in attendants (Fig. 5–7).

Most of my attendants are found through newspaper ads. They have been black and white, young and old, men and women. Present payment for 5½ days is $45/week or, if they just take occasional time off, $50. Weekend helpers receive $18 for the period between Saturday morning and Sunday evening, or $1.50/hour when only morning or night care is needed. My mother helps every other weekend. When my attendant wants a few hours off, various people from friends to neighbors are called upon to substitute. Some refuse payment, others are paid rates ranging from 50¢ to $1.50/hour.

The house where I live rent free belongs to my cousin, but I pay the taxes, utilities, insurance, and maintenance. A neighborhood boy mows the lawn for $4; spring and fall cleaning or other chores are done for $2/hour. Friends offer their individual talents as gifts. For instance, one friend painted the porch and porch furniture, another fixes electrical problems, one made new bathroom curtains, and still another laid a new kitchen and bathroom floor.

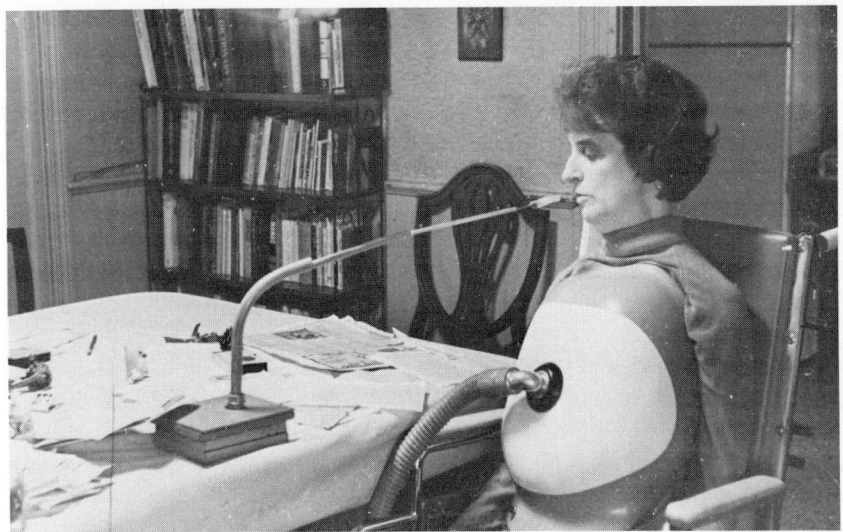

Fig. 5–7. Donna McGwinn lives with an attendant and is also helped by friends and neighbors. She uses a mouthstick when reading.

I live in a small village of 500 people where everyone knows everyone else. Most people are willing to help, but I try not to take advantage of their willingness. The local firemen are familiar with my respiratory equipment, and the rescue vehicle is wired to accommodate it. Many of my neighbors and friends know how to start my gasoline generator, get me in or out of bed, aspirate, or transport me. A large network of people keeps me functioning and I am grateful to them all.

My home is on a main thoroughfare and is easy to reach for the many people who stop in. The doors are rarely locked, even when I go away for a few hours. Some of my attendants find this free-flowing atmosphere hard to adjust to, but it serves to keep me in easy contact with people and is a safety factor if there is trouble in the house. If something should happen to my attendant at night when I am without access to the telephone, I can be reasonably assured that within 24 hours someone would call or come over. A walk-in policy also frees my attendant from having to answer the door. This is especially helpful during power failures when there is a lot to be done and we welcome the physical and emotional help of others.

One of the most important things I have learned from my living experiences is that almost any plan of life is possible. There are enough types of people in the world to be part of any scheme, no matter how wild or unprecedented. The secret to making the plan work is to have faith in it, and possibly to have a believer or two to reinforce your faith when it is sorely challenged.

I can type, dial the phone, and write with my toes (Figs. 5–8, 5–9, and 5–10). Almost everything else requires attendant assistance. The best type of attendant for me is one who does not mind being at home much of the time and with whom I can comfortably interact. By now I know what type of personality I can adapt

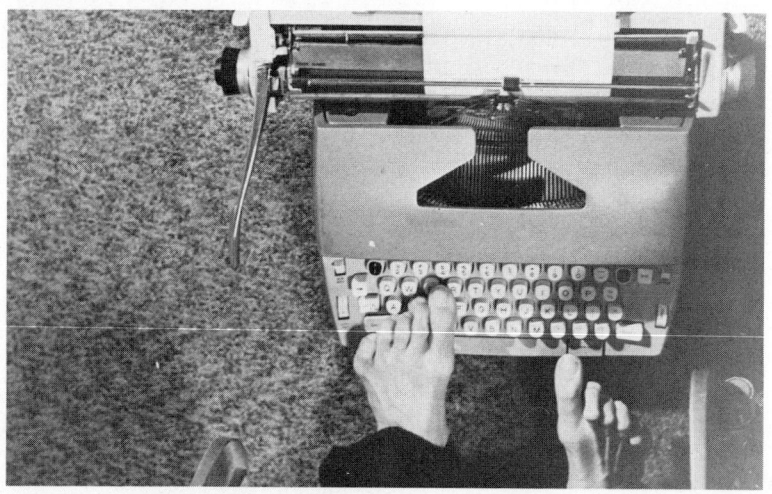
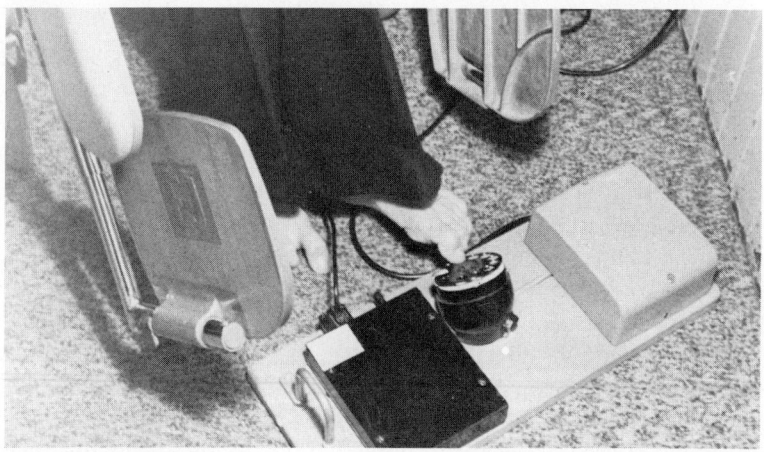
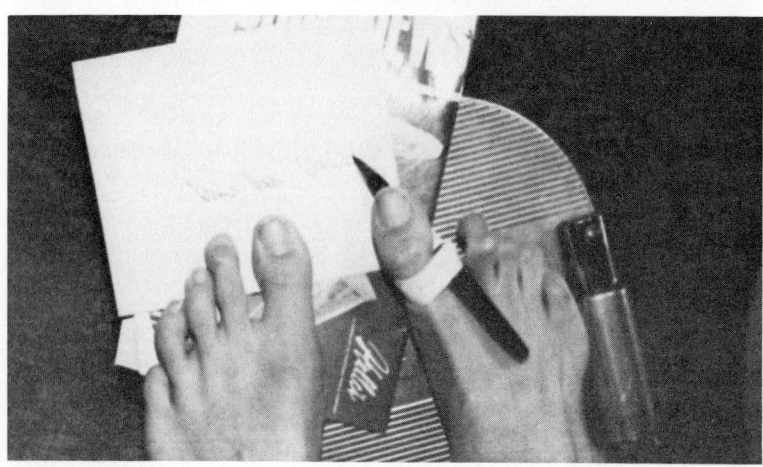

Fig. 5-8. Typing by toes. Donna can put paper in the typewriter, fold and put letters in envelopes with her feet.

Fig. 5-9. Dialing by toes. A bendable metal arm holds the ear and mouthpiece of Donna's phone so that she can push her wheelchair up to it. The dial and on/off switch are attached to a plate on the floor.

Fig. 5-10. Writing by toes.

to most easily. I can adjust to most types of people, with the exception of those with extremes of loquaciousness or silence and those who are largely irrational. The knowledge of what traits are incompatible was gained through a great deal of experience and emotional energy.

From the experience of living with two other people instead of one, I have learned that the fewer personalities I have to live with, the happier I am. I also realize that taking care of me and my home and working closely with just one other person full time is a demanding job for an attendant. However, my personality, limited funds, and total physical dependency make it the best arrangement for me thus tried. A recently devised signal system activated by a 12-volt battery allows my attendant to be upstairs and still in touch if needed. This gives us both more freedom and privacy.

Although it is very expensive, I keep a car to assure my mobility. My respirators run on the car battery, and the car must be carefully maintained. It is convenient to use for shopping or other errands.

Much of my time is spent writing. I am book editor and do other work for *Rehabilitation Gazette* and have had articles published in many magazines. I would like to write fiction. Although it might seem I would have a lot of time for reading and writing, both favorite indulgences, there are many people in my life, and each of them receives a significant amount of attention, energy, and time. For public service I am chairman of the annual collection drives in my area for research into cancer and birth defects.

My family, friends, and attendants have all helped to make me independent. Needing people for every physical need has initiated contacts I might never have made and generated friendships I might never have enjoyed. People are the means of my expression and continuance of life. I cannot help but appreciate and love them.

"Only through other people have I been able to survive out of a hospital."

Ruby Heine

6
Attendant Care
DONNA McGWINN

Many people with disabilities must have help with the necessities and enjoyments of life. Sometimes assistance is provided by family or friends. When this help is not available or the needs are too great for the number of people to answer them, outside help has to be hired. Requirements vary with personality and the degree of disability. People who are totally disabled need help with everything from personal care to lawn mowing, while those with less extensive disablement can get along with limited aid. Personality also makes a difference. Many people do not mind or even prefer staying alone for a few hours; others are nervous and insecure unless there is someone with them.

An attendant can easily be the most important person in a disabled individual's life. Without someone to activate his wishes and intentions, a disabled person can become a nonfunctioning invalid. The need for attendant care usually carries certain contingent problems. The most prevalent one is lack of money for attendant salaries. Most of the disabled have drastically reduced incomes at the same time they have greatly increased expenses. Some cope with precarious finances while others are forced on to public assistance rolls. The consequent small salaries they must offer attract few people, and of these many are marginal in mental or emotional stability, intelligence, or competence. The turnover is high, and the uncertainties for the disabled individual's safety and security are great.

Some applicants for attendant positions are themselves on public assistance rolls. Since additional income jeopardizes their continued standing, they do not like to work unless their employer agrees not to report their income. In most cases the person who is disabled needs an attendant urgently and is willing to agree to almost any terms. He breaks the laws that require the reporting of employee salaries and thereby eliminates for himself a sizable income tax deduction. The average short duration of an attendant's employ necessitates frequent advertising expense. All these expenses, unlike those associated with temporary illness, baby sitting, or housework, are as permanent as one's disability. They can amount to a formidable sum over the years.

The emotional expense of relying on a continually changing cast of attendants for almost every need can also be sobering. For the person not born with his disability there is first the arduous adjustment to the reality of another person taking care of his body, his personal possessions, and his home. Not only has he lost control of body movement, but of body maintenance. He is subjected to strange hands that can be too rough, too gentle, too awkward, too incompetent, too slow, too fast or, for the lucky among us, perfect in every way. His body and

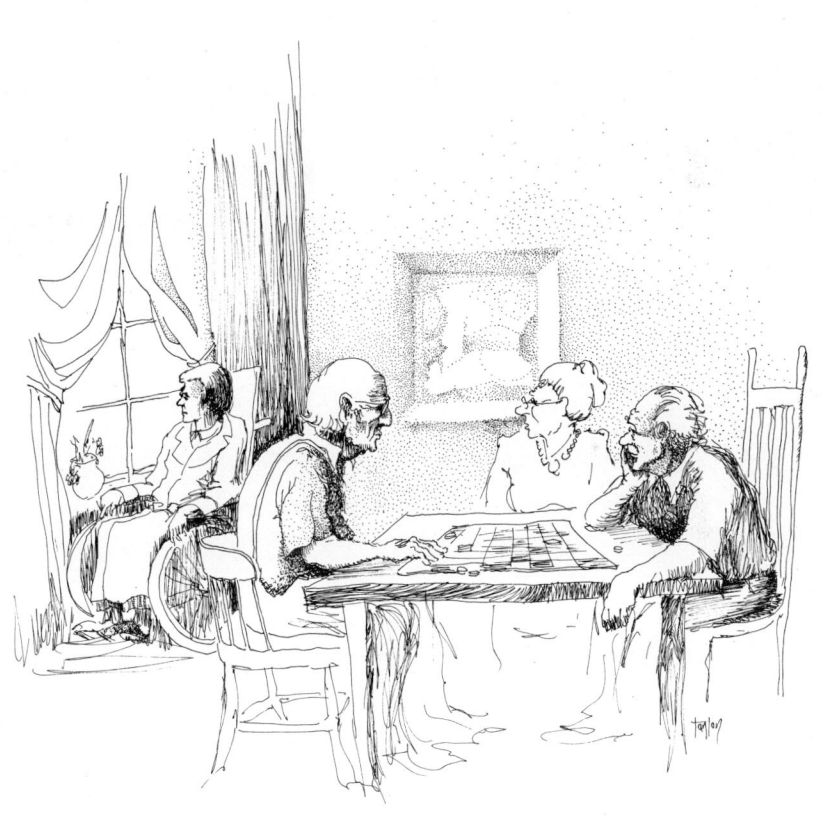

sensibilities are exposed and vulnerable to the unfamiliar and sometimes sadistic, corrupt, and hostile attitudes and scrutiny of a plethora of attendants. Fortunately, there are also in these ranks kind, warm, able, and devoted human beings who dedicate a large part of their time and energy to the employers they often regard as family or friends.

A person who is physically dependent must exert sustained effort to develop a sense of self and personal style. It is easy to become as psychologically passive as one is physically passive. The disabled individual is constantly being acted upon physically; his body is moved and positioned, and his tangible environment is moved by others. To retain control of his life and lifestyle under these dependent circumstances, the disabled individual must be almost constantly aware and able to direct his personal care and the running of his home, business, and social life. He has to be flexible and resourceful or he will have trouble interacting with the parade of personalities with which he must work and, in some cases, live.

There are generally two ways of relating to attendants. Some of the disabled keep the relationship easy but formal, and others regard their attendants as friends or part of the family. Which method is most successful depends upon the individuals involved. Those who feel uncomfortable using a detached manner of giving instructions prefer the friendly approach. Others prefer acting as employers for they feel guilty about asking persons considered friends or family to do things for them.

The wide range of personalities and attendant methods with which the disabled must work on an intimate basis can be stimulating or wearisome and discouraging. Most disabled people who have succeeded in conducting active, productive lives have managed to keep their own purposes and styles even though they have to operate through the hands of attendants who all have different backgrounds and techniques.

Predictable types of personalities are attracted to the disabled. Some have a desire to be needed. Some seek power over another, while others find an outlet for sadism. One type finds that association with the disabled diminishes their own problems, and another type discovers that a certain status is acquired by those in the position of helping humanity. The attitudes and actions projected from these motivations are not always palatable to a disabled individual, and certain tensions result. He may retaliate with a response derived from his own emotional problems and the relationship will become increasingly negative.

Some of the disabled have a series of attendants with whom they have unpleasant experiences, and they gradually become discouraged and depressed. It helps to define and discuss problems as they arise. Then both parties can decide if they want to work the problems out and continue the relationship. A good, positive relationship with an attendant can build confidence and security. Therefore, it becomes imperative for the disabled individual to determine exactly what type of personality he works best with and develop the perception to recognize it. The smooth execution of the basics of his life depends upon it.

Independent living is not fulfilling for all of the disabled. Some cannot cope, and some are afraid of coping with the responsibilities of daily dependent life. They prefer institutional life where their care is structured and supervised by others. Many persons now living with their families would rather enter institutions than live alone with attendants if their home arrangement should be changed by illness or death.

The attendant's view of his job is equally challenging. There are negligible monetary benefits. In most cases the attendant has to sublimate his methods and style to those of his employer. He has a physically primary but mentally secondary position, which some do not find satisfying. They feel that they are doing all the work and their employers are getting all the credit and attention. In a number of instances, attendants with little education are exploited by their employers. They are asked to work long hours and given uncomfortable sleeping quarters. If they live with the employer, they are required to conform to his sleeping and eating hours, menus, and the tempo and manner of his life, leaving them little time or opportunity to express their own tastes and inclinations. And always there is the pressure of having someone vitally dependent on them.

In a good attendant–employer relationship, however, the benefits can be the close, rewarding relationship itself, the satisfaction of doing personal, helping work with visible results, the importance of being needed, and sometimes a home and acceptance into a family.

HOW TO FIND ATTENDANTS

The first problem for a disabled individual who wants to live outside of an institution with his family or on his own is to decide how much help he needs and how much he can pay for it. For many it is cheaper to have someone live in and offer him room and board as part of his remuneration. Others manage more easily by having help with personal care mornings and evenings and relying on themselves or their families the rest of the time. Some of the disabled need help for a number of activities that are not performed on a daily basis, such as once or twice a week baths or showers, therapy, assistance with a business, trips outside the home, or nighttime attendance.

Once the appropriate amount of help needed has been determined, it has to be located and rates of payment set. Rates vary greatly even within the same geographic area. In the Cleveland, Ohio area, for instance, attendant help can be found for 90¢ to $6 hourly. The higher rates are for experienced and professional help such as nurses' aides and practical nurses. The lower rates are acceptable to an assortment of people of all ages and experiences. This writer has had competent attendants aged 11–80 and with disabilities from cerebral palsy to mental retardation. Mothers whose children are in school, senior citizens, men and women with one part-time job who would like another, high school and college students—in all these groups people willing to work as attendants can be found.

The most common way of looking for an attendant is through newspaper advertising. Wording of the ad depends upon an individual's taste and situation. Margaret Anderson, a quadriplegic from Minnesota who wanted a live-in attendant, put her ad only in the Sunday paper. She notes that advertising just 1 day is cheaper and brings as much response as running an ad all week. In her ad the top line is intriguingly worded: "Unusual Opportunity, Unique Job, Interesting

Change." The next lines are "No exp. Take care and keep home for active polio woman. Own room, TV, weekends off. Write particulars Box No."

Margaret says, "By letters you can tell a lot about a person. I pick first choice and write duties and salary, and tell them to come and try it out for 1 or 2 days. I can tell in a day if they will work out. Then I ask them to stay a few weeks. If they like the job, it is theirs." Margaret's rate of payment is $220/month.

Barbara Carter of California keeps her ad simple: "HOUSEKEEPER live-in 5½ days. Small happy home. Se habla español. 363-0000." This standard ad was arrived at after much trial and error. Barbara's disability is not mentioned because she does not want professional nurses or aides to reply. She feels these people are unwilling to do housework and would consider her a patient instead of a person. Details of her disability are avoided as much as possible on the phone, and she tries to project a voice image of a lively, vigorous, well person who just happens to be unable to walk. She automatically screens out those who are married, have children under 18 years of age even if living with a grandmother or other relative, and those who have to travel more than an hour by bus or half an hour by car on weekends. The Carters pay $40/week with regular raises.

Newspaper ads draw all types of people. Checking references is helpful to some extent, but should not be relied on completely. In many instances those who have had few or undesirable references have made satisfactory attendants, and others with high recommendations have failed in the role. This is true also of people referred by employment agencies. The main reason for this is the personal nature of an attendant position. An attendant is usually working with only one other person or within a family structure. If the relationship is good, there are fewer job problems than in a situation with several impersonal personalities. If the relationship is not good, a dozen excellent references from former employers will not make it better.

Social service agencies can be a source of attendants. Public assistance agencies, vocational rehabilitation services, Salvation Army, senior citizens groups, Catholic Charities, Jewish Vocational Service, mental health and retardation, and dozens of other organizations have contact with possible attendants. Many of the disabled find help through word of mouth and bulletin board notices in schools, hospitals, and churches. This writer found an efficient live-in attendant by writing letters to the pastors of several churches inquiring whether they knew of anyone wanting a live-in position. A pastor gave his letter to a college counselor who happened to know of a student looking for a job and a place to live. The student was a member of Alcoholics Anonymous and welcomed the opportunity to live in a home where drinking was not a regular part of daily life. This experience suggests that Alcoholics Anonymous is another source of possible attendant help.

The disabled individual should do his own interviewing, hiring, and firing unless he is unable to supervise his own care and the other details of his life. He is the one who must relate to the attendant and whose living problems the attendant is being hired to help. It is also a valuable psychologic asset for the person who is disabled to pay his attendant directly. This reminds the attendant for whom he is working and reinforces the employer's feeling that he is in control of his life.

The disabled who live alone with the help of attendants have to be very careful when hiring them. Some are undeclared drug addicts, alcoholics, or victims of illnesses that endanger themselves and their employers. It is wise for disabled individuals who live alone to have an emergency signaling system or friends or neighbors who will occasionally check to see if everything is harmonious during the trial work period. There are telephone recordings that, when activated, alert the local police or sheriff departments to an emergency.

DISABLED ATTENDANTS

Many of the disabled hire the disabled as attendants. There are numerous kinds of disabilities, but those with disabilities also have abilities. One disabled individual's abilities can make up for another disabled individual's disabilities. The blind can move for the disabled. The disabled can see for the blind and talk for the cerebral palsied. The mentally retarded can be the arms and legs for the disabled, and the disabled can explain to and organize for the mentally retarded. Whatever his disability, each person can help someone else in some way.

The disabled employer may have the same initial hesitancy to hire the disabled that the able-bodied employer has. There is skepticism as to whether someone with an obvious disability can handle the required work. It is only when we remember the surprise and doubt our own abilities have encountered that we become less prejudiced in considering a disabled applicant for attendant.

PHYSICALLY DISABLED ATTENDANTS

To draw again from personal experience, one of my most competent attendants, Phyllis Koch, was a woman with cerebral palsy. My paralysis from respiratory polio is severe; I cannot breathe without respiratory equipment or use my hands and arms. I can stand with help, although one leg is fairly weak. Everything must be done for me. Even able-bodied attendants sometimes have difficulty getting me in and out of bed or strapping on the chest respirator.

Phyllis's involvement was described as moderately severe. With great concentration and effort she could control her spasms enough to get me in and out of bed, feed and aspirate me, strap on my chest respirator and start the rope-pulled, throttle-controlled generator when the power failed. When Phyllis first began these duties, it would take her a long time to complete them. In time, she perfected them and could complete my care and housework routine as quickly as many able-bodied attendants. Once she handled a power failure completely on her own. I was on the rocking bed when the electricity went off; the bed stopped at an extreme angle. Phyllis leveled the bed by pulling on the fan belt, quickly strapped on my chest shell and hooked me up to the battery-operated respirator, set up my phone so I could call the electric company, started the generator and switched the cords from the house power to generator power.

In another emergency she performed not only competently but miraculously. One of the greatest problems Phyllis and I had was getting me in and out of bed. We were both very scared the first time we tried it. In getting me out of bed, the usual procedure was to turn my legs off the side of the bed and then in one turning and lifting movement of my upper body, missing the overhead reading rack, to stand me up. Phyllis could not bring her arms up high enough to lift very much, nor coordinate her movements to turn and lift at the same time.

The method we developed was to move my shoulders to one side and turn my legs off the bed so that I was lying horizontally across the bed. Holding my neck and shoulder, Phyllis slid me off the bed and pulled up just before my feet hit the floor. It was a precarious operation, but it worked every weekday for 3 years without mishap. It even worked one day when the odds against success were long indeed. That day my pant leg caught on the bed and I stood up on only one leg. I immediately lost my balance and, as Phyllis tried to steady me, she fell over backward. I continued to plunge toward the dresser, fully expecting to break my neck. That is when Phyllis miraculously managed to get up and stop my fall, holding me steady until our shouts brought a neighbor who released my pant leg. It might be noted that twice before able-bodied attendants had not been able to keep me from falling.

Phyllis brought a stability and dependability to my life that made it possible for me to do many things besides worry about who was going to help me. In return she received acceptance as a contributor to society, new confidence in her own abilities, social contacts, and a modest income. We each gained the other as a friend.

Attendants with physical disabilities might be located through vocational rehabilitation agencies, rehabilitation hospitals, groups and organizations for the disabled, and agencies whose purpose is to finance research and assist the victims of specific diseases, such as the Arthritis Foundation, National Easter Seal Society for Crippled Children and Adults, United Cerebral Palsy Associations, Muscular Dystrophy Associations of America, National Multiple Sclerosis Society, and American Foundation for the Blind.

MENTALLY RETARDED ATTENDANTS

Many mentally retarded individuals are well-suited for attendant positions. They are often dependable, proficient at routine work, amenable to the confinement involved with many cases, willing to follow instructions, conscientious and even-tempered. The mildly retarded are generally physically healthy and able-bodied. There is growing acceptance of their ability to help the physically disabled as more and more people in both groups attempt employment and independent living.

Robert Urie, PhD, writes in his *Rehabilitation Record* article on "Retarded Attendants for the Handicapped," "It has often been pointed out that it is not generally the inability of work skills that hinders the retardate in adjusting satisfactorily in society; rather it is the lack of social skills and/or the inability to take care of all the necessary activities of daily living (*e.g.*, purchasing, budgeting, cooking, etc.)." In most attendant positions these skills would not be required.

The Evaluation and Training Center in Fargo, North Dakota is one organization that trains the mentally retarded to be attendants. The Center arranges for potential attendants to work at job stations in maid service, kitchen work, laundry, nurse's assistance and cooking classes at the Home Economics Department of North Dakota State University. "From these varied experiences the potential attendants learn the variety of tasks at independent settings. The final stage of training is provided by an individual that needs an attendant and thus the training procedure is an amalgamation of many learning experiences," explains Paul Ornberg, Director of the Training Center.

Training can be done solely by a disabled individual. All that is needed are determination, patience, and the ability to give specific instructions. This is proved by the experience of Lynne Scroggins of Kansas City who found her attendant by contacting a state school for the retarded (Fig. 6–1). After inspecting Lynne's home, the school sent her Margie, a "trainable" retarded young woman. Margie arrived alone and scared, but with Lynne, who was equally scared, she worked out a relationship that, at the time of this writing, has lasted 3½ years.

Fig. 6–1. Lynne Scroggins found her attendant, Margie, at a state school for the retarded. They have learned to help each other. (Photograph by J. J. Maloney, Kansas City Star, 1974)

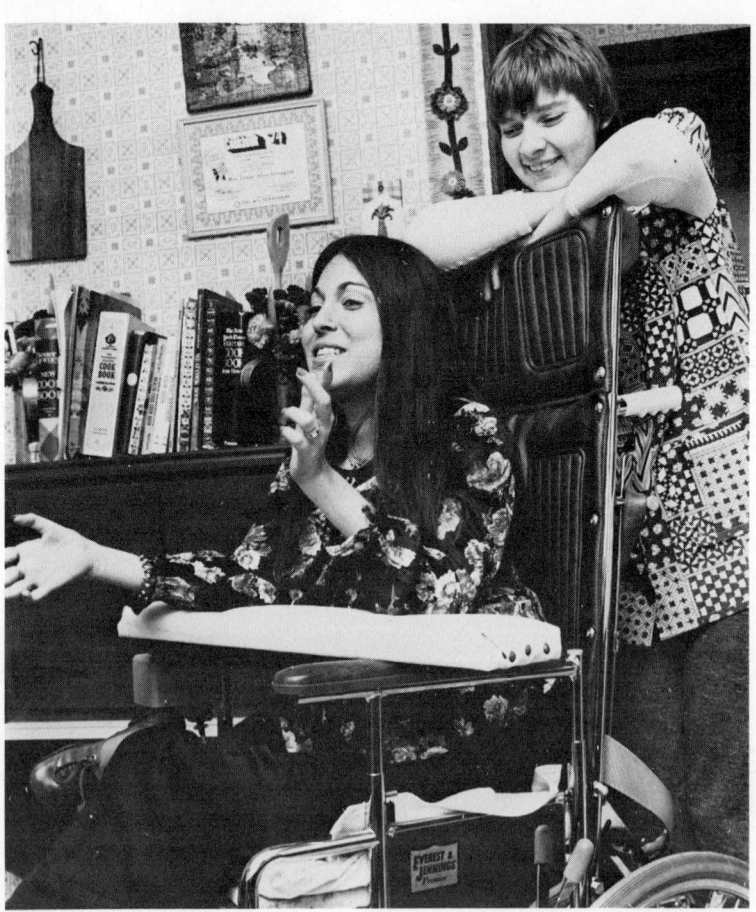

Lynne is disabled by amyotonia congenita, a form of muscular dystrophy, and needs help with all of her personal and home care. She had been in a nursing home for 6 years before she married John Scroggins. Between working and helping his wife, John became fatigued to the point of endangering his health. It was then that they decided to look for a live-in attendant.

When Margie first arrived, Lynne was worried that their relationship would not work. Margie would not talk because of her speech defect. She would not respond in any way, not even to indicate when she was hungry or had to go to the bathroom. But they both tried to help each other, and at the end of a week Margie was bathing, bedpanning, and dressing Lynne. It was not long before she learned to do the household chores and, with Lynne telling her how, to cook. They became so good a culinary team that they won a cooking contest and started cooking classes for the mentally retarded.

The relationship benefited both parties. Through Margie, Lynne had the physical means to be independent and have her person and home cared for in the way she wanted. Margie gained confidence and self-satisfaction at her new skills, and two people who loved, wanted, and needed her. Lynne says, "To put it rather coldly, I supply the brains and Margie supplies the muscle. We're a team. Between us, we make a whole person."

Lynne's comments on how she communicates with Margie may be helpful to others who work or plan to work with mentally retarded attendants. "I have to be thinking every moment. Dealing with Margie calls for extra explanations that another person wouldn't require. I have to use a lot of descriptive words. If I want a carrot or a stick of celery, I have to indicate clearly what I want because Margie gets them mixed up."

These two people are simpatico; Lynne understands Margie's disabilities and aversion to institutions, and Margie has compassion for Lynne's limitations. Margie never complains no matter how many requests Lynne makes.

Persons seeking mentally retarded attendants might contact vocational rehabilitation agencies, organizations, as well as city, county, and state schools for the retarded and high school counselors who work with educable mentally retarded students.

EMOTIONALLY DISABLED ATTENDANTS

Emotional disability is defined here as chemically or emotionally caused distortions in perception and behavior control. Many persons who are emotionally disabled are not in institutions. They can function well enough on their own or with drugs to handle the necessary demands of living. There are various categories of emotional disability, but no matter what the diagnosis, persons affected have trouble finding and keeping jobs.

Many of the emotionally disabled apply for attendant positions. They do so for a variety of reasons. Some cannot find other jobs, some feel that only someone else with a disability will understand and accept them, and some, if it is a live-in job, want a change from their home environment and someone with whom to relate. The employer–attendant relationship is the important variable upon which job success rests.

The most difficult emotional states in an attendant for a disabled individual to cope with are anger and hostility, withdrawal, anxiety and paranoia, and confusion and unreality. It depends on the personality and emotional health of the employer whether he can accept the emotional problems of his attendant. Equally important is whether the attendant can adapt to the confinement, routine, and disabilities of his employer.

Ben Meads of New South Wales, Australia has as his attendant a man with schizophrenia and an extreme anxiety neurosis. Disabled by a very rare disease, dermatomyositis, Ben needs help with all his daily activities. To provide this help he and his wife, Kath (who is also disabled), share their home with Jim, whom they met in the sheltered workshop complex where all three worked.

Jim has his own room and television set. In return for his room and board and acceptance by the Meads, Jim does all of Ben's personal care and gets him into the wheelchair and car every day. Upon specific request he will do other chores such as mowing the lawn and taking out the garbage. He has little initiative and undertakes few tasks on his own.

Ben recommends this arrangement to other disabled individuals. He and Kath would not be able to afford an attendant who worked only for money, and they know it is difficult to find a person who needs a place to live who would also make a suitable attendant. Jim fits into their life better than might a student who would want to go out often or a divorced or unwed mother whose children would present more challenges and adjustments for the Meads. Ben feels he can direct his own life and decide such things as when he will go to bed without the objections that might be forthcoming from a helper who had many competing interests.

There are certain extra expenses involved in the Meads' living arrangements, however. They are remodeling their house to include an extra kitchen for Jim's use, even though Kath will continue to prepare his evening meal. These alterations will cost about $2000 but are made necessary by the stress involved in sharing a kitchen with someone who doesn't have the motivation to keep things neat. Rather than complain and risk jeopardizing the peace of their home, the Meads decided the solution was a new kitchen.

The chief emotional expense is the sharing of their life with someone who needs to be constantly reassured that he is doing his work well and that he is well-liked, wanted, and needed. Ben considers that this is a price worth paying for reliable help and the opportunity of living outside an institution.

Possible attendants might be found at vocational rehabilitation agencies, rehabilitation and mental health hospitals, and halfway houses.

MORMON ATTENDANTS

Young men of the Church of Jesus Christ of Latter Day Saints, commonly referred to as the Mormon Church, are asked to give 2 years to missionary work. They usually go away from their home area and are not allowed to work or earn money.

Their efforts are to go solely toward informing others of their religious doctrine. Consequently, these young men have to live economically. They generally live with a family and pay little or nothing for room and board. This is an ideal arrangement for the disabled who need attendant care.

Ruth Davis, a respiratory polio quadriplegic in Cleveland, Ohio needed an attendant while her husband was at work nights (Fig. 6–2). She slept with a chest respirator, and there was the danger of power or equipment failure, fire, or other emergency. The Davises decided the best answer to their problem was to have someone share their home for a minimal fee in exchange for night attendance. They put an ad in the paper and found two young Mormons who were willing to try the arrangement.

The result was a living situation that was helpful to everyone. Most Mormon missionaries travel in pairs, and when the term of one was up, another was sent

Fig. 6–2. Keeping in touch with friends by telephone is an independent operation for Ruth Davis, who has a phone dial and switch mounted on her footboard. Ruth has found Mormon missionaries dependable and helpful as attendants.

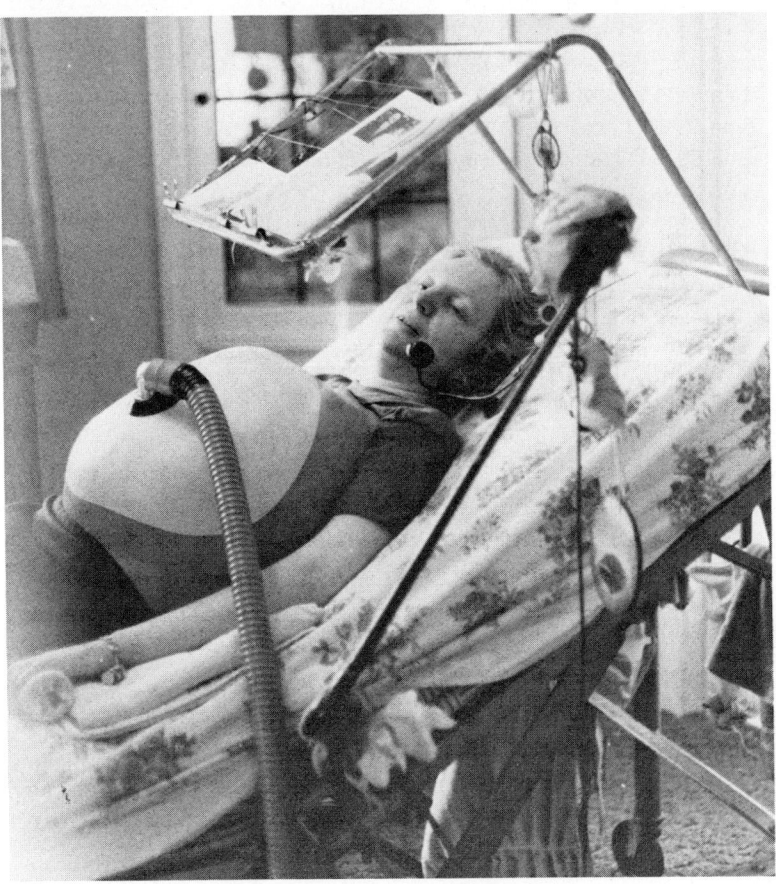

to take his place. The one who was left at the Davises would show the replacement what was to be done. Their services to Ruth were night attendance by at least one of the men, putting on and removing her chest respirator as needed, and transporting her to the doctor, dentist or other appointments.

The attendants paid a percentage of the light, water, and heat expense based on the percentage of the house's floor space contained in their room. They put in their own telephone because it was instrumental to their missionary work. After about 3 years Mormon missionaries were no longer sent to the Cleveland area, but the Davises continued having two male roomers as night attendants.

Sometimes young Mormon women also work as missionaries. Inquiry can be made as to whether Mormon men or women are working in a certain area anywhere in the world by writing to The Church of Jesus Christ of Latter Day Saints Mission, Salt Lake City, Utah 84100.

STUDENT ATTENDANTS

High school and college students provide a large and variegated pool of attendants. Young people are usually alert, easily trained, capable, adaptable, lively, and fun to have around. They can also be restless, undependable, emotionally dependent, and unskilled in homemaking tasks such as cooking, cleaning, and even bed making. Many will work for little compensation and some for room and board. Students can be contacted through school counselors, bulletin boards in stores, laundromats and youth centers, school or community newspapers, and churches.

Jean Vien, a quadriplegic who lives in Minnesota, is a homemaker who needs help only for bathrooming, bathing, and getting ready for bed when her husband is not home. The other chores she does herself. She prepares meals, does the laundry and ironing, washes dishes, and mops the floor. Her needs are simple but vital, and she finds the best attendants are high school girls who come in during their lunch hour and two evenings a week when her husband is away from home (Fig. 6-3).

Jean's attendant arranges her classes so that a study period is scheduled next to her lunch hour. This allows the student an hour and a half to walk the six blocks to the Viens', take Jean to the bathroom, have lunch, and walk back to school. When the weather is cold, Jean pays her attendant's cab fare. If the girl prefers to walk even when it's cold, Jean gives her money equivalent to the cab fare. The other recompense is lunch and $6.25/week.

Two nights a week when Jean's husband is away, her attendant comes about 5 P.M. and takes Jean to the bathroom. A Hoyer lift is used for all transferring. The attendant then leaves and returns when convenient for her. On one of these nights Jean has a bath. In the morning the attendant gets Jean out of bed, bathrooms and dresses her, a process that takes about 45 min. Payment for this night–morning service is $4, breakfast, and favorite snacking foods during the evening. The attendant's total income is about $57/month.

Jean's fringe benefits to her attendants are nightgowns, tennis shoes, clothes, or gifts such as plane fare to a special event. She and the girls who help her have

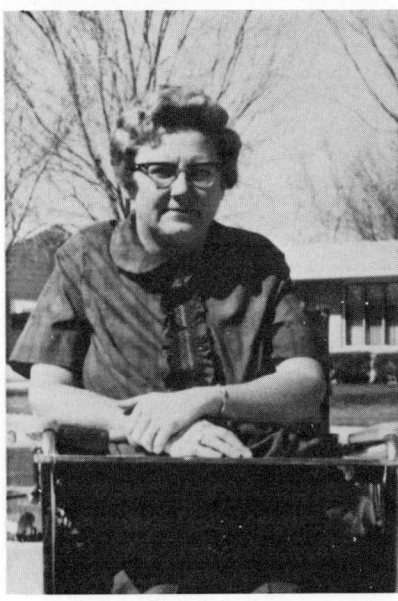

Fig. 6–3. Jean Vien has developed close relationships with the high school girls who have taken care of her attendant needs. She has found them to be kind and good company.

a mutual concern for each other. Most of her attendants stay an average of 3 years, starting in the ninth grade and continuing until they graduate.

Jean writes, "We used to go nearly crazy looking for new girls, but the past several years the girls have watched and waited until they spotted the 'right' girl to take their place. By the time they have been here so long, they are concerned and want to get just the girl that will take care of me, be kind, and be good company for me. This has been much more satisfactory in all ways."

ALIEN ATTENDANTS

Applications for alien workers are often rejected. Federal minimum wage scales pertain to applicants, and many of the disabled cannot afford these rates, some have imported aliens under false declaration of wages or purpose. Yet even those who can afford the minimum or higher rates cannot easily get government clearance.

One of the major assets of attendants from other countries is their positive attitude toward domestic work. It does not have the low status in many countries that it does in the United States. A primary disadvantage is the likelihood of a language difference between employer and employee. Bridging the gap can be either impossible or enriching and enlightening.

The procedure for applying for an alien attendant is first to know of a person willing to take the job. The next step is for the employer to prove to the local state employment agency that he is unable to find someone already in the country to fill the position. The employment counselor reviews the employer's income and the salary he intends to pay the alien, then sends it on for approval to the regional office of the Department of Labor. If the request is approved, a certified job order is sent to the United States Immigration and Naturalization Service. This agency sends forms to the employer that request information as to how many hours the employee will work, what his duties will be, hourly and weekly wages, how many hours allowed away from the employer's premises, previous work experience in the same area of work as that being applied for, and so on.

Some employers have had personality clashes or other problems with their alien attendants after they arrive. The usual solution is to help the attendant find another job. Two-weeks notice is required of both parties if either decides to terminate employment.

A quadriplegic woman, who shall remain anonymous, lives with her husband and two illegal Mexican aliens. One alien works as her attendant during the week and the other on weekends. The one who works during the week, who shall be referred to as #1, does the personal care of her employer and all the household chores. On her free afternoon time between 1 P.M. and 4 P.M., she does housework for neighbors. This brings her an extra $10–$12 weekly to add to her salary of $60. She has Saturday afternoon and Sunday off one week and Sunday afternoon and Monday off the next. Her starting salary 4 years earlier was $40/week.

Attendant #1 shares a room with Attendant #2. Attendant #2 does housework in other homes 35–48 hours a week and relieves Attendant #1 on her days off. She receives free room and board. Fortunately, the attendants are compatible. They work out arrangements for holiday coverage between themselves.

This disabled individual suggests that others hiring aliens practice close and constant supervision at the beginning of their employ. She says, "Some are unfamiliar with our tools, such as kitchen equipment and electrical appliances. Simplify equipment and routine. If you plan to use Hispanic help, learn how to speak Spanish. Chances are you have had more education than your helper and it will therefore be easier for you to learn. Besides, if your helper learns English, she will probably leave for a better paying job."

She continues, "Some problems might arise if your attendant is a country girl or from a poor family. She might sleep in her clothes on top of the bedcover, go barefoot, or not use a knife and fork. A kind explanation, patience, and time will take care of these problems. Also, if the girl is separated, divorced, widowed, or an unmarried mother, it is wise to have a frank talk about birth control as soon as it becomes necessary, for instance, when a male 'cousin' appears on the scene."

FOSTER FAMILY ATTENDANTS

The disabled who do not have their own home or a family member to live with, sometimes contract to live with a foster family. Arrangements are different in each case. Some families provide room, board, and personal care for a certain monthly sum. Others offer room and board, or simply a room, and the disabled individual hires attendants for personal care and other duties. Details of payment, service, and privileges are worked out between the involved parties. Both benefit, with the foster family receiving a regular income and the disabled individual a noninstitutional place to live.

Jack Prial of Baltimore, Maryland, found his foster family through a social worker. The family converted their dining room into a room for Jack. It is large enough for his electric bed, a large stereophonic record player, a television, books, and tapes. "I don't have to wheel to the bathroom to shave, comb my hair, or brush my teeth. Everything's in my room," says this contented lodger.

Jack is a C5–6 quadriplegic as a result of an automobile accident when he was in college. He was in a custodial hospital many years before he decided to start living an active, interested life again. Since February, 1973, he has been working as assistant public information officer at the Maryland Rehabilitation Center. He has now added to his responsibilities and income by becoming librarian at the Center. Before he could start his job as librarian, however, Jack had to find a place to live because residents were not allowed on the Center payroll. After searching for months, he found his foster family.

In return for room, board, and personal care, Jack pays his family $350/month. The wife of the couple acts as his attendant. Jack's personal care requires 1 hour in the morning and ½ hour at night. Two days a week he hires an attendant for morning care, and the husband of the couple or an attendant does his night care. Medicaid covers the fees for the relief attendants, and Jack pays for his other expenses from his salary and Social Security checks.

On the joys of being out of a hospital, Jack says, "I don't have to subjugate my daily routine to that of an institution. I wake up at 10 A.M. to breakfast in bed, wash up, get dressed, and am out of bed by 11 A.M. My cab driver picks me up at 11:30 A.M. I work from 1 P.M. to 9 P.M. and return home about 9:30 P.M. Then I read, listen to tapes, talk with the family, and go to bed about 10:15 P.M. There I eat a sandwich, read some more, listen to music or watch a late movie, and go to sleep about 1:30 or 2 A.M."

Of the family he lives with, Jack says, "Their financial subsistence depends on me. Without me, their standard of living is lower. This makes our relationship (which is really good) symbiotic. I need them, but they also need me."

Persons interested in trying foster family living might contact social service agencies, public assistance departments, or churches, or try newspaper advertising.

CONCLUSION

How a person with a disability arranges his attendant care depends upon his own situation, personality, goals, and resources. There are many people willing to help him. The more people he learns to work with successfully, the more freedom and independence he will have.

Ruby Heine, a quadriplegic since 1949, lives alone with attendants, and she observes,

Only through other people have I been able to survive out of a hospital. You can learn to have enough confidence in yourself and how to take care of yourself so that you can take a stranger off the street at a moment's notice and calmly, intelligently explain to that person how to take care of you in the rocking bed and pneumobelt, how to fold the wheelchair, and how to get you in and out of bed. You will feel like you're taking care of yourself through other people's hands. This way you will be able to let them go, to illness, old age, death, other interests, and still be able to function.

Bibliography

Retarded Attendants for the Handicapped. By Robert M. Urie, PhD and Donn Brolin, PhD. REHABILITATION RECORD, pages 12–14, September–October, 1973.

"Nobody should stay in an institution if his social or medical problems can be solved in other ways. . . . Lodgings can be provided, furniture can be bought, and home help can be found. Thus the individual's independence, a very precious thing in human existence, is saved—and always at a lower price than institutional care."

—*Margareta Nordstrom, Royal Social Welfare Board of Sweden*

7
Organized Home Services

HOME HELP SERVICES

In the old days of established neighborhoods, of large households in which there lived several generations, and of inexpensive domestic help, the family and the neighbors provided the services that cushioned illness and disability. When these helping hands disappeared with the current mobility, urbanization, and smaller families, governments and voluntary organizations all over the world had to develop organized home help services to replace them.

The International Council of Home Help Services defines home help as follows: "Home help is the aid rendered to the family under competent direction by persons qualified to undertake household and family tasks in instances of illness, childbirth, overly large families, chronic illness, old age, or other social problems." Typical of the dimensions of these services is the following description of England's part-time arrangements by the Hon. E. Carnegie–Arbuthnott, OBE, President of the International Council: "We are apt, with older people, to send the home help in two or three times a day. She will arrive at eight in the morning to help with washing and bathing, change bed linen and get breakfast. She (or another home help in the district) will come in to give the noon meal, or it may be delivered. She may come in to fix a cup of afternoon tea and again in the evening to get the evening meal or get the person to bed."

EUROPEAN HOME HELP PROGRAMS

Home help programs in Europe have a much longer history than those in the United States. Systematic social security has been a fact in most European countries since the nineteenth century. Home care has been an important part of European social institutions because of the Europeans' essential belief in the right of the individual to protection of his personal self in his own family environment in times of stress, crisis, or failing vigor.

In the early days the services were primarily directed at child care and the preservation of family life. As the large family all but disappeared and the population of the elderly and the chronically disabled increased, the need for home health services broadened. European governments became increasingly involved in home help services through legislation, training, standardization, supervision, and financing or subsidy. Now home help programs are considered essential. In

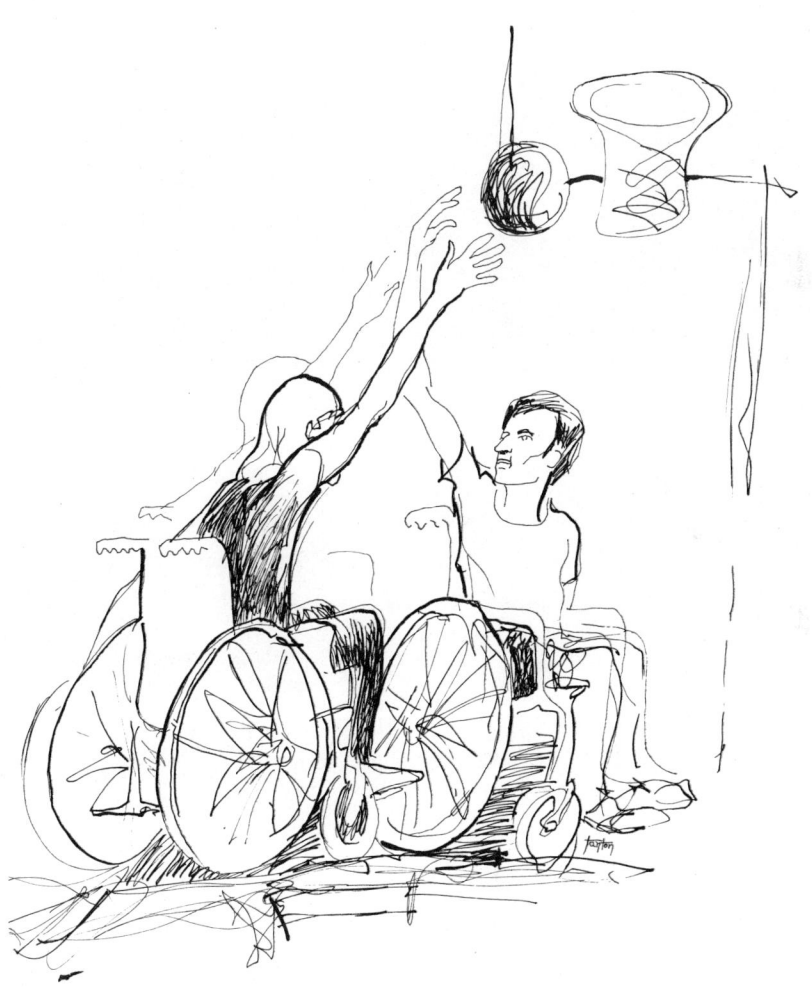

most countries, workers who are employed in the programs are respected and well-trained, and the field is generally regarded as one which is vocationally interesting and worth entering.

Sweden

The family aid (home help) services in Sweden have been in existence since 1920. Originally offered by the Red Cross and other private organizations, the Swedish services were taken over by the local authorities in 1943. The full-time aides are given extensive training in boarding schools to prepare them to handle a broad range of care in the home: caring for children, maintenance of the home, care of aged persons, cooking, and household management. In addition, married women are given brief courses in working with the aged and the long-term disabled as "family Samaritans" for several hours a day or a few hours a week; when necessary, 24-hour service is provided.

Other European Countries

Belgium's home help services were originally provided by religious orders; later they were subsidized by the government. Training is provided in accredited home help training centers. Finland, Denmark, and Norway have similar programs; Denmark pays family members to work at home and care for their disabled. The home help organization in Switzerland serves both the German and French populations, both lay and religious groups. Madame Viollet created Mothers' Aid in 1920 in France. After an era of voluntary activities, home help as a profession was organized. Today it is regulated by the French Ministry of Public Health and Welfare. The Netherlands' first services were intended to provide services only to the sick; now the emphasis is on those services which will maintain or reestablish healthy patterns of family life in the home. Home helpers are subsidized by the government.

European programs in general place a great deal of emphasis on training. The longest training period is required in West Germany, which provides 2 years of training—1 year in a residential school and 1 year in supervised institutional assignments and in the field. Most of the other countries require 6 months to 1 year of training. England, which uses more mature experienced housewives, requires only 2–3 weeks of training, plus short-term practical experience in institutes. Actually, it is more sensible to use the highly trained helpers when they must replace the mother and handle the entire responsibility of managing the family and to use the less trained workers with the elderly and disabled whose requirements are highly individual and who would prefer to direct their own care.

In all the European countries, the provision of home help services is closely tied to social and psychologic considerations and to supervision by the physician and district nurse. France, Switzerland, Finland, Sweden, and Germany appear to teach their home helps to provide a combination of the services that the United States public health nurses provide and/or teach family members to provide. England, Denmark, and The Netherlands appear to provide services that more closely parallel the United States definition of "personal care."

Home helps in all European programs are expected to perform those household tasks which are a part of the normal homemaker's routine. Heavy emphasis is placed upon those services which protect and increase the quality of family life and which instruct families in methods intended to achieve these objectives. The services include cooking, baking, shopping, cleaning, taking care of the children, laundry, ironing, mending, and personal care. In rural areas, they may also include preserving, canning, drawing water, fetching wood, and shoveling snow.

FINANCING THE EUROPEAN PROGRAMS

Although there are provisions for financial participation of the family in almost all programs, the ability of the family to pay for services is not an important element in any European program. If the programs are built into the social insurance system, anyone who is in need of the service may receive it, the cost being absorbed by state and local funding (England and the Scandinavian programs). In other countries the services are funded through combinations of government subsidy, private funds, and selected insurance benefits (France, Germany, Belgium, Holland, and Switzerland).

In England, Denmark, Sweden, Norway, and Finland legislation requires that home help services be established in local communities. The Ministry of Health and the local health authority are responsible for the English program. Funds are made available from the National Health Service Budget to each local health authority for the cost of the home health service. This pattern is followed in the Scandinavian countries, except that the Ministries of Social Affairs are responsible for services.

France, Belgium, The Netherlands, and West Germany have somewhat different patterns. France has a combination of government and religious and voluntary programs grouped in a national committee or Federation of Home Help Associations. In The Netherlands and Belgium the programs are administered by private organizations, most of them religious, with government subsidies. In West Germany, local governments and insurance benefits provide funds for home help services with some family payments (of which only 1% are full fee). In Switzerland, the Ministry of Health and Welfare regulates training, and the various cantons differ in their methods of funding services. Some are voluntary; some, completely public. Public subsidies are provided when the services are administered by private agencies.

England

Each local authority health service is required to supply the following supports for the aged: chiropody service, meals on wheels, home help service, occupational therapy, recuperative holidays, residential homes for mental health, home nursing, health visiting, ambulance service, day centers and clubs, and residential accommodation.

The present English comprehensive service system for disabled individuals is mandated by the Chronically Sick and Disabled Persons Act of 1970. Details of the services in the Act are included in the chapter on Great Britain. The emphasis of the Act is on providing services that help people to take a full part as members of their families and their communities, avoiding wherever possible the need for residential care and separation from family.

Canada

In Canada organized home care programs mobilize the resources of a large number of voluntary agencies and provide coordinated rehabilitation services that include medical and nursing care, physiotherapy, and related services to individuals in their own homes. Services are financed by government grants and private philanthropy. Included among the services are the provision of wheelchairs, meals on wheels, functional aids, prosthetic devices, homemaker and meal preparation services, assistance in mobility, day-care and drop-in centers, and travel programs.

The largest voluntary health organization, the Canadian Red Cross Society, operates some 22 programs, including home nursing and homemaker services. The Victorian Order of Nurses provides services to over 100,000 people annually through 16 coordinated home care programs located in all provinces except Prince Edward Island and serves as the principal home nursing service in urban areas. Specialized agencies, such as the Canadian Paraplegic Association, provide counseling, equipment, home adaptations, and the coordination of whatever services are necessary to the particular type of disability.

HOME CARE SERVICES IN THE UNITED STATES

The history of homemaker-home health aide services in the United States has been singularly marked by contradiction and paradox. As a culture, we profess unusual interest in the integrity of family life. Yet, for many decades, we have chosen institutional paths for our young, our dependent, our sick, and our aged: paths which stress separation and which undermine security. Unlike other Western cultures, there has been surprisingly little interest in the United States in the development of in-home services as an alternative to institutional care.

The above was written by Brahna Trager in 1973 in *Homemaker/Home Health Aide Services in the United States.* The situation has not actually changed much since then, though there is hope in recent legislation.

The first organized home care program in the United States, started at Boston Dispensary in 1796, had the following objectives:

1. The sick, without being pained by separation from their families, may be attended and relieved in their own houses.
2. The sick can, in this way, be assisted at a less expense to the public than in any hospital.
3. Those who have seen better days, may be comforted without being humiliated; and all the poor receive the benefits of charity, the more refined as it is the more secret.

The first visiting housekeeper programs in the United States were developed in the early 1900s by private charitable family agencies for the care of young children whose mothers were ill. Emphasis on child care, as the primary purpose of organized services, continued into the 1950s, although passing references were made to service for adults—particularly older persons with physical disabilities who might be able to remain in their own homes if supportive in-home services were provided. The enactment of the Kerr–Mills legislation providing medical assistance to the aged and, finally, the passage of Titles XVIII and XIX of the Social Security Act (Medicare and Medicaid) stressed the public responsibility for the health of persons over 65 and for financially dependent persons of all ages. These factors stimulated both the extension of homemaker services to adults in established programs and the development of new programs directed primarily to services for adults.

With the development of services to adults, the question of whether to provide personal care and housekeeping became a major issue. In 1968, the United States Public Health Service sponsored a 2-day workshop to clarify and resolve the issues; the representatives of the organizations attending adopted the principles that 1) homemaker-home health aides are a part of an array of services for care of patients in the home, 2) their training should include preparation for assuming the duties of both homemaking and personal care, and 3) professional supervision is basic to the delivery of their services.

In addition to homemaker-home health aide services, the most frequently provided services are professional nursing, professional social service, and physical and occupational therapy. Some agencies also offer speech therapy and nutrition services, and a few offer meals on wheels. The European "blitz clean" or mobile janitorial services are not provided in the United States. Equipment and transportation are rarely provided.

MEDICARE

This federal program of health insurance pays for the major portions of hospital care, physician's services, and care for a limited time in a skilled nursing facility or at home. In addition to those 65 and over, disabled people who have received social security disability benefits for at least 2 years and persons under social security who need dialysis or a kidney transplant became eligible after July, 1973. The home health care benefits cover up to 100 home health visits per year or per benefit period. They must be prescribed by a physician and furnished by an approved home health agency. This agency may be public or private and must specialize in giving skilled nursing services or other therapeutic services, such as physical therapy or speech therapy in the home. Other health service may include occupational therapy, medical social services, the use of medical supplies and medical appliances, and the part-time or intermittent services of home health aides. Home health aides may help the patient bathe and shampoo, go to the bathroom, get in and out of bed, exercise, and take self-administered medications ordered by the physician. Conversely, a patient who does not require intermittent skilled nursing, physical therapy, or speech therapy cannot qualify to have payment made under the program for any health services furnished.

MEDICAID

This federal/state program covers medical care to certain categories of persons entitled to public assistance under the Social Security Act. States may administer their own programs or may contract with private organizations for assistance in administering their programs. In addition, states determine Supplemental Security Income (SSI) criteria for Medicaid eligibility. Home health care agencies qualified to participate in Medicare home health care benefits program are qualified for participation in Medicaid. Any person eligible for skilled nursing home services, and for whom home health services are prescribed by a physician, is eligible to receive home health care. Medicaid home health services include, but are not limited to, nursing services on a part-time or intermittent basis, home health aide services, medical supplies, equipment, and appliances.

The Medicaid home health care benefits differ from Medicare benefits in that a person need not require skilled nursing care or physical or speech therapy to be eligible. Also, they do not provide for medical social services.

LIMITATIONS OF MEDICARE AND MEDICAID

Relative to Medicare and Medicaid, the November 1974 report prepared by the Subcommittee on Long-Term Care of the Special Committee on Aging of the United States Senate concludes,

While home health care is authorized under both Medicare and Medicaid, expenditures for home health care constitute less than 1 per cent of either program. Why? Under Medicare, benefits are limited to a narrow and restrictive definition of 'skilled nursing.' Under Medicaid, few states have made more than a token effort to make these services available.... One result of this failure is that the United States does not take advantage of the significant cost savings inherent in a viable home health program. Some 2.5 million seniors are without necessary care, which could postpone or prevent institutionalization if provided in a timely fashion. Moreover, it could allow elderly persons to live independently, in their own homes, where most would prefer to remain.

In considering this Senate report on aging, one should add "and the disabled" wherever the word "aging" is used because Medicare includes those on disability benefits for 2 years and Medicaid includes those on SSI according to the state's criteria. Though the lifestyles of older and younger persons may differ in many areas, their needs are similar in the areas of home care services, housing, and transportation. Neither group can afford the home health care needed. Neither group has its problems solved by Medicare or Medicaid: Medicare is limited by the word "skilled," and Medicaid is limited by the willingness of the states to participate. For instance, a May, 1974 report by HEW on the 1972 expenditures points out that the U.S. spent far less than 1% of Medicare's total outlay on home health expenditures. Medicaid coverage for Oregon included payments for only

12 people, totaling $3392; Missouri paid $4637 to 36 recipients; while the state of New York spent $15.5 million to cover 33,000 recipients (more than half of the total spent in the entire country).

SENATOR MOSS' SUGGESTIONS FOR REFORM

This Senate report on aging concludes with a letter from Senator Frank E. Moss, Chairman, Subcommittee on Long-Term Care, to the Chairman, House Ways and Means Committee. Dated August 15, 1974, the letter recommends that the long-term care needs of older Americans be considered in the National Health Insurance bill. In the letter Senator Moss makes the following suggestions for reform:

The American Association of Retired Persons, National Retired Teachers Association, and other senior citizen groups are unanimous that long-term care should be provided to all older Americans and not just to the poor. They are unanimous that Medicare should be the vehicle for extended long-term care coverage. Recognition of this fact was the most favorable aspect of Title II of the Kennedy–Mills bill, S.3286. The goal can be accomplished as follows:

1. Liberalize the definition of Medicare's nursing home coverage beyond "skilled nursing."
2. Include intermediate care as a covered service.
3. Liberalize the home health benefit beyond "skilled nursing," removing the word "skilled" or authorizing coverage for other levels of nursing, *i.e.,* "non-skilled" or "preventive."
4. Day care should be authorized as an optional substitute for some or all of the authorized home health visits presently offered.
5. Preferably, coinsurance amounts should be eliminated.
6. Funding should be from general revenues rather than further increases in regressive Social Security payroll taxes.
7. A residual Medicaid program would absorb premiums for the poor as well as providing the remaining four mandatory services, physician's care, x ray and lab services, hospital care and mental health care, as well as other voluntary services.
8) There should be some tie-in with the Areawide Agencies on Aging authorized under the Older Americans Act, which have been given the various areas of our states. Perhaps senior citizens centers could be established as screening centers in which the medical and social needs of the elderly could be assessed and then matched with medical services under agencies participating in Medicare or with services under Title III of the Older Americans Act.

LEGISLATION

Social Services Amendments of 1974: P.L. 93–647

This significant legislation amends the Social Security Act by adding a new Title XX to establish a program of federal aid to the states for social services. It was signed into law on January 4, 1975 and became effective on October 1, 1975. The new law calls for the states to provide at least one service in each of the following goal areas, except in the case of SSI recipients for whom at least three types of services must be provided:

1. achieving or maintaining economic self-support to prevent, reduce, or eliminate dependency
2. achieving or maintaining self-sufficiency, including reduction or prevention of dependency
3. preventing or remedying neglect, abuse, or exploitation of children and adults unable to protect their own interests, or preserving, rehabilitating, or reuniting families
4. preventing or reducing inappropriate institutional care by providing for community-based care, home-based care, or other forms of less intensive care
5. securing referral or admission for institutional care when other forms of care are not appropriate, or providing services to individuals in institutions

Services that are directed at these goals include, but are not limited to, child care services, protective services for children and adults, services for children and adults in foster care, services related to the management and maintenance of the home, day care services for adults, transportation services, training and related services, employment services, information, referral, and counseling services, the preparation and delivery of meals, health support services and appropriate combinations of services designed to meet the special needs of children, the aged, the mentally retarded, the blind, the emotionally disturbed, the physically handicapped, and alcoholics and drug addicts.

The federal government will pay 75% of the costs of services, up to the state's allocated ceiling, and 90% of family planning services. Title XX is planned both to ensure that the most needy have priority and to reach a wider range of economic levels than previous legislation. At least 50% of the expenditures must be made to persons who are eligible for SSI, state supplemental payments, Aid to Families with Dependent Children, or Medicaid. The states have the option of providing services to those whose incomes are between 80%–115% of the state's median income for families, adjusted to family size, if a fee related to income is charged; the services may be provided without charge to those with incomes below 80%.

One of the most important provisions of the legislation is the requirement that the states publish their comprehensive service plans at least 90 days prior to submitting them to HEW for approval. This mandates involvement by the public in the planning of the programs.

Social Services '75. A Citizen's Handbook is a pocket-sized 27-page guide to Title XX which is free from Social and Rehabilitation Service, U. S. Department of Health, Education, and Welfare, Washington, D.C. 20201. Request (SRS) 75–23038. It includes a summary of the services included in the program, public participation, allotments by state, median incomes by state, and a citizen's calendar.

NATIONAL COUNCIL FOR HOMEMAKER-HOME HEALTH AIDE SERVICES, INC.

The National Council, 67 Irving Place, 6th Floor, New York, New York 10003, is a nonprofit, tax-exempt membership organization, established in 1962 by the National Health Council and the National Social Welfare Assembly. It is composed of 256 agencies which employ and pay homemaker-home health aides, 297 individuals, and 155 organizations. Members include visiting nurse associations, public welfare agencies, voluntary social service agencies, family service associations, county welfare departments, and county health departments in the United States and Canada.

In order to clarify the terminology of services, the Council redefined the following separate and distinct services:

Homemaker-home health aide services means professionally directed personal care and home management services by trained and professionally supervised homemaker-home health aides to maintain, strengthen, and safeguard the functioning of eligible persons in their own homes where no responsible person is available for this purpose. The term professionally directed means individual assessment and implementation of a plan of care.

Chore service means services in performing minor home repairs, heavy cleaning, yard and walk maintenance which eligible persons are unable to do for themselves because of frailty or other conditions and which do not require the services of a trained and supervised homemaker-home health aide or other specialist. Chore services may include such activities as: help in lawn care, periodic heavy cleaning, simple household repairs, and running errands.

Many local agencies use various types of nonprofessional in-home services to supplement the core program of homemaker-home health aide services. The National Council encourages this trend. Supplementary services are not the professional services rendered in the home but they frequently supplement such services. They are provided by paraprofessionals and/or volunteers under the aegis of a professional health or social service agency that assumes responsibility for evaluating the need for the service and is accountable for the performance of personnel and the quality of the service delivered. Supplementary services—those nonprofessional in-home services other than homemaker-home health aide services—include, but are not limited to, chore services, meals on wheels, friendly visitors, telephone reassurance, household repairs, escort service, shopping services, and transportation.

Over the years, the Council has been involved in legislation to broaden and improve the quality of home care. Membership in the organization includes a newsletter and special bulletins that are an excellent means of keeping up with the latest developments in federal legislation concerned with home care.

HOME HEALTH CARE AGENCIES

Nursing

The Visiting Nurse Association, a nationwide nonprofit organization and a certified home health agency under state and federal requirements for Medicare and Medicaid, provides professional nursing and physical therapy. Its services are provided by the hour, during weekday working hours.

Public health nurses work with city or county health departments and provide home care without charge to those who are eligible.

The Yellow Pages section of any large city's phone book lists a half dozen or more agencies under "Nurses—Licensed Practical—LPN." Most of them furnish the entire range of helpers: registered and practical nurses, housekeepers, live-in companions, substitute mothers, nurse aides, home health aides, visiting home managers, and friendly home companions. Many of these agencies are nationwide; all employees are bonded and insured. Some are not reimbursable under Medicare or Medicaid; others are covered by Medicaid but are reimbursable under Medicare only if ordered through a certified home health agency such as a Visiting Nurse Association or a physician. Each agency has a different set of rules and charges for the specific type of service offered; some have a minimum of 3 or 5 hours, others work on 8-hour shifts only.

Church-Sponsored Respite Care Programs

Home Care Services for the Handicapped, Inc, St. John's Parish House at Lafayette Square, 1525 H Street, N.W., Washington, D.C. 20005 offers respite care through the the Outreach Committee of the parish. Care consists of innovative services for children that could be copied for all ages. Registered aides, motivated by a desire to serve, are screened individuals who are trained by specialists to handle behavior and medical problems of retarded as well as disabled children. The registrar makes every effort to match the registered aide to the child and the family. Parents are encouraged to preregister their needs rather than wait until the need for service arises. The fees are quite reasonable and may be arranged for periods of 3–24 hours and for weekends. Transportation is provided by parents or paid by the parents on a mileage or carfare basis.

Red Cross Home Aides Training Course

The St. Louis Bi-State Chapter, American Red Cross, 4050 Lindell Boulevard, St. Louis, Missouri 63108 has developed an instructor training course to teach men and women to train youths and adults to become home aides for the mentally and physically disabled. The course was developed by Mrs. Marcia Bregman, RN, author of *Assisting the Health Team: An Introduction for the Nurse Assistant.* Mrs. Bregman developed the course with the assistance of the United Cerebral Palsy Association and the St. Louis Association for Retarded Children. Following training, instructors organize community classes and teach a 10–12 hour course. Those who complete the course are certified as Home Aides for the Handicapped and are placed on lists at the agencies which service the disabled. Parents who need aides for respite care use the lists and employ the aides directly. The instructor training course includes basic first aid and home nursing skills. The course covers transfer techniques, safety in the home, feeding and assisting on various levels of need, and communicating with the families of the disabled.

Occupational Therapists' Home Service Programs

Independent Living for the Elderly, a project developed out of a neighborhood center in Madison, Wisconsin, was conceived by and is carried out by occupational therapists with funding from the Older Americans Act and United Way. It consists of three components: 1) adult education—12 class sessions on problem areas such as self-care from a wheelchair, living one-handed, housekeeping with sight limitations, and solving the problems of living with arthritis; 2) home consultation by an occupational therapist—evaluation as to safety and efficiency, referrals to needed services such as mobile meals, visiting nurse, homemaker help, or other services, prescribing equipment such as grab bars, shower seats, reachers, or kitchen aids; and 3) transportation to supermarkets and shopping centers, doctors, and other essential trips provided by volunteer drivers.

Although 95%–97% of the elderly live in the community, the therapists found that lack of transportation kept them from participating in the community around them. Another major need, information about services and equipment, was met by their courses and home visits. In addition, the therapists arranged with the public library to have special displays of building plans and kitchen and bathroom adaptations. The project, described in detail in the May–June 1973 issue of *The American Journal of Occupational Therapy* demonstrated that occupational therapy possesses a special expertise which, when made available to the community, can help the elderly (and disabled) live a more normal life.

Another interesting occupational therapists' homebound program was created at the Northwest Institute in Seattle, Washington. The program, planned to follow through on hospital treatment, had the following objectives: provide adapted equipment, interpret the disabled person's needs to the family, loan equipment for trial, and provide a telephone consultant service. The Institute equipped a van with a hydraulic lift, drill press, saw, and a sewing machine. The therapist could thus sew canvas and leather and could alter and repair equipment as needed.

Home Economists' Home Service Program

According to Professor Lois O. Schwab of the College of Home Economics, University of Nebraska-Lincoln, home economists are being trained to assess a disabled individual's capability for training and employment. Following assessment, training in independent living is given in a special facility or at home. If the individual's home requires adapting or remodeling, the home economist is trained to advise and supervise. The home economists are also taught counseling and learning procedures for serving the disabled, the blind, and the mentally retarded and emotionally disturbed.

Oklahoma's Unique Home Care Program

The 1970 changes in Title XIX (Medicaid) resulted in a creative program in Oklahoma. Its authorization for federal financial participation is found in the Code of Federal Regulations, February 1, 1970, 249.10 (b) (15) (vii) which states that payments can be made for "personal care services in a recipient's home rendered by an individual, not a member of the family, who is qualified to provide such services, where the services are prescribed by a physician in accordance with a plan of treatment and supervised by a registered nurse." The home care service is available for both the categorically needy and the medically needy. In every instance, the care must be recommended by the disabled individual's attending physician and authorized by the state agency's Medical Evaluation Unit.

The program in Oklahoma was developed by Lloyd E. Rader (Director, Institutions, Social and Rehabilitative Services, P.O. Box 25352, Oklahoma City, Oklahoma 73125) with the assistance of the Oklahoma State Nurses Association. The state supervisor of the program, Dora J. Stohl, RN, is a retired member of the Army Nurse Corps. The program furnishes care to more than 3200 disabled individuals in their own homes (Fig. 7–1). Without this service, the majority of these individuals would have been placed in nursing homes at a cost of $410/month. Instead, services are brought to them at home for an average monthly cost of $139.05 ($118.48 cost per recipient, $20.57 administrative cost).

The state is divided into six districts; in each district there is a registered nurse district supervisor, and an assistant, plus one or more registered nurses. There are

Fig. 7–1. Under Oklahoma's unique home care program, Nannie White is cared for in her own home by Willie Seldon, who has been trained to be a provider of services.

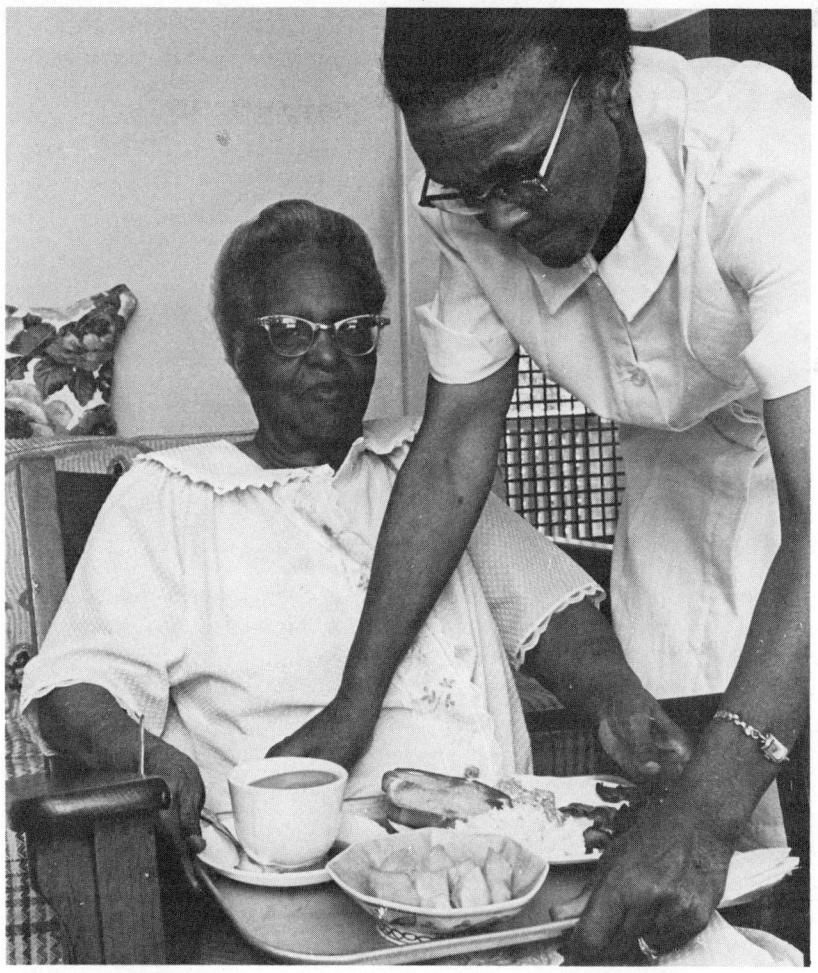

50 registered nurses and 10 licensed practical nurses who supervise 2383 attendants or "Providers" who provide the services in the homes. Each provider receives 20 hours of instruction, either a Red Cross Home Nursing Course or individual lessons. Their age range is from 15 years to over 75; about half of them are 45–65. They work from 1–12 hours/day; some live in the homes of the disabled individuals. The daily rate of vendor payment for care of one person in a home is $5.31. A new ruling makes it possible for some relatives to be providers. Any relative except a parent, son, daughter, son-in-law, or daughter-in-law, if he or she is living in the home only in order to care for the relative, may be an approved provider. A few mentally retarded persons, who can learn the simple tasks needed to care for some recipients, have proven to be very dependable workers.

The nurses who are involved in the training and supervision of the providers work out of the county welfare offices, as do the case workers from whom they receive their referrals and with whom they collaborate closely. They also work closely with the local physicians. They make home visits on a routine basis, visiting individuals receiving the home care services at least once every 3 months.

The 250-page manual for providers, *Handbook for Non-Technical Medical Care Aides,* by nurses of the Oklahoma Department of Institutions, Social and Rehabilitation Services, is available from L. E. Rader, the director. Written and illustrated in a clear and direct style, it covers every phase of homemaking, food, care of the bedfast or chairfast person, elimination, temperature and pulse taking, and home emergencies. An imaginative chapter covers homemade equipment such as using cardboard boxes to make a bed table, a tray, a foot support, a bedpan holder, or a back rest.

Additional information on the program appears in the article by Dora J. Stohl, RN, "Preserving Home Life for the Disabled," in the *American Journal of Nursing* of September, 1972.

Personal Care Organization, a "Model" Plan

The Levinson Gerontological Policy Institute, The Florence Heller Graduate School for Advanced Studies in Social Welfare, Brandeis University, Waltham, Massachusetts 02154 has developed a model plan for helping the aged and disabled to continue living independently within the community. The plan calls for a Personal Care Organization (PCO) which would assume responsibility for providing whatever service, or mix of services, are needed by disabled individuals in order to stay out of expensive 24-hour care institutions or hospitals. According to the model, the mix of services is tailored to the individual's specific needs— housing, transportation, house chores, shopping, personal grooming, whatever— and is available for indefinite periods of time. Varying combinations of family, neighbor, volunteer, and paid staff would be involved, depending on individual circumstances or need. A "case manager" would make arrangements and subcontract for services as necessary. The Institute envisions Medicaid or insurance companies negotiating contracts with PCOs, just as they do now with hospitals or nursing homes.

The PCO concept assumes that for the functionally disabled individual, personal maintenance is a basic requirement which deserves attention apart from other health or social service needs. The PCO will make personal maintenance its central concern and offer those services even in the absence of other service needs. Most fundamentally, PCOs are intended as an alternative to institutional care for persons with serious but not extreme functional disabilities and with limited need for professional medical attention. Although a PCO may be launched as an entirely new agency, it is perhaps more likely that it will be developed as an adjunct to an existing agency concerned with the elderly, disabled, or chronically ill.

It seems likely that the PCO will hire its own staff of nonprofessional home helpers who will form the core of the service. It is possible that specialized jobs like heavy housecleaning or home remodeling will be subcontracted. Either the PCO or a subcontractor will recruit, train, and supervise those persons who provide the practical helping services. In some cases, the PCO may choose to hire a member of the disabled person's family to provide basic services. The PCO will probably make extensive use of persons available for no more than 2–4 hours of work per day. In addition, many part-time personal care workers will be able to work close to home by serving disabled persons living in their own residential areas.

The "case planner" will work with the disabled person and his family in negotiating the level of funding through third party payments and will play something of an advocacy role by maintaining continuing contact. Volunteer services will be organized to assist with expressive or recreational activities.

In its basic form, the PCO is designed to assist the disabled person in making use of available programs in other sectors without itself assuming direct responsibility for those programs. The PCO, for example, might help the disabled person find suitable housing, with the rent to be furnished primarily through an income maintenance allowance.

State and City Information Centers

In New Jersey, Statewide Computerized Referral Information Program (SCRIP) is the product of the New Jersey Committee for the Developmentally Disabled, a coalition of six private, nonprofit agencies serving those disabled by mental retardation, epilepsy, cerebral palsy, and physical and learning disabilities. The SCRIP concept was developed out of the need for information on services, treatment, and facilities—including explicit knowledge of treatment facilities, locations, and availability of government services. With federal (HEW/DDSA) and matching funds, SCRIP was established in 1973. As of June 1974, the data base contained 1055 facilities, providing some 40 types of services for disabled individuals. The system is primarily a tool for the social workers of the four agencies in which computer terminals are located.

In Alabama, the University of Alabama (Mrs. Catherine Beasley, EdD, Office of Independent Study, Division of Continuing Education, P.O. Box 2967, University, Alabama 35486) provides a unique information service to disabled Alabama homemakers and the professionals who work with them. The service began in

1971 as a 14-part videotape series. After the tapes had been aired twice on both the Alabama and Georgia Educational Television networks the accompanying news sheet evolved into a 4-page monthly newsletter. The newsletter now has a circulation of 9213, including 1500 Alabama homemakers and professionals in 47 states and 5 countries. Bound and indexed yearly issues are available at a cost of $2 for the 1971 volume and $1 each for the 1972, 1973, and 1974 volumes. The project is a direct and subtle means of providing professional assistance to disabled homemakers. The subjects cover every phase of independent living, including homemaking and gardening hints for the blind, child care, clothing adaptations, family life, hints for retirement, resource material, and work simplification.

In New York City, Eunice Fiorito, director of the Mayor's Office for the Handicapped, has initiated an information and referral center for disabled New Yorkers who have questions concerning their rights or problems such as discrimination, housing, SSI, and Medicaid. The center, located at 61 Chambers Street, is staffed with experienced case workers who will offer assistance or advice. The center is open weekdays from 9 A.M. to 5 P.M. It is convenient to all subways and is accessible to wheelchairs. The telephone number is (212) 349–5205.

In Philadelphia, Bonnie Gellman is Director of Services of the newly formed Mayor's Office for the Handicapped (Room 428, City Hall Annex, Philadelphia, Pennsylvania 19107). The program has three divisions: 1) the Employment Program for Handicapped People has been a part of the city government for several years; it endeavors to find employment for the disabled in city government and private industry; 2) the Research Division develops data about the disabled population, keeps track of relevant legislation, and studies fund-raising sources; and 3) the Services Division serves an advocacy role, acting as an ombudsman for the disabled to ensure that all city agencies are responding to the needs of the disabled and keeping the community informed of their needs. In the near future, a Mayor's Advisory Council for the Handicapped will be appointed to make recommendations and supply information to the city government.

HOME SERVICE PROGRAMS OF VOLUNTARY ORGANIZATIONS

The National Center for Voluntary Action, 1785 Massachusetts Avenue N.W., Washington, D.C. 20036, a clearinghouse of information about ongoing volunteer activities, furnishes specific information on nationwide volunteer programs listed with the Center. Many of these programs are concerned with the home care of the disabled and elderly under the following categories: information and referral services, transportation, telephone reassurance services, meals on wheels, and recreational and social programs. The Center will provide free information sheets on programs in any of these categories, giving details and the name, address, and phone number of the person to contact, In addition, each information sheet contains a description of the program, how it began, how it operates, the general cost of operation, its goals and accomplishments, the number of volunteers, the kinds of work they do, and the training and supervision of volunteers.

MISCELLANEOUS SERVICES

In Maryland the Department of Medical Social Work of the Baltimore City Hospitals has developed a foster home type of alternative to nursing homes, known as "community care homes." The homes provide three levels of home nursing care, and the homeowner is paid accordingly. The homes are visited regularly by public health nurses, visiting nurses, and medical social workers.

Community Chronicare Centers, which would provide a broad range of health services for the chronically ill and disabled, have been proposed by the American Nursing Home Association.

Supported by local, state, and federal governments and supplemented by private donations, the National Institute of Senior Centers was organized by the National Council on the Aging, 1818 L Street, N.W., Washington, D.C. 20036. More than 4000 senior centers are operated in the United States under the sponsorship of churches, synagogues, clubs, and nonprofit corporations.

Home Health in Chinatown, a delightful 32-page booklet, describes the development of homemaker-home health aide services in San Francisco's Chinatown area. Under the leadership of a bilingual social worker and a bilingual nurse the language and cultural barriers are overcome and hundreds of elderly people are provided with much needed home services. The program, directed by the San Francisco Home Health Service, was effected through the cooperation of Self Help for the Elderly, a Chinese organization, and the Chinese Hospital.

A Resource Guide for the Disabled of Massachusetts is a comprehensive guide published by the Massachusetts Association of Paraplegics, Inc. A model that should be copied by every state, it includes information on housing that is accessible, as well as on transportation, service organizations, equipment, employment, travel, sports, and legal and tax information.

TALKING BOOKS

The Library of Congress will loan a free record player and send free recorded books and magazines to the blind and to the disabled who have problems turning pages because of relatively useless hands. The recordings cover a wide variety of subject matter, including Medicare and social security. Catering to all ages and many disabilities, the talking books are available in Spanish, German, Yiddish, and French. Of particular interest to the disabled is *ENCORE,* a bimonthly recording of selections from *Accent on Living, Paraplegia News, Performance,* and *Rehabilitation Gazette.* For further information, contact local libraries or write: Division for the Blind and Physically Handicapped, Library of Congress, Washington, D.C. 20540.

VACATION RESIDENTIAL EXCHANGE

HEW has started a new 10-day vacation program for senior citizens to give those who have limited incomes the therapeutic experience of a vacation in a new environment. In May, 1975, about 20 elderly persons in high rise apartments in

Denver exchanged apartments with 20 persons in similar circumstances from Minneapolis. HEW paid the air fare; the individuals paid $20 for insurance and took care of any personal expenses. In Minneapolis, the housing authority collected several thousand dollars from businesses and agencies to provide special activities for the Denver guests. At about the same time, the housing authority of Portland, Oregon, made arrangements for 20 senior citizens to exchange apartments with others from Sacramento, California. Seattle and Las Vegas groups made similar exchanges. HEW plans to develop the program on a nationwide basis.

Other home services that are being provided or tried around the country are 1) home maintenance, 2) purchase and installation of special equipment, 3) psychologic therapy and counseling, 4) interpreter services, 5) reader services, 6) nutritional services, 7) speech pathology and audiology, 8) sports programs, 9) spiritual counseling, 10) peer counseling, 11) recreational therapy, 12) wheelchair repair, and 13) physical therapy, including mobility training.

TRAVELING DEMONSTRATIONS

For many years, Sweden operated a bus with a specially equipped kitchen which traveled throughout the country demonstrating the possibilities of adaptive equipment. The Nebraska Cooperative Extension Service crisscrossed the state with a bus which functioned as a teaching and demonstration mobile unit until it wore out the bus. In addition to the model kitchen and bathroom in which the homemakers could see and try out new ideas, homemakers were given information on diets, care of children by disabled mothers, cleaning, and family care. In addition, clothes were displayed in the closets to show how clothing can be adapted to make dressing easier. For a time Nebraska had two buses, one for homemakers, the other for research projects and training students in the field of homemaker rehabilitation.

The St. Louis Hearing and Speech Center has been operating a 30 ft custom-built van as a mobile vision, speech, and hearing testing unit for the past 7 years. It is equipped with a waiting area, an explanation area, audiometers, and a sound room that weighs 12,000 lb. The van covers school age children daily and all ages in the surrounding communities three times a month. The technician driver and three volunteers staff the unit.

The May, 1975, issue of *HUD Challenge* reports that the Colorado Division of Services for the Aging is financing a 45-passenger bus which has been converted for use as a grocery store. The mobile store makes ten stops a week in low income neighborhoods and housing projects. A police escort protects elderly customers against possible attack by vandals.

Bibliography

Canada

THE FEDERAL MEDICAL CARE PROGRAM. Questions and Answers. Published by Health and Welfare Canada, Health Insurance Directorate, Health Programs Branch. 1974.

Great Britain

CHRONICALLY SICK AND DISABLED PERSONS ACT 1970. Chapter 44. London. Her Majesty's Stationery Office. 1970.

United States

ASSISTING THE HEALTH TEAM: AN INTRODUCTION FOR THE NURSE ASSISTANT. By Marcia S. Bregman, RN. $6.50 St. Louis, The C. V. Mosby Co., 11830 Westline Industrial, St. Louis, Missouri 63141. 1974.

HANDBOOK FOR NON-TECHNICAL MEDICAL CARE AIDES. Request from L. E. Rader, Director, Institutions, Social and Rehabilitative Services, P.O. Box 25352, Oklahoma City, Oklahoma 73125.

Home Care Programs. By Cecil G. Sheps MD, MPH, and Jack Kasten, MPH. REHABILITATION LITERATURE, Vol. 23, No. 5, pages 130–135, May, 1962.

HOME CARE PROGRAMS. With Special Reference to Hospital Based Programs. Selected References 1960–1967. Medical and General Reference Library, Department of Medicine and Surgery, Washington, D.C. October, 1968.

HOME CARE SERVICES OF THE CHRONICALLY ILL AND AGED. Selected Annotated Bibliography. Compiled by Mabel I. Edwards. 1967. Order from Institute of Gerontology, University of Iowa, Iowa City, Iowa 52240.

HOME HEALTH CARE BENEFITS UNDER MEDICARE AND MEDICAID. Report to the Congress by the Comptroller General of the U.S. 1974. Order #B-164031(3)from U.S. General Accounting Office, Room 6417, 441 G Street, N.W., Washington, D.C. 20548. $1.

HOME HEALTH IN CHINATOWN. Bureau of Community Health Services. Health Services Administration, HEW, Washington, D.C. U.S. Government Printing Office Washington, D.C. 20402. 1973. 50¢

HOME HEALTH SERVICES IN THE UNITED STATES: A WORKING PAPER ON CURRENT STATUS. A Summary of Proceedings from a Conference: "In-Home Services. Toward a National Policy." Prepared by the Special Committee on Aging United States Senate. Washington, D.C. 1973. Order from U.S. Government Printing Office, Washington, D.C. 20402. 50¢.

HOMEMAKER/HOME HEALTH AIDE SERVICES IN THE UNITED STATES. By Brahna Trager. Bureau of Community Health Services, Health Services Administration, Public Health Service, HEW, Washington, D.C. 1973. Order from U.S. Government Printing Office, Washington, D.C. 20402. $4.70.

Independent Living for the Elderly. By Betty R. Hasselkus, OTR, and Jean M. Kiernat, OTR. AMERICAN JOURNAL OF OCCUPATIONAL THERAPY, Vol. 27, No. 4, pages 181–188, May–June 1973.

NATIONAL HEALTH SYSTEMS IN EIGHT COUNTRIES. The health care systems of Australia, Canada, Federal Republic of Germany, France, the Netherlands, New Zealand, Sweden, and the United Kingdom. By Joseph G. Simanis. Office of Research and Statistics, Social Security Administration, HEW. 107 pages. Order from Superintendent of Documents, U.S. Government Printing Office, Washington, D.C. 20402. DHEW Publication No. (SSA) 75-11924. $1.80. 1975.

NURSING HOME CARE IN THE UNITED STATES: FAILURE IN PUBLIC POLICY. Prepared by the Subcommittee on Long-Term Care of the Special Committee on Aging, United States Senate. Washington, D.C. U.S. Government Printing Office, Washington, D.C. 20402. November, 1974. $1.85.

Occupational Therapist in Home Health. By Ellen Dunleavey. AMERICAN JOURNAL OF OCCUPATIONAL THERAPY, Vol. 28, No. 8, pages 484–487. September, 1974.

THE PERSONAL CARE ORGANIZATION: AN APPROACH TO THE MAINTENANCE OF THE

DISABLED IN THE COMMUNITY. By Francis G. Caro. 1973. Order from Brandeis University, Waltham, Massachusetts 02154.

Preserving Home Life for the Disabled, By Dora J. Stohl, RN, AMERICAN JOURNAL OF NURSING, Vol. 72, No. 9, pages 1645–1650, September, 1972.

PROCEEDINGS OF THE INTERNATIONAL CONGRESS ON HOME HELP SERVICES. Held in Paris, September 1962. English translation. Washington, D.C. U.S. Government Printing Office, Washington, D.C. 20402. 1965. 30¢.

A RESOURCE GUIDE FOR THE DISABLED OF MASSACHUSETTS. Request from Massachusetts Association of Paraplegics, Inc., P.O. Box 48, Bedford, Massachusetts 01730.

SOCIAL SERVICES '75. A CITIZEN'S HANDBOOK. Program Options and Public Participation Under Title XX of the Social Security Act. Free from Social and Rehabilitation Service, U.S. Department of Health, Education, and Welfare, Washington, D.C. 20201. Request (SRS) 75-23038. May, 1975.

"The time has come for disabled persons to participate more fully in the making of decisions affecting their lives. The needs of disabled Americans must be articulated by disabled Americans in a coherent and well-thought-out manner."

—Eunice Fiorito, President, American Coalition of Citizens with Disabilities

8
California Attendant Programs

Why does California have more recently developed experiments in independent living arrangements by and for physically disabled than any other state? The answer is simple: money in hand from state allowances for attendant care and the new federal-state Supplementary Security Income/State Supplemental Payment (SSI/SSP), plus community information services. Of course, many severely disabled are still unnecessarily in convalescent homes and hospitals, but the combination of attendant care and SSI/SSP has made it possible for many to leave institutions and achieve independent living in home situations of their choice with supportive services. This growing spirit of independence is further fostered by The Center in Independent Living, a unique comprehensive community information service created and directed by physically disabled and blind persons, and by a number of other advocacy groups of disabled persons.

Before tracing the developments that resulted in attendant care allowances, consider the present funding available to a severely disabled person in California with limited income.

1. Social Security disability payments are available nationwide for those who have earned sufficient credits from employment.
2. Supplementary Security Income (SSI) is a nationwide program that is available to anyone with limited income and assets who is over 65, blind, or disabled, without regard to past work history. The basic amount, which is correlated to the cost of living, is currently $157.50 for one person and $236.60 for a couple if both members are eligible. This federal program, started in January, 1974, replaces federal-state public assistance payments and is run by the Social Security Administration.
3. State Supplemental Payments (SSP) are made by California, among other states, to supplement SSI and bring its payments up to the previous level of public assistance payments. Currently, the SSI/SSP payment amounts to $292 for a blind person, $259 for a qualifying disabled or elderly person, and $488 for a married couple, if both are eligible. (This arithmetic discourages marriage.)
4. A recipient of SSI/SSP is eligible for Medi-Cal.
5. If there are no cooking facilities, an additional sum of $29/month per person for restaurant meals is available.
6. Homemaker/Chore Service is the most important service for severely disabled individuals.

For all the other services, eligibility for SSI/SSP is necessary. For attendant care service, one may have too much income for SSI/SSP, but not enough income to cover all the costs of attendant care; in that event, the state will pay a reasonable additional amount to meet the amount required for an attendant. The payments range from around $150 to a maximum of $505/month for those who are so severely disabled that they require 20 hours of care a week; the average is about $300. Most importantly, receiving any amount of care monies qualifies one for Medi-Cal.

The Homemaker/Chore Service (H/C) is also critical to less severely disabled persons, such as the elderly, blind, or ambulatory disabled. For these recipients, H/C can provide essential transportation, laundry, shopping, housecleaning, and cooking of major meals.

The Homemaker/Chore Service (Welfare and Institutions Code, Sec. 12303 and 12304) has two classifications of attendant care. Homemakers are provided for those who are unable to supervise their own care or define their own needs; chore service provides care for those who are competent to direct and supervise their personal needs.

Attendants are not required to be state employees, and most counties make direct cash payments to the recipients. The law states specifically that any severely disabled recipient has the right to receive a cash payment in advance for his attendants. The disabled individual then hires, fires, and pays his attendants directly. It is interesting that counties will not let a recipient pay much more than the minimum wage, but will pay much more to homemaking agencies ($4.-50–$6.55 an hour).

Both of these recently enacted services, which evolved from H.R.1 (1972. P.L. 92-603; 1973. California A. B. 134), are replacements for the attendant care legislation that had been in effect since the poliomyelitis epidemic days of 1957. Currently, the state pays 25% of the program's cost and the federal government pays 75%; however, budgetary problems of the counties may eventually necessitate more federal government participation. Utopia is not at hand, of course, and the advocacy groups have fought and worried through many crises when it was feared the program might be dropped, attendants assigned without any individual selection, or the funds curtailed. Nevertheless, SSI/SSP, Chore Service, and Medi-Cal now add up to enough support so that severely disabled individuals have begun to extricate themselves from institutions and to start living independently.

RANCHO LOS AMIGOS HOSPITAL HOME CARE PLAN

California's present attendant care program had its origins back in March, 1953, when a very successful home care plan was developed by Rancho Los Amigos Hospital, 7601 East Imperial Highway, Downey, California 90242, for 158 quadriplegic poliomyelitis persons using respiratory equipment. The plan was effected because the county realized that these patients were unnecessarily occupying $37/day hospital beds when they could be cared for at home with trained attendants and supportive services for $10/day.

Basically, the Home Care Plan was defined as the theoretical annexation of the patient's home to the hospital. The patient remained a patient of the hospital and all hospital services needed were provided, including occupational and physical therapy, social service, drugs, medicines, dental care, clinical lab, x ray, and respiratory equipment. Because county tax money was the principal resource for financing the Home Care Plan, admission to the program was limited to Los Angeles County residents. Per diem rates were calculated and bills rendered on the same basis as inpatients. After an amendment to a Los Angeles County ordinance governing the indebtedness for medical care, this patient group was billed only according to their "current ability to pay."

One of the most creative aspects of the Home Care Plan was the hospital's cooperation with the patient's own community physician. The patient's personal physician was placed on a Polio Physician's Panel, giving him status with the hospital and making available the hospital staff for consultation on a 24-hour basis. The physician filled out forms that served both as reports and invoices of all house calls. Transportation was always ready to return the patient to the hospital for any special clinics, such as orthopedic or ENT.

Most of the patients required attendant/housekeeping help beyond that which could be provided by families. The recommendation for hours needed was made by the Home Care staff. The attendant/housekeepers were selected by the family and, though they were paid by county warrant, they were not county employees. Training was provided by the hospital nursing instruction staff; nonprofessional persons trained in the care of a particular patient were found to be most satisfactory.

Medical Social Service worked out financial and other social problems with the patient and his family, encouraging the use of community agencies and making plans to attain the greatest degree of independence possible. Physical therapists were recruited from the community or paid overtime by the hospital to provide treatments in the home and to instruct the family in physical therapy maintenance programs. Occupational therapists provided and trained the patients in the use of assistive and adaptive devices.

Most of the respiratory equipment provided for home service was owned by the hospital; inpatient equipment was owned by the National Foundation—March of Dimes. Depending on need, the equipment furnished included cuirass respirators (chestpieces), tank respirators (iron lungs), rocking beds, suction machines (aspirators), and autostart generators. Minimum physical standards for the home, such as generator wattage, width of doorways, and support of flooring were established. A preventive maintenance check and service of all equipment was provided once a month and emergency service was available 24 hours/day. A repair truck, large enough to hold an iron lung or rocking bed, was equipped with a hoist; on-the-spot repairs could be handled with the truck's workbench and supply of repair parts.

The Polio Panel Physician was given special prescription forms which allowed the prescription to be filled at a contract pharmacy and billed to the hospital. The more common drugs, medicines, and nursing supplies were dispensed by the hospital's pharmacy and central supply via messenger service.

Arrangements were made with Public Health Nursing agencies to provide skilled nursing supervision. Monthly reports of visits were requested and became part of the hospital record.

Discharge planning was started as far in advance as possible and included consultations and psychologic counseling with the patients and their families. Vocational counseling was given to help determine a feasible vocational plan. An indication of the patient's needs at home was made by the medical, orthopedic, ventilation, physical therapy, occupational therapy, and nursing departments. Trial visits over weekends prepared the patient and his family for the final move. To ease the way, the Home Care Nurse and maintenance man accompanied the patient home on the day of discharge, and the patient was usually met by the Public Health Nurse.

According to an evaluation dated January, 1958, the results of the program were significantly successful for the 158 patients whose care at home would have been extremely difficult, if not impossible without such a home care plan. The Home Care staff increased from 9 to 19 persons, but in spite of the increased staffing, the Home Care Plan remained very economical. Fifteen patients without homes were carried as home care patients in contract sanitariums. Sanitariums were also used for short-term placement when families needed rest periods or went on vacation.

The Home Care Plan represented a significant savings to the taxpayer. The inpatient per diem of the late 1950s was $37.87, and the cost of the Home Care Plan was $10.80/day. This represented a savings of $27.07/day. The inpatient per diem at Rancho Los Amigos Hospital in the mid-1970s is $175; attendant care under Chore Service still averages about $10/day.

In addition to the actual savings, there were many other benefits. Most important, of course, the patients became people again in their own homes and resumed their roles in the family and in the community. Later, the program was expanded to include other severe disabilities.

1975 FOOTNOTE

Seventeen years later, Rancho Los Amigos Hospital is still showing its concern for 57 of its former poliomyelitis patients living in Los Angeles County. In the spring of 1975, Rancho Home Health Service assumed the responsibility for managing their Dial-A-Ride program and for certifying eligibility for a supplemental payment from revenue sharing funds of $100/month which was earmarked for the use of former Rancho poliomyelitis patients who live at home and who need 7 day a week live-in care. The revenue sharing funds had been secured for this purpose through the efforts of a group of former patients. They had formed the organization, Totally Disabled Helpers Association, 315 North Sierra Vista, Monterey Park, California 91754, for the purpose of solving their transportation and attendant problems.

AN EXAMPLE OF RANCHO-PLANNED HOME CARE

The 1964 issue of the *Gazette* (then called the *Toomey j Gazette*) published the account of two young ladies severely disabled by respiratory poliomyelitis who demonstrated that two can live much more cheaply together in their own home than in a hospital. Mrs. Enid B. Callahan, Home Care Coordinator of Rancho Los Amigos Hospital, worked out every detail with the active participation of the two individuals. Both in their 20s, they had spent nearly 10 years in the hospital. One used an iron lung at night, the other used a chestpiece; they were both almost totally paralyzed. With the help of Mrs. Callahan they rented a lodgelike house with one bedroom for an attendant and a living room that was large enough for the iron lung and had an open-beamed ceiling and a huge fireplace. They comment:

We each receive a monthly check from the state, which pays for living expenses such as attendant care, rent, utilities, groceries, and transportation. We handle all of this ourselves and find it easier, financially, for two people to live together instead of separately. This living arrangement has proven to be very successful.

We employ three girls to take care of us. We prefer girls around our own ages, as we have more in common; older women tend to be "motherly." We also prefer to train the girls ourselves because we like things done our own way. The day girl works Monday through Friday from 8 A.M. to 3:30 P.M. She fixes breakfast, gets us up into our chairs, and cleans the house. The live-in girl's job is to cook supper, wash and iron the clothes, and put us to bed at night. She, of course, sleeps the same time we do and if we need anything, we just holler—sometimes in vain! The third girl works weekends from 8 A.M. Saturday until 8 A.M. Monday while the other girls are off.

THE SPASTIC CHILDREN'S FOUNDATION

Founded in 1944 as a training center for spastic children, the Spastic Children's Foundation (SCF), 1307 West 105th Street, Los Angeles, California 90044, now provides a total range of care, including residential facilities in apartments, for the physically and mentally disabled of all ages. In describing the scope of the program, Mrs. Anne Wendt, executive director, said, "People need people—especially the disabled and elderly. No one is too poor, no one is too disabled for our program. . . . Everybody is somebody."

The urban neighborhood in which the center has been located for nearly thirty years has undergone many changes, becoming completely integrated, with a wide range of ethnic groups. The center offers workshops, a thrift shop, physical and occupational therapy, speech therapy, counseling, an indoor swimming pool, recreational facilities, and dining room service. The dining room service is included for those in residential facilities as well as for 55 multihandicapped children on a 5-day program. Those in the 5-day program range in age 2–18 years and go home for weekends with their parents. The cost per person per day, including personal assistance, basic living support, recreation, and activity programs is $24. The center's range of services includes apartment-living facilities and a new facility in the suburb of Chatsworth for 48 persons who need lifetime care; eventually it will be extended to 160 in cottage type facilities.

As each child becomes an adult, he has available an appropriate "Design for Living"—a choice of lifestyles in one of four residential programs with central auxiliary services.

DEPENDENT DORMS

The 55 residents of this program are severely involved, multihandicapped adults with a wide range of mental abilities. They are housed in a two-story dorm building attached to the main facility and opened in 1967. It contains large recreation rooms, small sitting rooms, bathing areas, and nursing stations. The staff is composed of ten attendants on duty at all times, floor supervisors on each floor, an RN on duty 7 days/week with nursing aides assisting, and a full-time program coordinator. Auxiliary services at the center are available to the residents.

According to an SCF brochure,

This program is funded with Medi-Cal monies at the rate of $16.23/day. In certain cases individuals reside in the program unfunded. This program should be moving in the direction of funding through SSI monies supplemented with regional center's funds. The present license and requirements of a medical nature created by it are inappropriate due to the fact that the residents are not ill, but healthy individuals that have a physical disability. Presently, Medi-Cal monies are the only source of funds that approach the cost of care of individuals in need of complete care, programming for life style development and maintenance therapy.

SEMIDEPENDENT 6-UNIT APARTMENT HOUSE

In 1971 the 6-unit apartment house adjacent to the center was acquired for a program to give young adults the opportunity to discover their potential for independence by living in a controlled environment. Five of the two-bedroom units house 20 residents; the sixth unit is lived in by a training supervisor on 24-hour call. In addition, there is one other full-time training supervisor. They train the residents to set up and clean their own apartments, do their own washing, shopping, and caring for their clothes and personal hygiene. The highly structured program is planned as a stepping stone to more independent living, offering training in the purchase of services necessary for one's needs, i.e., food service, transportation, recreation, etc. Residents take part in the center's activities, eating all their meals in the dining room there. Cost per month per individual, including staff counseling, is $250. The program, funded through SSI monies, has been filled constantly since its opening.

SEMIINDEPENDENT LIVING

The second mortgage on 55 apartments located across the street, a half block from the center was donated in 1973. Designed as a therapeutic community with all kinds of people living together, helping each other, it includes people with developmental disabilities, staff, foster grandparents, and private citizens. The range of independence in the program is broad, but basically it offers two things to everyone living there: social interaction and staff on call for emergencies. Thirty of the units are rented to the disabled; all those in wheelchairs or on gurneys live on the first floor. All tenants connected with the Spastic Children's Foundation pay a discounted rate. Staff and nondisabled tenants must agree to act as emergency attendants to replace any attendant who does not show up. In such a situation, the disabled resident contacts the resident manager, and he locates someone to take over the responsibility.

The apartments are set up like any apartment building with a manager who provides coordination for attendant care, an assistant manager, a maintenance man, security staff, and custodial staff. The program coordinator makes sure that the needs of the residents are being met, working out problems, calling upon SCF and community resources as necessary, and coordinating special training, socialization, counseling, and environmental modifications.

The residents are quite heterogeneous: no age limits, all types of disabilities. Some go to college, some go to high school, and others work at the center's workshop or participate in its activity program. Some live alone, others with friends or attendants; some are married. They manage their lives as they wish, with whatever assistance they may need from the center. They may cook their own meals or eat at the center. A residents' council meets regularly and makes all group policy decisions.

The one-bedroom apartments rent for $115/month and the two-bedroom for $135. Those who move from the residence at the center go off Medi-Cal when they leave and go on Supplemental Security Income (SSI) which, with the state's portion, (SSP), amounts to $259/month; in addition, each one has $33 spending money. If an attendant is needed, the state's attendant allowance is usually an additional $350/month. Finding attendants has been no problem; the center helps with both locating and training them.

When the apartments were being renovated, some adaptations for wheelchair living were made. A few bathroom doorways had to be widened and grab bars were installed in the bathrooms when needed; nothing special had to be done to the kitchens. For the resident on the gurney, a wall was knocked out between the bedroom and the living room to give him more free space.

Transportation is an integral part of the planning. The center has its own vehicle and driver; both are available day or night, whenever needed for social activities.

INDEPENDENT APARTMENTS

Several of the physically disabled adults are dispersed in apartments throughout the community but continue under the umbrella of the SCF services. They may require help only with first time situations, or they may regularly seek the help of the SCF employee who also resides in the building. The apartment dwellers may cook their own meals or go to the center for meals and activities. The understanding is that whenever SCF is needed, its services and facilities will be available; in a sense, SCF plays the role of the surrogate family.

AUXILIARY SERVICES

The auxiliary services are provided to all residents of programs operated by SCF. Any individual is eligible to purchase one or all of these services. The Social Service Department takes care of all intakes and placements. It operates as a liaison with other social workers, government agencies, and funding sources. When appropriate, it can provide counseling, parent conferences, and special evaluations.

The Therapy Department is licensed as an inpatient and outpatient clinic. It has a staff of registered physical therapists, occupational therapists, speech therapists, and psychologists. This department is considered a separate vendor for Medi-Cal reimbursement. Besides individual and group prescriptive therapy, the department operates programs in movement, recreation, swimming and special events such as the annual wheelchair games and special olympics.

The Activity Center has a staff composed of a director and a number of aides who coordinate resident activities such as the Resident Council for Communal Living, the newspaper, outings to special events such as concerts, dinners, wine-tasting tours, etc. The department schedules regular trips for shopping, sightseeing, and visits to libraries and schools. Classes at colleges in the area for residents are coordinated through this department, as well as continuing education classes held at the center. Classes in dance, singing, geography and money management are held regularly to meet the requests of the residents. The workshop program is operated, supervised, and manned by residents of programs of SCF. Presently it is a small workshop doing contract work. Job training programs which include not only residents of SCF, but students in the special high schools in Los Angeles, operate within SCF. Placements in outside workshops are coordinated by the Activity Department also.

The Transportation Department handles all transportation to events, shopping, clinic appointments, etc. Individual or small groups of residents may schedule transportation from the department at a minimal charge subsidized by SCF. This is to encourage residents to interact outside the immediate community.

The Spastic Children's Foundation concludes: "The people who live in these programs have developed interests and individual ways of social interaction in forms of assimilation and confrontation with society on their own. They are mature, responsible adults. The lifestyles chosen and developed by these people are their own. Our purpose is to enable this to happen."

CENTER FOR INDEPENDENT LIVING

The Center for Independent Living (CIL), 2539 Telegraph Avenue, Berkeley, California 94704 is the most effective self-help service program in the United States. It is an innovative and comprehensive program created and directed by and for persons who are severely physically disabled or blind. Dedicated to greater mobility, opportunity, and independence of those it serves, the organization offers a wide range of supportive services to a target population of 30,000 physically disabled and blind individuals in northern Alameda County.

The Center for Independent Living is not a residential center. CIL members are dispersed in homes and apartments throughout the community. Founded in 1972, every step of the center's growth demonstrates unusual creativity and sensitivity. It came into being as a logical outgrowth of the Physically Disabled Students' Program (PDSP) at the University of California's Berkeley campus. PDSP had been created in 1970 by two doctoral candidates, John Hessler, a C5-6 quadriplegic, and Ed Roberts, a respiratory poliomyelitic quadriplegic, who were then living in Cowell Hall, the student hospital, and attending the University of Berkeley.

Their successful proposal for federal monies to support the initial program of PDSP was accomplished in an innovative manner: the university set up a course called "Strategies Towards Independence of the Physically Disabled" to help with the writing. From the 3-month course came the rough draft of the proposal. The finished product was the result of the research and writing of about 20 students, both disabled and nondisabled. Three students, plus one faculty advisor, did the final writing.

During its first 3 years, the student program provided services which enabled students to live in off-campus apartments for the first time. Quadriplegics, who had been completely waited upon, learned when they lived in the community that they could do many things, such as cook their own meals, if they set up their apartments adequately. Many of them shared cooking arrangements; for instance, two or three quadriplegics hired someone to do the shopping and cooking for four or five meals a week and went to restaurants, cafes, or friends' houses for the other meals.

From its inception, the entire program was directly run by disabled students and former students, with the assistance of nondisabled volunteers. The most dramatic results of the quadriplegics sharing their knowledge concerning medicine, equipment, and supplies were in the field of preventive care: the incidence of pressure sores and urinary infections dropped to almost zero for the 78 quadriplegics living in the community and the 10 at the Cowell Residence Program. The PDSP answered inquiries, helped disabled students to be accepted in the university, gave advice about transportation, repaired wheelchairs, oriented students to the campus and the community, provided help in finding attendants and housing, and served as a meeting place and center of exchange of ideas—a subtle form of group therapy. PDSP did not provide financial aid, but information as to sources of assistance and methods of tapping them.

With the success of the student program, disabled and blind people in the area began work on a similar program geared to the needs of all the disabled in Berkeley and the adjoining communities. To determine the number of people needing services, the types of services wanted, and from what agencies these services were available, the fledgling CIL organization received a small federal planning grant. Working out of makeshift quarters, a core staff laid the groundwork for the present staff of several dozen disabled and blind persons in a conveniently located downtown Berkeley office building.

CLIENT SERVICES PROGRAM

This CIL program provides an integrated approach to meeting the needs of the blind and severely disabled. It acts as a clearinghouse for information on other agencies, both public and private, and as a source of services not otherwise available. It also provides peer group support, a vital element in enabling the disabled individual to acquire first the motivation and then the ability to achieve functional independence.

COMMUNICATIONS

One of the CIL's prime concerns is communicating the needs and options of the severely disabled and blind to the entire community. This is accomplished through lectures, articles, press releases, attendance at conferences and symposia, and special events. The communications department publishes an attractive and forthright quarterly, *The Independent*. Distributed nationally, it contains articles of interest both to the disabled and the professional personnel with whom they deal. It is a bargain at $2/year.

Two CIL radio documentaries about physical disability, titled *Stigma I* and *Stigma II*, have been broadcast over hundreds of stations in the U.S. and Canada. The first program presents frank and casual discussions of subjective reactions to disability and its effects on family, friends, and lovers; the second deals with the importance of organization by the disabled, tracing the development of the disabled community in Berkeley from a loose confederation to a tightly structured action force. Counselors have found the tapes to be invaluable teaching aids, particularly for those who are newly disabled. Tapes are available from CIL for $11.50 to counselors, hospitals, and schools and for $3 to blind and disabled individuals.

COMMUNITY ENVIRONMENT

This branch of CIL focuses on the community, its systems, facilities, and services. As a result of cooperative effort between CIL, government, and businesses, the target community is swiftly becoming a model environment which allows full access and mobility to its entire population, disabled as well as able-bodied. For example,

1. The city of Berkeley is practically barrier-free as a result of a 3-year program to install wheelchair ramps and safety measures on city streets.
2. The city of Oakland has begun a similar barrier removal program.
3. The Bay Area's rapid transit (BART) system already contains many of the safety measures which allow the disabled and blind to use it; more are being installed.
4. Building codes are being modified to increase the number of dwellings accessible to the disabled.
5. Government job classifications are being redefined to permit hiring of the disabled, and employers are being urged to help the disabled find appropriate, challenging jobs.

SUPPORTIVE SERVICES

Supportive services of CIL include

1. Counseling the families of the newly disabled with emphasis on the economic as well as psychic benefits of independence for the disabled member of the family.
2. Counseling the blind. Despite some differing needs, the CIL staff believes that only by working together can the two groups solve their common problems. The staff mobility instructor helps blind people learn to use the white cane safely and effectively. She also orients them to new neighborhoods, bus lines, and the BART transit system. The counseling staff locates good readers to help with shopping, reading mail, or personal care.
3. Attendant pool. CIL offers assistance in locating, training, financing, and managing attendants. The staff members interview prospective attendants and maintain a file of prospective attendants from which the disabled may make their own choices.
4. Housing. The search for adequate housing is unceasing and involves not only the keeping of listings but also making arrangements for home modifications.
5. Wheelchair repair. It would be impossible to overestimate the importance of the power chair to the severely disabled individual. However, it requires a skilled mechanic and someone who knows electronics to keep it going. One of CIL's most valuable services is its wheelchair repair shop where an expert mechanic fixes manual and electric wheelchairs, as well as all kinds of orthopedic aids and prosthetic devices. In addition, the repair shop installs adaptive aids such as key holders, special door handles, small ramps, and grab bars.
6. Advice and advocacy regarding rights under social welfare and health programs. CIL explains the almost incomprehensible regulations that cover public assistance and the workings of the various agencies. Acting as ombudsman, the organization is prepared to appeal any case that appears to need it.
7. Personalized counseling by peers leading to self-reliance in personal care and management of bodily function. There are no experts more familiar with the needs of the disabled, more aware of inadequacies in existing services, or more experienced in providing realistic solutions to problems than those individuals who have developed successful techniques for achieving functional independence.
8. Psychologic assistance. Early outreach and identity reinforcement, as well as crisis counseling, are available from trained psychologists on the staff. After evaluation and counseling sessions, referral is made to health and other specialized facilities as necessary.
9. Specialized medical clinic. Efforts are being made to set up a Disabled Community Health Clinic which would have active input by disabled persons and which would focus on preventive care of the problems associated with paralysis, such as skin breakdowns and urinary infections.
10. Transportation. Lift-equipped vans service the wheelchaired within the target area and provide feeder service to BART and other public transportation systems.

FUNDING

CIL has gained the support of private individuals, foundations, and government agencies. Private donations have made it possible to purchase vehicles for the transportation program as well as other equipment, and grants from the county of Alameda, the city of Berkeley, the San Francisco Foundation, and others have helped to implement programs. Some programs can be self-supporting (i.e., wheelchair repair and specialized transportation), but most will continue to be offered free to all disabled. These will have to be funded by concerned individuals and corporations and the local, state, and federal governments.

On the national level, CIL received funding in 1975 from the Rehabilitation Services Administration. The federal agency is funding CIL's research division to study the following programs with a view to implementing them nationally: 1) $125,000 for a Research and Demonstration Project, renewable for 3 or 5 years, to work with disabled individuals who have not responded to established rehabilitation practices; 2) $50,000 to train professionals in Region 9 (Hawaii, California, Nevada, and Arizona) to deal with severely disabled individuals; and 3) $50,000 to set up an IBM computer program to train and employ severely disabled individuals.

THE ALPHA PLACE

The founder and director of Alpha Place, 1024 Walnut Woods Drive, No. 1, San Jose, California 95122, W. E. "Ernie" Armstrong, has created an independent living facility for himself and about two dozen other severely disabled persons in an apartment complex that was being foreclosed at the time he began his project in 1973.

After an attack of poliomyelitis in 1929 when he was 6 years old, Ernie walked with the aid of braces and crutches. He ran an insurance and real estate business until "crutch paralysis" resulted in severed nerves in his arms and he became a dependent quadriplegic. When loss of family forced him into a convalescent hospital, he planned ways of achieving independent living for himself and the others there who were unnecessarily institutionalized. He began by returning to school, with the backing of the State Department of Vocational Rehabilitation, and obtaining a Convalescent Administrator's License. With the encouragement of the Valley Medical Center, which had considered forming a young adult residential program for years, he searched for low-cost housing developments until he found a 98-unit complex owned by interested investors. Ernie talked the investors into letting him have two first floor apartments rent-free for 4 months. He and a friend and an attendant moved in and renovated them. After becoming incorporated in September, 1973, the project gathered momentum and attracted other adventurous disabled persons.

By early 1975, Alpha Place had rented 22 apartments (some were used for the central kitchen and dining room, office, and attendants' quarters); a total of 24 severely disabled individuals were living there independently and cooperatively. The fourplex apartments consist of two apartments on the first (or ground) floor and two on the second. The disabled live on the first floors, and the attendants and five families from the community live on the second. The two first floor apartments were connected by cutting a door through coat closets; thus the four people who live in the two apartments have two kitchens, two bathrooms, two living rooms, and four bedrooms—ample space for wheelchairs and for various arrangements of living spaces, such as a quiet room for studying. The apartments are furnished with gifts from the community; they need painting, but they are carpeted. A number of the other units in the complex are still empty and direly in need of renovation.

Grab bars were installed in the bathrooms for the five or six who needed them. Since Medi-Cal will furnish equipment such as lifts and electric wheelchairs, all who really need them have lifts to use in the bathroom and electric wheelchairs. The kitchens are large and well arranged, and most of the bathroom doorways are wide enough, except for one or two where the doors had to be removed and replaced by curtains. Small ramps were built over the one step at the entrances.

Most of the residents came from convalescent hospitals or VA hospitals. Their disabilities include poliomyelitis, birth injury, mental retardation, amputation, cerebral palsy, arthritis, and spinal cord injury (40%). Many of the residents are enrolled in local colleges. There have been two marriages and a number of congenial couples arrangements.

Most of the residents receive disability benefits from social security; some receive $259 from SSI. All of the severely disabled receive the California attendant care allowance which ranges from $150–505/month, depending upon need. The apartments rent for $80/month, and food averages $155/month; each resident chips in $75/month for communal food. Ernie says it costs about $1000/month for food for the community dining room; residents may eat together in the communal dining room, take prepared food from the community kitchen to their own apartments, or cook their own meals in their apartments.

The residents pool their attendant care allowance, and Ernie hires the staff. By pooling, they can have 24-hour coverage in 8-hour shifts. The rate per hour is about $2.10. There are 14 full-time attendants; three or four work on each of the two day shifts, and one person, who sleeps there, is on call at night. Two of the attendants are students. Most of the attendants have been found through newspaper ads. The attendants do the housekeeping as well as personal care. Four of the residents own vans, and they share them with the other residents. A resident registered nurse is on duty during the day, and Medi-Cal pays a doctor to be there a half day twice a month.

Ernie and his assistant work full-time, without pay, to handle all the details of food purchasing, menu planning, attendants, transportation, maintenance, furniture scrounging, and money raising, as well as acting as surrogate parents to residents and attendants. "There are many problems," says Ernie, "greed, selfishness, ill-prepared individuals who try independent living before they are ready, overprotective parents . . . It all takes a strong person to keep on top of everything."

According to Armstrong, the arrangement would be highly practical if they could own the apartments and derive profit from the complex. They are working on proposals to get backing and on new legislation, such as the Housing and Community Development Act, which might make purchase possible. They are seeking an "angel" with $10,000 or $12,000. It costs almost $500 to bring a resident in, renovate his apartment, and set him up with furniture. Armstrong would like more staff so he could "go out and dig up projects to bring home to employ the residents. . . . We get so many referrals that we could double every 3 months if we had sufficient money; now we can only accept about one person per month."

GLASS MOUNTAIN INN, INC.

In 1968, Dorothy Gassage, severely disabled by rheumatoid arthritis, dreamed of building the ideal home and employment facility for disabled individuals. A vibrant person, she organized Glass Mountain Inn, Inc., (GMI) 3401 Del Monte Drive, #13, Anaheim, California 92804 with other disabled persons, many of whom lived in convalescent homes. Growing to a group of 145 members, they met monthly and worked for about 5 years to raise money for the dream. They bought two vans with hydraulic lifts to provide transportation to meetings, school, medical appointments, and recreation.

Gradually their focus changed and evolved toward assisting individual members to grow in self-determination and to realize their potentials. Their new goals are stated in their newsletter, *Feedback Journal:* "Members are challenged to think and act for themselves, and to explore every opportunity for education, rehabilitation, employment, and participation in the life of the community. The organization offers a source of information, strength, and moral support to the handicapped."

Meanwhile, one of the members, Jennie Rotherham, severely disabled by osteogenesis imperfecta ("brittle bones"), who had been living independently for several years with a student attendant, wanted to move nearer to college. She found a large and accessible apartment with a cooperative landlord, but it was too costly for two. One of the other GMI members, disabled by cerebral palsy, then moved in to share expenses and attendant.

Within a year, a move to independent living had been made by eight more members of the group; they came from their own homes and from convalescent homes and hospitals. Currently ten disabled, both men and women, and five attendants rent five apartments. Most of the disabled and the attendants attend college. There have been many regroupings and one marriage. A close-knit "family" has developed; they are quite supportive of each other. They share shopping trips, attendants, personal problems, and weekly barbecues. They have had both good and bad luck with attendants; at least six have quit or were fired because they were immature, unstable, lazy, or unsuitable.

New apartment members are screened carefully, trying a few weekends at one of the apartments to see if the arrangement is mutually satisfactory. The members help the newcomer locate and train an attendant and assist with the moving. Often there is a reluctance on the part of parents to let their adult child become independent, and the "old-timers" talk with the parents to reassure them. A few did not fit in; they moved away from home too soon, while they were still overwaited upon, before they were ready for so much independence, before they knew what they could and should do for themselves. There are all the usual problems of communal living, but there are committees and rules and strong group leadership.

The president of GMI and the leader of the apartment group, Jennie Rotherham, summed up their thinking.

Our discussions indicate that our goal should be oriented toward individual self-awareness, personal growth, and development. People cannot respond successfully to a program until they know and understand the self, and realize what they can do. Perhaps a housing facility is an idle dream until we begin to know ourselves and each other, until we can determine what we want in our own lives.

We must get away from the concept of institutional care. In my opinion, if GMI builds its own facility, it will prove nothing more than moving people from one institution to another. When you get any large group of people living together, you have to create rules and regulations for them to live by, and, automatically, you wind up with another institution. I think, instead, in terms of two or three disabled living in their own apartment, working toward self-help, helping each other. This would be a beneficial living environment. It would also allow for GMI's easy expansion all over the country. Small groups could be accommodated in apartments, or in large houses, with able attendants sharing in the living situation. This brings an extended advantage, too. It puts the disabled into the community, rather than isolating him.

Many laws will have to be changed, or created, before the disabled can hope to live conveniently on their own. That is why GMI needs an active legislation committee to research bills, write letters, try to encourage adequate assistance through welfare and rehabilitation agencies.

THE FARM HOUSE MOTEL

In February, 1975, the Farm House Motel, 1435 University Avenue, Riverside, California 92507, began a group living program with seven disabled persons. The motel, located on what is known as 'Motel Row', is within wheeling distance of many restaurants, about 1 mile from the University of California and Riverside City College campuses, and about 10 miles from the scheduled VA spinal cord injury research and outpatient facility in Loma Linda. The motel has 27 units, a dining room, a swimming pool, and a van with a hydraulic lift. The seven disabled individuals, three women and four men, have large single rooms. Their attendants, a married couple, have a two-room apartment with kitchenette.

The expenses for each individual for room, board, attendant care, and transportation (one of the attendants drives them in the motel van) total about $350/month. The owner, George Taylor, said that welfare pays their individual expenses, which vary according to whether they receive "chore money" attendant care of from $300–$505/month; by pooling their allowances, they pay for the attendants and the transportation.

RSVP AT RIPPLING RIVER

This 150-unit "community" for physically impaired persons is the result of the dynamic determination and resourcefulness of its founder and administrator, Mrs. Elaine Castro, whose son is cerebral palsied. The project was first conceived in

1962, when physically disabled persons of the Monterey Peninsula area and their nondisabled friends started the organization, Rehabilitation Services and Volunteers of the Peninsula (RSVP), P.O. Box 525, Carmel Valley, California 93924, to eliminate barriers to an active life for the disabled; by 1967 it had become incorporated as a nonprofit organization and the members were raising funds by operating a clipping service.

In the next few years, they found 10 acres of land in Carmel Valley with eight accommodations already on the property, plenty of room to build a big swimming pool, large dining rooms, kitchen, and physical and occupational therapy workrooms. Mrs. Castro says:

> The Good Lord certainly was on our side, as we would never have had the property if we had not been "led" to it, and the loan through Weyerhouser Mortgage Company was unheard of; they actually asked us if they could finance our project for 40 years! That, of course, helped convince HUD to insure our loan for 40 years under their 231 program. If we had known all of the problems to be encountered perhaps we would never have gone ahead. I am glad that we never lost our enthusiasm. . . . We will be able to help other organizations not to make the same mistakes and to help with some of the shortcuts we had to learn the hard way.
>
> For instance, we had endless conferences to get the state to agree to license us as an adult residential care facility and a home health agency rather than a nursing home. Our residents are not sick and do not need expensive care. Then, our problems with the architects were incredibly time-consuming, as they had no conception of our requirements and fitting them under HUD regulations. We satisfied HUD's requirements after our feasibility study showed that there were many physically impaired who needed this type of care rather than convalescent hospital care.
>
> Weyerhouser Mortgage proved its faith in us; we did not have too much trouble convincing them that our project would be a success. Our worst problems were putting our ideas and needs over to architects and raising money to pay the architects was an even bigger problem. From the very beginning our whole area has been cooperative and accepting of the project. We have a long list of local people who want to work as attendants; in addition we have two retired Army nurses who live in the valley and will help with the care; further, we will have several Licensed Vocational Nurses and a Public Health Nurse on our staff.

The current prices are $325/month for paraplegic type people who can live fairly independently with minimum services; and $350–$400/month for quadriplegic type people who need extensive assistance. The monthly charges include minimum personal assistance in bathing, dressing, eating, personal shopping, general housekeeping, tray services if authorized by a physician, laundry and a center for personal laundry, 24-hour telephone connection with the office, draperies and carpeting, three meals daily, private room and bath, physical therapy in the covered swimming pool and in the adjoining therapy room, vans for recreational transportation, protectorship services if requested, and rehabilitation counseling.

All residents are urged to join the Residents Association to participate in house government, planning social activities, and handling complaints and suggestions. The office staff will handle all financial arrangements for residents on SSI and Home Health Service.

HANDICAPPED INDEPENDENCE PROVEN (HIP)

HIP, 5333 El Cajon Boulevard, San Diego, California 92115 is a business project created by a local contractor/realtor, Harry E. Hinton, and his disabled friend, Don M. Rice, who serves as coordinator. They convert existing facilities into duplex units that include resident attendant and housekeeping staff for small groups of disabled persons.

Working together on the project since 1973, the two have ironed out the problems of ramps, door widths and handles, bathrooms, adding grab bars and showers, lifts, and other conveniences and necessities, as well as the financial arrangements and attendants. They have been so successful with the duplexes for six residents that Hinton has plans to provide similar wheelchair-accessible residences for small groups near shopping centers, colleges, and hospitals.

Hinton regards the project as good business.

The economics of handicapped housing—that is, the application of the formula "income after expenses and debt service to determine the percentable rate of return on investment" —shows disabled housing to be as good an investment as any other residential income property. There are, however, several responsibilities that must be met by the producer of disabled housing that are not required in the production of basic residential income properties. These responsibilities are as follows: 1) extensive predesign planning in terms of geographic location and configuration, 2) building plans must maximize floor and land area usage, and 3) strict adherence to building plans means full-time construction superintendence.

A fourth responsibility listed by Hinton covers willingness on the part of the landlord to become involved with the problems of his tenants beyond the usual landlord–tenant relationship.

You will be dealing with a minimum of at least two public agencies on a long-term basis —the State Department of Public Health, the agency that makes funds for independent living available to the disabled; and the County Department of Public Welfare, which administers these funds. Finally, you will assist your tenants in locating, selecting, and hiring their attendants. With respect to the attendants, you function in the dual relationship of landlord, because the full-time attendants live in and are on 24-hour call, and employer because, rather than have each of your tenants go to the trouble and expense of becoming registered with the various governmental agencies and purchasing the required employer insurances, you perform this service for them as part of your landlord function.

Don Rice, who has been quadriplegic since a 1960 automobile accident, is a non-service-connected disabled veteran. At various times he has been in a nursing home and a veterans' hospital and has shared accommodations with two other quadriplegic friends. The majority of the other five residents are university students. One is a retired businessman with a PhD in engineering psychology who had a major stroke resulting in total deafness; two are quadriplegic because of spinal cord injuries, a young woman who had been in a nursing home and a former motorcycle racer; and two are quadriplegic because of poliomyelitis, one young lady in an iron lung.

To help others in their planning, Don has made a perceptive summary of their experiences to date in the areas of costs per resident and costs for staff.

COST PER RESIDENT

Total cost per resident per month is $705. This amount is arrived at by adding $125 for room, $75 for groceries and consumables, $505 for complete care. At HIP, this leaves a typical quadriplegic college student approximately $75/month to spend for personal needs. This is more personal spending money than we would have if we were staying in any nursing home. California will allow a similar person $25. Since all of us, except one, have similar needs for a maximum number of attendant hours per month, we all pay the amount indicated above.

Following are examples of two different, but typical, HIP residents. Resident A is a quadriplegic who receives maximum disability benefits from the Social Security Administration (including SSI and SSP). The maximum amount for students is $275/month. Since the physical condition of the resident is severe, she requires from 40–50 hours/week of attendant care. This makes her eligible for the maximum amount of financial assistance allowed by the Homemaker/Chore Services. This maximum amount is $505/month. Her total income is therefore $780/month.

Resident B is also quadriplegic and qualifies for maximum disability benefits (SSI/SSP). His severe disability also requires from 40–50 hours/week of attendant care. However, this resident also receives a disability pension from the Veterans Administration of $300/month, which is deducted from the Homemaker and Chore Services allowance.

Mr. Hinton is a qualified attendant and is identified as such on the formal documents of the San Diego County Department of Public Welfare. The funds for the Homemaker/Chore Services are provided by the federal and the state levels of government. It is at the county level, however, that the responsibility lies for the administration of this program. The County Department of Public Welfare determines original eligibility, and periodically verifies continuing eligibility, for this program. At the end of each month, the department also verifies that the Homemaker/Chore Services specified for each eligible recipient have been performed. Each eligible resident at HIP then receives a check to cover the cost of the attendants' salaries. Each check is made out jointly to the resident and to Mr. Hinton. This is done to safeguard the residents in case any of the staff leaves suddenly. It also minimizes the county paperwork required each time we have a change in our staff. When the check is received by the resident, he signs it and gives it to Mr. Hinton who, in turn, makes the necessary payroll deductions and pays the salaries of the staff. The Department of Public Welfare is, in effect, contracting with Mr. Hinton to ensure that we residents receive the required attendant care.

STAFF SALARIES

The primary reason that so few severely physically disabled persons live alone with a single attendant is that this is a luxury which they cannot afford financially. This, of course, is the same reason that so many end up in nursing homes. In small groups, lack of sufficient money is still a problem. However, by sharing common expenses, it is possible for us to function successfully. There is another advantage to living in small groups in a program such as HIP, which is sponsored by an involved and competent businessman. Mr. Hinton has made provision for staff living quarters in his overall plan. He, therefore, is able to employ higher caliber persons and pay them a more moderate salary because he is also providing them with room, board, and utilities.

One serious disadvantage remains: San Diego County only allows the attendant employers to barely exceed the minimum wage. If one cannot provide room, board, and utilities as part of a package agreement, the caliber of prospective attendants deteriorates. Many of us who are disabled know too well that we usually get what we can afford to pay for; also, the attrition rate of the lowest wage-scale employees is very high. To date, due to our unique arrangement, we have avoided this problem.

Part-Time Staff

Although we have employed most age groups from young teenagers to mid-70s, we prefer college students. We use them on a regular basis during peak workload periods, especially early morning and evening hours and on weekends. They assist in dressing, transferring to wheelchairs, grooming, and preparing and serving breakfasts in the mornings. In the evenings, they assist in transferring to beds and undressing. They are used in numerous other capacities, and their wages vary from $2–$5/hour, depending on their duties and experience.

Full-Time Live-In Weekend Staff

One of our three full-time staff is our weekend attendant. She is on call from 6 A.M. Saturday until 6 A.M. Monday. She helps supervise the part-time staff, assists in dressing, undressing, transferring, and grooming. She is also responsible for the meal preparation and serving, and some light housekeeping. One evening during the week she takes over after the evening meal has been served and is on duty until midnight. For these duties she receives room, board, utilities, and a monthly salary.

Full-Time Live-In Weekday Staff

The two who share this responsibility are both licensed vocational nurses. They are on call from 6 A.M. Monday until 6 A.M. Saturday, except for one evening from dinnertime until midnight. They are responsible for meal planning, grocery shopping, food preparation and serving, housekeeping, laundry, and yard upkeep. They handle bowel care, catheterization, catheter irrigation, bathing, grooming, dressing, undressing, transferring, and answering the call buzzers in case of emergencies. They attend to minor medical problems such as preventing decubitus ulcers by constant skin examination and care of such ulcers if they develop. Their medical background is an asset to all of us and is especially helpful in training new staff members. It is beneficial to know why certain medical procedures are necessary in addition to knowing how to perform them. For these services they receive room, board, utilities, and a monthly salary.

PROBLEMS TO BE SOLVED

We are aware of many problems which remain to be solved. Two of them with a high priority are as follows.
  First, we need an attendant pool. Locating competent and responsible attendants is a chronic problem for the severely physically disabled. It is also, however, a problem for the elderly and the convalescing, and this makes it a widespread community problem. A city-wide, centrally located office may prove to be the solution. Such an office could provide attendants of many types, such as companions, drivers, housekeepers, specialists in various disability fields, and nurses.
  Second, we need our own transportation service. At the beginning of the coming fiscal year we intend to apply to the California State Department of Transportation for a wheelchair-accessible van.

Bibliography

ATTENDANT/SSP PROGRAM

Attendant Care Programs vs Homemaker Programs For the Very Severely Disabled. By Ted Tanaka. THE SPOKESMAN, Vol. 13, No. 4, pages 8–12, 1973.

Don't Look Back. Government Administered Special Services. By Greg Sanders. THE INDEPENDENT, Vol. 2, No. 1, page 9, 1974.

RANCHO LOS AMIGOS HOSPITAL HOME CARE PLAN

The Home Care Plan of Rancho Los Amigos Hospital. By D. J. Perkins, J. E. Affeldt, and E. B. Callahan. Unpublished Report. 1958.

"Before Patients Go Home." By A. L. Horner and J. Jennings. AMERICAN JOURNAL OF NURSING, Vol. 61, pages 62–63 June, 1961.

Extending Hospital Services into the Home. By E. B. Callahan. AMERICAN JOURNAL OF NURSING, Vol. 61, pages 59–62 June, 1961.

Realistic Arithmetic: Removing Quads From Hospitals Saves Dollars, Makes Sense. By Gini Laurie. *Toomey i Gazette,* Vol. 7, pages 7–9, 1964.

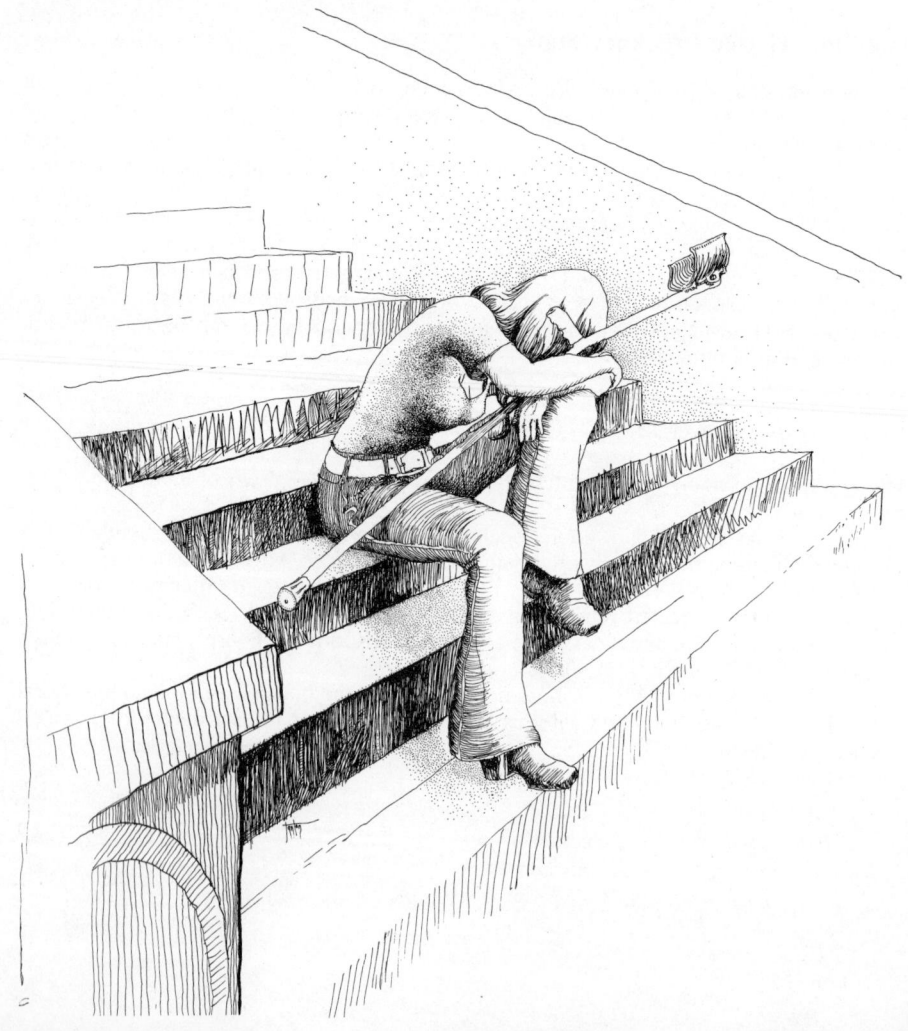

"Nobility through suffering is tripe. You're not a better person—only a different one."

—Peter Marshall, poliomyelitis quadriplegic, in "Two Lives"

9
Transitional Projects

In a sense, most modern living is transitional. On the average, one-fifth of the families in the United States move every year. Families and individuals move in a pattern dictated by age, income, employment, or fancy. These opportunities to make choices along the way of life are unavailable to many disabled individuals. Yet they, too, should have a choice of the locale or lifestyle that is right for each stage of development and maturity, should be able to move or stay put at will, should have living situations with built-in potential for change and growth.

In an attempt to set up a starting place for a normal life of change the concept of a "transitional" facility for the disabled has gained popularity recently. It was called a "halfway house" in rehabilitation parlance until this term became stigmatized by its use to describe a residence for former alcoholics, drug addicts, or convicts.

The transitional facility is the most frequently planned and the most infrequently completed facility. The usual pattern has been to start by designing a building, estimating the cost of attendant care, and figuring the amount of income of the potential residents. The totals are so frustrating that most planners soon give up.

The next step has often been to investigate the use of existing facilities, specifically, the creation of a "youth wing" in a nursing home. Those that have been tried have been dismal failures. The noisy exuberance of the young does not mix with the cotton-wrapped nursing home atmosphere, and the aides cannot change from giving orders to elderly patients to taking them from young people.

In spite of all the difficulties, a few transitional facilities have been built. Ironically, with the exception of the Paraplegic Lodge in British Columbia, Canada, which has a majority of persons actually in direct transition from a hospital among its 18 paraplegics and 6 quadriplegics, most of the residents of the existing facilities are "retreads"—that is, traumatic quadriplegics or other severely disabled individuals who have been wheelchaired for many years and have been living with their families or in nursing homes.

Recently, new trends in transitional living arrangements have been developed, replacing the original build-a-building approach. A wide range of supportive services to disabled individuals in the community has been created by a group of severely disabled individuals at the Center for Independent Living in Berkeley, California. The use of existing apartments, scattered throughout the community, with centralized supportive services, evolved from the Swedish Fokus plan (see Sweden, Ch. 18). Good examples are the projects developed by the Eastern Paralyzed Veterans Association (EPVA) in New York and the Texas Institute for Rehabilitation and Research (TIRR) in Houston. Then there is the use of adaptable mobile homes for practice living near hospitals and rehabilitation centers.

Both the old and new style facilities have the same red tape problem: lack of money to use wherever it is needed for independent living. In Boston, for instance, a hospital is receiving $111.50/day for each one of nine quadriplegics living there while they attend college. It is a safe bet that if much less were paid directly to the disabled student he could hire an attendant and live on his own or with friends, providing he had guidance from an umbrella organization, a resource center such as the Berkeley Center for Independent Living, the EPVA in New York, or the TIRR project team.

The flexibility of using existing apartments is a great advantage. The count of potential residents has always been a problem in planning, since it is impossible to predict how many severely disabled persons in the area will or will not need transitional assistance at any given time. Further, it is extremely time-consuming and difficult to set up the financing arrangements for each one with vocational rehabilitation, SSI, Medicaid, Medicare, or welfare.

It sounds simple to put 20 to 25 people together with the common problems of adjustment to severe disability and solve the problems wholesale. It does not work out that way. The problems of peopleness multiply by some unknown and astronomic factor within the abrasive confines of community living. The emphasis on solving transitional problems must be on an individual basis as a normal part of living. Transition does not take place in a vacuum, in an institutional setting. It is not a matter of mere passage of time. Transition is accomplished by experiencing real life situations. The housing projects organized and run by the disabled that are operating satisfactorily have one strong character in charge who acts as mother/father, referee, Solomon, manager, organizer, fund-raiser, bookkeeper, purchasing agent, dietitian, hostess/host, and psychologist in residence. It is almost a full-time absorption.

Rather than buildings labeled for transition, persons who are severely disabled need many more residential rehabilitation centers similar to the Woodrow Wilson Rehabilitation Center (WWRC) and a system of resources developed through them similar to the former respiratory centers. At WWRC transition starts with initial treatment and continues through hospitalization and rehabilitation. Disabled individuals are trained to progress within the center as they learn the techniques of independence and the skills of self-care and of directing others. They are taught to cope with their disability through trial home visits and contacts with the community. They are evaluated and assisted with vocational and educational goals. After such training, the majority are able to adjust; no separate place of transition is necessary. For instance, more than 6000 spinal cord injured persons have gone from WWRC back into their communities.

The emphasis must be on more support for more specialized residential programs in colleges and universities and on more residential training programs and vocational guidance for quadriplegics. WWRC estimates that, for every $1 spent on rehabilitation, a spinal cord injured individual returns $10 in earnings.

The emphasis must be on financial support during all stages of transition. Currently, vocational rehabilitation agencies support an individual through college or training and for a short time following, but not during the critical transition period of early employment when earnings do not cover the extraordinary expenses of disability. During all transition, a per diem allowance for attendant care should be available to supplement other income and make it possible for an individual to live as independently as he chooses.

IN-HOSPITAL TRAINING FOR INDEPENDENT LIVING

Stoke Mandeville Hospital in England, the pioneer of spinal cord injury centers, introduced the idea of a facility in which the disabled individual and his family try out living in an apartment set up at the hospital before leaving for home.

The Canadian Paraplegic Association added a model apartment suite to Lyndhurst Lodge, their new spinal cord injury center in Toronto. Here disabled individuals develop and practice the skills of independence. For example, the kitchen equipment is standard in every respect, and the disabled are taught techniques which allow them to manage with any equipment without drastic changes.

The first model home for the disabled in the United States was built by Dr. Howard A. Rusk. Known as the Functional Home for Easier Living, the home was constructed in 1959 on the grounds of the New York University Medical Center, adjacent to the present Institute of Rehabilitation Medicine. The home was designed to serve as a model for patients at the Institute, their families, and others interested in building or remodeling. Over the years, it has also demonstrated time- and energy-saving features of importance to the nondisabled public as well as the disabled and elderly, showing that the elimination of narrow doors and hallways, slippery floors, and unfunctional furniture makes life more efficient for everyone.

In addition to the model home on the grounds of the Institute of Rehabilitation Medicine, two kitchens have been constructed within the Occupational Therapy Department. The Department strongly recommends using two kitchens for training, one a typical normal kitchen and one designed especially for the wheelchaired. In this way, the therapists can stimulate ideas and show the homemaker how to work in her own kitchen if it is impossible to change it, how to change it in varying degrees, or how to work out the ideal kitchen for her individual needs.

RESIDENTIAL REHABILITATION CENTERS

WOODROW WILSON REHABILITATION CENTER

Woodrow Wilson Rehabilitation Center, Fishersville, Virginia 22939, is an outstanding example of intrinsic progression to normal living (Fig. 9–1). The entire program is geared to developing independence, to achieving maximum potential. The optimistic spirit of the director, Dr. J. Treacy O'Hanlan, pervades the center. Nearly 2000 people are served annually, with disabilities including spinal cord injury, brain damage, cerebral palsy, poliomyelitis, spina bifida, epilepsy, speech and hearing defects, and mental retardation. In addition, the Center offers an adult deaf training program.

Fig. 9–1. Woodrow Wilson Rehabilitation Center. The average daily enrollment is 455; of these 10% are spinal cord injured and 7% are brain damaged. **A.** Long gradual ramps at the vocational training building. **B.** Attendant activities building. **C.** Men's dorm. **D.** Auditorium. (Photographs courtesy of Woodrow Wilson Rehabilitation Center)

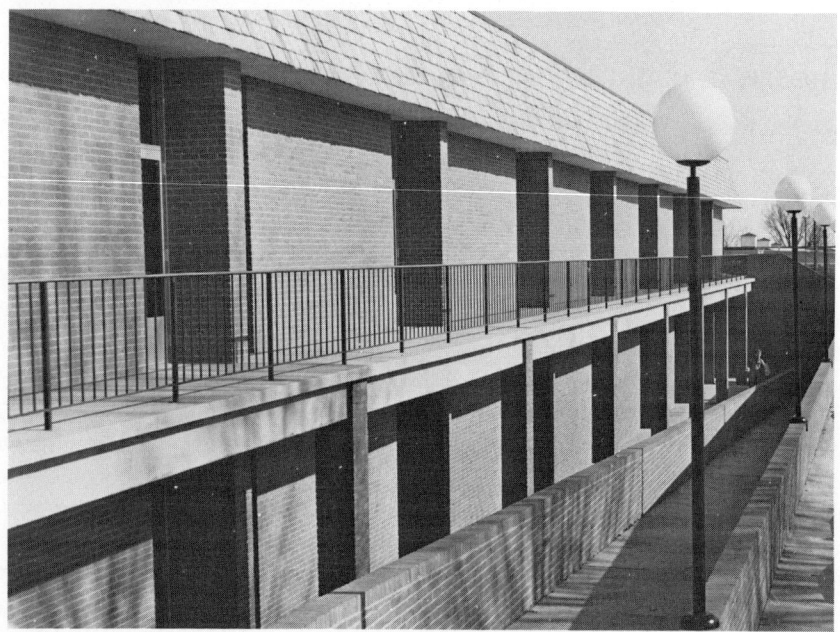

A

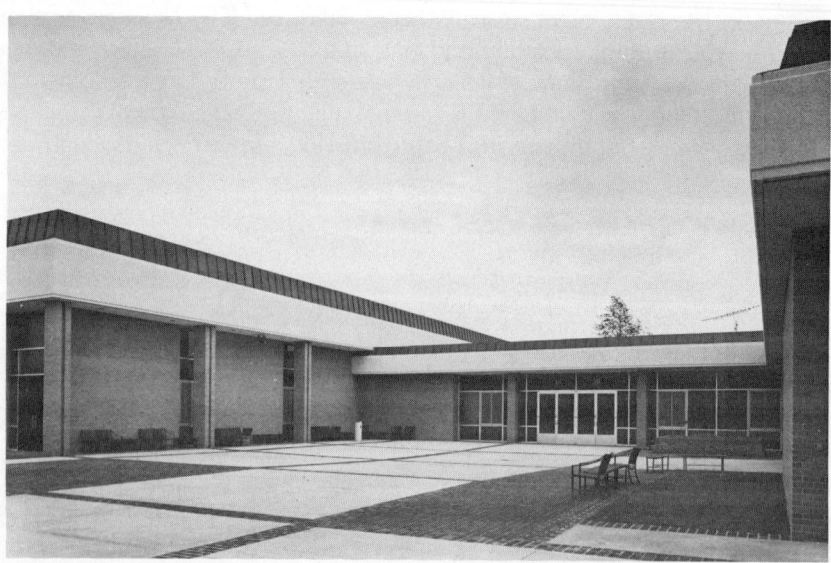

B

Transitional Projects 143

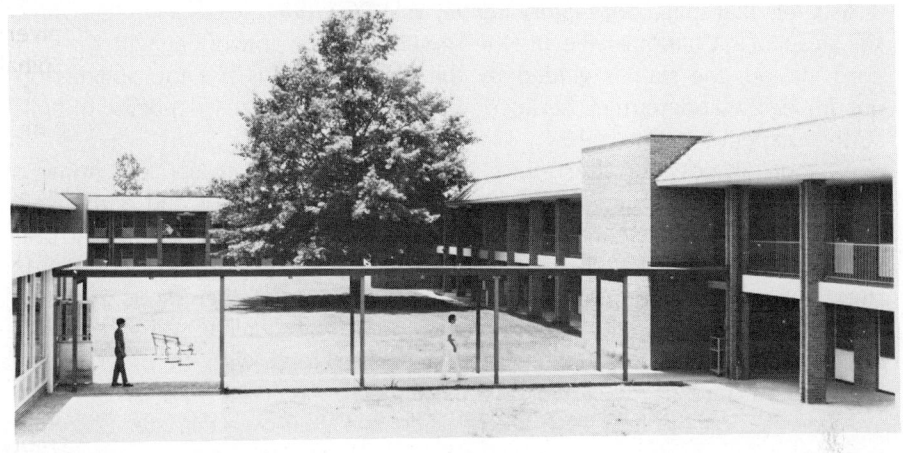

C

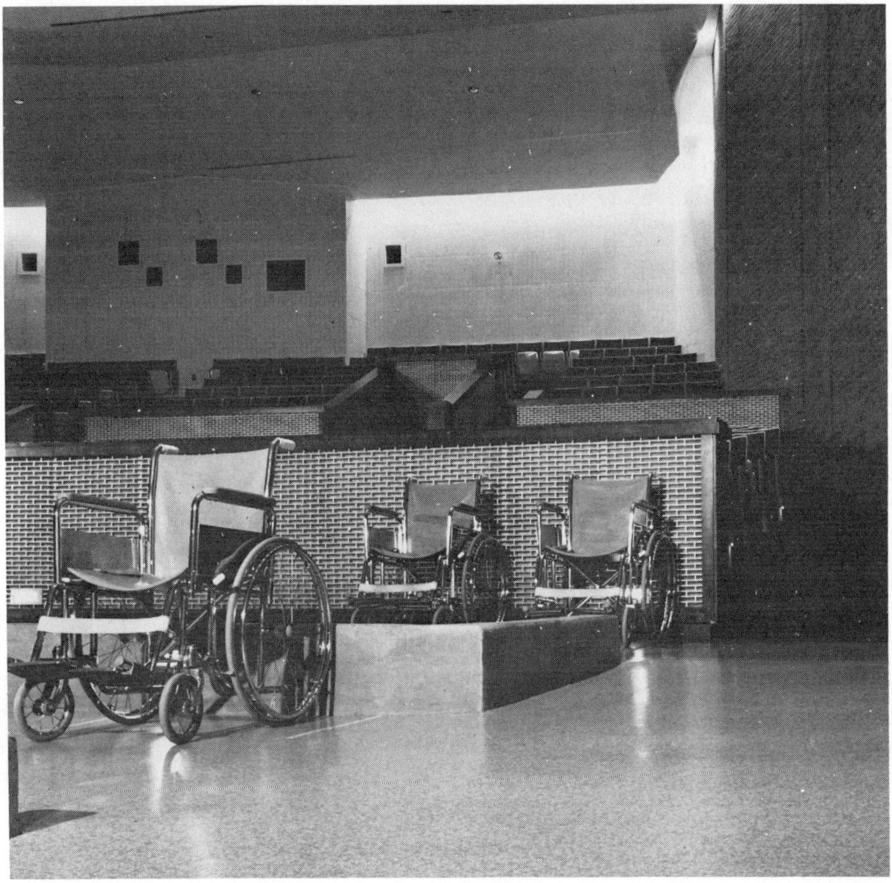

D

As a regional spinal cord injury center, WWRC works closely with the University Hospital in Charlottesville and the Towers Hospital. In working with the spinal cord injured, the staff is guided by the belief that it is not the abilities of a quadriplegic that determine his accomplishments, but what is expected of him—so they expect a great deal.

As soon as possible after injury, the students (patients) are sent home on weekends so they will start to realize the problems of adaptation and learn to meet them. Shortly after they are up in a wheelchair, they are taken to town to learn to tell people how to handle them. The first few times, they are left alone on the street in front of a store; they must learn to ask people to open doors and to ask clerks who wait on them to get the money out of their wallets. When they have learned to handle these situations, they may go to town with the other students and eat and drink in the restaurants and bars.

At WWRC quadriplegics are taught to change their own catheters, to empty their urinal bags, to deal with their own bowels, and to instruct any person to help with any bathrooming and dressing problems that they cannot manage by themselves.

The housing arrangements are subtly planned to teach and encourage independence. Initially, a cord injured student is assigned to the infirmary, which has rooms that can accommodate two, four, or six students. Here are those who need extensive nursing care.

As he develops the techniques of independence, a student moves forward to the intermediate wing (a halfway house). Here, the students are grouped in units of six in attractive two-bed rooms. Each room has an intercom to the nursing station, which handles 32 individuals. Students are expected to direct their own care and to make appointments with a nurse for specific help. The cost per day, including tuition, is $42 in the infirmary and the intermediate wing. This cost includes therapy and medical care.

The final progression to housing independence is reached when a student's functional level enables him to move into the dormitory suites. Here he has a maximum of independence. The costs here are $18/day. Therapy is an extra charge. The staff is minimal. The student is in complete charge of his own care.

Vocational training courses include computer training, keypunch operation, bookkeeping, calculating, courses specifically geared to employment as a payroll clerk or a shipping and receiving clerk, typewriting, radio and television repair, car servicing, furniture refinishing, welding, and woodworking. Recreational activities include music and art appreciation, languages, and all types of wheelchair sports, including bowling, archery, swimming, canoeing, and camping. The greatest emphasis is placed on counseling at all stages of rehabilitation.

According to Dr. O'Hanlan, one of the greatest obstacles to employment for the disabled is the problem of getting to and from work. WWRC therefore concentrates on teaching spinal cord injured persons to transfer from wheelchair to automobile and to drive. The driver-training program, with its 12 driving simulators, is one of the most popular courses.

WWRC works on the theory that a well-trained quadriplegic will never need a highly skilled attendant; he can work with any pair of willing hands. Independence is achieved by carrying out procedures oneself, or by learning them so well that one can tell another person how to do them. When a student is ready to be discharged, a referral is sent to his local public health nurse and to his field counselor of rehabilitation; both work very closely with the student and the center staff. To encourage this interaction, the center sponsors public health nursing workshops four times a year.

If needed, a team of two physical therapists and two occupational therapists will visit the student's home. As a rule these visits are unnecessary because the local public health nurse has taken complete charge and arranged for any adaptations necessary.

MARYLAND REHABILITATION CENTER

The general approach at the Maryland Rehabilitation Center, 2100 Argonne Drive, Baltimore, Maryland 21218, is very similar to that at Woodrow Wilson Rehabilitation Center. There are some interesting variations, such as apartments for married couples and a special program for blind people. In a model apartment, blind residents learn to cook and clean. The specially equipped kitchen is arranged with groceries in particular places and includes gadgets such as a braille timer.

Funded by the State Division of Vocational Rehabilitation, the Center is of particular value to the disabled from isolated rural areas who can live there while being trained. The Center includes a fully equipped woodworking shop, printing presses, and graphics equipment. There is also full training in such fields as cosmetology, dental technology, business, engine repair, and whatever new fields show employment potential. Designed for every group of disability, the Center evaluates and trains about 450 individuals at a time.

OTHER RESIDENTIAL CENTERS

Other centers in the United States with similar residential training programs are: Georgia Rehabilitation Center, Warm Springs, Georgia 38130; Hot Springs Rehabilitation Center, P. O. Box 1358, Hot Springs, Arkansas 71901; Pennsylvania Rehabilitation Center, 727 Goucher Street, Johnstown, Pennsylvania 15905; and West Virginia Rehabilitation Center, Institute, West Virginia 25112.

Further information on these and other centers, is included in the very attractive booklet, *Selected Rehabilitation Facilities in the United States—An Architect's Analysis* by Thomas Fitz Patrick, which is available for 90¢ from the U. S. Government Printing Office.

LAKESHORE REHABILITATION FACILITY

Through a unique joint relationship, a nonprofit corporation and a state vocational rehabilitation agency are developing a comprehensive rehabilitation center which will have a wide variety of residential arrangements, training facilities, and supportive services. The nonprofit agency is the Lakeshore Hospital, 3800 Ridgeway

Drive, Birmingham, Alabama 35209, a former tuberculosis hospital, located on 50 acres in a wooded area in Homewood, a suburb 3 miles from downtown Birmingham. The agency is the State Vocational Rehabilitation (SVR) agency. After a Rehabilitation Service Administration Planning Grant to evaluate its possibilities as a rehabilitation campus, the hospital became licensed in November 1973 as a rehabilitation hospital.

The joint effort has led to the existence of two administrations on campus. Lakeshore Hospital continues to operate the hospital unit and provide nursing care and therapy. The State Vocational Rehabilitation agency has financed substantial renovations and provides funding for disabled individuals and for staff to initiate vocational evaluation programs.

The hospital and the rehabilitation facility are currently offering the following services:

1. Hospital services. The hospital has 45 beds; presently 40% are sponsored by SVR, and the remainder are sponsored by other third parties.
2. Transitional living unit. The unit opened in July, 1974, with 5 residents; presently there are 14 residents. Eventually there will be 30 to 35 young men and women. Most of the rooms are double rooms, with two large four-bed rooms. The majority of the residents are spinal cord injured, though the facility is open to those with all types of disabilities, progressive or nonprogressive. Policies have not been set as to age limits or length of stay, except that one must be participating in a rehabilitation program. The cost per diem is $17.50 for those requiring little or no attendant care and $25 for those requiring a good deal of care; the cost includes room, all meals, and attendant care.

    The bedrooms and counseling offices are located on the second floor of the wing (there are two elevators); the first floor is occupied by the dining room, kitchen, community room, and occupational and physical therapy departments.

    The staff consists of one liaison counselor, two evaluators, one social worker, one training counselor, and two secretaries, plus the director and administrative assistant.
3. Vocational evaluation service. The present capacity is for about 12 persons at a time. All residents receive vocational evaluation and whatever basic training, on-the-job training, and work adjustment are necessary. Some residents are enrolled at various schools and technical institutions or studying for General Educational Development (GED). Others are in programs at Goodwill and Easter Seal facilities.
4. Training. Training presently includes clerical work and microfilming. The current capacity in the microfilming program is four persons; two are now in training. Eventually, one of the buildings will be converted to micrographics and possibly computer science programs. It is planned to provide training which will lead to homebound, sheltered, and competitive employment.
5. Transportation. SVR has provided two vans and one bus for transportation around campus and into the surrounding communities. Transportation is provided for any shopping necessary.

6. Recreation. A recreation director accompanies residents on excursions and provides on-campus entertainment. The residents play wheelchair basketball on the Birmingham team, and a gymnasium on the campus is in the dream stage.

Plans for the future include additional medical service spaces, a social activities center, additional vocational rehabilitation spaces for training and evaluation, and a workshop. Further plans involve adding an extended care level of service to the hospital and a separate building for the transitional living unit with facilities for 100 or more. Long range plans include building special apartments or condominiums for independent living.

The entire project is an exciting one, particularly because it is evolving gradually in response to the needs of the disabled individuals and the community. As an example of this fluid approach, the director, Donald Patrick, PhD, stated:

> The housing services proposed will be surveyed and scrutinized over the next several years. It is not the intent to construct yet another institution that would be terminal in nature, but one that would be enabling in nature with the ultimate objective of total movement of severely disabled back into the community to participate in a full range of life activities. . . . Obviously, substantial planning will be necessary, however, in order to make this dream a reality. Transportation services, attendants and ancillary medical services, social, recreational and vocational innovations, will have to be developed.

LIVING ARRANGEMENTS IN COLLEGE

Many of the severely disabled individuals who are now happily married, employed, and living in apartments or homes of their own made the discovery at college that they could live independently of their families by finding other students to take care of their daily needs.

The first college to make extensive adaptations for wheelchaired students was the University of Illinois at Urbana–Champaign. There, in the early 1950s, Professor Tim Nugent started a "temporary" rehabilitation program for a handful of disabled students. The handful has grown to hundreds yearly, and the facilities and activities have grown to include a special services building, a fleet of buses with hydraulic lifts, champion-level sports, and a fraternity. The program has been a model, continually evolving to meet developing needs. Both residential arrangements and attendant care are worked out on an individual basis; independence is developed with a fierce concentration. Among the more interesting setups is the commune type arrangement, Tanbrier, in an old, three-story house just off the campus in Champaign. Five male quadriplegics share costs of rent, maintenance, and help. The upper stories have apartments and rooms for college students who help with attendant care.

Another university in Illinois, Southern Illinois University at Carbondale, has also had years of experience with disabled students. The present blind and physically disabled population at SIU totals 600; of these 200 are in wheelchairs (75 of them because of spinal cord injury). Among the innovations are the arrangements for a student to earn two credit hours per semester for being a good attendant; the evaluation is done by the disabled person and two counselors. Most of the attendants are funded by the state vocational office; the current rate is $58 for 20 hours of care per week. To lighten the responsibilities of the attendants, most of the spinal cord injured students check in daily at the Health Center for catheter check and change.

One of the most important services at SIU is a wheelchair repair shop, especially for those with electric wheelchairs. To prevent total grounding when one of them is out of order, the rules stipulate that anyone with an electric wheelchair must also have a manual chair to use in emergencies.

Apartments for the disabled are either in the dormitory buildings or scattered throughout the community. Nearly every dormitory building has several accessible apartments on the first floor. Before a student can move into one of the apartments he must take a course that includes cooking, laundry, shopping, and managing an apartment. Additional courses cover other essentials such as basic sewing, dressmaking, and grooming.

Still another example of a totally accessible college is St. Andrews Presbyterian College, Laurinburg, North Carolina. It has developed a well-rounded program for disabled students under the direction of Robert M. Urie, Rehabilitation Services Director, who is wheelchaired himself. Assistance is given to disabled students in the form of roommate–aides, pushers, readers, and trained adult aides who do bathing, bathrooming, and dressing. In addition, adaptive educational courses offer individual and group programs of development in swimming, bowling, pool, weightlifting, and driver's training.

Many of the colleges that first made their facilities available to the disabled are located in California, where the Spanish influence resulted in more stepless architecture than in the ivied and turreted Eastern colleges. One of the first was the University of California at Los Angeles which developed a program shortly after World War II for disabled veterans. Many other California colleges have welcomed wheelchaired students—Berkeley, Riverside, Stanford, and a host of community colleges. In the Midwest and South, Wayne State in Detroit, Wright State in Dayton, the University of Missouri, and Earlham College in Indiana were among the pioneers.

Wheelchaired students have tackled most of the older colleges and universities and forced many of them to add ramps and make adaptations. The newer colleges are likely to have conformed to American National Standards Institute (ANSI) standards. Many of them are completely accessible and can assist with special services. At colleges around the country, disabled students have organized to work for accessible facilities and supportive services; the next logical step is a national association of disabled students.

Though a well-motivated disabled individual can make it at any college in a wheelchair by being carried up and down the steps, pushed up and down curbs, and making his own arrangements for attendant care off-campus or on, an accessible campus with organized special services makes life smoother and saves the time and energy spent on coping with barriers.

HEW has commissioned Abt Associates in Cambridge, Massachusetts, to make a nationwide study of the facilities for disabled students in colleges and universities. Until this study is completed, one can find helpful information in a study made in the mid-1960s, *Mobility for Handicapped Students,* which listed 189 accessible colleges. It is available free from Social and Rehabilitation Service, U.S. Department of Health, Education, and Welfare, Washington, D.C. 20201.

BOSTON CENTER FOR INDEPENDENT LIVING, INC.

In 1974 a residential program in Boston University (BU) dormitories for nine severely disabled college students who require attendant care was started by Paul J. Corcoran, MD, of the Boston University Medical Center, Robert McHugh, Massachusetts Rehabilitation Commission's Supervisor of the Severely Disabled, and Frederick Fay, PhD, consultant. It is the Boston Center for Independent Living, Inc., 745 Commonwealth Avenue, Boston, Massachusetts 02215.

The facilities are double rooms, located in BU's Theology and Towers dormitories. The Center is centrally located at BU so that residents can commute to classes; the Massachusetts Rehabilitation Commission (MRC) provides transportation to other schools.

Charges for room and board, based on university rates, are paid by SSI, personal funds, and MRC. Personal care attendants are students in the health sciences from Sargent College. Consultants available include a physician, occupational therapist, physical therapist, and rehabilitation nurse; a group counseling program is also available. Medicaid pays $20/day for attendants and consultants ($12 for the attendant and $8 for consultation, management, and medical backup).

WELLINGTON HALL

With similar support from the Massachusetts Rehabilitation Commission and Medicaid and Medicare, another program for nine severely disabled college students has been set up at Wellington Hall, the Spinal Cord Injury Unit of Middlesex County Hospital, Trapelo Road, Waltham, Massachusetts 02154. The unit coordinator, Richard Gould, is a traumatic quadriplegic who is currently working on his Master's degree in counseling. The rooms in the unit are all private rooms; the facilities also include a study, lounge, kitchen, and dining room. The costs per day of $111.50 are paid by Medicaid or Medicare; transportation costs are paid by MRC.

HOUSTON'S COOPERATIVE LIVING PROJECTS

After 4 years of concerted effort, an independent living project for 18 young disabled adults was opened in Houston in 1972. Begun by David D. Stock, ACSW, Director of Medical Social Work and Outpatient Care at the Texas Institute for Rehabilitation and Research (TIRR), 1333 Moursund Avenue, Houston, Texas 77025, the project involved the services and financial support of the staff and auxiliary of TIRR, the Texas Rehabilitation Commission, the Houston Housing Authority, HEW, and HUD.

BACKGROUND

Over the years, personnel of TIRR had made many attempts to initiate modified living arrangements for TIRR's patients but neither funds nor an interested agency had been found. In 1968, a community-wide conference was sponsored by TIRR and the Community Welfare Planning Association of Greater Houston to explore establishing living arrangements for several disabled young adults. The need was well documented by the community agencies present and a recommendation to pursue the project was made. However, local financing could not be mobilized and a stopgap measure was indicated. Therefore, a local nursing home was approached to set aside one wing of its facility for young disabled individuals. The arrangement was established in March, 1968, and a semblance of it exists today. It failed miserably because of the unaccepting attitude of the staff, lack of positive thinking, penalty for vocational activity, and an atmosphere of futility.

Next, planning turned to a 150-unit facility along the lines of the Center Park Apartments in Seattle (see Center Park Apartments, Ch. 13). The group spent months making a survey of the county to document the need to HUD. Questionnaires were sent to 162 persons known to TIRR between the ages of 18 and 40; 130 responded that they would be interested. Of these, 35 lived with an attendant or in a nursing home, and 95 lived with relatives or friends; 103 had incomes below $3200/year; 66 needed maximum physical assistance; and 34 were independent. The project limped along, getting no place for lack of finances, until December, 1971, when a ready-made building was purchased by TIRR and made available to the group by Dr. William A. Spencer, medical director. The building, called the Annex, was the Priester Foundation Hospital which had been built for persons with respiratory problems.

The Annex is located near the medical center and close to downtown Houston in a declining section of town slated for urban renewal. It consists of two patient wings, each with 18 units, one on each side of the building, and an inner patio and living and lounge areas. One half of the building was suitable for the housing group, and the other half was needed as an intermediate care unit for an extension of the Institute's rehabilitation program. Architecturally, the Annex was ideal since everything had been planned at wheelchair level, including the light switches. Some of the special features included wide doors and wide halls, wrist-operated door latches, and emergency power designed for respirators.

The coordinator of the project, David Stock, endeavored to develop a multiagency involvement including: 1) the Houston Housing Authority to set up a rent supplement program; 2) the Texas Rehabilitation Commission to provide vocational evaluation and training services; and 3) the State Department of Public Welfare to assist with financial support.

The wheels of government bureaucracy turned slowly for many months while the Institute negotiated for funding. In late December, the Auxiliary to TIRR held a successful fund-raising event, the Vega raffle, and donated $9500 which enabled the residential unit to open. On January 17, 1972, the dedication ribbon was cut by the manager, Rodney Shaw, a quadriplegic, and the unit opened with 12 severely disabled individuals in residence, most of whom were in school or about to begin employment.

In the following month the entire concept was in jeopardy because the Texas Department of Public Welfare would pay $436/month for each eligible resident only if the Annex were established as a nursing home. The Department would not consider the Annex as a resident's own home but instead interpreted it as a room and board situation. In a room and board situation, the cost could not exceed $125/month. Also, the Department could not meet the costs of attendant services under its guidelines.

HEW STUDY GRANT

In the fall of 1972, TIRR was awarded $75,000 for one year's operation and research by the Social and Rehabilitation Service, HEW, with support for the second and third year depending on demonstration of project goals. Support for subsequent years depended on the amount of demonstrated need. Titled "The Cooperative Self-Support System for Severely Disabled Young Adults," the grant was awarded to prove the benefits of establishing opportunity-oriented living facilities for people with severe mobility handicaps.

A SYSTEM OF SHARED SERVICES

The Cooperative Living Concept involves sharing attendant services, meals, and transportation. Most of the annex residents were quadriplegic because of spinal cord injury and were aged 18–30. During the first years of the project the expenditure per resident per month amounted to $462. The monthly cost charged to each resident was $348. This cost included: room, $88; meals, $60; attendant, $180; and transportation, $20. General financial support was provided by TIRR and the grant from HEW; individuals received assistance from the Texas Rehabilitation Commission, SSI, rent subsidy, and individual earnings or family support.

Cooperative Living at the annex was governed by a Resident Management Council of four elected representatives. The council managed the attendant and transportation services as well as hiring new staff members, choosing new residents, maintaining financial records, and working with service branches of TIRR.

The staffing pattern was scheduled to meet the needs of the residents, the largest staff during peak activity periods from 6 A.M. to 10 A.M. and from 8 P.M. to 12 P.M., with a minimal staff at other times. The 16 members of the staff were primarily college students who had had no previous training but were trained by the residents, who directed their own care. The service needs of the residents were coordinated into a schedule through activity lists, such as get-up sheets, evening activities lists, and shower lists. Each resident signed up for the specific times he wanted services performed.

Food service was provided by TIRR. Residents ordered food on a meal-by-meal basis, ordered food from outside, or ate out. TIRR's food service is located in the building.

A van and driver were available for transportation to school, work, clinic appointments, recreation or shopping trips. A flat fee per month was charged each resident. In addition, several residents had their own cars equipped with hand controls, others owned vans, and nondisabled friends provided transportation or drove the residents' vans.

Almost all of the residents made progress toward their educational or vocational goals. They reported that living in the project "among other young persons leading active lives had aided in their motivation to attend school or work and had also been helpful in teaching them new ways to deal with the logistical problems connected with these activities."

CHANGE IN CONCEPT

According to Stock, the Annex was never visualized as a transitional facility. It evolved naturally into a transitional model. During the first years the project was considered to be temporary until there was funding to build the planned 150-unit facility. However, by early 1974, Stock had visited a number of European facilities and had become convinced that having a mixed population and a number of small facilities in the community was preferable to having a single large facility. At the same time, several of the residents had achieved self-confidence through their experiences with independent living at the Annex and were ready to move on into more independent living arrangements. When the Annex was closed in September, 1975, 40 people, aged 19 to 33 years, had been residents during the three years of its existence.

VALUE OF THE COORDINATING TEAM

Not only has the initial facility at the Annex functioned successfully as a training ground for independent living, but from it have evolved other projects and plans which have even more possibilities for independence, such as a cluster of six or eight satellite apartments in the vicinity of the University of Houston.

Dr. Spencer and the project team, David Stock and Jean Cole, have a delicate harmony with the disabled leaders of the projects, the community, federal government agencies, state legislators, and state rehabilitation agencies. The team, viewing the projects in the context of the whole environment, works to effect legislation that would change licensing procedures to include cooperative living arrangements by the disabled and to bend the rules of state welfare agencies to make independent living by the disabled as feasible as nursing home existing. Further, to achieve environmental unity, they have built transportation systems into every project at the very beginning. TIRR's project team has provided the expertise and corporate strength needed to establish community and governmental participation and has worked closely with the disabled residents so that they have free rein to express their needs, to train and schedule their attendants, to handle food services as they wish, and to develop additional living situations as they progress to higher levels of independence.

As a further plus, not only do the extensive data that are being collected by Stock and his staff prove the value of the project to these individuals in terms of increased independence, employability, educational achievements, and social and leisure activities, but they will be available to others who need such factual leverage to work out similar projects. The final report will be a "How-To-Do-It Action Guide" that will spell out how others can develop housing solutions and communicate with state legislators.

In a brief report in the 4th quarter 1975 issue of TIRR's publication, *The Promethean*, Jean Cole reports optimistically on the developments of the Cooperative Living projects and on a new program. The projects demonstrate that severely disabled people who know their own needs can use nonprofessional attendant services and that the costs of sharing attendants and services are far less than in a nursing home or an individual home situation. Residents gain self-confidence about what they can do and they learn from each other. The new program will provide a 2 to 3 month transitional live-in experience and extensive contacts with disabled individuals who are active in their communities.

According to Ms. Cole, "The Cooperative Living program taught us that there is no one best way to do things. People are individuals and what is best for one is certainly not best for another. We need to work on a diversity of options."

PROJECTS BEING PLANNED

MADISON HOUSING AUTHORITY

The Housing Authority of the City of Madison, P.O. Box 1785, Madison, Wisconsin 53701, is working on plans to construct a transitional facility on a site in the Triangle Urban Renewal Area. To assist the Housing Authority, a Technical Advisory Panel was formed in the spring of 1975. Members include potential residents, a clinical psychologist, a physician, a professor in the Department of Engineering at the University of Wisconsin, a landscape architect, nurses, social workers, and other interested professionals.

The panel envisions the project as an apartment building containing 20 two-bedroom units. Each unit would house one disabled person and one attendant, or perhaps two disabled persons. The residents would be "severely disabled young adults, between the ages of 18 and 35 years, who require wheelchairs, are emotionally independent, and are employed, employable, or intending to further their education or training."

The Housing Authority received a loan from the Wisconsin Department of Local Affairs and Development to cover architectural consultant fees for the preparation of preliminary plans, specifications, and cost estimates for the project.

A number of financing arrangements are being explored: 1) construction—discussions are underway with HUD to determine if the project is eligible for a Section 202 direct loan; 2) permanent financing—discussions are also under way with bond underwriters and representatives of the Wisconsin Housing Finance Authority (WHFA); 3) rent subsidy—it appears likely that rent subsidy will be obtained under Section 8 of the Housing and Community Development Act; and 4) other financial assistance programs such as SSI, vocational rehabilitation, Workmen's Compensation, and medical assistance, are being investigated.

This will be an interesting project to follow, not only because it has had such outstanding professional advice but because some of the disabled residents in the Madison area oppose the urban renewal location, considering it too remote from a normal shopping and residential area to be suitable.

MEXICAN EXPERIMENTS IN INDEPENDENT LIVING

Guadalajara, Mexico, has become the site of unscheduled experiments in independent living by hundreds of disabled veterans and civilians from the United States and Canada. The experiences of these disabled individuals of all ages, all types of disabilities, and varied backgrounds and incomes demonstrate that, with minimal income, quadriplegics and other severely disabled individuals can choose their own lifestyles, arrange for transportation, direct their own attendants, and manage in a wide variety of accommodations.

EXODUS OF DISABLED TO MEXICO

The exodus of the disabled to Guadalajara, Mexico's second largest city, began casually in the 1960s when two paraplegic veterans rented houses there and invited other disabled friends from the United States to be their paying guests so they could keep themselves supplied with poker players. In those preinflation days, the prices were enticing: food, lodging, laundry, and attendant care averaged about $150/month; the added luxury of a personal attendant cost $32/month more. Since then prices have risen steadily so that present prices are more than double what they were then. Nevertheless, costs are still less than those for comparable accommodation and attendant care in the U.S.

In addition to the several hundred disabled individuals, Guadalajara has become the home of 10,000 retirees and the location of one of the largest chapters of the Paralyzed Veterans of America (PVA). Guadalajara's climate is gentle. With two medical schools, its medical care and hospital facilities are excellent and inexpensive.

SPECIALIZED RESIDENCES RUN BY DISABLED

Severely disabled individuals own or operate the seven or eight residences, supervising all details of the meals, shopping, housekeeping, maintenance, and hiring and training of attendants. The residences, scattered throughout the city and suburbs, vary from converted motels to small single homes, have from 20 to a handful of residents (some for men only) and are operated in a manner from regimented to disorganized.

A MATTER OF CHOICE

Living in Mexico is a possibility only for writers or those with fixed incomes, since tourists may not secure a work card to engage in paying activities. Most of the disabled residents go down first as "snow birds" for a winter vacation. They usually start at one of the specialized residences they have heard about or read about in one of the publications for the disabled. When they meet other North American disabled at the various residences, they discover that there are many other ways of living. Many make several moves before finding the most satisfying residence, seeking a way of life and people that are congenial. As independence develops, some find group living is a strain and they team up with one or more other wheelchaired persons and move to a house or an apartment, hire their own attendants and cook/housekeeper, and share expenses.

For some short-term visitors, their vacation in Guadalajara is their first opportunity to see how other quadriplegics manage and to discover their own possibilities for independence and self-direction. For them, the visit may serve as a transition to further independence and productive living back in the U.S.

EXPERIENCES OF DISABLED VISITORS AND RESIDENTS

A writer and an artist, cerebral palsied Gil Nagy of New York State, has lived in Guadalajara for a number of years. He emphasizes the need to adjust to existing conditions: "If you decide to 'go Mexico,' don't expect to find all the so-called comforts of a nursing home or hospital. You will have to tolerate certain inconveniences. If you are in the frame of mind to accept trivial annoyances, and fasten your attention on the sunny, warm climate, the freedom of movement and action, and the charm and beauty of a foreign land, then you will LOVE Mexico."

Several respiratory poliomyelitis quadriplegics, who require rocking beds or chestpieces at night only, have reported that they had difficulty breathing on their own in Mexico City's 7000-ft altitude, but had no trouble in mile-high Guadalajara except for the surprises of occasional nocturnal irregularities in the electricity. W. G. Robertson, Jr., who uses a pneumobelt or chestpiece 24 hours daily, drove with his parents on several extended trips throughout Mexico, including long stays in an apartment in Guadalajara. An engineer, he made careful plans for every emergency so that there were no problems with batteries or electricity, although he has a vital capacity of only 650. "The electric current in Mexico proved most reliable," said Robertson, "but its voltage sometimes varied anywhere from 100–135 from hour to hour. An Acme Voltage Transformer, Type T10307, with input of 75–145 volts and output of 115, was used in conjunction with the Thompson and Monaghan respirators; the rest of the equipment withstood the fluctuations."

The atmosphere and the feeling of independence are vitally important, according to Walter C. Pinsonnault of New York State, who is disabled by Friedreich's ataxia. He wrote after his first visit,

At Kegan's Hacienda Las Fuentes the atmosphere is friendly, informal, and unrestrictive. You can do what you want and, if you need help, you can get it.

The people I met down there were unlike any others I have ever come across. They were very friendly, and their handicaps and difficult lives made me feel akin to them. The stories I heard were almost unbelievable, and yet they told them almost nonchalantly. In their company I felt not like an abnormal person but like one of the gang.

Another point which I thought of when I was pondering about Guadalajara and why I enjoyed it so was the independence and lack of supervision that I felt. In some things I need help. But if I can do things myself, even though slowly and clumsily, I would rather than have someone do them for me. There I organized my days and I ran my life and I feel all the better for it.

About ten of the guys staying there had their own cars, so getting around was no big problem. You can hire an aide if you need one; a few aides are provided to assist those without personal aides. We went shopping, to drive-in movies, to restaurants and night clubs, sightseeing, and the local PVA Club, where they have bingo.

TRANSPORTATION AND ARCHITECTURAL BARRIERS

As Pinsonnault states, transportation is not a big problem. Many of the permanent residents drive their own cars with hand controls, often accompanied by their personal aides, and they share their cars with others. Taxis are relatively inexpensive, and the drivers offer physical assistance. Most of the owners of the residences will make arrangements for in-coming guests to be met at the airport with a car and an aide if sufficient notice is given.

Architectural barriers are eliminated by "people power," the strength and willingness of the aides as well as the taxi drivers, shopkeepers, and the average Mexican. They are not inhibited by union regulations or the fine print of insurance policies and are accustomed by their culture to hauling great loads. They will wrestle wheelchairs into trunks of taxis or race up stairs with both chair and occupant sedan-chair style.

RED TAPE

Shots and vaccinations are no longer necessary and passports are not required. Only a Tourist Card is necessary for entry. This may be secured in advance from a Mexican Consulate in the United States by an individual or any travel agent or airline. United States citizens need only carry proof of citizenship in the form of a birth certificate, voter's registration card, or a passport.

Complete information on these details as well as city maps, accommodations, money exchange, highways, and generally helpful facts is available in the American Automobile Association's annual guide. A postcard to Sanborn's, P.O. Drawer 1210, McAllen, Texas 78501, will net a list of books and information on the necessary automobile insurance, as only Mexican insurance is valid.

LISTING OF GUADALAJARA RESIDENCES

The following four residences have been in existence for many years and would be recommended starting places, either for a winter vacation or permanent residences. Inflation is sending prices soaring throughout Mexico, too, so be prepared for increases and make inquiries and reservations before going down.

1. Kegan's Hacienda Las Fuentes, San Antonio 67, Las Fuentes, Guadalajara, Jalisco, Mexico. Phone: 21-13-44.
2. La Morada, Cubilete 147, Colonia Chapalita, Guadalajara, Jalisco, Mexico. Phone: 21-07-69. (Men only.)
3. Sun Haven, Euclides 3177, Guadalajara, Jalisco, Mexico. (Men only.)
4. Villa del Sol, San Antonio 45, Las Fuentes, Guadalajara, Jalisco, Mexico. Phone: 21-09-40.

For all the latest listings, address an airmail request to American Consulate General, Guadalajara, Jalisco, Mexico. Also, write to Service Officer, Paralyzed Veterans of America, Las Palmas 226, Ciudad Granja, Jalisco, Mexico.

VETERANS ADMINISTRATION TRANSITIONAL LIVING

HOSPITAL-BASED HOME CARE

Mrs. Essie Davis Morgan, Chief, Socio-Economic Rehabilitation, Spinal Cord Injury Service, VA Central Office, 810 Vermont Avenue, N.W., Washington, D.C. 20420 has pioneered a program that provides house calls to facilitate the transfer from hospital to home. The service involves a physician, a social worker, a nurse, and an administrative person as a core troop with other professional persons added as needed. Individuals receive the same specialized services in their homes that they would receive in the hospital.

INPATIENT TRAINING PROGRAM

Many of the VA spinal cord injury centers around the country have added apartments within the hospital in which the disabled veteran and his family can practice living together under the guidance of therapists. The kitchens and bathrooms are built with standard equipment, and the veterans are taught how to circumvent the inconveniences.

The Castle Point VA Hospital has gone a step farther in a pilot project to train quadriplegics and their families to handle the details of daily living. The project is a joint operation with the Eastern Paralyzed Veterans Association. The VA has rented and furnished an apartment about 20 miles from the hospital and adapted it to wheelchaired living by widening the doorways and adding a roll-in shower. Before he has been discharged from the hospital, a quadriplegic and his family may live there for 3-4 weeks and discover the problems of adapting and coping while the staff members are available to help.

ROGOSIN HOUSE—APARTMENTS WITHIN THE COMMUNITY

The evolvement of the plans of the Eastern Paralyzed Veterans Association (EPVA), 432 Park Avenue South, New York, New York 10016, from a specialized building to individual apartments within the community typifies the development of services and housing of the last dozen years. According to the EPVA *1972-1973 Annual Report,*

During the early 1960s, those people who were the leaders of EPVA had a dream of building one apartment building specifically for paraplegics and quadriplegics. They knew that if they could find a philanthropist to provide a fairly substantial grant, they could perhaps acquire additional funds for completion of the project from the federal government. Well, they found that generous benefactor in the person of the late Israel Rogosin. And with Mr. Rogosin's grant, EPVA of New York House, Inc., was formed, and the project had a beginning.

The ball really started to roll in the mid-1960s, when the New York City Housing Authority granted a site for the paraplegic housing project in the Bronx. . . . Unfortunately, funds from the federal government for housing were cut back drastically at the height of the Vietnam conflict, and the EPVA of New York House was denied federal monies.

During the years that followed, the philosophy of housing for paraplegics and quadriplegics changed within our organization: it was now felt that any realistic housing program must integrate disabled individuals with the mainstream of society, and the "transitional" housing concept could fulfill this role while simultaneously providing a necessary final step in the rehabilitation process. And so, the birth of Rogosin House.

The following details were presented by Joseph Chasin of EPVA at the April, 1974, conference, Housing Alternatives for Handicapped Adults, in New York City.

Rogosin House was officially reactivated on May 1, 1972. The concept now was for a halfway house program in which a turnover of residents could be achieved every 9–12 months, thereby making the apartments available to a greater number of individuals. Such a program would offer advantages that were impossible with the earlier idea. The economics would be well within our means, and the program could be enlarged or reduced to fit the indicated need. Unlike the permanent housing concept, where a stable population would exclude newly rehabilitated patients from the opportunity to test their wings outside the hospital, the transitional approach gives anyone who wants to try it a ready-made opportunity.

On November 1, 1972, we opened our first apartment in Mt. Vernon, N. Y. Since then we have activated three more. Each one is leased in the name of Eastern Paralyzed Veterans Association. Each is equipped completely with all necessary furniture, appliances, utensils and linen so that the wheelchair-bound veteran is not faced with these expenses when leaving the hospital. With the approval of the landlord at the time of leasing, we also make the necessary minor modifications, such as widening a doorway, installing a special shower, or any other to complete a barrier-free environment. . . . We rent two-bedroom apartments because, 1) we think the buddy system adds a sense of security and is essential to the success of each experiment, and 2) it contributes to the reasonable economics of the plan.

A Rogosin House apartment gives the resident an opportunity to get on his feet financially, since his rent is adjusted to his ability to pay. Of vital importance, a Rogosin House apartment provides the security of supportive services. Periodic visits are made to each resident by staff personnel of EPVA. Any necessary medical, nursing, social, psychologic, or dietetic services are delivered at each apartment by the Veterans Administration's Hospital-Based Home Care Program. There have been some emergencies and they have been handled with prompt and efficient care.

Selection of our residents is completed by interviewing all spinal cord injured patients at the Bronx and Castle Point VA Hospitals to determine need and interest. A patient selection committee at each hospital, composed of a staff physician, psychologist, and social worker, and two staff members of EPVA of New York House, then make the final decisions.

Residents of Rogosin House apartments are responsible for rent, food, housekeeping, telephone, and electricity costs, exactly the same responsibilities faced by any other individual in the community. Our Rogosin House staff has helped and will continue to help residents acquire suitable permanent housing to which they will move when they are ready for the transition. During his stay in the Rogosin House apartment, the resident will do the things necessary to establish himself: find a job, go to school, or whatever. Our services encompass counselling and practical assistance in every area necessary to get him going again.

An interesting sidelight is that not every resident has successfully made the transition. Perhaps he was not yet ready, but the program gave him the opportunity to find out for himself. If he finds that the problems of living on his own are more than he can cope with, physically, emotionally, or for any reason, the VA guarantees his return to the hospital.

In the year and a half since our first apartment was opened, we have graduated six from our program and currently have seven residents, several of whom will soon be moving on to permanent housing. One of the apartments is occupied by a paraplegic and his wife and young child. They had been living under extremely difficult conditions in an apartment with stairs and a destructive family relationship. Rogosin House has given them the opportunity they needed to live in peace and plan their future. They are working on plans for a wheelchair-accessible house.

Another EPVA member, Terence J. Moakley, a quadriplegic, says that the apartment housing plan "is completely practical. A cooperative landlord, a lease in the name of EPVA of New York House, Inc., some minor modifications which can be restored at the end of the lease, and appropriate furnishings are all that are needed. . . . There are men living in VA hospitals who could hold down a job, or go back to school, and get back to the business of living if they had a place to live."

VETERANS ADMINISTRATION BENEFITS

702 OR WHEELCHAIR HOMES

Under Title 38, United States Code, Chapter 21 (the original statute was P. L. 702) specially adapted wheelchair or 702 housing is available for veterans whose service-connected disability, due to war or peacetime service after April 20, 1898, entitles them to compensation for a permanent and total disability that has left them dependent upon the aid of braces, crutches, canes, or a wheelchair. Further, the veteran must be medically able to live in the house, the house must be adapted to his needs, and, with the help of the grant, he must be able to afford it. The grant may be used for a new home on land purchased for the purpose or on land already owned by the veteran; it may also be used to remodel his existing home or to apply on the unpaid balance of a specially adapted home that he acquired previously.

To apply for a wheelchair home, the veteran should contact the VA office where his claim records are located. A determination will be made as to the veteran's basic eligibility and whether it is medically feasible for him to reside in a specially adapted home. If the grant is approved, a representative of the VA field office will visit the veteran and help him to obtain a 702 home. The VA representative will give the veteran a selection of plans from a file of adapted houses, assist him to locate a building site, and help him choose an architect, obtain bids for construction, and arrange for financing.

For details as to the requirements for special adapted housing, request VA

Pamphlet 26–69–1, Revised January 1973. Among the requirements are 1) ramps: one for entry, one for exit, fireproof material, nonslip 8° slope, 3 ft 6 in. wide; 2) doorways: 36 in. wide; halls: 48 in. wide; 3) bathroom: generous floor area, nonslip floor, grab bars, covered water pipes, raised toilet if necessary, protected hot pipes; and 4) wall switches and outlets: 18 in. minimum, 48 in. maximum from floor.

The Veterans Housing Act of 1974 (P. L. 93–569), which was signed on the last day of 1974, increased the guaranteed loans for wheelchair homes from $17,500 to $25,000, as well as liberalizing a number of loan restrictions. Further, it increased mobile home manufactured housing guarantees from $10,000 to $12,500 for single-wides and from $15,000 to $20,000 for double-wides and extended loan maturities to 20 years. For the first time, the VA now has authority to guarantee loans on used mobile homes and on lots upon which to place mobile homes owned by veterans. In addition, Federal Credit Unions are authorized to make VA-guaranteed mobile home loans.

AUTOMOBILES

Veterans' and Servicemen's Automobile Adaptive Equipment Amendment of 1974 (P. L. 93–538) increases the grant from $2800 to $3300 for purchase of specially equipped automobiles; permits VA to repair, replace, or reinstall adaptive equipment; removes restrictive line-of-duty criteria presently imposed on service-connected veterans; and provides driver training by the VA.

Bibliography

A Better Life in Mexico. By Walter Pinsonnault. REHABILITATION GAZETTE, Vol. 13, pages 42–43, 1970.

By Car Through Mexico. By W. G. Robertson, Jr. REHABILITATION GAZETTE. Vol. 12, pages 54–56, 1969.

Comprehensive Rehabilitation Center: Woodrow Wilson Rehabilitation Center, By Gini Laurie, REHABILITATION GAZETTE, Vol. 15, pages 3–5, 1972.

Cooperative Living Moves into Community, THE PROMETHEAN, 4th Quarter, pages 4–5, 1975.

Cruise in Sunny Mexico. By Gil Nagy. REHABILITATION GAZETTE, Vol. 14, pages 80–81, 1971.

Driving a Camper Van. By Joe Laurie. REHABILITATION GAZETTE, Vol. 17, pages 7–8, 1974.

Selected Rehabilitation Facilities in the United States. An Architect's Analysis, By Thomas K. Fitz Patrick. U. S. Government Printing Office, 1973.

"As in all housing there should be a wide variety of good, well-designed choices available to the disabled of all economic levels because no single facility in a city would fulfill all of the requirements for all of the disabled."

—Dorothy Bladey Columbus, MEd. The Physically Disabled and Housing, *A Philadelphia Study*

10
Apartment Living Arrangements

Apartments offer a visible flexibility of prices, locations, sizes, and room arrangements. Most importantly, a trial project is not "cast in bronze" in a building that could become obsolete as ideologies evolve or a project grows or shrinks. A project that has spent itself can evaporate with the expiration of the lease and be moved elsewhere or abandoned. A successful project can grow with equal ease.

Apartments provide excellent opportunities for integration. Apartment dwellers are likely to be students, single working adults, young marrieds, transients, or retirees—the types of people that have less settled patterns than homeowners and more tolerance toward others. Apartments avoid the isolation of a house or hostel specifically labeled for the disabled. There are constant opportunities for normal integration in the elevators, halls, laundry, garage, and yards.

The numbers of units and the services of attendants or houseparents can be expanded or contracted to meet the needs of disabled individuals who are actually at hand. Degrees of independence can be achieved within the apartments according to the amount of supervision. Apartments can be arranged and rearranged to include communal cooking, dining, and recreation or totally independent individual cooking and living arrangements. Responsibilities for living can be gradually increased without changing physical settings. Apartment living in a group can be the springboard to further independence in an apartment or house totally unrelated to the group.

Another consideration of great importance is the avoidance of the stringent nursing home-oriented local fire and building code regulations that have wrecked many projects planned for groups in older homes and hampered plans for hostels. If apartments are leased by individuals, the fire and code regulations for groups do not apply.

The comprehensive 29-page booklet, *An Apartment Living Plan To Promote Integration and Normalization of Mentally Retarded Adults,* should be required reading for all apartment project planners. Written by Margaret Fritz, Wolf Wolfensberger, and Mel Knowlton, it was published in 1971 by The Canadian Association for the Mentally Retarded, Kinsmen NIMR Building, York University, 4700 Keele Street, Downsview, Ontario, Canada M3J IP3. (Price: 50¢.) The authors cover every phase of apartment living, including degrees of assistance and supervision, integration into the community, improvement of the cost–benefit ratio, selection of apartments, residents, staff, financing, and residents' activities.

The authors' recommendations for staff are particularly helpful: use a couple with children when more supervision is needed and working persons or college students (preferably of the social sciences) for less supervision; maintain back-up personnel, such as citizen advocates or other volunteers, and prepare the staff for their roles by encouraging positive attitudes.

The following examples of apartment living arrangements in the United States are divided into 1) those with supportive services for individuals who cannot live independently without attendant and housekeeping services and 2) those without supportive services for those who can live independently in housing that is accessible and usable. A third and very important project, 2100 Bloomington, is a maverick: it is barrier-free, both accessible and adaptable; it is planned by the disabled for the disabled and their families, thus it is both segregated and integrated; and it is in the process of working out the social services that are needed to suit the needs of the current tenants.

INTEGRATED APARTMENT LIVING WITH SUPPORTIVE SERVICES

INDEPENDENT LIFE STYLES

Westbury Country Village Apartments, 5152 South Willow Drive, Houston, Texas 77035, is a well-documented project of 31 modified ground floor apartments with a complex of two-story garden style apartments for older people. It is an outgrowth of the TIRR Annex project (see Houston's Cooperative Living Projects, Ch. 9). By the summer of 1974, Rodney Shaw and a number of the other severely disabled residents who had initiated the project at the TIRR Annex felt the need to progress from its transitional rehabilitation to a more integrated and independent lifestyle. Forming a corporation, Independent Life Styles (ILS), they contacted the builder of the Westbury Country Village Apartments while they were still on the drawing board and worked with him to include modifications that would make them accessible and functional.

Modifications

Thirty of the two-bedroom units on the ground floor are available to ILS, plus one for its office. Sixteen units are together; the rest are dispersed throughout the complex. Modifications to the 30 apartments include a roll-in shower, a wheelchair height vanity and washbasin, single lever hardware for bath, kitchen, and all doors, lower light switches, wider doorways for walk-in closet and bathroom, and indoor–outdoor carpeting for smooth rolling. Also contained in each apartment is an intercom, activated by pulling a string and connected to the ILS staff office. The system is used by the residents to request assistance on a 24-hour basis. (It is significant to note that the builder reported that he had saved money on the ILS units because the roll-in showers were less expensive than bathtubs.)

Additional modifications and future improvements will include wider sidewalks, ramped apartment entrances, curb cuts or curb ramps, covered parking, a bell system in the drive area, a club room, and a small store.

Purpose

1. To provide living accommodations for severely handicapped young adults who require physical assistance in performing some of the activities of daily living.
2. To make available a coordinated system of homemaking services which can be purchased on an individual contract basis by any resident desiring such services.
3. To create a noninstitutionalized living situation for the handicapped citizen that will be conducive to maximum activity, productivity, and independence.

Medical Review

All residents requiring any of the services available through ILS will be required to present a doctor's statement describing the resident's general condition. The statement should also include a recommendation by the doctor verifying this type of living situation as adequate to meet that person's basic needs.

Resident Population

Admission criteria are 1) those persons confined to wheelchairs who require assistance in performing daily activities and require the benefit of special architectural design; 2) those of adult age and capable of entering into contractual agreements for services rendered; 3) medically stable persons with physical limitations requiring assistance to perform certain activities of daily living but not requiring constant supervision or regular medical treatment; 4) persons capable of assuming financial responsibility for all services rendered to them by ILS.

As of early 1975, the residents ranged in age 20–41. There were eight unmarried females, three married and nineteen single males. Of these, five were working, five were receiving veterans benefits, and the rest were university students. Their disabilities included arthritis (1), muscular dystrophy (1), spina bifida (1), paraplegia (1), respiratory polio quadriplegia (1), traumatic quadriplegia (all the rest).

Costs and Services

The average cost per month is $430. This includes rent, attendant care, transportation, meals, and housekeeping services. The Texas Rehabilitation Commission (TRC) has worked out different arrangements with each individual. After figuring income from Social Security, Supplemental Security Income, pensions, insurance, or trusts TRC makes up the difference. All special services, such as transportation, attendant care, and meals are available to each resident on an individual contract basis under the exclusive supervision and management of ILS. Residents may purchase the entire system of services or one or more of the services on this contractual basis.

Medical Care

A number of medical personnel happened to reside within the apartment complex and offered their services on an emergency basis; they included a physician, a registered nurse, and a licensed vocational nurse.

Attendants

Three shifts cover the total 24-hour period. As a permanent standby, one female lives in the complex with her disabled husband and is on 24-hour emergency call. The corporation pays her rent of $245 and a salary of $30/week. The attendants are drawn from a variety of sources. Some are university students, and seven were former nursing home attendants. They are paid $2/hour. The living/dining room of the ILS office apartment is used as their headquarters and call station.

Four attendants are on duty from 6 A.M. to 2 P.M.; three from 2 P.M. to 10 P.M.; and two from 10 P.M. to 6 A.M. The corporation has divided attendant care into three categories, based on the average amount of time per day required. Each resident pays only for the assistance he needs based on the following formula: $60/month for 1 hour/day; $120 for 2 hours; and $180 for 3 hours.

Meals and Transportation

Most of the residents manage to have their shopping and meals taken care of, though the shopping center is not within rolling distance. A program of prepared meals is available for about $60/month, including shopping and preparation.

The Texas Rehabilitation Commission donated a rural school bus that seats four adults and stows eight in wheelchairs. Transportation costs are based on a decreasing cost per mile basis. The bus has a hydraulic lift on the side and a folding ramp at the rear.

Legislative Effort

In order to secure more feasible alternatives to the inadequate availability of housing for the severely handicapped individual in the community, a concentrated effort will be made to introduce new legislation in 1975. The Texas Institute for Rehabilitation and Research and ILS are in the process of collecting information and drafting new legislation to include the consideration of controlled and regulated housing situations for the handicapped adult.

This housing would allow for self-contained living units combined with supportive services necessary for independence in daily activities. The purpose of such legislation would be to create provisions for licensing of facilities that provide minimal nonprofessional attendant assistance for those handicapped individuals with stabilized medical conditions.

FREE LIVES, INC.

Independence Hall, the 292-unit apartment complex for the elderly and handicapped sponsored by Goodwill Industries in Houston, opened in 1973 (see Independence Hall, Ch. 13). By the summer of 1974 approximately one-sixth of the residents were in wheelchairs. As it gradually filled, the management sought groups of disabled to fill a wing or a portion of a wing.

Bob Geyer, a traumatic quadriplegic, conceived the idea of pooling resources with other disabled while he was a resident of the Annex, TIRR's transitional unit. With five others, he formed a corporation, Free Lives, Inc., and in July, 1974, they moved into the end of a wing on the first floor of Independence Hall. Four of the other traumatic quadriplegics had been living in nursing homes, and Danny Brown, a polio quadriplegic, had been living with his father.

All of the six residents receive $157.50/month from Supplemental Security Income. At first, each put half into the general fund and kept half for food and other expenses. Under FHA Section 236, the apartments cost $95.25/month; the attendants cost $200. Originally the Texas Rehabilitation Commission made up the difference, about $220. "It is much cheaper," says Brown, "to have us in a group than to fund us individually. TRC will fund us while we are in college and continue while we are looking for jobs. Our counselors have been helpful and understanding." Eventually, Goodwill Industries, through Independence Hall, took over the responsibility for both food and attendants.

CREATIVE HANDICAPS, INC.

In the spring of 1975, a group of 18 quadriplegic young people, most of them from nursing homes, and several concerned professional persons, set up a nonprofit corporation, Creative Handicaps, Inc. (Mrs. Irene Sarbor, RN, Project Supervisor, 7001 Hillcroft, Houston, 70036), to share expenses in the Springtree Apartments in southwest Houston. The 14 apartments, all on the ground floor, required little modification except the installation of an intercom system.

The attendants consist of five full-time employees, four of whom live in, and three part-time employees. In addition, Homemakers/Chore Service, sponsored by Medicare, is available to 17 of the residents.

All of the disabled residents are on SSI; four of them receive social security disability payments. All 18 are on the food stamps program, and they all share food purchases. The group is trying to get the Houston Housing Authority to sponsor rent supplements; the present rents are $155 for one-bedroom apartments; $185 for two-bedroom, one-bath apartments; and $190 for two-bedroom, two-bath apartments.

Only three of the residents are involved in university studies and qualify for assistance from the Texas Rehabilitation Commission. Many attend "The University Without Walls," and many more are trying to attend the university. The group has a number of ideas for cooperative enterprises, but they lack seed money.

Transportation consists of two vans with hydraulic lifts that were given to Creative Handicaps, Inc. Most of the drivers are volunteers.

ATLANTIS COMMUNITY, INC.

Denver has become a Mecca for young disabled because of its medical facilities as well as its accessible universities. The Denver disabled population includes former patients at the Veterans Administration Hospital, Craig Rehabilitation Hospital, Children's Hospital, Sewall Rehabilitation Hospital, University of Colorado Medical Center, and Spalding Rehabilitation Center. The Community College of Denver, the University of Colorado in Boulder, and Metropolitan State College have well-organized services for their disabled students.

The result of such a concentration of disabled has been a woeful scarcity of housing and transportation facilities. Consequently, young people have been forced into nursing homes for the elderly. Though "youth wings" have been tried at two nursing homes, they have not been successful. After the newness wore off, problems erupted in the areas of funding, staffing, meals, recreation, and general morale.

Eventually the stultifying life at some of the nursing homes drove the young disabled residents to become a cohesive unit determined to achieve independent living and create opportunities to lead a meaningful life. Joining with members of other organizations for the disabled, such as the Denver Chapter of the National Paraplegia Foundation, United Cerebral Palsy Association, Muscular Dystrophy Association, Heritage House Youth Wing Council, Young Disabled Adults from Life Center, Mobility Among the Disabled, Multiple Sclerosis Society, the Denver Community Design Center, and the Mayor's Commission on the Disabled, who shared their convictions, they formed the organization, Atlantis Community, Inc., 619 South Broadway Boulevard, Denver, Colorado 80223.

Atlantis Community hopes to make disabled individuals as independent as possible and to assist them to live in the community. They are first experimenting with satellite apartments with attendant care. The long-term goal is to have a proportion of all apartments designed so that they are accessible.

The Atlantis Early Action Program (AEAP), under the direction of Ingo Antonitch, Chairman of the Board of Directors, spent a year working out details to rent seven apartments for 14 young disabled persons. The three-bedroom first floor apartments, leased from the Denver Housing Authority, are located in a 186-unit apartment complex, Las Casitas, at 11th and Federal (Fig. 10–1). Atlantis Community signed a one-year lease with the Housing Authority for the seven apartments at $83/month each. The apartments are located in the southwest part of the city, in a low income urban renewal area. They are a short distance from downtown Denver and immediately adjacent to scheduled bus service. The complex has shaded court areas between the buildings and a large recreation area which includes a basketball court. The Westside Neighborhood Health Center is located one block away. The Residents' Council of Las Casitas has met with representatives of Atlantis Community, Inc. and wholeheartedly supports the AEAP.

A screening committee, composed of both disabled and nondisabled persons, selected the residents on the basis of the individual's potential to adapt her/himself to a living environment outside of an institution. The screening committee

168   Housing and Home Services for the Disabled

Fig. 10–1. A. Atlantis Community, Inc., has rented seven satellite apartments in the one-story units of the Las Casitas complex of the Denver Housing Authority. **B.** Kitchen in one of the Atlantis Community satellite apartments. (Photographs by Dana Stanton)

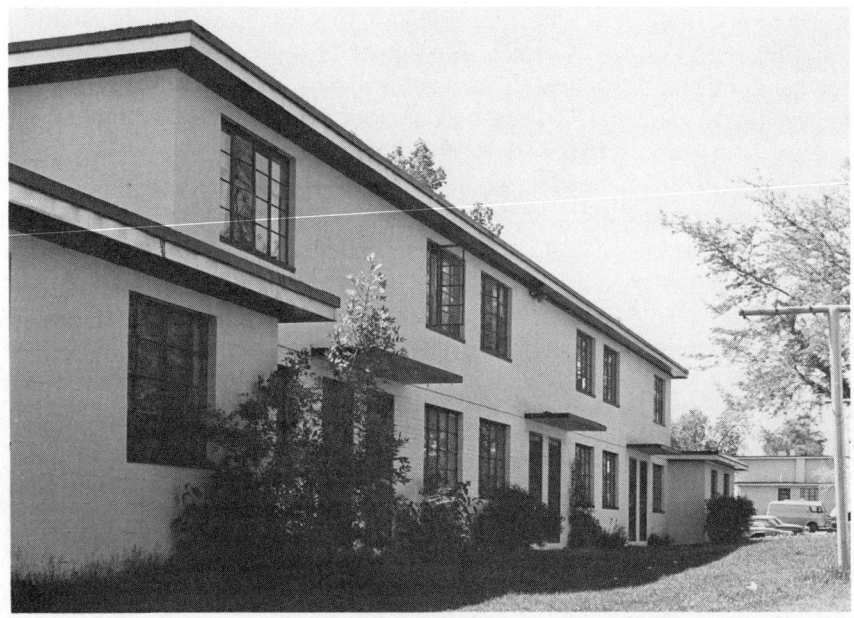

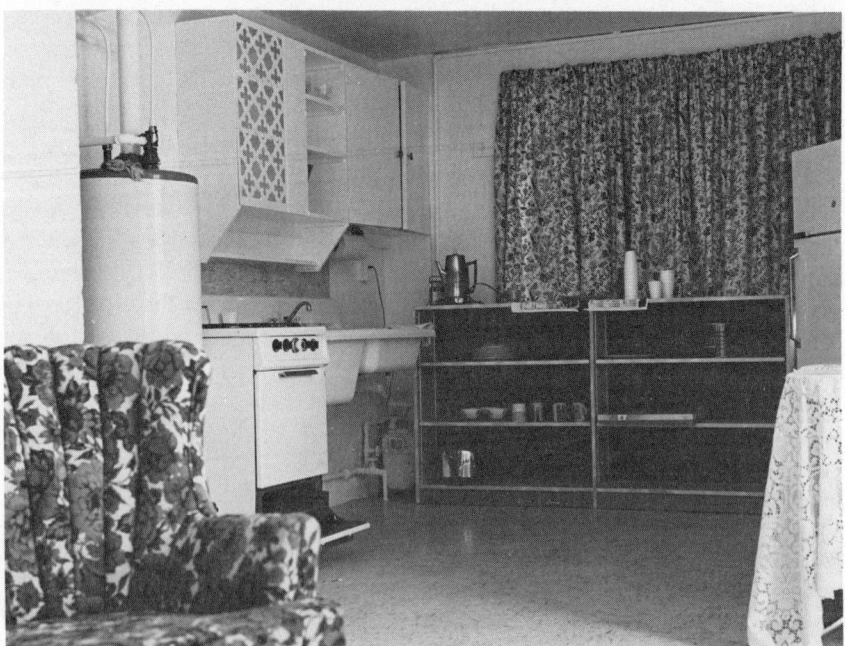

included representatives of the Colorado Department Social Services, the Division of Vocational Rehabilitation, the Denver City Council, the Denver Police Department, area rehabilitation centers, and neighborhood residents from the Las Casitas area.

The Denver Housing Authority allocated $14,000 for the renovation of the apartments, and Atlantis Community gathered furniture by public appeals and a matching grant from Colorado State Rehabilitation. The apartments, in clusters of two or three in different one-story buildings, were redecorated and made accessible with ramps. Each apartment houses two people. Each resident has a private bedroom; the third bedroom is used as a storage area for lifts and wheelchairs.

A pool of attendants is on call on a 24-hour basis with three shifts of 8 hours each. The amount of attendant care is determined on an individual basis. Each disabled person calls on the attendant pool only for the hours of service needed and is billed according to the actual time used.

Atlantis worked out arrangements with the welfare department to include home care services so that, with SSI payments, each resident has a total income of $360/month. To assist with attendants, United Way made a grant of $2400.

In addition, Atlantis Community has written proposals for a van with a raised roof and lift to take residents to their rehabilitative training, employment, schools, and for general mobility and emergencies; for an intercommunication system among the units for emergency calls for an attendant; and for special telephone equipment to set up a hotline for the Denver area, a number any severely disabled person could call for information or for emergency service.

As of the summer of 1975, Atlantis Community received a preplanning grant of $80,000 from HUD for a paid professional staff to plan a central housing and information facility. After Ingo Antonitch resigned as Chairman of the Board of Directors to become the Director of the Denver Mayor's Commission on the Disabled, Dana Stanton became chairman. Dana, who has been disabled by respiratory poliomyelitis quadriplegia since 1955, has worked for years with different groups to solve housing and attendant problems.

This combination of an umbrella organization, composed of a cohesive group of disabled individuals and representatives of community agencies, an information center, and apartments scattered in the community, has great potential.

PROJECT INDEPENDENCE

In 1972, a group of disabled young adults, most of whom lived at home and worked at a cerebral palsy center, formed the corporation, Independence for Impaired Individuals (III), 1528 Inglehart, St. Paul, Minnesota 55104. In 1974, the corporation purchased a 4-unit apartment building and converted it into two second floor rental apartments and one ten-room first floor apartment. Four of their disabled members and two student attendants moved in during the spring of 1975.

The chairperson of the corporation, LeAnne Nelson, 571 Como Avenue, St. Paul, Minnesota 55103, described the $5000 gift from the White Bear Lions Club for the down payment as the magic that made the project a reality. In addition to this gift, the corporation put on two benefit concerts which netted about $1000 and solicited donations to pay for the repairs and remodeling. Except for the plumbing, most of the work was done by volunteers. The major remodeling involved knocking out a wall between the two first floor apartments to make the ten-room apartment, installing a roll-in shower in one of the bathrooms, and building a ramp.

The house is located in a good residential district, near a shopping center and close to several colleges. Transportation to work is furnished by the United Cerebral Palsy van. The staff consists of a housekeeper who comes in during the day to clean, cook, and do the laundry and two live-in student attendants. The residents, disabled by cerebral palsy, range from ambulatory to wheelchaired and using a talk board.

The purchase price of the fourplex was $37,500. The monthly payments, including taxes, are $373; insurance is $252/year; and the vacancy allowance (1/12 of a month's rent) is $20/month. The rental income from the two second floor apartments totals $240/month.

The total cost per person for all living expenses (house payments, maintenance, utilities, attendants, housekeeper, food, and laundry) amounts to about $528/month. (Previously the state had been paying $600/month per person in nursing homes.) This includes $140 for housing, $214 for food, and $314 for attendants, part-time help, and housekeeping. The two live-in attendants are each paid $300/month, plus room and board; 32 hours a week of part-time help costs $3.50/hour; and the housekeeper is paid $3/hour for 15 hours/week. The attendants are paid by welfare through the Homemakers Service program.

All the residents receive SSI payments, food stamp allowances, and medical assistance as well as the attendance allowance.

INDEPENDENT LIVING FOR THE HANDICAPPED, INC.

The Richard S. Weinberger Fund, Inc., 9 Winthrop Street, Brooklyn, New York 11225, was started in the 1960s by the parents of disabled children "to give life to their years, not years to their lives." The Independent Living program began in 1970 when the mother of a disabled man died and he wanted to stay on in their apartment, with attendant care services, rather than being institutionalized. The Weinberger Fund eventually convinced the New York City Department of Social Services that it should fund the man and another friend who was disabled for a total of $51/day ($25.50 each) for the two of them rather than a total of $112/day ($56 each) for hospital care. (This same hospital care has more than doubled, but the men are still receiving their initial $51/day grant.)

The Weinberger Fund staff developed the experiences with these two men into a coordinated program, titled Independent Living for the Handicapped. The program is a service program to help people live as they choose. It does not involve a specific building or even specific apartment units. The staff consists of a program coordinator and two part-time employees who drive its van. Although the organization operates on an annual budget of less than $20,000, it has sponsored 22 apartment units spread throughout New York City. A total of 37 people live in these apartments, and of them only two, a married couple, decided they wanted to live in a building exclusively for the elderly and disabled. Of the 37 people, 80% are under 40.

The program fosters total integration because, according to Nick Pagano, former coordinator, "it is so much easier for one person in a wheelchair to make friends with people who are not in wheelchairs if he is the only one in that building who happens to be in a wheelchair."

Pagano defines the Independent Living program: "It is the coordination of basic community and social services in such a way that the severely physically disabled and mentally alert person can live as a member of the community of his choice." The organization provides the following services:

1. Counseling advocacy service
2. Friendly visiting
3. Personal assistance. The organization acts as an ombudsman to expedite a personal assistance program. The New York State Medical Assistance Program, Medicaid, provides that anyone who needs a housekeeper or home health aide can get one by establishing the need through a doctor's certificate and meeting financial eligibility requirements. Need must be reviewed biannually by the Visiting Nurse Service. Many of the aides are found among the foreign born who are looking for a job and a place to stay and who are willing to work at low salaries.
4. Emergency aide service. The disabled tenants compiled a list of friends, volunteers, and nursing services in the city that can be counted on in acute emergencies.
5. Transportation. The Weinberger Fund provides a subsidized livery service for $1 round trip that costs the Fund $20.
6. Group therapy sessions. Tenants meet periodically to discuss ways of becoming more independent.

BIRD S. COLER HOSPITAL PILOT STUDY

In this pilot study at Bird S. Coler Hospital (Ronald F. Green, MD, Bird S. Coler Hospital, Roosevelt Island, New York 10015), patients were discharged to Goodwill Terrace apartments in Queens, New York, a low rent specially adapted apartment building combined with a sheltered workshop in the basement, and four moved to modified apartments in a public housing project. The patients, ranging in age 39–64, were disabled by hemiplegia, amputation, peripheral neuropathy, and quadriparesis; they had all been hospitalized for periods of up to 2 years.

Before the patients were discharged they were evaluated by a team consisting of a physiatrist, an occupational therapist, a physical therapist, a social worker, and a psychologist. In addition to making the evaluations, the team visited the apartments, and modifications were carried out as needed.

172   Housing and Home Services for the Disabled

One year after they had been discharged, the patients were reevaluated. Factors considered included social readjustment, use of special equipment, including prosthetic and orthotic devices, changes in medical status, and maintenance of functional level. With the exception of one patient who had to return to the hospital for treatment of a progressive disease, all had continued to function successfully in their apartments and had maintained or improved their functional levels. None desired to return to the hospital.

The study concluded that the provision of suitably modified living facilities for physically disabled persons within the community appears to be a promising alternative to long-term institutionalization.

HANDICAPPED ADULTS ASSOCIATION, INC. IN CO-OP CITY

The disabled residents of Co-op City formed a nonprofit educational and charitable organization in June, 1973 (Anna Capell, 100-5 DeKraif Place, Bronx, New York 10475). They are apartment dwellers of Co-op City, the largest cooperative housing development in the world (Fig. 10–2). Interspersed throughout the area are 35 high-rise apartment buildings, 28–33 stories high, and about 200 townhouses. The three community centers, which are entirely accessible, contain shops, health services, libraries, and meeting rooms.

Fig. 10–2. Co-op City accommodates 60,000 residents in 15,000 apartments. The 300-acre development contains extensive parks and is accessible through graded curb crossings and level terrain and entrances.

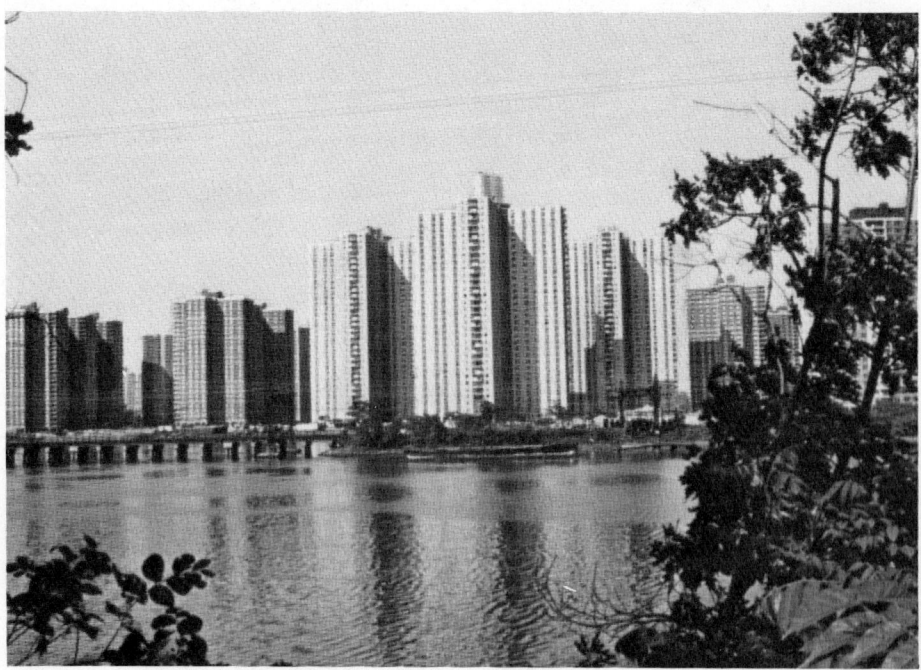

The Handicapped Adults Association consists of 75 active members with a wide assortment of disabilities: multiple sclerosis, muscular dystrophy, epilepsy, cerebral palsy, blindness, diabetes, and arthritis. Some require attendant care and receive assistance from public or private agencies. The organization concentrates its efforts on achieving legislation to attain public homemaker services for the homebound, suitable public transportation, tax considerations, and barrier-free architecture.

PUBLIC HOUSING

Beginning in 1970, public housing authorities were enjoined by HUD to provide some design features for the disabled in 10% of the units of all projects built for the elderly (PG46—Minimum Property Standards for Housing for the Elderly, with Special Consideration for the Handicapped). The relevant HUD directive reads as follows: "Fixtures in bathrooms of at least 10% of the living units of each type . . . shall be arranged and space provided to permit access and use by a person in a wheelchair."

HUD also requires a minimum of 10% of "Turnkey" units, under which most federal public housing is being built, to follow PG46 and to have accessible public areas and accessible bathrooms. No provisions are made for other special design features. The requirement of accessible bathrooms and public areas, however, applies only to facilities which are designated for occupancy by the elderly or the disabled, have an elevator, and consist of 25 or more units within a single structure.

Public housing has both advantages and disadvantages for the disabled. The best feature, of course, is the low rent. However, integration with the elderly is more satisfactory when the disabled are middle-aged rather than when they are in their 20s and there are the normal conflicts between generations. Further, it can be traumatic if a young disabled person must move out as soon as he has completed his training and starts to earn a living that is beyond the income limitation.

Basically, public housing is designed for elderly and disabled people who can live independently. However, the experiences of the housing authorities with all ages of people have been that a range of social services is a necessary component of all housing. Some housing authorities allow considerable leeway to take into account the expenses of disability. For instance, if a person needs attendant care, some or all of the amount may be deducted before calculating income and some housing authorities furnish a bedroom for the attendant. Nevertheless, there should be a nationwide increase in the allowances for disabled individuals to compensate for the expenses that accompany disability.

MASSACHUSETTS PUBLIC HOUSING AND SERVICE PROGRAMS

The cooperation of state and federal agencies with the Boston Housing Authority and the Massachusetts Council of Organizations of the Handicapped (MCOH) has resulted in an innovative program adapting public housing for the elderly to the disabled and providing a range of services. Concurrently, legislation effective January, 1971, providing that a minimum of 5% of state-aided housing built for the elderly must be designed and made available to disabled persons, regardless of their age, has resulted in several hundred accessible units all over Massachusetts. Much of the credit for this legislation goes to the very important cooperation of the Massachusetts Coalition of the Elderly and Handicapped (MCEH), which was formed through the melding of common interests of the Legislative Council for Older Americans, the MCOH, and other organizations of the disabled.

The story behind the Boston Housing Authority (BHA) program is told by Harold Remmes, former president of MCOH, in *Rehabilitation Record* in 1972. According to Remmes, the program began when Glen E. Gresham, MD, assumed the position of project director of the Tufts–New England School of Medicine Research and Training Center (R&T-7) in Boston. His vital interest in the problems of the disabled led him to the Massachusetts Association of Paraplegics and their work with MCOH towards solutions of housing problems.

The first step was a committee consisting of representatives from HUD, Social and Rehabilitation Services, MCOH, BHA, the Department of Public Welfare, the Massachusetts Rehabilitation Commission, and other concerned agencies. A three-pronged project was initiated: 1) identify persons living in BHA facilities who have mobility or functional impairments; 2) select a small number of families to relocate in BHA facilities made accessible through funds from R&T-7; and 3) study the lifestyles of selected families before and after the removal of architectural barriers.

After more than a year of negotiating between BHA, MCOH, and R&T-7, it was agreed that R&T-7 would provide the funding for the staff and for the physical changes in the selected apartments, while BHA would provide staff time and painting of the apartments.

The identification of those in BHA with mobility problems was conducted through the mail by sending 15,000 letters, in both Spanish and English, to the tenants of BHA facilities. The tenants were asked to contact the R&T center if he or members of his family had mobility problems. Following tenant response, those who seemed eligible were screened by telephone and were then visited in their homes. Of 150 responses, 10 were considered to have qualifying mobility problems.

A Unique Plan

"What is unique about this plan," says Remmes, "is that it documents for the first time a rationale for allowing the local housing authorities to request additional funds in their operating budgets to service the needs of their disabled tenants (for changes in the physical plant). . . . Since the project requires the cooperation of several departments, it serves to move the authority one step further away from the 'bricks and mortar' tradition and into line with their current policy of providing ameliorated services through cooperation with outside local service providers."

Handicapped Services Center

By December, 1973, the Boston Housing Authority had established a Handicapped Services Center at 1701 Washington Street, Boston, Massachusetts 02118. The office has two full-time staff members, both of whom are wheelchaired: Harold Remmes, Handicapped Services Specialist; and Vivienne Thomson, Handicapped Services Aide. The facility is adjacent to public transportation and completely accessible, with parking space in the rear. Here applications are taken, interviews conducted, and supportive services coordinated. All applicants are processed by BHA's Handicapped Services Center; eligibility is determined, application filed, medical documentation secured. Rent computation and assignment to a facility are then processed by the Tenant Selection Department.

Criteria of Eligibility

The criteria of eligibility are 1) the disabled person or his family must benefit from the specific types of housing, supportive services, or equipment available; 2) the applicant must be able to function independently or have an attendant; 3) the individual must meet the usual income limitations with extra exemptions for special needs related to the degree of handicap; 4) it must be certified by a physician that the physical or mental impairment is of continued duration and will improve or remain stable in suitable housing; and 5) the applicant must qualify because of at least one of the following impairments: use a wheelchair, walker, braces, or crutches; walk with difficulty because of arthritis, spasticity, or pulmonary or cardiac conditions; be insecure because of impaired sight or hearing; be so frail he needs special housekeeping services; or have addictions, frailties, developmental disabilities or emotional disturbances which make it impossible to live independently in conventional housing.

The program at the Handicapped Services Center moves quietly forward, meeting problems on a one-to-one basis. Much of the success is due to the creativity, resourcefulness, warmth, and enthusiasm of the two directors of the program; BHA, though constrained by regulations, is making a sincere effort to meet the needs of its disabled tenants through innovative methods. To date, the program has had numerous exciting success stories; for instance, a 22-year-old who had spent most of his life in a rest home for the elderly is now attending college and taking care of his own needs; a wheelchaired housewife no longer requires a homemaker because she can now cook her own meals on a lowered electric range; and a single man can get himself in and out of bed with a hydraulic lift and maintain himself in his own apartment with a minimum of assistance.

The directors of the Handicapped Services Center report that the average age of the disabled whom the program has placed in apartments is 23. Paraplegia and cerebral palsy are the most common disabilities. Though they have observed a tremendous divergence in the lifestyles of the young and elderly, the young have tried to conform to the majority. The directors are looking forward to better housing alternatives when it will no longer be necessary to put young disabled persons in an elderly environment.

Conclusion

The Handicapped Services Center has been instrumental in placing 150 disabled persons in the one-bedroom wheelchaired apartments; adaptations and equipment furnished have included entrance ramps, hydraulic lifts, raised toilet seats, lowered stoves, cabinets, and sinks, closed circuit TV, and grab bars. In addition, maximal advantage is taken of available medical and homemaker services from local institutions and agencies. These physical adaptations are financed by the BHA and installed as a part of the construction cost.

Meanwhile, the Massachusetts Department of Community Affairs, which is responsible for enforcing the law requiring at least 5% of all low rent housing for the elderly to be available to disabled persons, reports that it has made 400 specially designed units available to the disabled and hopes to have a total of 600 completed by the close of 1975. The Department of Community Affairs emphasizes that the best way for a disabled person to find suitable housing is to contact his local housing authority to determine if he is eligible for suitable housing and to get his name on the waiting list early.

HANDBOOK FOR HOUSING THE HANDICAPPED IN PUBLIC HOUSING FACILITIES by Harold S. Remmes. The purpose of this informative little booklet is to acquaint local housing officials with some of the specialized requirements of the disabled. It should be required reading for all local housing officials. The booklet suggests administrative actions to alleviate the housing problems of the disabled: 1) liberalize income requirements to balance the extra expenses caused by disability, 2) assign knowledgeable staff to deal with the disabled, and 3) make all future construction accessible to and usable by the disabled.

NEW COMPLEX WITH 40% FOR THE DISABLED

"On May 7, 1975," according to Remmes, "the Massachusetts Housing and Finance Company approved funding for a 124-unit housing complex in Brookline. The building will cost several million dollars and 40% of the apartments will be for the disabled. This will be a building (nonelderly) with an economic mix of low, middle income and market price units (Section 236). Developer is the Tamboni–Bennett Corporation of Reading and the partner, without financial responsibility but with income from the project as well as providing expertise, is the Massachusetts Council of Organizations of the Handicapped."

TANYA TOWERS

Tanya Towers, 620 East 13 Street, New York City, New York 10009, is the accomplishment of Tanya Nash, retired executive director of the New York Society for the Deaf. She conceived the project because the deaf are excluded from facilities built for the elderly. The 136-unit apartment building, sponsored by the New York Society for the Deaf, was financed through a city Mitchell–Lama mortgage for aged deaf of moderate income. The developer found the site for Tanya Towers ideal for the project: the parcels of land were vacant lots; it is a slum area, zoned for urban renewal; and it is near its sponsor. It was the first and only project to be given a 100% mortgage guarantee. A private minibus is proposed to overcome transportation problems; it needs improved internal and external security measures, as well as more involvement by local community centers and cultural and health services.

INTEGRATED APARTMENTS WITHOUT SUPPORTIVE SERVICES

PRIVATELY BUILT APARTMENTS

In 1962, a private builder, Rose Associates, included 14 specially designed apartments in a middle-income housing project, Evergreen Apartments, 955 Evergreen Avenue, Bronx, New York 10472. In addition to several studio apartments there are one-, two- and three-bedroom units. The living rooms are airy and spacious; the bathrooms are extra large and equipped with handrails; the kitchens have low work counters and refrigerators; and all doors are wide enough to accommodate wheelchairs.

LEASED HOUSING UNDER SECTION 8

Disabled individuals or groups of disabled considering cooperative arrangements should contact their local housing authority to find out what is available with rent supplements, not only in apartment buildings built for the elderly but in a wide variety of accommodations. Many of the housing authorities around the country have been both helpful and creative in working with groups of disabled to meet local needs.

Under the Section 202 direct loan program authorized by the Housing and Community Development Act of 1974, all 202 developers must apply for and receive rental subsidies. Section 8 (formerly Section 23), authorizes HUD to provide housing assistance payments on behalf of eligible persons for occupancy of new construction, rehabilitation of older housing, or existing rental housing. Payments are made directly to owners (who may be private owners, nonprofit entities, cooperatives, or public housing agencies). This payment will make up the difference between the HUD-approved rent for the unit (at fair market value) and the amount the tenant must pay, which is not less than 15% nor more than 25% of the tenant's adjusted income. Eligible tenants are those who, at the time of the initial renting, have total family incomes not more than 80% of the area median income.

To sum up, if a prospective tenant is at least 62 years of age or disabled and meets the income and other requirements, the housing authority may rent an apartment or house at the going rate, which must be within the limitations set by HUD. The landlord has three options under which he may rent to the housing authority: the landlord selects the tenants; the authority selects the tenants with landlord approval; the authority rents to anyone it selects. HUD pays the full amount of the rent to the landlord, and the tenant pays 15–25% of his adjusted income to the housing authority. Example: an individual has an adjusted income of $4000; he pays 20% or $800 a year rent on a $150 a month apartment and the housing authority pays the difference between the $66 a month and the $150.

As an example, the Housing Authority of Portland, Oregon, has made creative use of the former Section 23 and present Section 8 programs to provide rent payments for groups of young disabled in private buildings scattered throughout the city rather than in identifiable housing for the disabled. The Authority works closely with the local Easter Seal Society and Cerebral Palsy Association. The voluntary agencies raise the funds to cover the rehabilitation/remodeling costs to make the various buildings accessible and adaptable to the needs of the disabled. In return the Authority arranges for the rent assistance payments and gives the agencies priority in placing their disabled young people, usually under age 35, thus bypassing the 5000 people on the waiting list for existing housing.

United Cerebral Palsy Association of Oregon has set up a number of similar group home programs for independent living. The agency utilizes outside resources such as public welfare and visiting nurses and holds weekly classes at which the staff occupational therapist instructs the tenants in matters relating to their independent living experiences, such as checking accounts, food buying and preparing, and budgets.

The complexities of Section 8 are clarified in the publication, *Answers to Questions on Section 8 Lower Income Housing Assistance Under the Housing and Community Development Act of 1974. A Guidebook,* by Thomas A. Duvall and Edward White. The 65-page book is available from the National Association of Housing and Redevelopment Officials (NAHRO).

SUBSIDIZED 236 HOUSING

Housing facilities built under Section 236 provide housing for those with a variety of economic backgrounds. In each of the subsidized programs, there are specific eligibility requirements relating to income, family composition, etc. To qualify, a tenant must not exceed the income limits established for the particular community. The tenant's contribution is based on a proportion of adjusted gross income. Although one of the eligibility factors is physical disability, the apartments are not necessarily suitable for wheelchair use.

Lakewood Plaza

Lakewood Plaza, 5631 Tidewater Drive, Norfolk, Virginia 23509, is a privately owned 14-floor high-rise for the elderly whose first floor apartments have been reserved for the disabled. Occupancy is open to those who are 62 or older and the disabled. There are only two types of apartments, one bedroom ($214.84/month or $74 under rent supplement) and the studio ($179.80 or $62 under rent supplement). Rent includes kitchen equipment and all utilities. All the bathroom and bedroom doors are wide enough for a wheelchair; the walks are ramped; and there are emergency call systems from every apartment and a closed circuit TV to check callers in the lobby. All the apartments have an oversized balcony with views of the adjacent river or park. The apartments are unfurnished, and there are no special services available within the complex.

Elmwood Park Tower

Elmwood Park Tower, Chene at Lafayette, Detroit, Michigan, is an 18-story apartment tower for the elderly which opened in November, 1974. Located in the midst of a shopping center, it has 202 one-bedroom apartments with 12 apartments per floor. Two on each floor are designed for the disabled. These special units have wide doors to admit wheelchairs and grab bars in the bathrooms. All apartments have special alarm switches in the baths and bedrooms. Built under the Section 236 subsidy program, persons with moderate income pay only one-fourth of their monthly incomes.

Wyandotte Co-op Apartments

When the tenants of the Wyandotte Co-op Apartments have a complaint, they get action because the tenants are also the management for the 11-story, 161-unit building opposite the Wyandotte General Hospital. The apartments were built by Cooperative Services, Inc., a Detroit-based nonprofit consumers' cooperative established in 1942. All the tenants are members of the cooperative. To join, an individual buys into the cooperative's businesses with a $1 entrance fee, and for an additional $100, which can be paid over a 10-year period, becomes a voting member. The apartments are financed on low interest federal loans under a special citizens program and rents average $66–$77 for a studio apartment, and $77–$89 for a one-bedroom apartment. All services including lights and heat are included in the rent payments. The cooperative has been so successful that another apartment building has been built in Wyandotte, and proposals to build similar apartment projects in southwest Detroit, Highland Park, Allen Park, Wayne, Royal Oak, and Kalamazoo are being studied. In addition to the apartment, the cooperative operates a low cost optical service for its nearly 12,000 members.

Ocean Village

This complex of 11 apartment buildings, managed by U/A Management Corporation, 1921 Mott Avenue, Far Rockaway, New York 11691, is located on the Atlantic Ocean, on Rockaway Beach Boulevard between B.56th Place and B.59th Street at Far Rockaway. A dramatic construction by Carl Koch & Associates, Inc., it has a campuslike atmosphere with shopping facilities, landscaped walkways, and children's play areas. The housing program was developed by the New York State Urban Development Corporation, which was created by the State of New York to provide housing and community facilities in cooperation with local governments and/or nonprofit community organizations.

Built under the Section 236 program, the Ocean Village apartments provide housing for families of varied economic backgrounds under their 70-20-10 formula: 1) 70% of the housing is reserved for families whose adjusted income is approximately $9000–$17,000/year, who pay 25% of their income as rent but no less than the basic 236 rent; 2) 20% is reserved for families whose adjusted income is less than $10,000, who pay 25% of their income for rent, and who are disabled or at least 62 years old—thus an efficiency apartment whose 236 rental is $172 could be rented for $51 for a single person with an income of $6000; and 3) 10% for those 62 or over who will pay rent based upon their income.

ACCESSIBLE HOUSING IN ROSWELL, NEW MEXICO

Ralph Markward, a veteran, has been wheelchaired by traumatic paraplegia for 24 years and rheumatoid arthritis for the last 5 years. When he moved to New Mexico in 1970 he found Roswell extremely difficult for a wheelchaired person and decided to change the environment. He worked with the Zia Chapter of the Paralyzed Veterans of America (PVA) and James Macfarland, a nondisabled retired foreign service officer; they concentrated on state legislation and publicity through newspaper articles written by Macfarland.

According to Markward,

"Roswell now has over 60 ramps built by businessmen. It has three accessible motels—Motel Six, Frontier Motel, and Roswell Inn, and 17 restaurants a wheelchaired person can get into alone from the parking lot, although not all the rest rooms are accessible. . . . It is possible now to do one's own thing without people staring. In other words, people in Roswell accept you for what you are. Roswell, in the last election, elected a postpolio quadriplegic to the New Mexico House of Representatives.

While senior citizens apartment complexes are fine for the elderly and those young people who desire them or have no other choice, they leave a lot to be desired for young people in their 20s. I am 49 years young and have lived with senior citizens most of my disabled 23 years, so I have learned to adjust.

Here are some senior citizens apartment complexes in Roswell:

Sunset 1600 Apartment complex, 1600 Sunset Avenue, Roswell, New Mexico, 88201, is a 60-unit, one-story garden type complex for senior citizens and the disabled. It is privately owned with a FHA-guaranteed loan. Ten percent of the apartments were designed for wheelchairs and while they are not perfect, they are accessible. The subsidized rent for an efficiency apartment is $100 unfurnished and $117 furnished, if the income for a single person is no more than $4700; otherwise the rent would be $132 without subsidy.

Sunny Acres apartment complex, 1414 South Union Street, Roswell, New Mexico 88201, is a 97-unit complex with one-, two-bedroom, and efficiency apartments (Fig. 10–3). All are accessible; residents must be 62 years old or be disabled. For an extra charge, the apartments are rented furnished.

Roswell Housing Authority, 2 West Byrne, Roswell Industrial Air Center, Roswell, New Mexico 88201, manages the 785 one-, two-, three-, and four-bedroom homes at the former Walker Air Force Base, which was closed in 1967. Most of these homes are accessible in that they all have 32 in. wide bathroom doors (somebody goofed). These homes rent $95–$140, including all utilities.

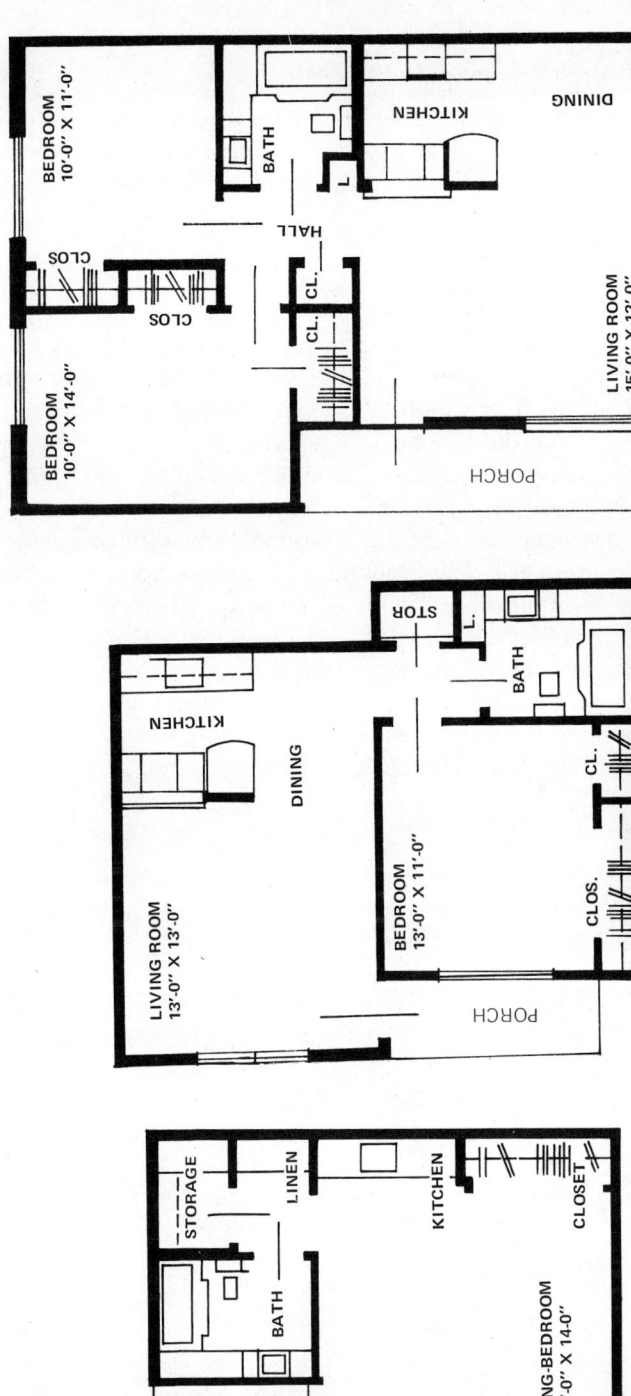

Fig. 10-3. Sunny Acres Senior Center in Roswell, New Mexico.

182   Housing and Home Services for the Disabled

Information on help and attendants and costs may be obtained from Chaves County Home Health Service, Inc., 216 East Jefferson, Roswell, New Mexico 88201. The local newspaper is the *Roswell Daily Record,* 2301 North Main Street.

BARRIER-FREE APARTMENTS

A 90-unit accessible and adaptable apartment building at 2100 Bloomington Avenue, in Minneapolis, Minnesota 55404, is one of the best organized projects in the country (Fig. 10–4). Its nonprofit sponsor is backed by the United Handicap Federation, 1951 University Avenue, St. Paul, Minnesota 55104. The major credit for the project is due to the architect, John A. Myklebust, 400 Clifton Avenue, Minneapolis, Minnesota 55403, who orchestrated the specialized design, the financing, and the organization of the sponsoring nonprofit corporation.

The project is an outstanding example of cooperation from the Minneapolis Housing and Redevelopment Authority, which cleared the land for development, and the Model City Physical Environment Corps, which approved additional bonus funds for many of the special design features.

The sponsors of the project are: 21st and Bloomington Nonprofit Housing Corporation (backed by United Handicap Federation), the Greater Minneapolis Metropolitan Housing Corporation (GMMHC) (established in 1971 by the Min-

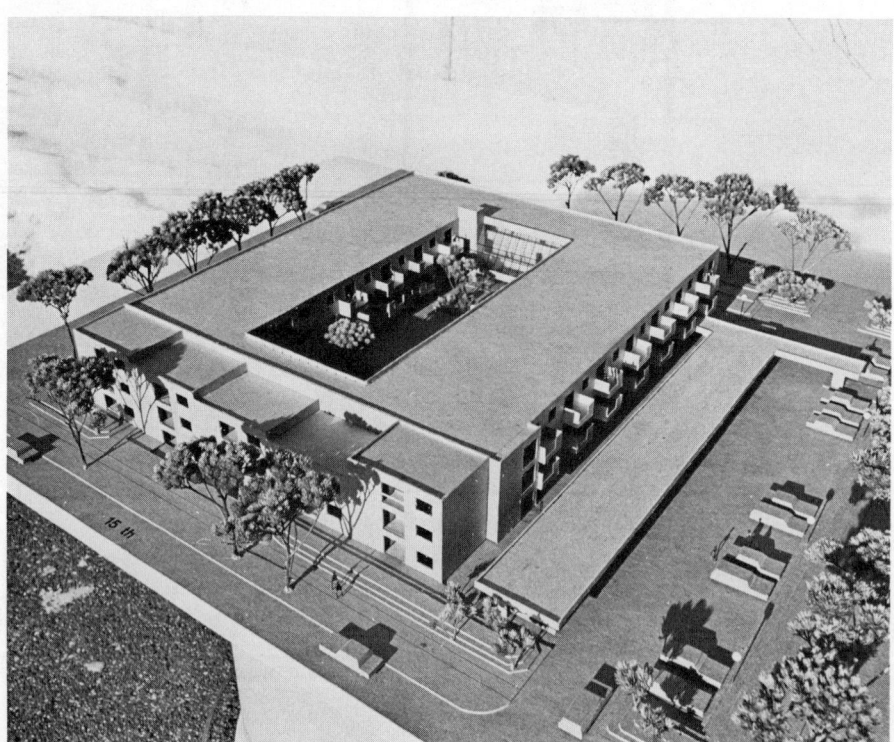

A

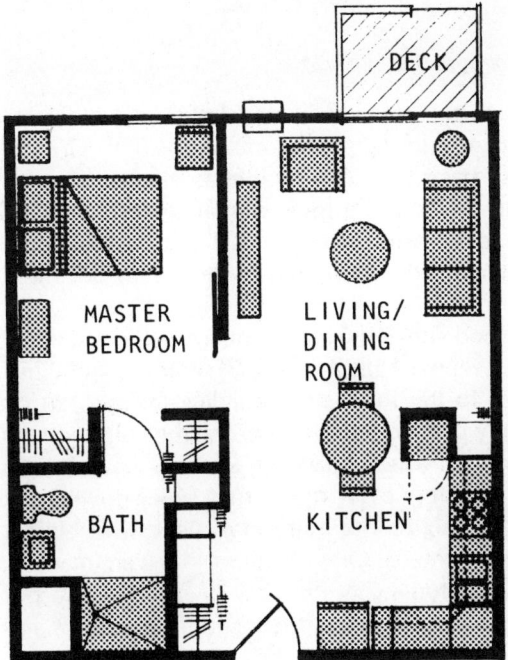

One Bedroom Unit

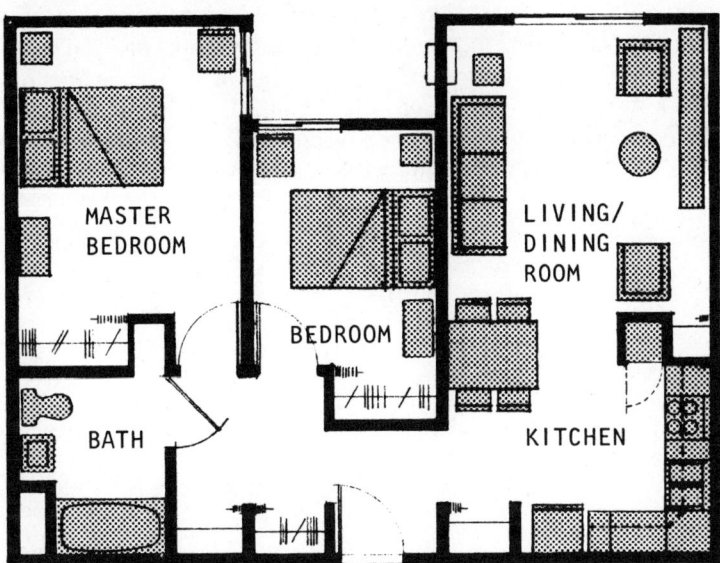

B ## Two Bedroom Unit

Fig. 10–4. A. The United Handicapped Federation, a coalition of over 3000 disabled persons and 30 organizations, backed the non-profit sponsor of this 90-unit accessible and adaptable apartment building, which was opened in the summer of 1975. **B.** The project is geared to those with low to moderate incomes in excess of the public housing limitations. With 236 subsidy, the 61 one-bedroom apartments rent for $145 month; the 29 two-bedroom units rent for $170 month. (Plans and photographs supplied by JA Myklebust, Architect)

neapolis business community to generate low income housing), National Housing Partnership, and Dan J. Brutger, Inc. (general contractor). Both GMMHC and National Housing Partnership have the considerable assets that were essential to the implementation of the project. The total estimated development cost is $1,976,402. The financing was arranged through the Minnesota Housing Finance Agency, with GMMHC providing the "front-end" money to get the project started.

The brick building with a wood veneer is situated on a one block parcel of land surrounded by Bloomington Avenue, 15th Avenue, 21st Street, and 22nd Street in south Minneapolis. Access to the three-story building includes an elevator, special wide stairs, and a gently pitched indoor ramp. All the units in the building are accessible and usable from a wheelchair. The kitchens have open spaces under the range, sink, and counter; oven doors that swing to the side; and counters that are adjustable in height. The bathrooms have wheel-in showers, adjustable mirrors, and special bathtubs. Other features that were made possible through the bonus funds of the Model City Physical Environment Corp include the security system, power-operated doors, carpeting in the corridors and living units, and the addition of the community room.

A nonprofit management group, called Cooperative Management Services, manages, maintains, and provides the social services of the housing project.

In the spring of 1975, the individuals behind the development of United Handicap Federation–Apartment Associates, Inc. (UHF–AA), formed a nonprofit corporation called the National Handicapped Housing Institute, Inc. (NHHI) for the purpose of establishing barrier-free multifamily housing under the Section 8 program of HUD. According to Michael J. Bjerkesett, the dynamic paraplegic staff director, the corporation plans to develop high density housing in two other cities in Minnesota in 1975 and eventually to develop projects in other parts of the country.

Bibliography

Accessible Housing for Boston's Disabled. By Harold S. Remmes. REHABILITATION RECORD, Vol. 13, No. 6, pages 24–26, Nov-Dec, 1972.

ANSWERS TO QUESTIONS ON SECTION 8 LOWER INCOME HOUSING ASSISTANCE UNDER THE HOUSING AND COMMUNITY DEVELOPMENT ACT OF 1974. A GUIDEBOOK. By Thomas A. Duvall and Edward White. 65 pages. National Association of Housing and Redevelopment Officials, 2600 Virginia Avenue, N.W., Washington, D.C. 20037. $8. (NAHRO members, $5). 1975.

HOUSING ADJUSTMENTS FOR DISABLED PERSONS. By Harold S. Remmes. 1974. Order from Massachusetts Department of Community Affairs, 100 Cambridge Street, Boston, Massachusetts 02202. Free.

Housing for the Disabled: A Follow-Up Study, By R. F. Green, M. Silver, C. Hinterbuchner, ARCHIVES OF PHYSICAL MEDICINE AND REHABILITATION 55:10 447–449, Oct 1974.

Individual Apartments, Long term. By Nick Pagano. HOUSING ALTERNATIVES FOR HANDICAPPED ADULTS. Conference on Housing for the Handicapped sponsored by New York City Chapters of National Association of Social Workers and National Rehabilitation Association. pages 55–57 April, 1974.

Tanya Towers, By Benjamin Gastel, HOUSING ALTERNATIVES FOR HANDICAPPED ADULTS. Proceedings of a Conference, New York City, pages 20–22, April, 1974.

Utilizing Sec. 23 to Provide Housing for the Handicapped in Portland, Oregon. By Judith Londahl. PROCEEDINGS OF NATIONAL CONFERENCE ON HOUSING AND THE HANDICAPPED. Bethesda, Maryland, Health and Education Resources, Inc., 1974.

"Wherever there are human wills and emotions, differing personalities, varying degrees of maturity and spiritual desire, there will be problems. It's how we work them out that counts."

—Donna Rosen, disabled resident of Christian League for the Handicapped

11
Long-Term Residential Facilities

PROJECTS BY DISABLED INDIVIDUALS

The following two projects, one by a disabled individual and the other by an organization of disabled individuals, represent an incredible amount of determination and independence of spirit. Both are privately funded by scrounging for donations and by fighting for monies through endless sales, bazaars, raffles, and fairs. Between them they have 33 years of experience in group psychology, problem-solving, and tightrope walking. They are invaluable sources of practical information.

FREEDOM GARDENS FOR THE HANDICAPPED, INC.

Freedom Gardens, Strawberry Road, Lake Mohegan, New York 10547, attests to the extraordinary fortitude and zest of its founder, Mrs. Lillian Petock Crowley, who is disabled by muscular dystrophy. The project had its beginnings in 1958 when Mrs. Crowley, facing institutionalization because of her mother's death, gathered a small group of adults and formed a nonprofit organization to establish a home for severely disabled persons in which they could share the costs of attendants. Their money-raising activities involved telephoning friends and neighbors to ask for discarded clothing and household materials which could be picked up, repaired, and sold.

By 1962, they had raised enough money to make a down payment on a former resort colony of nine frame buildings on a 6-acre piece of land that included a swimming pool and a brook at Mohegan Lake. (Eventually, one acre of land with two bungalows had to be sold to pay off a mortgage.)

Then began the first of a series of setbacks: the rejection of a request for a special use permit by the local zoning board. After 11 months and a Supreme Court ruling, the group received a favorable verdict with the proviso that the home be run as a cooperative apartment complex, not a nursing or convalescent care home, and that all structures comply with codes relating to multiple type residences.

Another major setback was the refusal by the state welfare office to place any persons receiving welfare funds in the facility because the buildings were not fireproof. However, this ruling was relaxed when Mrs. Crowley cited several examples of disabled people on welfare living in wooden buildings. As a compromise, it was agreed that the social workers will not inform a client about Freedom

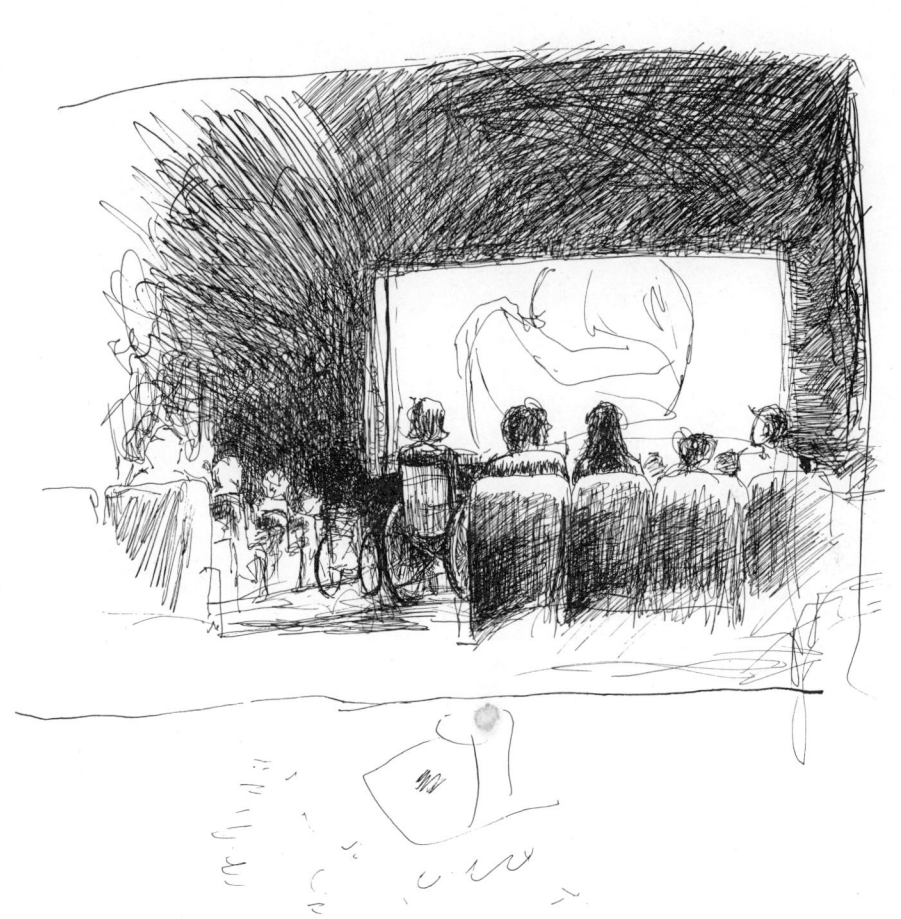

Gardens, but they will not prevent a client from moving there if he so chooses.

At present, ten of the apartment cottages are being used; eight are rented, one is used as a communal recreation room, and one is an office. The present tenants are disabled by poliomyelitis, emphysema, muscular dystrophy, nervous disorders, and back conditions. Rents are $155/month for the studio apartments and $225 for the two-bedroom apartments. Attendants are $3/hour for each working hour. Food purchases are pooled and no average amounts are available.

When Mrs. Crowley was asked what advice she would give to others who might be planning a housing project, she said,

Don't! There are too many problems. Money is the biggest: I had to create all this atmosphere so I could be earning my salt. If I had had the money for an attendant I could have stayed peacefully back in Yonkers instead of "working" without a salary 7 days a week on Freedom Gardens since 1958.

People are the next big problem: first, the neighbors fought having Freedom Gardens here—"a home for the poor disabled is a fine idea—some place else." Then, the tenant-to-tenant relationships can be awful. The polios don't want to live with the cerebral palsied; the earlier tenants glare at the newer tenants and say about each other, "that person doesn't belong here, she should be in a nursing home."

We also have a big problem with attendants, especially those paid by the state. As far as I know I am the only disabled person in New York State that does the vouchering for my own attendant. If the state pays for attendant care, the individual has nothing to do with the payment. A vendor paper is filled out and the attendant sends it to the state to get the money. It is a mess. The attendant must wait 4 weeks for the first payment even if he did not work out and left after only 1 week. I negotiated all the way up until I became a vendor and could pay our attendants myself.

If a disabled person in New York State submits to a nursing home, payments by the state range $900–$1500/month. The maximum allowed this same disabled person outside the nursing home is $206/month plus up to $20/day for an attendant, provided that a doctor will certify that 24-hour care is necessary and provided that someone can be found who will be satisfactory for that amount. Home Health Aide services could be made available, but obtaining them is so complicated that the effort requires superhuman maneuvering. For instance, a licensed sitter service charges about $30/day for 24-hour attending. Organizations like Upjohn charge $35–$40/day.

My final conclusions: there should not be so much emphasis on housing, but on attendants under civil service. Under the Lillian P. Crowley plan, you would have an attendant corps throughout the U.S. just as you have a police corps. You would use this corps, just the way you call the police, and a nice uniformed person would appear on your doorstep and bathe and dress you. Sometimes I wish I had started a home for the mentally retarded, they are so much easier to please than the so-called "normal" disabled people who expect you to provide an individual Utopia; their tastes vary considerably and their needs (or what they think they need) become costly beyond imagination.

For any future Freedom Gardens to become successful, a disabled child has to start to learn to function as a human being, he has to know about hygiene, budgets, shopping, and the moral laws of an adult. I've found myself many times saying, "I am not your mother, I am your landlady." I cannot stress strongly enough that parents and teachers have the choice of conditioning any child to dependence or to expect the child to become a head of a household. Some of today's disabled adults have been protected, sheltered, and ignored for so long the best they can do is "play house."

188 Housing and Home Services for the Disabled

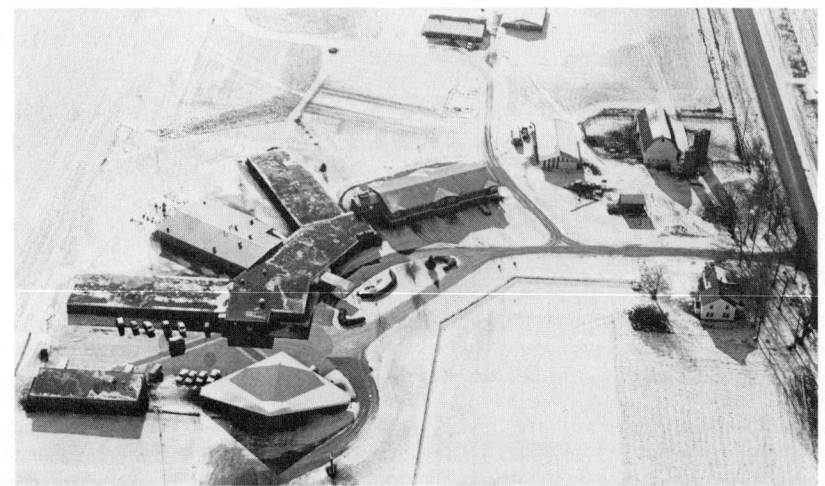

A

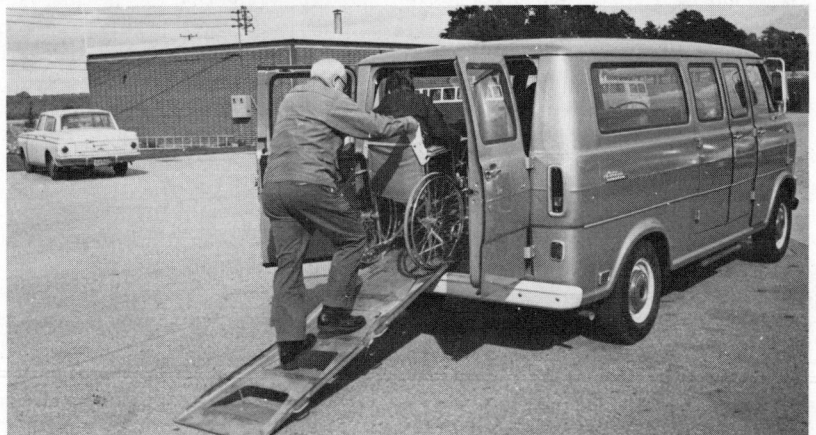

B

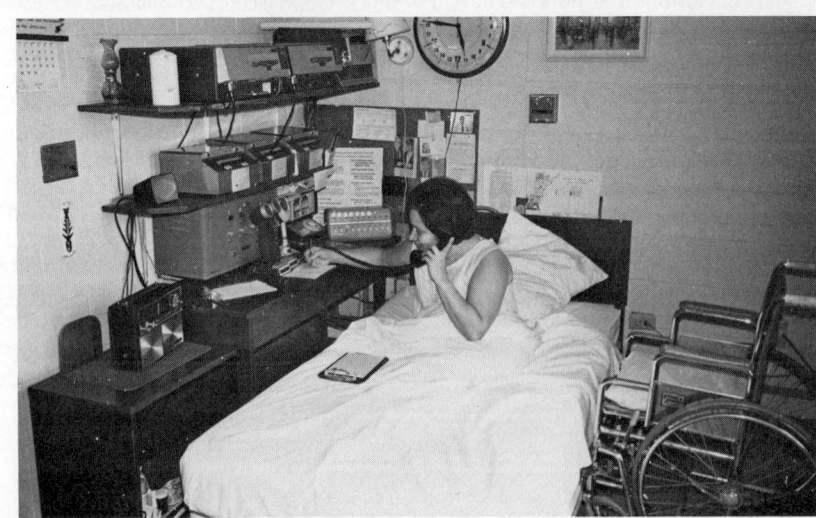

C

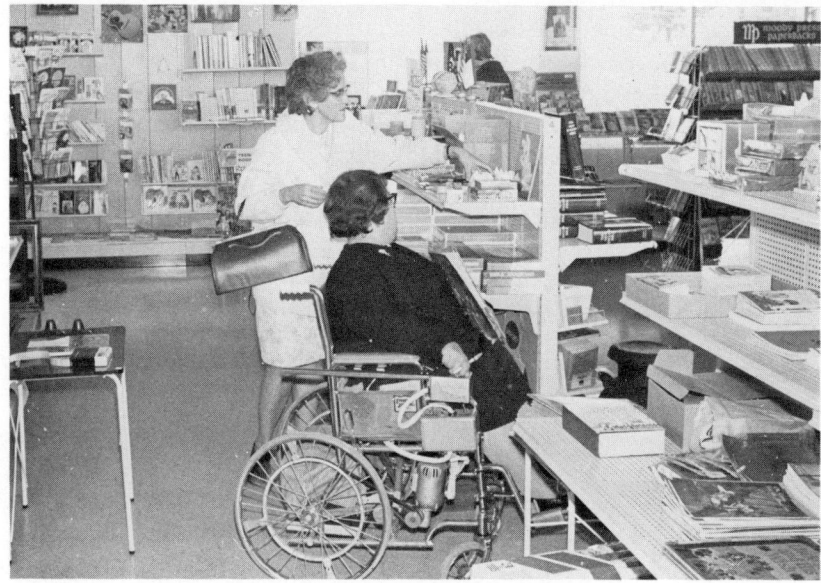

Fig. 11-1. A. An overall view of the residence building, workshop, store, apartments, therapy building, barns, and farm house of the Christian League for the Handicapped in Walworth, Wisconsin. **B.** Transportation is provided to church, shops, or entertainment. **C.** A 24-hour answering service provides employment for several of the residents. **D.** Clerk in a wheelchair waits on a customer in the gift shop. (Christian League Bulletin 12(1), 1974)

OCCUPATIONAL HOME AND APARTMENTS

Christian League for the Handicapped, P.O. Box 98, Walworth, Wisconsin 53184, is a nondenominational independent organization whose mission is the total rehabilitation of the physically disabled. Under the direction of Charles E. Pedersen, formerly a pastor with the Independent Fundamental Churches of America, its program includes Christian living, fellowship through local chapters, recreational programs, job training, and work opportunities. Founded in 1948 in Chicago, it moved to Walworth, Wisconsin, to start a camping program. Later, the organization purchased a house and church in the town of Walworth to be shared by a handful of disabled residents. The first gift shop was also opened at that same site.

In the next decade, the organization's programs were gradually developed to fill the evolving needs of its members. Without government grants or denominational support, the organization raised funds from local church groups, foundations, and bequests which enabled it to purchase 160 acres of farm land and an old frame farm house in 1959. The property is located in the midst of the wooded resort area of nearby Lake Geneva. In 1964 a resident facility for 68 persons was constructed there, along with an apartment wing and a gift shop. Later, an indoor swimming pool, a therapy wing, and an outdoor picnic patio were added (Fig. 11-1).

At present an educational and inspirational center with 27,000 sq ft of functional floor space is under construction, with the boost of a $25,000 gift from the Kresge Foundation. Week-long study camps for adults have been arranged for years at reasonable rates in the Walworth area as well as in New York and Pennsylvania. The new Walworth complex will permit the expansion of the camping program as well as the sophistication of services to the Division of Vocational Rehabilitation.

The 34 bedrooms, both single and double, are arranged with a large bathroom between; monthly rates, including meals, are $210 for double occupancy and $305 for a private room. The entrance age limits are 18–50. Attendant nursing care is available up to a maximum of 1 hour/day at a maximum charge of $100/month.

The facility is licensed as an Intermediate Care Facility, and three members of its staff (one disabled, two nondisabled) have become Nursing Home Administrators licensed by the state of Wisconsin. Meanwhile, the expansion of the project is toward more independent living apartments because the state nursing home regulations are becoming too restrictive for the young healthy disabled individuals accommodated in the bedrooms.

There are 16 apartments in the a two-story wing of the main building, served by an extra large elevator. They are unfurnished, but include stoves and refrigerators. They are leased on a lifetime basis for $12,000 or $15,000 depending on size. Maintenance costs are $52.50/month. During the summer of 1974, eight new two-bedroom apartments were added to the complex. More apartments will be built as need is indicated. All of the services and privileges offered to the home residents are available to persons living in the new apartments, including limited help or personal care through a visiting nurse plan.

Transportation is by bus or van, and the fee depends on the distance. Interaction with the nearby communities has always been encouraged through attendance at churches and through the book store and gift shop which supply Sunday and Bible School materials to about 50 congregations as well as religious books, records, music, and handcrafted gifts to the general public.

With the cooperation of the Wisconsin Department of Vocational Rehabilitation the organization maintains a sheltered workshop where contract work such as packaging, assembly, small machine operation, and inspection is done for a number of companies. Wage and hour laws are observed, and all jobs are rated to give the workers comparable wage potential. About half of the 85 residents are self-supporting through either the book store, the workshop, office work, an answering service for fire and police calls of neighboring towns, or laundry and food preparation services. Feeder cattle are raised and sold or used to supply meat for the home's table.

During its 17 years of operation, the Christian League has found it necessary to add a variety of services to meet the needs of its residents. A psychologist/minister offers specialized help at the home, and the plan is to supply year-round living quarters at the new center for temporary residents being treated. The physical therapy department has recently added a regular therapy program. Three times a week the nearby Gateway Technical Institute sends two teachers to lead a free study program which ranges from elementary to college level. Other programs include bowling, night school courses at the local high school, chess tournaments, and a fine arts program of music.

A documentary film, *Undefeated,* on the activities and ministry of the Occupational Home is available for loan to churches and civic groups; it will be mailed on a free-will offering basis. The 16-mm color film runs for 30 min. The monthly publication, *The Christian League Bulletin,* reports the activities of the home and camp as well as of the 20 local chapters that are located in Pennsylvania, New York, Ohio, Illinois, Wisconsin, Minnesota, and Missouri. Anyone interested in living at the Christian League would be able to form a clear impression of the League from the film and the free monthly bulletin.

Donna Rosen, who has spent 3 years as a resident in the home and 6 years in one of the apartments, shares some of her thoughts about living there:

Do I like it here? Yes! I say that with enthusiasm, at the same time remembering that "This isn't Utopia." Life here is not free from problems. But I like it in spite of problems that do exist. Wherever there are human wills and emotions, differing personalities, varying degrees of maturity and spiritual desire, there will be problems. It's how we work them out that counts. Yes, I like it here.

I like the convenience of living without steps or other architectural barriers. I like being as independent as I can possibly be. I have muscular dystrophy and am very limited physically. Because I have to depend on someone else for so many of my needs, convenience is superimportant. The little gal who is personal assistant has a learning disability, but is capable of doing many things completely on her own, and other things with guidance and direction. She is cheerful, willing, and helpful, and I am aware that much of my personal satisfaction with life is that I have someone like her. . . .

I like the spiritual emphasis here. It is not just an administered thing, but a spontaneous reaction from the residents who are Christians and who care. . . . The fellowship here is great. This is a friendly place, and many good friendships have been formed. For some it is the first time in their lives they have really had a chance to make friends, to go places and do things. I like being involved with the Resident Council, and I enjoy helping to plan some of the projects and activities.

I like being a part of a place that is work-oriented. Admittedly there is a gap between the goal of each person being gainfully employed and the way it actually is, but I'm thankful for those who are, for those who try to find work the handicapped can do. I'm thankful that I am able to work and enjoy the atmosphere of the place where I am employed (the book store–gift shop).

PROJECTS BY NONPROFIT ORGANIZATIONS

These projects also represent work and determination, for most of them are privately funded by drives, solicitations, donations, and bequests.

THE VIRGINIA HOME

The Virginia Home (formerly known as The Virginia Home for Incurables), 1101 Hampton Street, Richmond, Virginia 23220, was founded in 1894 by Miss Mary Tinsley Greenow with a capital of $36 and one patient. Miss Greenow, a paraplegic, had been thrown from a horse when she was in her early teens; she founded the Home for severely disabled people who had no place to live. Now in an imposing seven-story brick building, the Virginia Home continues to offer long-term care to severely disabled residents of Virginia. The median ages are 50 for males, 63 for females; the principal diagnostic classifications are cerebral palsy (27), arthritis (22), and multiple sclerosis (14). According to the 1973 brochure, the cost of care was $531/month; 96 residents were on public assistance and receiving Medicaid. The attractive brochure describes a wide range of services and activities, many of them directed by an active volunteer corps.

NEW HORIZONS WING

The management of New Britain Memorial Hospital, 2150 Corbin Avenue, New Britain, Connecticut 06050, has been extraordinarily understanding and cooperative with New Horizons, Inc., an organization of its severely disabled patients. When it opened a new wing in October, 1960, it arranged for the New Horizons group of resident members to be moved into their own unit on the ground floor. Called the New Horizons Wing, it has large rooms and expansive window areas looking out on the countryside or into the picnic patio; a raised fireplace in the wing's lounge is decorative and inviting, though not usable because of fire regulations. The wing has been freed of hospital type regulations and has been decorated with happy colors and furnishings to give it a feeling of warmth and friendliness.

The hospital donated space for an office and for the well-stocked store that the residents of the wing operate for the patients, staff, and volunteers. The residents are quite free to clutter their rooms with hobbies and books and decorate their walls. Some of the residents have telephone jobs and maintain regular working hours; a number have taken correspondence courses.

The costs per diem, as of April 1975, are $49.50; most of the residents have their expenses paid by Medicare/Medicaid.

After the following paragraph appeared in a 1970 issue of the *Rehabilitation Gazette,* the hospital received requests from disabled readers all over the United States. Twenty individuals actually made the move from their homes or other hospitals or nursing homes to live in the hospital's wing.

HOSPITAL RESIDENCE FOR THOSE ON WELFARE ANYWHERE IN THE U.S. According to Mr. Elmer G. E. Johnson, administrator of New Britain Memorial Hospital, New Britain, Connecticut 06050, any disabled person on welfare anywhere in the U.S., who wishes to transfer from his present state to New Britain, Connecticut, is an eligible candidate. The procedure is to write to the Connecticut Commissioner of Welfare in Hartford. Others who wish to apply can be referred through their physician and many do—from all over the world. The hospital has a "New Horizons" wing and a dynamic program for its severely disabled permanent residents.

As of the spring of 1975, Mr. Johnson confirmed that the offer is still open and he will welcome new residents to the New Horizons Wing.

McLEAN HOME

Opened in 1971, the McLean Home, 75 Great Pond Road, Simsbury, Connecticut 06070, was a gift to the State of Connecticut from the late Senator George

Payne McLean. In his will, McLean specified the home should be built for "the worthy, indigent, infirm or incurable, mothers, widows, single women and other persons," so long as they be residents of Connecticut. Anyone over 14 years of age is eligible; though many of the residents are elderly, there is a good mix of ages.

Situated on 53 acres, the complex is planned around the Activity Center in the manner of a New England village square as the hub of activity; the center includes a lounge with a dramatic fireplace, dining rooms, a game room, talking books room, a quiet room, beauty and barber service, arts and crafts center, sewing room, laundry, and a practice kitchen. Physical, occupational and speech therapy rooms and clinical facilities are all included in the complex.

The comprehensive care facility has space for 122 individuals in three separate levels of living. The residence accommodates 33 who can live independently, including having their own cars. Costs range $19–$20/day, depending on whether the individual has a private or semiprivate room and bathroom. The Rest Home, with nursing supervision, is designed for 31 persons who need occasional assistance. Costs range $18–$24/day. The third level, the Nursing Home, is occupied by 58 persons who need skilled nursing care and constant medical supervision. Costs range $27–$37/day. The three levels of living make it possible for residents to transfer to an appropriate level as needed. McLean Home is not related to any religious organization. About 50% of the residents are Medicaid (State) residents.

Each room of the two-story triangular facility has a sliding glass door opening onto a terrace or balcony with a view of the surrounding woods. More than a year of research went into details such as having wardrobe drawers with a flip-down drawer front to permit the contents to be seen from a wheelchair. Special attention was given to the bathrooms: a sink was purchased in England that was specifically designed for use from a wheelchair; the sink faucet has an easily operated blade that replaces the knob which was imported from Canada; the toilets stand 19 in. from the floor, 5 in. higher than normal.

The Day Center program provides recreation and therapeutic opportunities to local residents and provides the McLean Home residents with the opportunity to meet them. In addition, volunteers of all ages are recruited to work in the home, and the facilities of the entire complex are available to the community for meetings and social gatherings. "The Home," said Executive Director Howard S. Pfirman, "is not an end for its residents; its primary responsibility is to rehabilitate."

COURAGE RESIDENCE

The residential care facility of Courage Center, which opened in late 1975, is the culmination of the years of planning and fund-raising that began with a survey in 1966 of the housing needs of physically disabled young adults. The residence program is the fourth service to be included in Courage Center, the new rehabilitation facility developed by the Minnesota Society for Crippled Children and Adults, Inc. (MiSCCA), 3915 Golden Valley Road, Golden Valley, Minnesota 55422. The

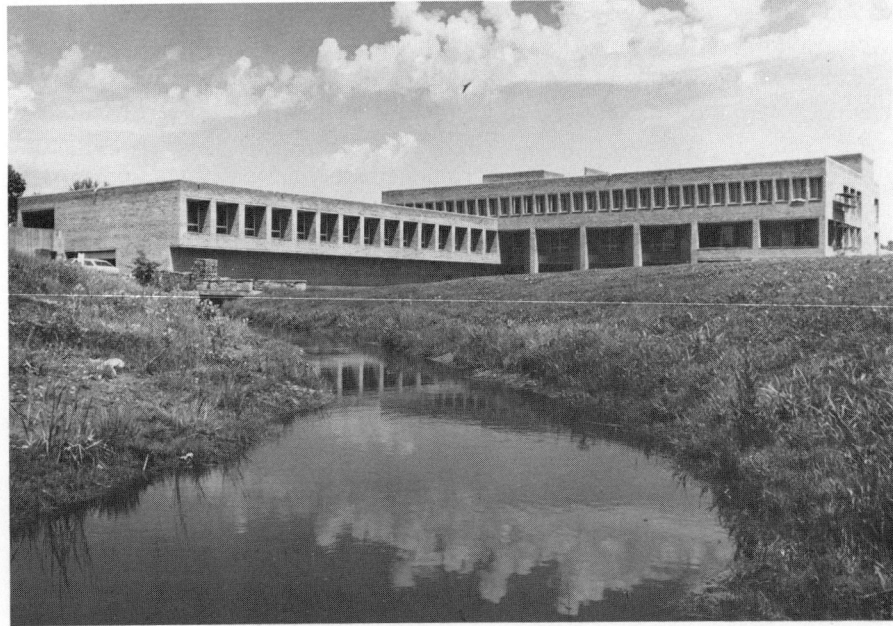

Fig. 11–2. Courage Center, headquarters of the Minnesota Society for Crippled Children and Adults. The new residence for 64 disabled young adults is attached to the complex.

Fig. 11–3. Margaret Anderson, a respiratory poliomyelitis quadriplegic, is the administrator of the residence at Courage Center. A talented artist, she holds the brush between her teeth to paint and to create original needlepoint designs.

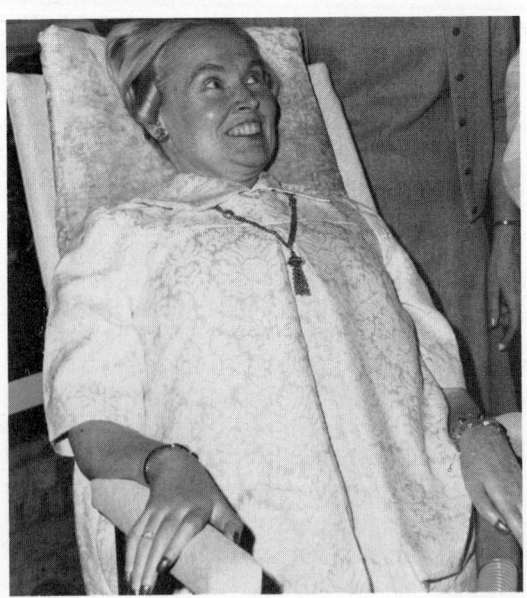

Center is located on a 7½ acre site adjacent to a golf course and the Golden Valley Health Center, in a suburb of Minneapolis (Fig. 11–2.).

The complex contains the Curative Workshop, gift shop, gymnasium (used for wheelchair basketball as well as for square dancing and as an auditorium), therapeutic preschool program, speech and hearing clinic, adult occupational and physical therapy, administrative offices, cafeteria, dining rooms, employment training, craft area, the amateur radio group known as Handi-Hams, and an indoor swimming pool.

The residential area has access to all the services and programs of Courage Center as well as a beauty shop and laundry facilities. About two-thirds of the residents are transitional residents receiving vocational training or physical restorative services; the rest are long-term residents, employed in some area of MiSCCA. The 30 double occupancy bedrooms of the two-story residence have private bathrooms and open onto a patio or a balcony. Each floor has a kitchenette and an activity room. The main lounge has a fireplace, and there is a quiet room for escaping the pressures of community living.

Fig. 11–4. Inglis House, founded nearly 100 years ago as The Philadelphia Home for Incurables. Main entrance.

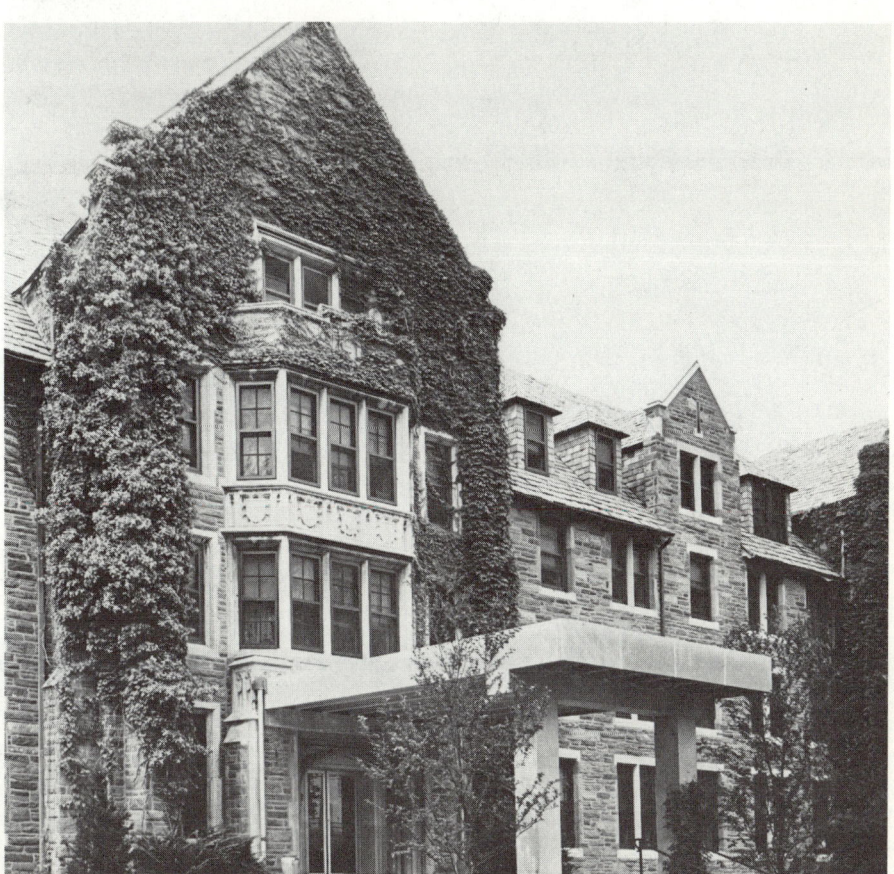

Fig. 11–5. The Esther M. Klein Apartments contain 16 units for independent disabled. **A.** The building is located on the grounds of Inglis House and overlooks the golf course. **B.** Floor plan of the efficiency unit. **C.** Cecilia Salvatore, an Inglis House resident, tries out the new wall oven. **D.** A wheelchair wash basin and a lowered medicine cabinet.

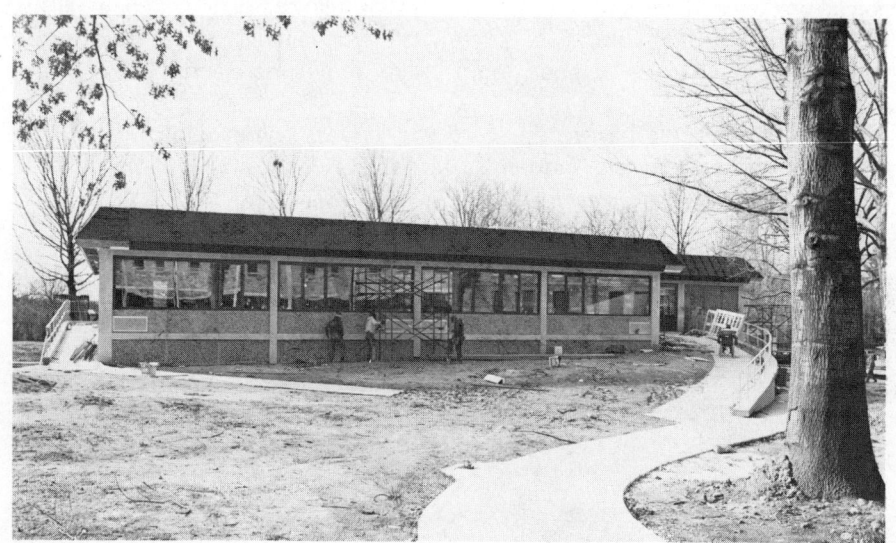

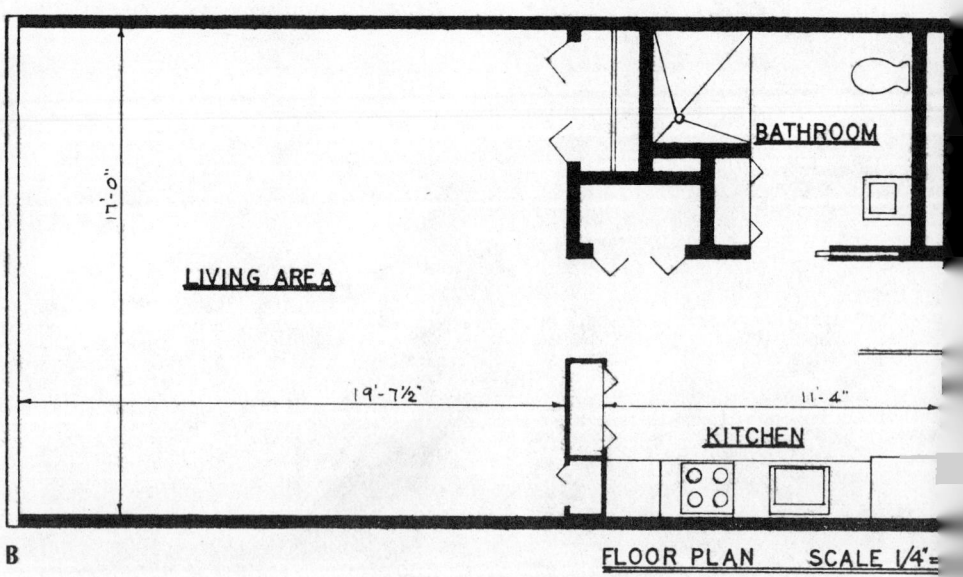

Long-Term Residential Facilities 197

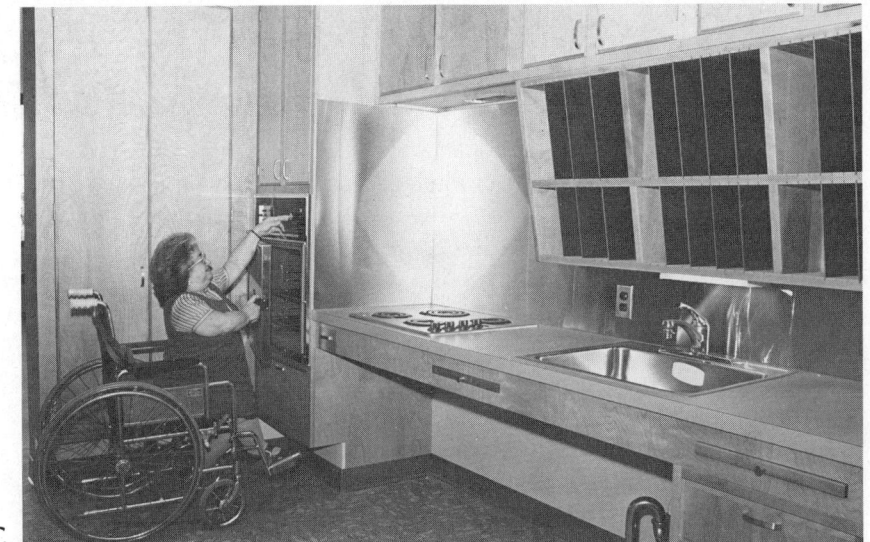

C

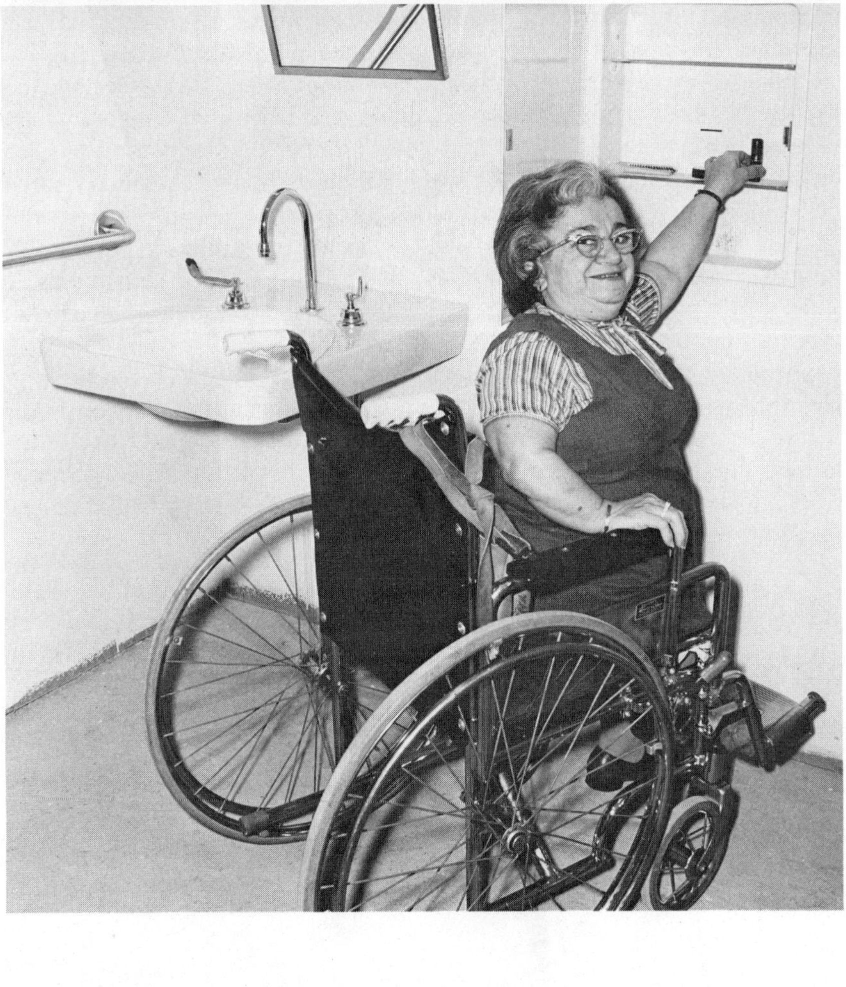

D

Since it is licensed as a skilled and intermediate care facility, the costs are covered by public welfare for those who are eligible or by the residents' own earnings or income, supplemented by scholarship funds. Transportation and all degrees of attendant care are provided.

The dynamic administrator, Mrs. Margaret Anderson, a respiratory poliomyelitis quadriplegic since 1953, uses a chestpiece as a breathing aid (Fig. 11-3). She was the originator of the annual art show at Sister Kenny Institute for disabled artists. She has been active on the residence planning committee since its inception. In the summer of 1974 she completed training in nursing home administration. She is a wise choice; her warmth and charm will ease many of the growing pains.

INGLIS HOUSE

Inglis House, 2600 Belmont Avenue, Philadelphia, Pennsylvania 19131, offers complete medical and nursing care to its 290 chronically ill and severely disabled residents (Fig. 11-4). Fees are on a sliding scale, ranging from the amount public welfare allows for skilled nursing home care to the actual cost of care. Its 7 acres of grounds are located on the edge of the Bala-Cynwyd Country Club in a residential section of Philadelphia near a shopping center. Services include transportation in a bus with a hydraulic lift, active volunteer involvement in cultural and recreational activities, a general store and thrift shop, beautician and barber, religious services, and participation in the Residents Council. Additional services include temporary care and a day resident program.

As part of its program to increase its services to young disabled persons, Inglis House has added a residential facility, the Esther M. Klein Apartments. The 16-unit apartment building, was privately financed and is operated independently of the institution. Architecturally designed for wheelchaired persons who can live independently, it was opened in early 1975 (Fig. 11-5). Each efficiency unit includes an intercom system. The all-electric kitchen includes a garbage disposal, refrigerator, and self-cleaning oven. Each floor has a utility room, laundry room, and trash chute. A multipurpose room is available for entertaining, and there is ample parking space. Rents are $95/month, plus electric utilities of about $50/month.

GOODWILL INDUSTRIES OF AMERICA

Recently, many local Goodwills have responded to the needs of their trainees and workers and entered the housing field, thus extending their services beyond their traditional role of providing vocational training and employment. With the exception of two large projects, Goodwill Terrace Apartments in Queens, New York, and Independence Hall in Houston, Texas, most of these Goodwill projects are small transitional facilities for 20-30 disabled individuals who are physically able to take care of their own daily needs and who are receiving rehabilitation services at the local Goodwill.

To coordinate the existing projects and plan for future developments, Dean Phillips, the President of Goodwill Industries, sponsored a seminar on housing in October, 1973. The participants were the 13 Goodwill executive directors who had initiated housing projects and representatives from HUD and HEW. Much of the following material derives from the ensuing report and from follow-up correspondence with the participants.

1. Abilities & Goodwill, Inc., 803 Forest Avenue, Portland, Maine 04103. Two facilities are in operation, and one is being planned. Ingraham House, a transitional home with a 12-month maximum length of stay, has a capacity of 31 persons who live there while their rehabilitation potential is being evaluated; the program is funded by the Maine Bureau of Rehabilitation. Carleton House is a long-term care home for adults with low employment potential. The Maine Department of Health and Welfare finances the 14 person project. A third facility that will feature barrier-free design is being planned.
2. Christ Mission Goodwill Industries, 2747 Belmont Avenue, Youngstown, Ohio 44505. A dormitory for 18 persons is located within the plant building; it is supervised by two housemothers who work on a rotating basis. An adjacent structure to house 40–50 workshop employees is being proposed. Recreational resources would be increased; management would be in the hands of a husband and wife team. Funding would be carried out through federal and/or state sources.
3. Goodwill Industries of Des Moines, Inc., 2550 East Euclid, Des Moines, Iowa 50316. A residential rehabilitation facility in a former nursing home has been in operation since 1972 for 114 psychiatric patients.
4. Goodwill Industries of North Central Pennsylvania, DuBois, Pennsylvania 15801. Concerned with the problems of rural rehabilitation, this Goodwill has purchased a number of old houses for group homes.
5. Goodwill Industries—Suncoast, Inc. 10596 Gandy Blvd., St. Petersburg, Florida 33733 A residence is provided for persons who are in evaluation, adjustment, or training programs. Round-the-clock supervision is maintained with a minimum of two professionals on duty during evenings and weekends.
6. Goodwill Terrace Apartments, 4–21 27th Avenue, Astoria, Queens, New York 11102. Located near the Triborough Bridge, this 206-unit, 15-story apartment building was built specifically for the disabled. It serves all types of disabled, the physically or emotionally disabled and the mentally retarded. Most of the residents are elderly, but all ages are accepted—if they are able to care for themselves. The studio apartments rent for $56, if the individual's income is under $5800, or for $124 if the income is $5800–$9000; the one-bedroom apartments are proportionately higher. Though it was built for the disabled, many of the existing features are inconvenient for the wheelchaired. Among the problems are bathrooms that are too small and do not have roll-in showers; the 36 in. high sinks and ranges are too high, and the storage is inaccessible; the closets have bifold rather than sliding doors, and the rods are too high; drinking fountains and elevator buttons are too high; and the double-hung windows are difficult to operate.

7. Goodwill Industries of Western Connecticut and Sheltered Workshop, Inc., 165 Ocean Terrace, Bridgeport, Connecticut 06605. The Wahlstrom Goodwill Residence was financed by a $470,000 gift from Mr. Magnus Wahlstrom, with matching gifts from the community of Bridgeport. The residence, completed in 1971, comprises 21 double and 8 single rooms for 50 persons who are participating in Goodwill programs. Day-to-day activities are under the supervision of a house parent.
8. Independence Hall, 8200 Jensen Drive, P.O. Box 21185, Houston, Texas 77026 (see Independence Hall, Ch. 13). It is particularly noteworthy because it is evolving so smoothly, adding supportive services such as transportation, wheelchair repair, a snack bar, and attendants as needs crystallize.
9. Wall Street Mission Goodwill Industries, 312 South Floyd Boulevard, Sioux City, Iowa 51102. Goodwill Residence Hall accommodates 80 persons, both workers and trainees, especially those with problems of mental health, alcohol, or drugs. War Eagle Village consists of 10 buildings with a population of 101 persons. The facilities range from one-bedroom to four-bedroom apartments and townhouses. The disabled are among several categories of persons entitled to preference; seven units have ramp access. Amenities include an attractive setting, nearby bus transportation, and imaginative play areas for children. Rents are fixed below prevailing commercial levels. Financing is through the FHA.

FEDERALLY AIDED NEW TOWN—ROOSEVELT ISLAND

The new town concept is the ideal way to create a totally barrier-free environment for the disabled and elderly, to integrate them naturally in a proportionate number of special units, to locate shops and recreational facilities within walking or wheeling distance of living accommodations.

The Roosevelt Island project, backed by the New York State Urban Development Corporation (UDC), will include apartment buildings ranging from 4–22 stories containing 5000 dwelling units, more than half of them for low and moderate income families. Existing hospitals, occupying 21 acres, are expected to provide jobs for about 5000 of the 7500 people who will work on the island. Schools, shops, and other facilities will be integral parts of the residential buildings. Parks, promenades, open space, and streets will take up more than half of the island's land.

In an effort to free themselves of unnecessary institutionalization, three patients represented their fellow patients from the two hospitals for the chronically ill on the island, Goldwater Memorial and Bird S. Coler, at the Board of Estimate hearings back in 1969. They requested that 1000 units be assigned to hospital-related housing and that all construction on the island be made barrier-free. In the final plans, 250 units were designated for the disabled, 750 units for hospital employees, and 300 units for the elderly.

Unfortunately, there have been delays in construction, uncertainty about supportive services, and increases in the rents. By early 1975, only 49 units for the disabled had been built, and the rest are several years behind schedule. One plus:

all units will have 32 in. doorways so free movement between all apartments will be possible.

PROJECTS BEING PLANNED

NAPH FARM–HOME, INC.

For the past 8 years, a group of members of one of the nationwide clubs of disabled individuals, the National Association of the Physically Handicapped (NAPH), 6473 Grandville, Detroit, Michigan 48228, has been planning a village complex with employment facilities. During all this time, the chairman of the project, M. W. Munns, has not lost his determination despite a series of setbacks. One of the problems has been the lack of an exempt rating from the Internal Revenue Service; another has been deciding on a site. The site has now been moved from southeastern Michigan to 25 acres of land in Ulster County, New York, that would be donated for the purpose.

In 1968–1969 the planners sent out a questionnaire to the 35 NAPH chapters. There were 700 responses: 506 individuals were interested in the idea; 200 would give serious thought to moving in if it were built. An architectural firm in Detroit has drawn plans and has been acting as a housing consultant in contacts with HUD. Most residents of the proposed complex would be NAPH members and able to live independently; nonprofessional aides would be available for others.

NEW HORIZONS, INC.

New Horizons, Inc., New Britain Memorial Hospital, 2150 Corbin Avenue, New Britain, Connecticut 06050 had secured a state license to build a 60-bed facility, a lender, a preliminary and conditional approval from FHA, a fund raiser (FHA requires $250,000 for granting firm commitment), an architect, and an impressive brochure. The proposed project would be staffed by a director of nurses, 3 registered nurses, 5 licensed practical nurses, 12 nurses aides, and 9 male aides, salaried at $190,000. The projected building is star-shaped with five wings and includes space for a shop and physical therapy facilities.

WINNING WHEELS, INC.

Winning Wheels, Inc., P.O. Box 121, Prophetstown, Illinois 61277, was started after the death of a young quadriplegic who had spent 12 years in five different nursing homes. In 1970 a group of citizens, both disabled and nondisabled, organized to build a care center for 72 severely disabled, nonretarded, wheelchaired persons. Plans for the facility include medical care, physical and occupational therapy, recreational activities, work opportunities, and spiritual and psychologic guidance.

The driving force behind the project is Paul S. Yackley. The membership includes 1500 people, of whom about 250 are in wheelchairs. Over $130,000 has been raised through benefits, bazaars, auctions, raffles, memorials, memberships, and contributions; a combined Radiothon and Wheel-A-Thon in October, 1974, netted in excess of $20,000. In May, 1974, a Hill–Burton grant in the amount of $381,356 and a loan guarantee of $469,774 were awarded toward the estimated cost of $1,500,000.

Twelve acres of wooded land have been purchased and a building design drawn that is also a star-shaped building with five wings—a typical nursing home design. All rooms are planned for single occupancy with a private bath. If it is licensed as a skilled nursing care facility, the costs may run $525–$550/month.

FRIENDS OF THE CHESHIRE HOME IN NEW JERSEY

The project of the Friends of the Cheshire Home, Red Cross Building, One Madison Avenue, Madison, New Jersey 07940, to establish a Cheshire Home in the United States was given its launching boost in 1971 by Ronald Travers of the Cheshire Homes in England. The committee plans a permanent home for physically disabled young adults of normal intelligence in a familylike environment. After a survey and several years of work, the planning committee is still hampered by state requirements because its plans do not fit into any established pattern for facilities providing care.

OUR WAY, INC.

Our Way, Inc., 2500 McCain Place, Suite 112, North Little Rock, Arkansas 72116, was begun by five young people, four quadriplegics and one nondisabled, who are planning an extended care facility for 50 mentally alert adults aged 18–50. The president, Jerry McMahen, has been a quadriplegic since 1959 and has lived in nursing homes for over 5 years. By the spring of 1976, they had received two grants, totalling $67,739, from the Arkansas Regional Medical Program. With the grants, they have completed a management training program and arranged for a feasibility study and preliminary architectural plans. With another grant from Urban Mass Transit Authority and the Arkansas Highway Department they have purchased a van equipped for wheelchairs. During the planning stage, they are developing advocacy and awareness programs.

PARAQUAD, INC.

(14 North Newstead, St. Louis, Missouri 63108.) Since 1970, Max Starkloff, a quadriplegic, has been working toward a residential and commercial complex for both physically disabled and nondisabled individuals. The complex would have dwelling units near commercial operations and shops. Max, founder and executive director, has raised funds from local foundations and individuals to have an unusually extensive market study made by Team Four, Inc., planning design and development consultants. Currently, of the 4000 questionnaires sent out, 500 have been returned and are being analyzed. Later, a detailed follow-up questionnaire will be sent. The architect of the proposed project, Laurent Jean Torno, Jr.,

is working out technical design features with his students at Washington University School of Architecture and several disabled individuals.

CONTEMPO CARE

Contempo Care, 12831 Maclay Avenue, Sylmar, California 91342, is an extended care facility located on 14 acres of land in the foothills of the San Fernando Valley. It is planned for 214 nongeriatric patients and is licensed to accept disabled persons for the amount the state pays under the Aid to the Disabled program. The rejuvenated facilities include a swimming pool, game room, library, music room, therapy rooms, and auditorium. They are all available to community organizations which aid the disabled. The rates per day are $45 for a private room and bath, $27 for semiprivate with bath, $19 for a three-bed room, and $17.50 for a four-bed room. The owners, Mr. and Mrs. Irving Feld, have plans for a residence for disabled individuals who can take care of themselves.

KEY PALM VILLA

Key Palm Villa, 4200 N.W. 18th Street, Lauderhill, Florida 33313, is a 1000-unit complex of apartments which has been checked out by the Paralyzed Veterans Association (PVA) of Florida, Inc. as being accessible for wheelchairs and adaptable to modifications for special needs. All the buildings have ramps and elevators, and the kitchens and bathrooms are usable. The facilities include four tennis courts, a volleyball court, an olympic pool, shuffleboard, and a club house with a restaurant, lounge, pool tables, ping-pong tables, and saunas. The complex is located one-quarter mile from a large shopping mall. Though no attendant care program presently exists, members of the PVA group feel that it could be developed. A physical therapist has taken a tentative lease on two adjoining apartments and is planning to set up a clinic and gymnasium. The rental range is $180 for studio apartments, $210 for one-bedroom apartments, and $235 for two bedrooms and two baths.

RAMBLING PELICAN GARDEN VILLA CONDOMINIUM

Rambling Pelican Garden Villa Condominium is being planned for December, 1976, occupancy by Ruth and Murray Fein of Rambling Tours, Inc. To be located in Coral Springs and priced at $25,900, the one-bedroom, two-bath units are designed for accessibility. Brochures are available from the Feins at 618 Palm Drive, Hallandale, Florida 33009.

12
Mobile Homes

Today's mobile homes constitute about the only truly low cost and flexible housing available in the United States. Their increasing popularity is reflected in the 1974 sales figures: mobile homes comprised 43% of all single family housing sold at any price and 95% of all single family housing under $20,000. Their increasing safety and standardization are reflected in the broadening of the mobile home loan programs of both HUD and the VA and the growth of the industry's self-regulation.

The mobile home industry is in the process of changing its name to "manufactured housing," a more accurate name since only 10% of the homes are ever moved after they have been set up initially.

DISADVANTAGES AND ADVANTAGES

The Council of Better Business Bureaus, Inc., 1150 17th Street, NW, Washington, D.C. 20036, with the technical advice of the Manufactured Housing Institute (MHI)—formerly the Mobile Home Manufacturers Association—has prepared an informative free publication, *Tips on Buying a Mobile Home*. The pamphlet includes a summary of the advantages and disadvantages of mobile home living as well as a listing of a half dozen inexpensive all-about-mobile-homes books. Anyone vaguely considering a mobile home should start with this free pamphlet and study it carefully, then send for some of the other booklets and books.

First, the disadvantages. Mobile homes are only theoretically mobile. They must be moved by professionals, and a long distance move may be too expensive and too complicated to be considered. If the move is over 500 miles, the average costs are about $1/mile; if under 500 miles, the minimum charge varies. Many of the homes in various climate zones of the country are designed to resist specific area wind velocities or snow loads and may not be suitable for other climate zones. This information will be indicated on a map and posted inside homes built to the national standards.

Further, many cities and towns have zoning regulations that severely restrict where a mobile home can be located. Parks rarely offer the protection of a long-term lease so there may be rapid rent increases.

The price of a home is just the beginning. It does not include the site, which must be rented or purchased separately. In addition, most new parks require extras which will add at least another 15% to the cost of the home: skirting, steps, shrubbery, awnings, and anchoring systems which must be installed by a reputable firm. If the home is placed on private property, it is necessary to check the zoning laws and to arrange for installation of the pad on which it will be set or for excavation and foundations, as well as water and utilities, all of which may run $2500 or more.

Price and flexibility are the most attractive advantages. Mobile homes offer low initial costs as well as low maintenance costs. In 1974, the average price was $9130, including furnishings, carpet, furniture, and appliances. The national average monthly mobile park rental was $55. The most common and economical size is the single-wide unit, 12 or 14 × 66 ft. This offers up to 14 × 62 ft. of living space, or 868 sq ft. (The length of the towing hitch is usually quoted in the overall dimensions and should be excluded when measuring actual living space.) More than 36 states now permit 14 ft wide mobile home homes to be moved over highways, but the others do not. This should be checked with a local dealer before deciding on the width. As a rule, the basic purchase price will only include transporting the mobile home to a nearby site, within a stated area, and the setting up for initial operation. It is wise to inquire whether this is included in the price and have it written into the sales contract.

Many mobile home retailers have their own financing programs, but the buyer should shop around and investigate the financing possibilities of banks, commercial finance companies, credit unions, and savings and loan associations. Many of these organizations have special programs for mobile home loans. Generally, terms for financing a mobile home are for shorter periods and are less favorable than for conventional housing; mobile homes tend to depreciate in value rather than increase with use as is the case with conventional homes and lots. The quality of the park determines the rate of depreciation.

Under certain conditions, the Federal Housing Authority (FHA) or the Veterans Administration (see the VA Housing Benefits, Ch. 9) will guarantee loans for mobile homes and for sites, as well as preparation costs. A federal loan guarantee has the advantages of a lower interest rate and an extended period in which to repay the loan. Complete details are available through the nearest HUD Area Office or HUD–FHA Insurance Office. To qualify for FHA or VA loan programs, mobile homes sold in any state must meet the national standards established by the American National Standards Institute, ANSI Standard A119.1, and the National Fire Protection Association, NFPA 501B.

THE NEW MOBILE HOME PARKS

Experienced mobile home residents suggest selecting the park before buying the home because in many areas lots in the choice parks are in such demand. The more than 22,000 parks now in operation range from overcrowded, low rent parks to lavish mobile home estates with large landscaped lots that include such amenities as swimming pools, club houses, tennis courts, paved streets, and wide sidewalks. Services include garbage disposal, fire and police protection, home repair service, ample electricity, and tie-downs.

To secure a list of parks, write to Manufactured Housing Institute, P.O. Box 201, 14650 Lee Road, Chantilly, Virginia 22021. Request the name and address of the particular state mobile home association (manufactured housing). The state association will send the latest list of parks and their quality ratings.

The American Association of Retired Persons (AARP) has been making an in-depth study of criteria for the development of mobile home communities around the country. The Association has been analyzing a high-quality pilot program known as Hawthorne at Leesburg (Colonial Penn Communities, Inc., P. O. Drawer "T", Highway 27 South, Leesburg, Florida 32748). The homes, sold furnished or unfurnished, feature a call system to summon assistance, carports, porches, and utility rooms. The park includes 1300 home sites, five small lakes, a club house with heated swimming pool, saunas, shuffleboard courts, a putting green, billiard room, library, and a boat basin with marina facilities. A committee of elderly residents has been making recommendations relating to transportation and services such as medical, social, recreational, and educational. The park management advises that the following adaptations for wheelchairs can be provided: a ramp at the entrance, wider interior passageways, and an opening at the dressing table.

FACTORY-MADE ADAPTATIONS

Wheelchaired individuals as well as the elderly are attracted by the low price and flexibility of mobile homes. In the past, for only a small additional charge, they could order changes made at the factory to suit their particular needs.

Among the enthusiastic residents of mobile homes are Jim and Herb Hooper of Lima, Ohio. Jim, in his 40s, is severely physically disabled by cerebral palsy; Herb, his father, has been retired for a number of years (Fig. 12-1). After the death of Mrs. Hooper, they made drastic changes in their lifestyles, selling their old family home, purchasing a van with a lift, and buying a home in a mobile home park. They found an attractively landscaped park, Indian Village, at 3050 DeLong Road (at I-75 and Breese Road), Lima, Ohio 45805 and ordered a Royal Oak 60 × 12 ft two-bedroom home made by Fawn Homes, P.O. Box 803, Middlebury, Indiana 46540.

Herb's description of the relatively inexpensive changes made at the factory to suit their needs demonstrates the adaptability of mobile homes.

We had our home lengthened 5 ft with two extra feet in the master bedroom and three extra feet in the living room. The hall is 3 ft wide; all inside doors are wide and sliding. The only carpet is indoor/outdoor in the living room, and the rest of the floor covering is the new embossed nonskid which won't need waxing. We asked for a shower stall instead of bathtub, and we have a platform in the shower with a small ramp up to it so I can wheel Jim in the shower in a shower chair.

Jim chose this floor plan because it has a door directly into the bathroom from his bedroom. This is the only plan we saw with that because of the placement of closets or bathroom fixtures. We had the floor plan reversed from the living room on back so both outside doors are on the same side. We have our Wheel-O-Vator porch elevator at the rear door, and the awning is 12 ft wide for 20 ft in the rear so we can drive our van with side lift under that part of the awning and wheel his chair up to the elevator and stay in the dry.

Pauline Penkivich, an Air Force wife who found mobile homes a solution to her housing problems, writes

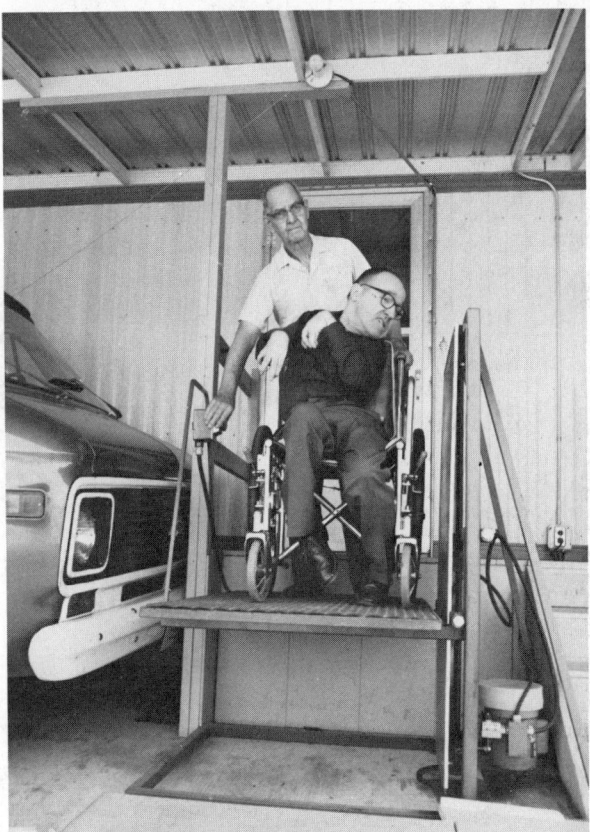

Fig. 12–1. Herb Hooper and his son, Jim, who is disabled by cerebral palsy. The elevator is placed at the rear door under the awning so they can load into the van under cover.

I have been a quad for 31 years. At the age of 17 I dove into shallow water and dislocated the 7th cervical. I have partial use of my hands, arms and shoulders, but no grip in my fingers. . . . I am married to a school chum who made the military his career. . . . We have three teen-age daughters, each born in a different state—but all in a state of chaos. . . . We lived in two mobile homes for 14 years. I designed both for my wheelchair, after trial and terror with second floor apartments. The first one was 8 × 42 ft. Can you imagine five people in one that size? The second one was 10 × 60 ft, three bedrooms, built-in stove and oven, and built for travel with three axles instead of the normal two. Now my husband has retired from the Air Force, and we are living in a big older house in a suburb near O'Hare Airport with doors wide enough for an elephant to get through. I'm working on an article on how not to buy a house.

A retired Californian, Thomas E. Keenan, who is hemiplegic as the result of spinal fusion surgery, writes of their mobile home.

We have been in our home for nearly 3 years and we are quite satisfied, especially with the barrier-free park which allows me to get out and about in a power chair. This park, Swan Lake, in Mira Loma, has ground level facilities and even a pool with steps. We found that our Brettwood home, made by Viking, provides great freedom of movement. We

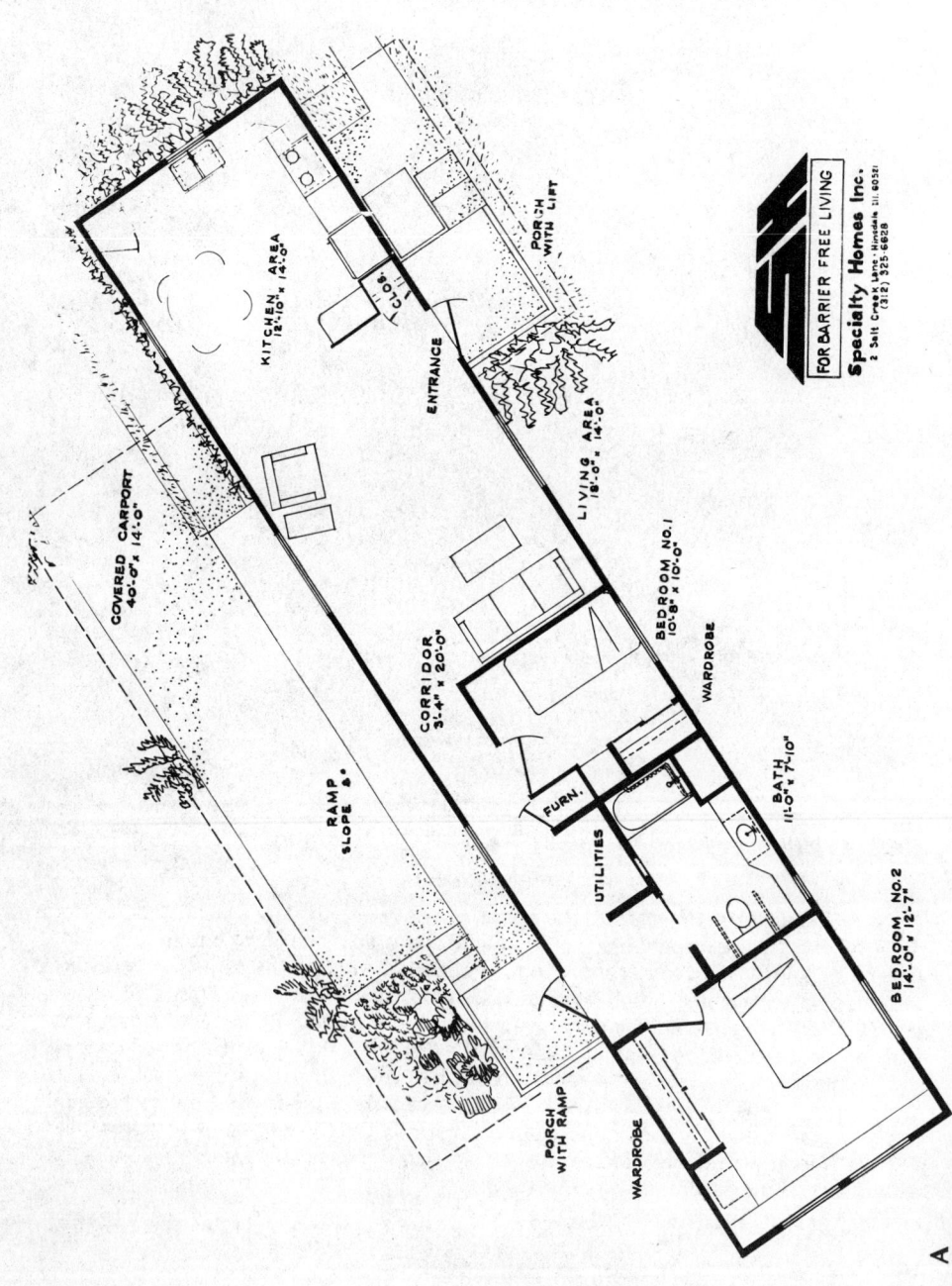

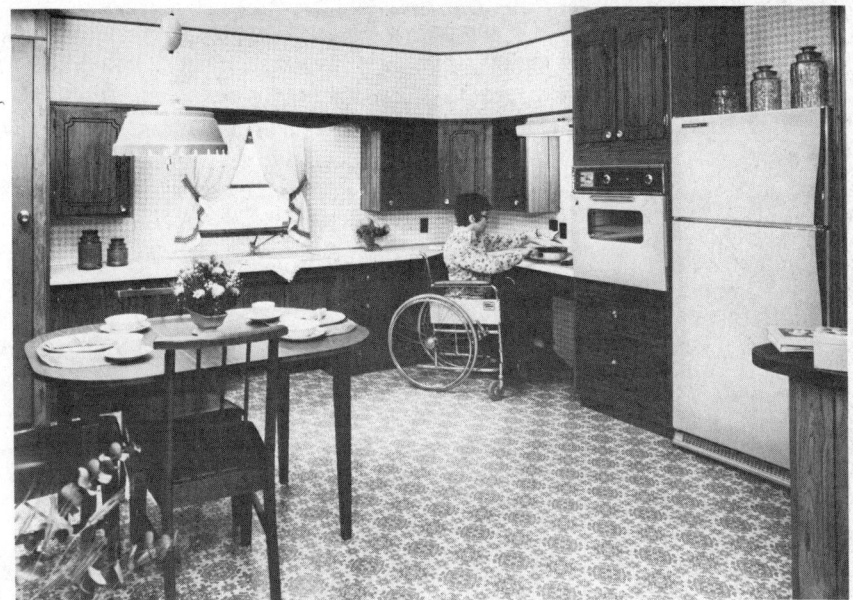

Fig. 12-2. Specialty Homes, Inc., produces a wheelchair model of a mobile home. **A.** Floor plan. **B.** The kitchen includes a number of special features.

added a ramp instead of steps. . . . I can negotiate the 5 × 8 ft bath with the door opening inward, but I prefer a room 6 × 8 ft with a sliding door. If a buyer requires a roll-in shower, the whole room must be constructed of waterproof materials, including waterproof light fixtures and switches, to meet the California building code requirements. If a tile floor is wanted, it will be done at the home site to avoid breaking in transit.

SPECIALLY DESIGNED HOMES

A series of coincidences resulted in the forming of Specialty Homes, Inc., 2 Salt Creek Lane, Hinsdale, Illinois 60521, to market factory-built adapted units. In 1972, Dr. Harold P. Lyon, director of an insurance rehabilitation program, consulted Beitler and Associates regarding the use of mobile homes for wheelchaired persons. He shared the information with *Rehabilitation Gazette,* which published a brief article about the possibilities of mobile homes for the disabled and gave Beitler and Associates as a source of information regarding their adaptability. As a result of the article, the firm received numerous inquiries from insurance companies, occupational therapists, and individuals across the country. These inquiries prompted the Beitlers to start researching the possibilities of adapted homes built at the factory.

In September, 1974, a letter was written to all the people who had made the original inquiries to see whether they were still interested; the response was quite favorable, with additional suggestions that the homes be used not only for individuals or groups, but also in conjunction with rehabilitation centers as halfway houses.

The Beitlers consulted with a number of experts, including Professor Timothy Nugent of the University of Illinois, several of his staff members, National Easter Seal Society, Peter Lassen of the VA Construction Project, and the National Paraplegia Foundation. With their assistance, the Beitlers worked out specifications to adapt a mobile home to wheelchair use. In early 1976, they selected a home made by the DeRose Industries, Inc., and they have established a network of mobile home dealers around the country who will handle the orders for homes built to fit individual needs (Fig. 12-2 A and B). Free brochures are available from Specialty Homes, Inc.

There are two factory-built models, 14 × 66 ft. The standard model has a kitchen with 36 in. high counters. The special wheelchair model, built to ANSI standards, has 31 in. high counters. Its other special features include lower overhead cabinets, knee space under the kitchen sink (with protection from hot pipes), easy reach pantry shelf, and roll under work space next to refrigerator and stove. A useful extra is a chopping block cart with castors that can be used between stove and table or between refrigerator and sink; it is 31 in. high and can also be used as a cooking surface.

Other special features are sliding doors on the closets, reachable shelves, and low rods. The bathroom is equipped with grab bars; a tub is standard, though roll-in showers will be available eventually. There are wide hallways, wide doorways, and safety devices such as smoke detectors.

The approximate cost of the unit is $13,500–$16,000. Lifts, ramps, awnings, carports, or other amenities are additional.

NURSING HOME WITH MOBILE HOME UNITS

The Pleasant View Nursing Home, R.R. #2, Wabash, Indiana 46992, has purchased 85 mobile home units and located them adjacent to the nursing home building. They are occupied by patients who are mobile, whether ambulatory or using walkers or wheelchairs. Ramps are added for those in wheelchairs.

The homes are the Holly Park model manufactured by Gerring Industries. They have dimensions of 12 × 60 ft, a large front porch, and a front and rear bedroom which makes each unit suitable for two patients.

Each home has a phone connected to the nursing home switchboard. The nursing home complex has a full-time registered nurse on duty to provide medication, a doctor on call, and 73 employees. The cost of meals in the restaurant/dining area adjacent to the park is included in the overall charge.

HUD-SPONSORED MOBILE HOME STUDIES

In 1974, a $200,000 contract was awarded to St. Andrews Presbyterian College, Laurinburg, North Carolina 28352, to develop design guidelines for the modification of mobile homes to make them suitable to the needs of the disabled. The project director, Dr. Rodger Decker, is evaluating the possibilities of converting mobile homes for occupancy by the disabled. The project began with the renovation of four standard mobile homes from the HUD disaster housing stock; a group of disabled students moved into them in the fall of 1974 to test various living arrangements and adaptations.

The study allows 1 year to study the problems and 1 year to develop solutions. A fifth surplus home, developed as a demonstration unit, will incorporate the most desirable design features. The project team is giving special attention to safety factors, as well as doing psychologic testing to determine the effects of the increased independence and responsibility.

The new ANSI standards relating to the disabled, which are being updated by Dr. Edward Steinfeld, School of Architecture, Syracuse University, will include updating the existing standards for mobile homes.

According to *HUD Challenge,* January, 1975, the use of mobile homes is part of the effort by HUD under the 1974 Housing and Community Development Act to make housing available for low income families. The December 1975 issue of *HUD Challenge* features two articles on mobile homes: *Mobile Home Standards. The Federal Role* by Bonnie Beckman, an urban intern in HUD's Office of Mobile Home Standards, and *Fannie Mae Installs Mobile Home Program* by Russell Clifton, Vice President for Mortgage Programs, Federal National Mortgage Association.

"If there is no local interest, no local action, no local sponsor, no local effort to alert the public to grievous need, there will be no housing."

—Marie McGuire Thompson, DSS, HUD Consultant, Housing for the Elderly and Handicapped

13
HUD-Assisted Housing Projects

Between 1967 and 1974, eight HUD-assisted facilities with 1085 units were designated and designed for housing the disabled. Between 1958 and 1974, more than 500,000 HUD-assisted dwelling units were specially designed and set aside for persons 62 years or older. (Of these units, 10% include minimum provisions for the disabled: an accessible entrance and mobility through the principal rooms.) Why the vast difference? Probably because of the misconception that the disabled were "special" and needed very "special" housing with very "special" equipment.

Valuable lessons have been learned from building and managing these eight projects. The disabled are not stereotyped; they are as diverse as all other people; all need services more than special accommodations; some need personal assistance with daily living activities; all need transportation to employment, schools, training, medical appointments, recreation, sports, entertainment, or shopping; some need social services, house-cleaning services, meal preparation services, or meals on wheels services. Most importantly, all need to be able to choose where they want to live.

How can HUD facilitate housing the disabled? Primarily, by being more attuned to their needs and by clarifying its programs. Local HUD offices should have at least one staff member trained to understand the needs of the disabled. More individuals who are disabled should be hired. Simplified guidelines to HUD programs should be published.

All federally assisted housing, whether publicly or privately owned, should be made accessible and a proportion should be made adaptable.

The income limits in public housing should be increased for the disabled to allow for the additional expenses of disability. The asset limits should be removed.

Local housing authorities should be educated to the necessity of individual adaptations and services. The Boston Handicapped Services Center might well be a model (see Massachusetts Public Housing and Service Programs, Ch. 10). Whatever the method, trained individuals, disabled or nondisabled, should be available to prescribe or furnish—without red tape—raised toilet seats, hydraulic lifts, wheelchairs that raise and lower, wheelchair narrowers, ramps, utility carts, portable ovens, portable burner units, extension cords, and lever door and tap handles.

Nonprofit organizations wishing to develop small transitional or permanent housing arrangements should be encouraged and helped with information about funding. They should be advised to experiment through Section 815 which provides $10 million of HUD research funds for demonstrating various types of housing to meet special needs. Start-up funds should be available to help in preparing loan applications.

Rent subsidies and tax incentives should be utilized to attract private developers to build and remodel accessible and adaptable housing. Home ownership by disabled individuals should be encouraged through liberalized financing and tax incentives.

Good omen! In the spring of 1976 HUD named "Elderly and Handicapped Housing Coordinators" in their ten regional offices. For the name and address of the nearest coordinator, write to Mrs. Helen F. Holt, Assistant to the Secretary, Programs for the Elderly and Handicapped, HUD, 7th and D Streets, S.W., Washington, D.C. 20410.

VISTULA MANOR

Address: 615 Cherry Street, Toledo, Ohio 43604
Sponsor: Toledo Metropolitan Housing Authority
Date Opened: 1967
Number of units: Total 164: 15 2-BR, 80 1-BR, 69 efficiencies
Cost: $3,800,943
For: Elderly and disabled
HUD program: Low rent public housing

Vistula Manor is of particular interest because it was the first public housing project in the U.S. to be designed for the physically disabled and elderly and because the final report of the research by the University of Toledo was most significant (Fig. 13-1). The project was conceived in 1960 by a disabled couple, Mr. and Mrs. Gerald Carey, who learned of the apartments on Hans Knudsens Plads in Copenhagen that had been especially built for the disabled and who tried to duplicate them in Toledo. They energetically contacted a wide range of people, eventually interesting the Toledo Metropolitan Housing Authority, which secured a research grant in 1964 of about $100,000 to study the social, architectural, and medical factors related to designing, constructing, and operating specialized housing.

The primary research team was composed of a sociologist, a physiatrist, and an architect. The initial phase entailed a social survey of 1100 names submitted by a number of Toledo organizations serving the disabled. When the time for occupancy arrived, only 17 families and individuals were allocated apartments because of physical disability; the rest failed to meet the income levels, changed their minds, or died. Ironically, among those who failed to meet the income levels were Mr. and Mrs. Gerald Carey.

Ultimately, for the purposes of evaluation, 65 individuals were classified as disabled by including those who had originally been admitted because of age but who also had disabling physical conditions. The group consisted primarily of unattached, adult, white, retired females, 50 years of age or over, with less than a high school education. The major disablements were heart disease, arthritis,

Fig. 13–1. A. Vistula Manor in Toledo, Ohio, the first public housing project designed specifically for the disabled. **B.** The Vistula Manor bathrooms were fashioned after the model home at New York University. **C.** Kitchen in Vistula Manor demonstrated by the late McClinton Nunn, who was director of the Toledo Metropolitan Housing Authority during construction.

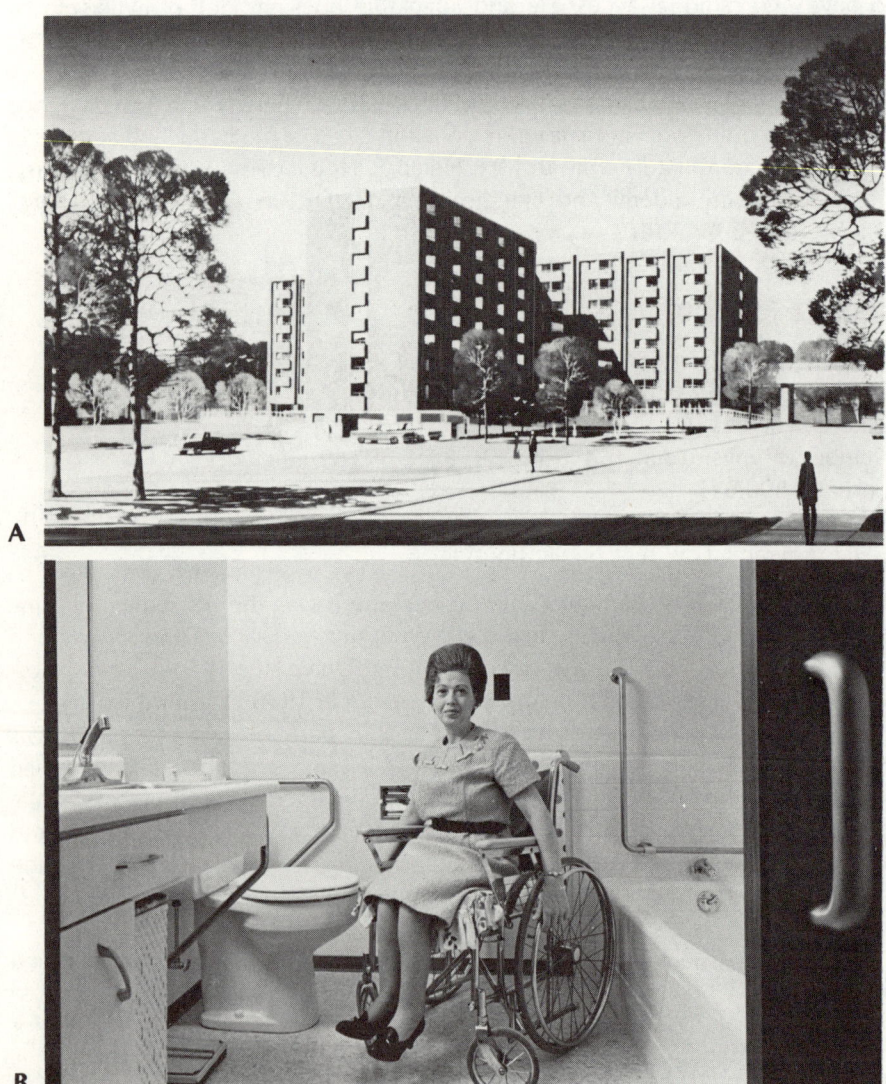

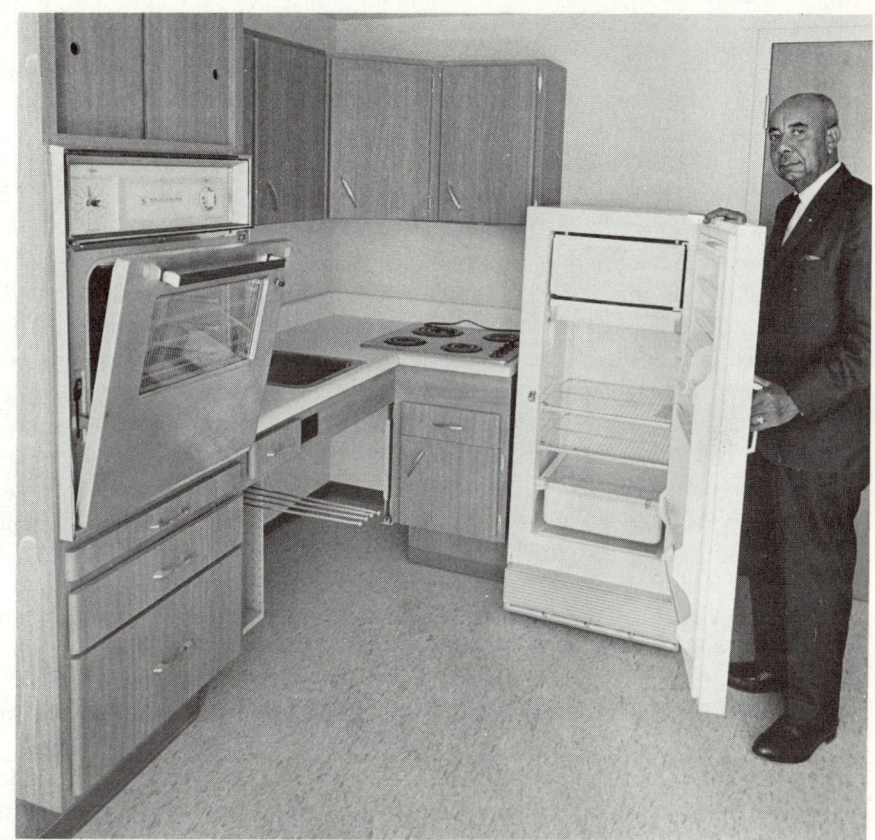
C

and sight loss. Four used wheelchairs, six used crutches, and six used walkers.

New York University's Institute of Rehabilitation Medicine directed the planning of the special architectural features, with special attention to the kitchens and bathrooms. Additional rooms and services include a large multipurpose room, social space, coin-operated laundromats on every other floor and a garage. A number of desirable features had to be eliminated because of the economies of public housing: air conditioning (installed later at an inflated price), garbage disposals, kitchen exhaust fans, an intercom system, and a third elevator.

By the summer of 1974, the proportion of elderly and disabled, which had been planned to be 50–50, had reached only 25% disabled. The average age of the elderly was 70 and of the disabled was 45–50; arthritis was the principal disability. Most of the residents were female; there were 16 or 17 couples. The majority were unemployed; four were working and one was in training at Goodwill.

The building, located in a downtown urban renewal area, has a feeling of isolation, since there is no established residential community with possibilities for integration nearby. Though there are two other projects for the elderly only a block or so away there has been no coordination of recreation or social activities. The residents are very conscious of the need for safety in the area, carefully bolting their apartment doors. The halls and the social areas are wide, empty, and bleak.

Each year it has been necessary to add more and more social services through Welfare and City Recreation Departments and the Board of Education. Presently, the Red Cross is available 1 day/week to take residents to the grocery store three blocks away; Visiting Nurses call regularly; Mobile Meals brings dinner, plus the makings of breakfast, to 10 or 12 residents; the Welfare Department arranges for maintenance and cleaning and has a case worker on call for assistance to individuals; a worker from the Board of Education runs a rehabilitation program 4 hours/day, 5 days/week, that includes assistance with shopping; the City Recreation Department directs activities such as ceramics and candle making and a nutrition program that includes a 25¢ meal. The only transportation available is the local cab company. Management consists of a part-time project manager, who is a combination social worker, factotum, and a part-time office manager.

The final report, *Vistula Manor Demonstration Housing for the Physically Disabled,* prepared in 1969 by Leon A. Pastalan, PhD, is fascinating reading. It is available from National Technical Information Service, 5285 Port Royal Road, Springfield, Virginia 22151, for $3. Order OHIO LIH D-2 (No. P.B. 194 363).

The report indicates that the residents studied were improved in health and in self-sufficiency. On the other hand, they visited old friends less frequently and spent more time in solitary activities, such as television viewing. They were nearly unanimous in their enthusiasm for the architectural modifications.

The Appendix contains 14 pages of clear and comprehensive lists of recommendations for architectural details. Some of the items are of special interest: a cork floor is a successful compromise between carpet for elderly and hard surface for disabled persons; smooth wall surfaces are recommended; full-length mirrors are important for encouraging good grooming; acoustics are most important; sliding or bifold doors to storage areas should go all the way to the ceiling; a successful compromise work surface height would be 2 ft 10 in. for both elderly ambulant or wheelchair users; for safety reasons electricity is recommended for cooking; elevator buttons should be used instead of touch-light controls; and elevators should not have automatic closing devices but be manually closed after entry and activated by a button.

PILGRIM TOWER

Address: 1207 South Vermont Avenue, Los Angeles, California 90006
Sponsor: Pilgrim Lutheran Church of the Deaf
Date opened: June, 1968
Number of units: Total 111
Cost: $1,723,000
For: Deaf and Elderly
HUD program: Section 202 Direct Loan

Reverend Arnold T. Jonas, pastor of the Pilgrim Lutheran Church of the Deaf, and Jack A. Falkenberg, loan consultant, guided Pilgrim Tower (Fig. 13–2) into being after years of planning and work by the parishoners. The loan application for 100% financing under HHFA's 202 was made in 1965, and the first tenant moved in during June, 1968. Located next door to the church, the 13-story building contains 111 apartments which rent for $83–$130/month; rent includes utilities, carpeting, draperies, stove, refrigerator, and disposal.

Currently there are 117 deaf tenants, 4 of whom are also blind. The building is staffed with personnel who can communicate in sign language and who are ready to furnish a variety of services, such as making telephone calls and accompanying the residents to doctors and social security offices to act as their interpreters. The unique communications system is based on light signals; the doorbell is connected with lights, and the elevator has a light signal and a telephone. Each apartment has a bright light flasher and a special TV channel connected to a closed circuit projection in the manager's office; when the light is flashed, the tenant turns on the TV and sees the manager giving a message in sign language.

A Tower Council, composed of the tenants, coordinates all of the social activities, which range from 1-day excursions to card parties, bazaars, and holiday celebrations.

Fig. 13–2. Pilgrim Tower for the deaf uses a communications system based on lights.

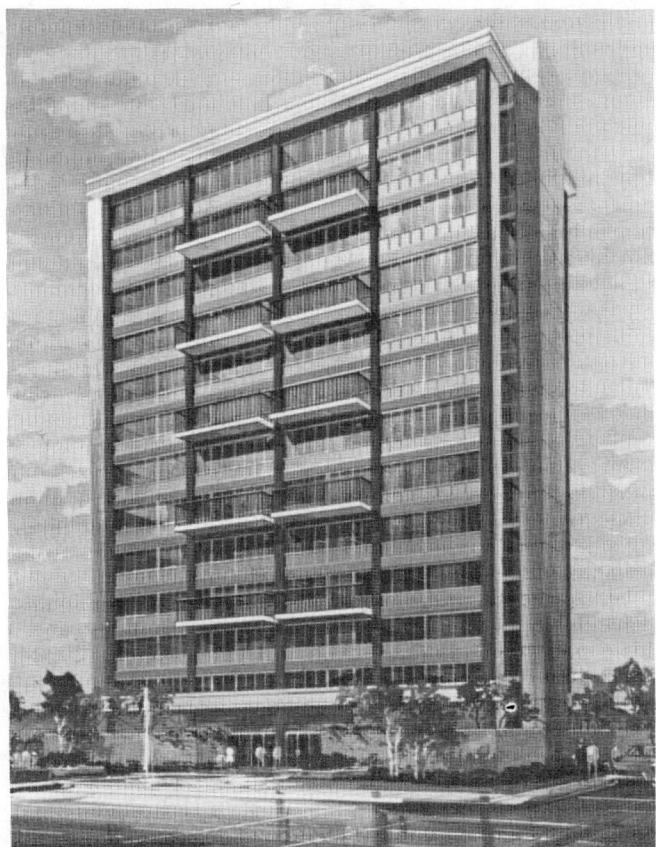

Fig. 13–3. A. Center Park Apartments, Seattle Housing Authority's 150-unit apartment building for low income disabled. **B.** The 7 foot long flower boxes outside large sliding windows are a source of pleasure to garden-loving residents.

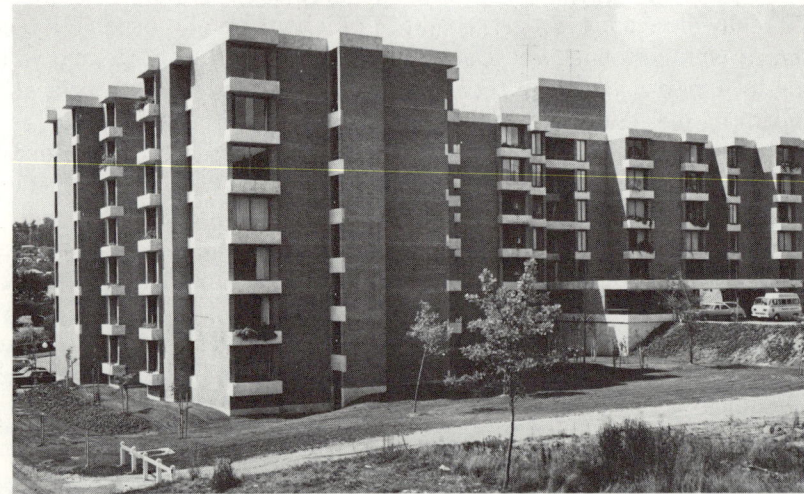

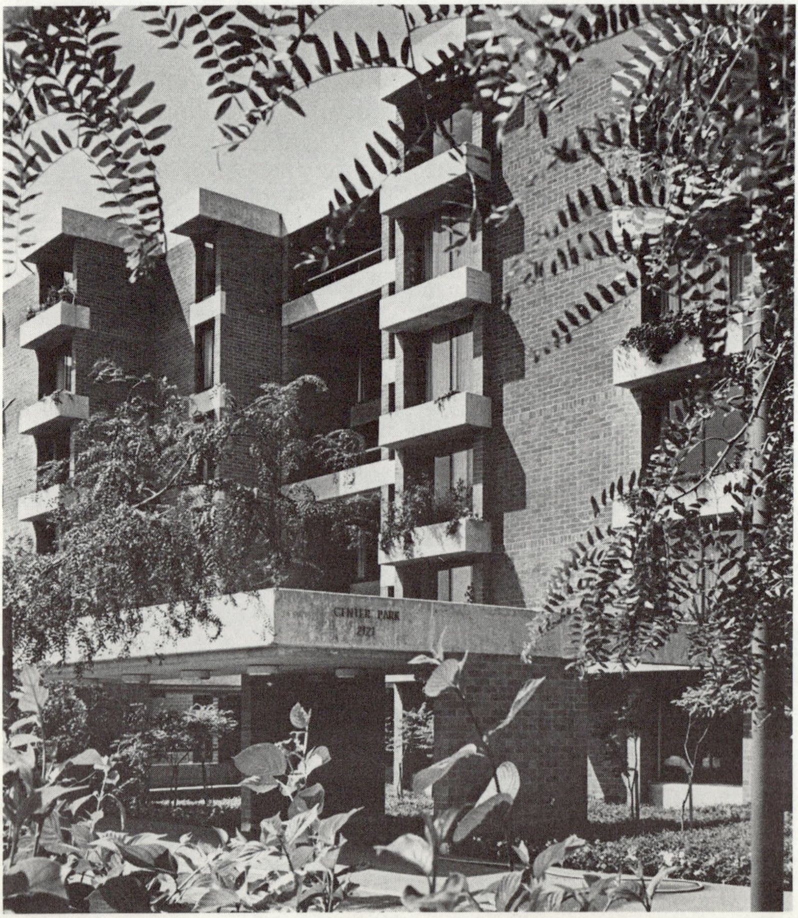

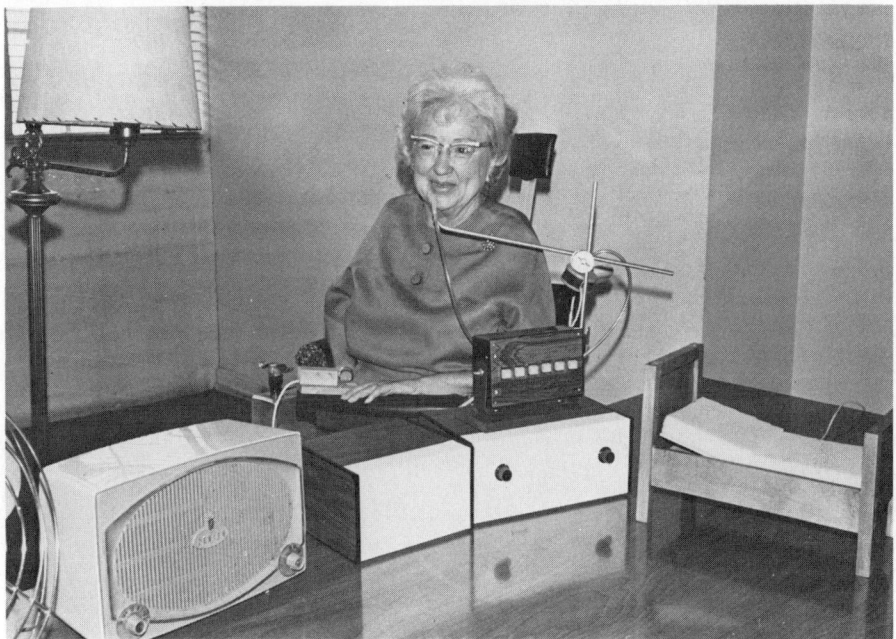

Fig. 13–4. Mrs. Ida Daly demonstrates a mouth-operated remote control system, Genie, with which she can operate a number of electrical appliances.

Reverend Jonas and his parishoners see the need to develop additional facilities to aid the deaf of all ages: facilities for congregate living, a convalescent facility, a rehabilitation program, and a referral information center to give whatever assistance is necessary.

CENTER PARK APARTMENTS

Address: 2121 26th Avenue South, Seattle, Washington 98144
Sponsor: Seattle Housing Authority
Date opened: 1969
Number of units: Total 150: 6 2-BR, 18 1-BR with movable room dividers, 126 1-BR with solid walls
Cost: $2,596,421
For: Elderly and handicapped
HUD program: Low rent public housing
Architect: Kirk, Wallace, McKinley & Associates, Seattle

Center Park Apartments (Fig. 13–3), a high-rise apartment and community building, evolved from the dreams and hard work of the Seattle Handicapped Club, a social and rehabilitative organization of disabled persons, which founded the Seattle Handicapped Center in 1957. The director, Mrs. Ida Daly, quadriplegic because of muscular dystrophy, spearheaded both the center and the apartment project (Fig. 13–4). The story is delightfully recounted in her autobiography, *Adventure in a Wheelchair.*

The apartment building has an irregular design, with three wings varying from six to seven stories. It is located on the site of a temporary war housing project —Stadium Homes. The site lies between two main north–south arterial highways, 10 min south of the central downtown business area. Unfortunately, the sidewalks and streets nearby are unimproved, and the area is a muddy barrier to wheelchairs. Further, there are no shopping or community facilities close to the apartments.

The original plan was for a complex of services for the disabled near the apartment facility. Unfortunately, the Seattle Handicapped Club was not able to build an adjacent multiservice center because of lack of funds. Consequently, the Club abandoned its plan to build there and purchased an older downtown building. This left the apartments without recreation and rehabilitation programs until August, 1974, when the Seattle Housing Authority opened the adjacent Community Building (Fig. 13–5)

KITCHENS AND BATHROOMS

The Seattle Handicapped Club members involved themselves in the planning of the kitchens and bathrooms by having models built in the dining room of the Center so that members with various disabilities could try them out and make suggestions. The kitchens have some excellent special features: the counter, with drawers, sink, and cooking units can be raised or lowered; above-the-counter cupboards are lower than average; ball-bearing drawers are self-closing; shelves are adjustable; sink faucets are at the side of the sink; there is extra wheel-in storage; a counter range or a plug-in oven/broiler can be used on the countertop or on top of a rolling cart; range controls are located in front; a pull-across folding screen divider closes off the kitchen area (Fig. 13–6).

The bathrooms are fairly large. All bathrooms have bathtubs and a special wheelchair lavatory. A large shower, with both overhead and hand sprays, is located on each floor. So many of the grab bars had to be changed to suit individual tenants that it would have been better to install them only as needed.

The poor features of the kitchens and bathrooms are relatively minor, since the architects profited by the experiences of Toledo's Vistula Manor and the club members' ideas. The freezer at the top of the refrigerator is unreachable, however, and the cut-out in the bread board pull-out is fine for one-handed cooks (though the cut-out should be on the side instead of the center) but a nuisance to others. The toilet bowls are too high for some wheelchaired but convenient for those who have difficulty rising.

PROS AND CONS

The front and rear doors from the parking garage are extremely difficult to open, and there is a lack of security in the garage. The building has an intercom security

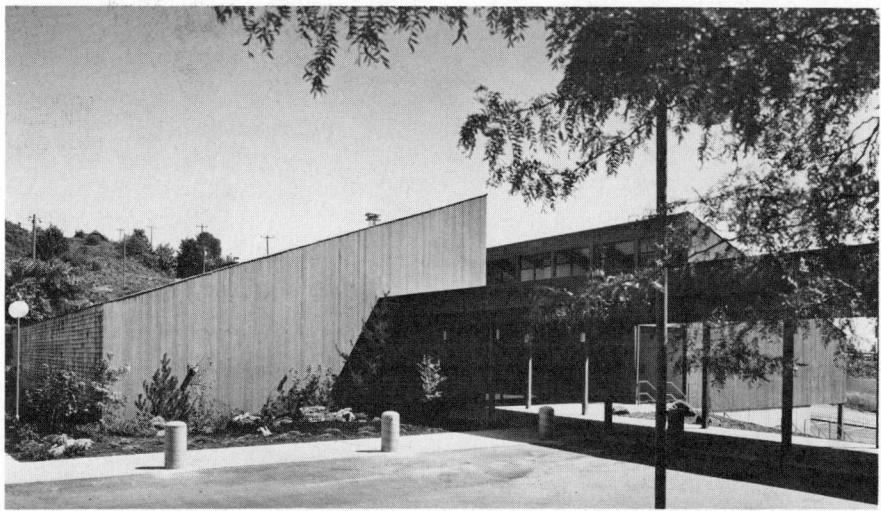

Fig. 13–5. The new Community Building, erected by the Seattle Housing Authority, provides the recreation and social facilities that were lacking during the first years of the Center Park Apartments.

Fig. 13–6. Kathé Young, a wheelchair sports star, tries out a friend's kitchen at Center Park.

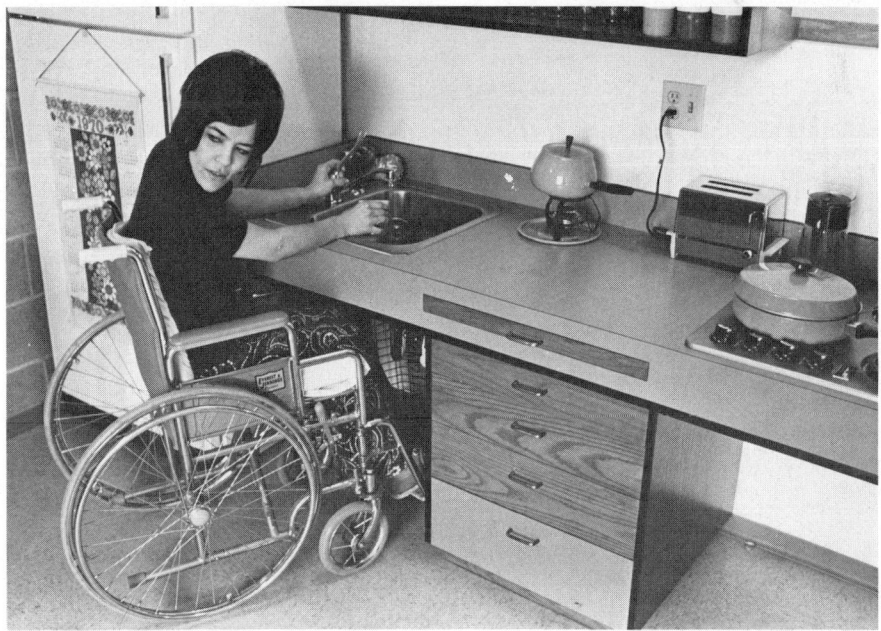

system located above the outside directory that enables visitors to call the apartments for clearance. In all units there are smoke detectors and an emergency alarm system that signals distress with a gong and panel lights.

Also on the positive side are wide elevators that accommodate a stretcher, hold six wheelchairs, and have low button panels; folding closet doors; high electric outlets; three balconies on each floor; lever door handles; and a large recreation plaza on the roof of the covered parking area that can be used for sunning, barbecueing, square dancing and enjoying Mt. Ranier and the surrounding hills.

There are also poor features, however: no external elevator indicator; no handrails in the halls; small sleeping areas in the efficiencies; and unpleasantly rough interior brick.

RESIDENTS

Admission priority was given to persons with an orthopedic or neurologic disability. The Seattle Housing Authority set up special eligibility requirements that were reviewed by an Advisory Committee consisting of doctors, physical therapists, the staff of the Handicapped Center and others working with the disabled. Initially, admissions were sporadic, although the units were all filled eventually. The present age range is from 21 to the mid-80s. Out of 155 disabled residents, there are now 113 in wheelchairs. The two most common disabilities are arthritis and multiple sclerosis.

STAFF AND SUPPORTIVE SERVICES

Because of the predominance of orthopedic and neurologic disabilities, the service needs are extensive and the staff inadequate. The staff consists of a manager who is there three times a week and two live-in custodial men. A public health nurse, homemakers, and home health aides are available at set hours. About a half dozen of the residents have their own live-in attendants, paid for by public welfare. (Only six apartments have two bedrooms, so there is little provision for live-in attendants; more two-bedroom units should have been included.) The new Community Building, connected to the apartment building by a covered walkway, has provided needed recreation and social facilities such as classes, hobby work, crafts, and lunches 2 days/week.

During the first few years of the project's operation, Mrs. Daly was the resident director. (Ironically, when she retired as resident director because of her age, she could no longer live there because of the income limitations.) Activities initiated by Mrs. Daly which still continue include weekly game night, classes, trips, tours, outside entertainers, and weekly grocery shopping and delivery. Church services, held in the lobby, are ecumenical, and include all major faiths. She also started a system of floor monitors; two residents in each wing watch unobtrusively for signs of any illness or accident, such as milk or papers that are not taken into an apartment, and report to the manager's office.

In 1973, after 4 years without any regular transportation for residents, Metro

Transit in Seattle permanently assigned one bus with a lift, and space for 11 people including 6 in chairs. In the first year, it covered over 45,000 miles, providing 5866 trips to clinics, work, school, and social events. In the summer of 1974, the availability of the bus was cut from 12 to 8 hours/day, curtailing evening use, but the residents indicate they still find the service helpful and convenient.

PROBLEMS

Mrs. Daly summarized the problems at Center Park Apartments in the August, 1971, issue of *Archives of Physical Medicine and Rehabilitation:*

Major problems have occurred in the areas of health, personal care, and housekeeping. Less critical but exceedingly important is a need for transportation for medical appointments, shopping, and recreation. Many health emergencies which require expensive ambulance trips to hospitals could be attended to by a system of interns and/or nurses stationed in the building in three 8-hour shifts. Many residents find bathing either in the tub or in the showers too difficult. Some health aides are supplied to Public Assistance recipients, but others must pay more than $5 for each bath. Hair care and barber needs are also problems. Public Assistance pays for housekeepers twice a week and live-in attendants for those unable to cook or care for themselves. However, this allowance is so small that it is difficult to find competent attendants. Housekeepers from the community are available at an hourly rate; those not on Public Assistance cannot afford this often enough.

These problems and recreation are outside the ordinary responsibilities of a housing authority. It has been suggested that one solution would be the formation of an independent entity, either of residents or an outside agency, which could handle all of these affairs, leaving housing staffs in charge only of management maintenance and overall supervision.

One of the residents reports her feelings, "In spite of the problems and fears that it would become a segregating 'island', Center Park is a nice place to live." It is unfortunate that it is located where it is, far from shops or community life, surrounded by muddy roads and lacking in transportation and other supportive services.

WALTER B. ROBERTS MANOR

Address: 1024 South 32nd Street, Omaha, Nebraska 68105
Sponsor: Omaha Association for the Blind
Date opened: 1969
Number of units: 42
Cost: $422,900
For: Blind and elderly
HUD program: FHA Section 221(d)(3)

Walter B. Roberts Manor is a four-story project for the blind which has few special built-in features; the floors, door names, and mail boxes are indicated only by Dymo tape in Braille, and the elevator has no sound cues as to floor. The rooms are furnished, and there are central dining facilities with three meals a day available.

The age range is 19–90: 2/3 are blind; 1/3 are elderly; there is a waiting list of 25. With the exception of a few young blind persons, most of the residents are retired. All of the blind eat in the dining room, but the elderly prefer to cook in their own apartments; some of the residents have a community service clean their apartments. Most residents are not interested in entertainment; the older people prefer to stay in their rooms and enjoy TV, and the young people go out for their entertainment.

As to special facilities for the deaf and the blind, Dr. Morton Leeds, Director, Special Concerns Staff, HUD, expressed the opinion at the National Conference on Housing which was held in Houston in 1974 that if persons benefit from the presence of others with the same disability, such as the deaf, they should be grouped together; but if they are handicapped by the presence of others with the same disability, such as the blind, they should not be grouped together.

HIGHLAND HEIGHTS APARTMENTS

Address: 1197 Robeson Street, Fall River, Massachusetts 02722
Sponsor: Fall River Housing Authority
Date Opened: Fall 1970
Number of Units: Total 208: 98 1-BR, 110 efficiencies
Cost: $2,942,204
For: Elderly and handicapped
HUD program: Low rent public housing
Architect: Charles Associates, Brookline, Massachusetts

After Seattle's Center Park Apartments' problems with isolation and lack of services, HUD's project the next year in Fall River, Highland Heights Apartments, swung to the other end of the pendulum (Fig. 13–7). It was closely allied to

Fig. 13–7. The Highland Heights Apartments were planned from the beginning to provide community medical and social services.

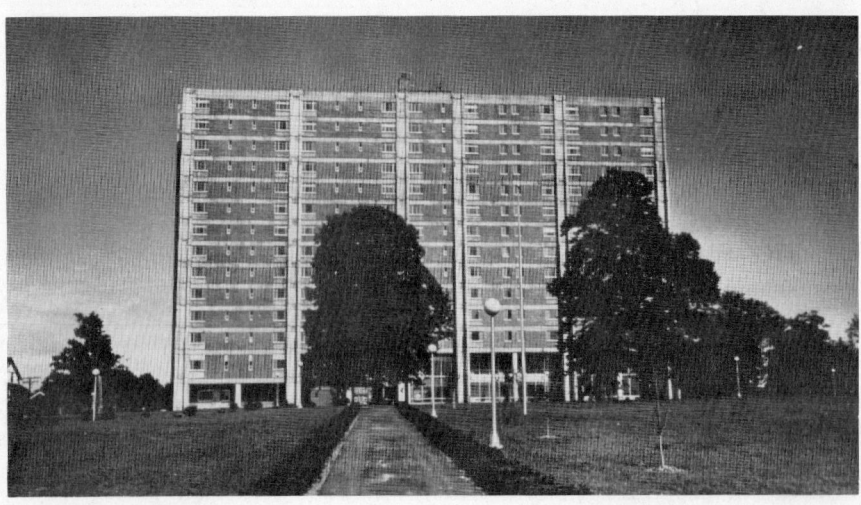

existing community services, connected by a tunnel to a municipal chronic disease hospital, and designed for low income physically impaired adults in need of supportive services.

The project was conceived by Dr. David S. Greer, medical director of the Hussey Hospital, because too many of his disabled patients could not return home after rehabilitation without assistive services and, consequently, were unnecessarily forced into nursing homes.

The 14-story building is located on top of a hill with an imposing view in a residential area of large old single family homes, across from a drug store and a bank and three blocks from a shopping center. The services include physical and occupational therapy, speech therapy, social work, and outpatient treatment. The unusual feature is the alarm system. An emergency switch in the bedroom and the bathroom activates a light outside the apartment and a gong in the clinics in the building and at the hospital. It also unlocks the apartment door.

During the first 4 years, the rehabilitation division of the hospital was located in the clinic or basement floor of the apartment building. In December, 1974, the Hussey Hospital was phased out because the city found it financially impractical to operate. The Visiting Nurse Association temporarily took over the rehabilitation space until arrangements were completed with another nearby hospital to take over the full rehabilitation division services.

The majority of the 248 residents are elderly (75% are age 62 or older), but their ages range 21–92. There are about twice as many women as men. An approximate count of the disabilities includes: about 52 wheelchaired by disabilities such as spinal cord injury, multiple sclerosis, or muscular dystrophy; about 20 severely limited in mobility by arthritis or other disabilities; about 10 blind and a half dozen deaf; the rest disabled by amputation, diabetes, strokes, or cardiovascular, kidney, or orthopedic problems.

SERVICES

The hospital's therapy and clinic services, visiting nurses, and home health care services were in operation immediately after opening, but social and other services were much slower to develop. Within 6 months after its opening, Tenant's Association (required by HUD) had been formed. Church services were brought into the building, and volunteer recreational services, a barber shop, and counseling services for tenants with critical problems were added. Shortly thereafter, a beauty shop, luncheon congregate dining, and some case-finding services became part of the facility.

The District Nurse Association covers 7 days, 24 hours/day, with at least one nurse on duty at all times and another to help with the overload. At least 24 Homemaker Home Health Aides work regularly with the residents, spending 1–8 hours per resident. The Fall River Council on Aging is located in the building and handles arrangements for hot meals (a local nutrition service furnishes a 50¢ noon meal to about 75% of the residents), use of surplus commodities, as well as other supportive services. Services in the community are available from many other agencies, including individual counseling from the Massachusetts Rehabilitation Commission and Romero Aid to the Elderly (RATE), a branch of the Family Service Society dedicated to helping the elderly maintain independent functioning for as long as possible.

The first floor is arranged to provide for a broad range of services and to act as a magnet for use by the community; it contains meeting halls, a dining room, craft rooms, game rooms, a coin-operated laundry, and a library.

Transportation is one of the unconquered problems; within the first year, two 12-passenger jitneys, equipped to handle wheelchairs, were available to residents and the community at large only for medical care transport. Efforts continue to be made to use the jitneys in the evenings for social functions or to acquire a van for that purpose.

ACCESSIBILITY FEATURES

The accessibility features are standard for a specialized facility: wide halls and doorways, plus handrails in the halls. Kitchens have low counters and cupboards with space beneath the sink, but there are complaints about having an electric oven and gas burners and the fact that the ovens are so low they are hard to reach from a wheelchair and almost impossible if using crutches. In the bathrooms the showers have grab bars, but there is a bump on the outer edge; the toilets are wheelchair height. Apartments were planned to be assigned according to whether one transfers from left or right, for half are one way and half the other.

RESEARCH REPORT

The research report comments that "particularly for persons with vision, hearing and speech impairments, the architectural features per se of the apartments do not seem to offer benefits beyond that of conventional housing." Since only 52 are in wheelchairs, it would have seemed that the kitchens and bathrooms are overdesigned for most of the residents and that the low ovens and counters would be actually inconvenient for the nonwheelchaired; however, the elderly discovered that they liked to sit down at the counters and work.

The lagniappe of the project is the final report of research on the impact of the facility and its services on the residents and on the economy of such a facility compared to a nursing or a long-term care facility. The 108-page report, *The Highland Heights Experiment,* by Sylvia Sherwood, PhD, of the Hebrew Rehabilitation Center for the Aged, and David S. Greer, MD, medical director of Hussey Hospital, is available from the U.S. Government Printing Office for $1.25. Supported by HUD, the Public Health Service, and the Fall River Housing Authority, the study not only developed screening techniques to select the residents and to identify their medical and social service needs but, in fact, actually stimulated the development of services.

The study of the impact of the milieu on the residents was divided into 1) a short-term study of the early effects of the facility on the health and well-being of its residents and 2) a substudy of 22 long-term care patients who had left institutions to become residents.

The short-term study included 420 persons—235 in the resident pool and 185 who were on the waiting list, who had been offered an apartment but refused, or who had canceled before being offered one. (Over 90% of the impact study sample were not gainfully employed.) The results of the study were a mixture of expected and unexpected:

1. Residents were more satisfied and in much better housing than if they had been left on their own.
2. Residency resulted in a beneficial change in lifestyle that would not have happened had they remained in the community; there was no feeling of being in a "health ghetto."
3. In terms of morale, the beneficial effect began when the resident was placed on the waiting list and remained the same during the first 9 months of the study.
4. Residency did not seem to increase the level of informal social activity over what it would have been had the person remained in the community. This surprised the researcher who had assumed that "these people have something in common, and this unity of understanding should go a long way towards breaking down the barriers that often hinder the handicapped in their attempts at achieving a satisfactory level of social involvement."

Comparative Costs

Totaling the costs of the 22 residents who had been institutionalized before, the report states, "The Highland Heights specialized housing provided a dramatically lower comparative cost than institutional care—a total of $4489/month ($204 each) at Highland Heights as compared with $18,135/month ($824 each) if the resident had remained in the institutional setting. An analysis of the data reveals that, on the average, the cost of institutional living is over four times greater than the cost of residing in Highland Heights for this group when both basic living costs and comparable service utilization costs are taken into consideration."

Conclusions

The data from this study support the proposition that many persons residing in long-term care facilities require only some of the services offered within the institution and could probably be successfully maintained in a more independent setting within the community were such services available.

Data from this substudy . . . clearly indicate that sheltered housing—consisting not only of mortar and bricks but also of ancillary medical and social services—is a viable alternative for some types of persons who tend to be institutionalized. Furthermore, by providing this type of housing alternative for selected persons from the elderly and physically impaired population, there is a more efficient utilization of medical care facilities and services and a reduction in unnecessary and excessively costly institutional care.

NEW HORIZON MANOR

Address: 2525 North Broadway, Fargo, North Dakota 58102
Sponsor: Fargo Housing Authority
Date Opened: July, 1972
Number of Units: Total 100: 80 1-BR, 20 2-BR
Cost: $1,947,875
For: All disabled
HUD Program: Low rent public housing
Architect: Mutchler, Twichell & Lynch, Fargo, North Dakota

New Horizon Manor has been under a lucky star since its inception in 1967, when three disabled members of the Red River Valley Handicapped Club, Ruth Erickson, Edna Hudson, and Mary Kodelka, began to plan a barrier-free motel along the lines of the Motel 66 in California. Eventually, their concept was endorsed by an orthopedic surgeon, an occupational therapist, an architect, and the mayor. When Fargo received an allocation of 250 low rent units in 1970, the mayor convinced HUD that 100 of these should be in a project specifically designed for the disabled.

The location is excellent for melding into the community scene: across the street from a regional shopping center, a bowling alley, restaurants, park, service station, within a residential area, and near two city parks that are especially designed for the disabled.

In terms of physical design and thoughtful planning, New Horizon Manor is the best of all the HUD projects for the disabled (Fig. 13-8). Its perceptive and creative architect, Seth Twichell, spent 3 months researching designs including visits to the earlier HUD project, Center Park Apartments, in Seattle. Throughout the planning, he was attuned to the requirements of the wheelchaired residents, consulting them on special details.

Twichell found that the cost of the special kitchen was almost the same as a standard kitchen; the only extra cost was having an oven separate from the range. He would have liked a different kind of refrigerator. He does not feel that it is absolutely necessary to have wheel-under-space under the countertop burners; most people can work sideways to stir or brown food.

As to bathrooms, Twichell stated that bathrooms for the wheelchaired need an extra 20 square feet of space (standard: 40 square feet in a 5 × 8 ft. bathroom). The special bathroom equipment cost $390 more than a standard bathroom (grab bars, $150; fold-down seat, $25; adjustable shower, $40; wall-hung toilet, $30; and sliding door, $20). Showers are more expensive to install than tubs in a high rise because of the precautions necessary to prevent flooding.

High-rise apartments offer many advantages to the disabled, according to the architect; they do not have to walk or roll so far to see each other as they would in dispersed units, and the elevator is a good social mixer. As to fires, Twichell said that they could not spread from floor to floor, and since there were only 11 units per floor, the residents could easily be evacuated by the firemen.

Expressing the viewpoint of a resident, Ruth Erickson says,

HUD-Assisted Housing Projects   229

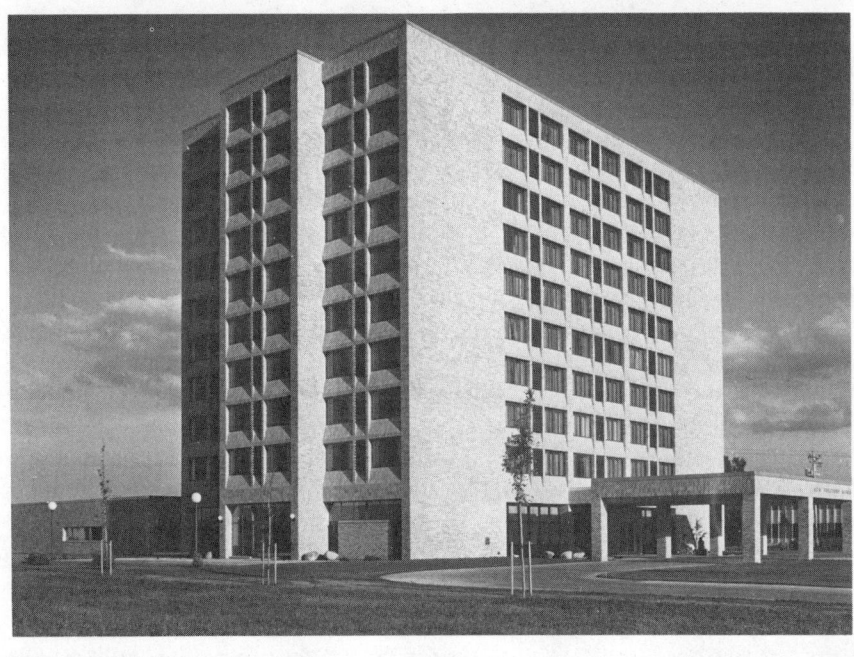

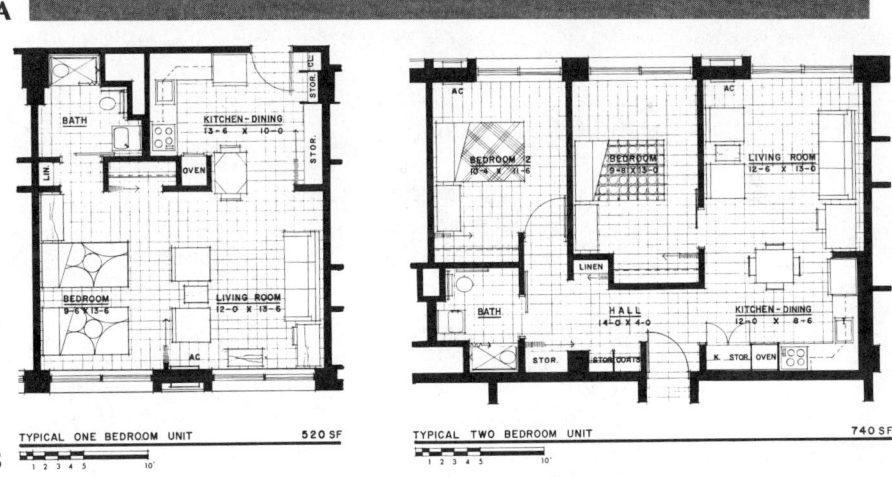

Fig. 13–8. New Horizon Manor, sponsored by the Fargo Housing Authority. **A.** The architect, Seth Twichell, kept a wheelchair on site during construction to use as a yardstick and a reminder of the future residents. **B.** Floor plans of typical units. (Plans and photographs supplied by S.W. Twichell)

As one approaches the main entrance, the door slides open and we can walk or roll in. . . . Our main floor consists of a lobby/lounge, two elevators, three offices (secretary, manager, and custodian), two custodian's apartments (accessible for wheelchairs), craft room, work shop, activity room, extra large party kitchen (from which we have one meal a day), storage space, public rest rooms, compacter room, and a lovely patio (which needs furniture). We started with one hobby room, then found that you need two, one for "clean" crafts like weaving and ceramics and one for "dirty" crafts like woodworking. The activities room is a little crowded for the number of people who use it. In the evenings we gather for a social hour or two to play cards or bingo or just an old-fashioned gab session. Many groups are interested in our new home and come to visit or entertain us.

The community facilities are excellent.

As a compromise on the usual shower vs tub controversy, showers were built in each apartment and three tub rooms were placed on three different floors. Erickson says the tubs have not been used because the residents could not get into them and they have become accustomed to the showers in their apartments; recently a hydraulic lift was added to one of the tubs to make them more usable by attendants and visiting nurses.

The rooms in all the apartments are ample and the bathrooms are large and well-planned (Fig. 13-9). The bathroom doors are sliding; the shower has a fold-down seat and a thermostat-controlled shower head that can be moved up or down or held in the hand. The height of the toilet seat was changed to wheelchair height; nevertheless, it is an annoyance to some who find it either too high or too low. Grab bars are well-located. The architect put particular thought on planning the cupboards, building mockups for the residents to try, then rede-

Fig. 13-9. The bathrooms are especially well-planned. **A.** Each bathroom has a special wheelchair lavatory and conveniently low cabinet. **B.** Unfortunately, the showers are not roll-in showers because HUD forced the use of a 4 inch curb to prevent flooding. (Plans and photographs supplied by S.W. Twichell, Architect)

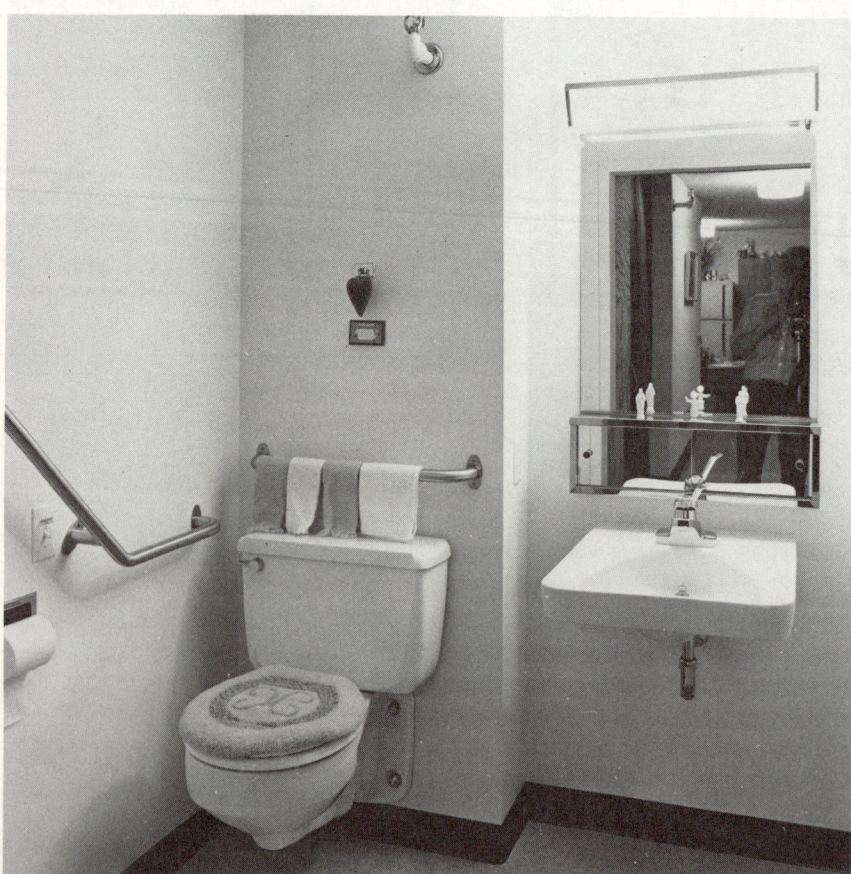

signing them all with adjustable shelves until they were suitable for the majority of disabilities.

Ruth Erickson reports,

> Our kitchens have a counter, sink, and work area all in one (Fig. 13–10). Under this area is a vast open space for wheelchairs. There is no need to stretch to use the sink because the sink was turned sideways and the lever type faucets are on the side of the sink, not the back. All cupboards have touch latch openings so a slight tap makes them spring open. What a wonderful feeling to open doors without a struggle! Light switches are low and outlets are high (though I wish they had not omitted ceiling lights, lamps are difficult for arthritic hands) . . . The counters are fine but the cupboards above should have been adjustable, too, because they are too high for many of us to reach; the corner diagonal unit has a lazy Susan. There are "panic" (alarm) buttons in the bedroom and bathroom, one would have been a comfort in the kitchen too.

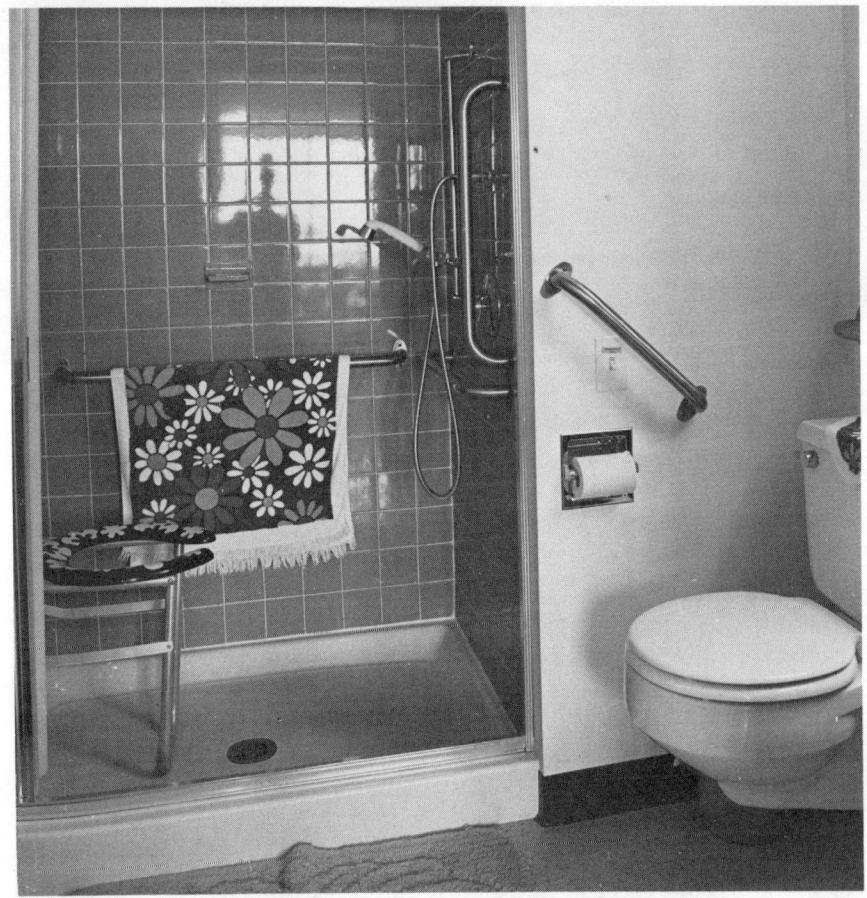

B

The ovens are a revised Westinghouse unit with a special side-opening door similar to a unit designed by an Alabama outfit (assiduously sleuthed by the architect) and a pull-out shelf below the door of the oven, in addition to the usual cutting board with the mixing bowl cut-out. The refrigerator is top-loading; unfortunately, it is not self-defrosting.

Miscellaneous features include an enclosed 24-car garage with headbolt heater outlets for open parking; all doors used by the residents are lever type. A complete sprinkler system, intercom system, and smoke detectors are in all apartments. Very light wood slat closet doors are opened or closed by pulling a loop. Front and back doors are locked against intruders but open to keys after 10:30 P.M. There is an overcrowded physical therapy room on the second floor. The building is completely air conditioned.

All of the tenants are disabled; their disabilities include multiple sclerosis, arthritis, cerebral palsy, poliomyelitis, paraplegia, and blindness (majority: multiple sclerosis and arthritis). Their ages range 17–85, with most of them in their 40s or 50s. The young paraplegics, whose numbers have been increasing, do not participate in the group activities, such as pot luck suppers. Most of the live-in attendants are mentally retarded and have been trained by the Vocational Training Center; finding the right one is a matter of trial and error, patience, and luck. A "Floor

Fig. 13–10. The counter, sink, and work area can be lowered or raised 6 inches. (Photograph supplied by S.W. Twichell, Architect)

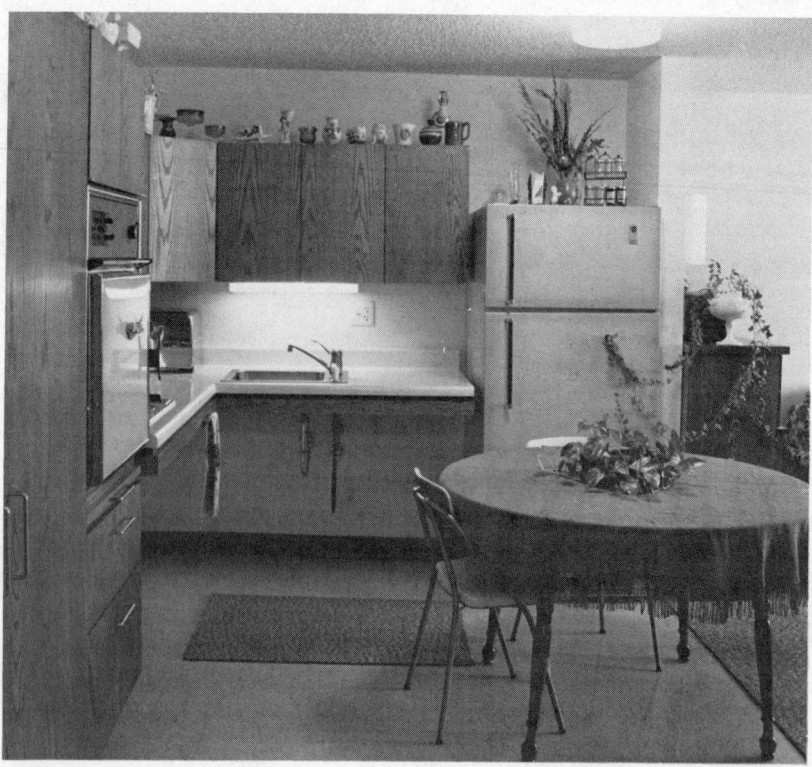

President" on each floor is responsible for investigating a call for help on the alarm system and then notifying the custodian, if necessary.

Eligibility is based on the local public housing formula: income for a single person may not exceed $3400 and for a couple, one of whom must be handicapped, $3600. There is an asset limitation of $12,000. Rents are based on 22% of income and include light, heat, water, and garbage removal charges.

Transportation was a frustration until in 1975 the residents and the Red River Valley Handicapped Club collected enough coupons to purchase a van with a hydraulic lift. Drivers are paid by the city; one-way prices range from 50¢ to $1.50; scheduling is done by volunteers and return trips are arranged by CB radio.

The problem areas have been in services and operation, not in the building design or equipment. Most of the problems are being gradually solved as more agencies in the community become involved.

INDEPENDENCE HALL

Address: Airline Drive at Burress Street, Houston, Texas 77022
Sponsor: Goodwill Industries
Date opened: 1973
Number of units: Total 292: 20 2-BR, 128 1-BR, 144 efficiencies
Cost: $3,179,800
For: Elderly and disabled
HUD program: FHA Section 236

The previous public housing projects were designed for the lowest income elderly and disabled, while Independence Hall was built for lower and middle income groups under the Section 236 formula. Goodwill Industries of Houston, under the leadership of Mr. William A. Lufburrow, sponsored the project (Fig. 13–11).

Incredibly, the entire project was designed without any knowledge of previous projects for the disabled. The special features were all worked out anew by a panel of disabled people from the Goodwill workshop who submitted their own ideas for an accessible and workable environment. As a result of the varied assortment of disabilities, the adaptations cover a wide range—those for the blind, elderly, little people, and amputees, as well as those for people who use crutches and wheelchairs. According to Lufburrow, "The hardest part was convincing planners and builders that there is not a *typical* disabled person . . . We felt it was better to have built and goofed than never to have built at all."

The 292 units virtually fill the 10-acre site on the northern outskirts of Houston. The 12 two-story residence buildings and the administration building form three quadrangles, all interconnected at the points. The first floor of the administration building contains a brightly decorated two-storied living room with a corner fireplace. Though last minute drastic economies reduced the size, it is a warm and inviting meeting room. A large window-walled entrance lounge, a hall with individual post office boxes, and the reception office make the whole first floor a gathering area. In addition, there is an organ, a stereo, and color TV.

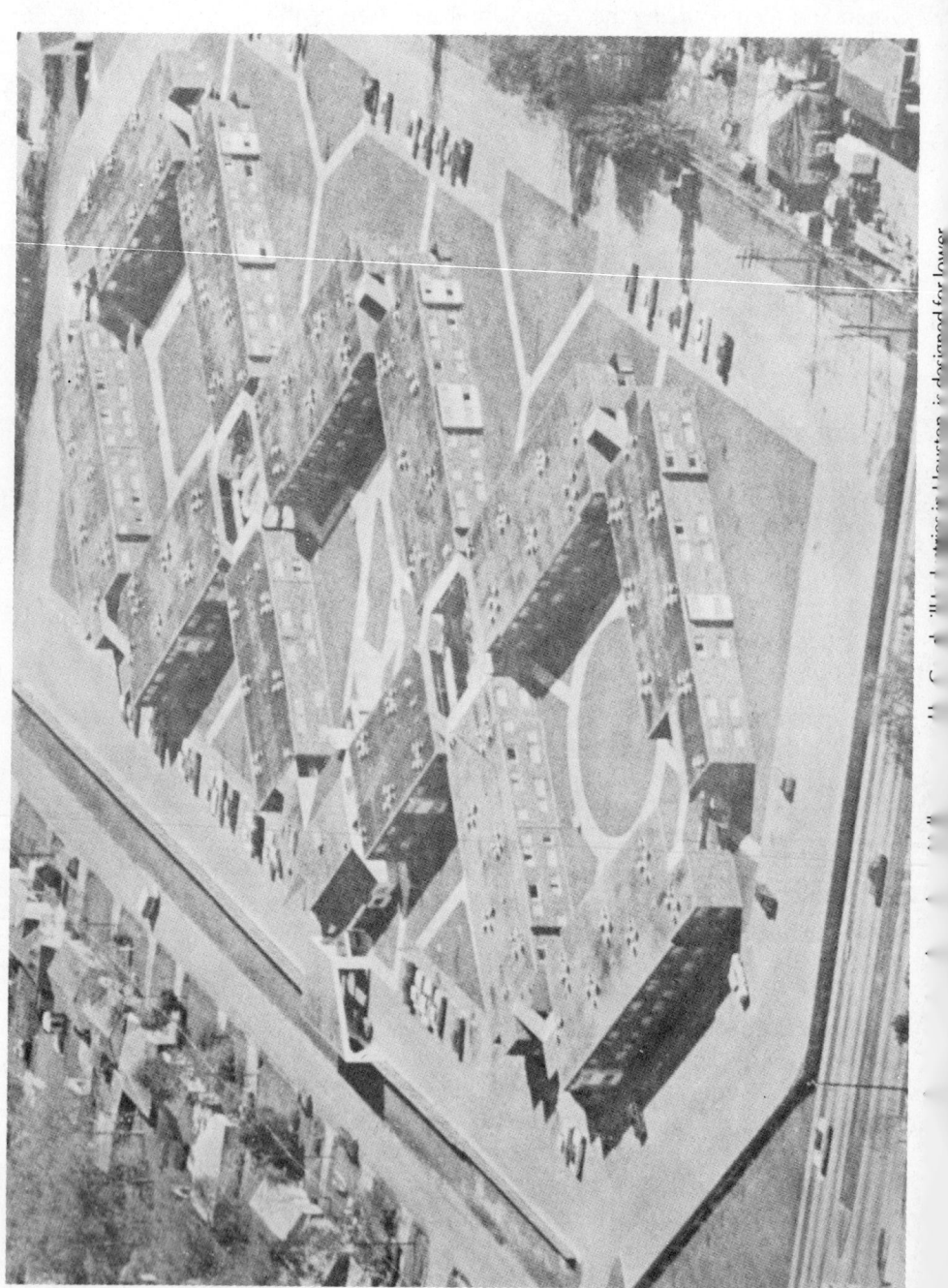

HUD-Assisted Housing Projects

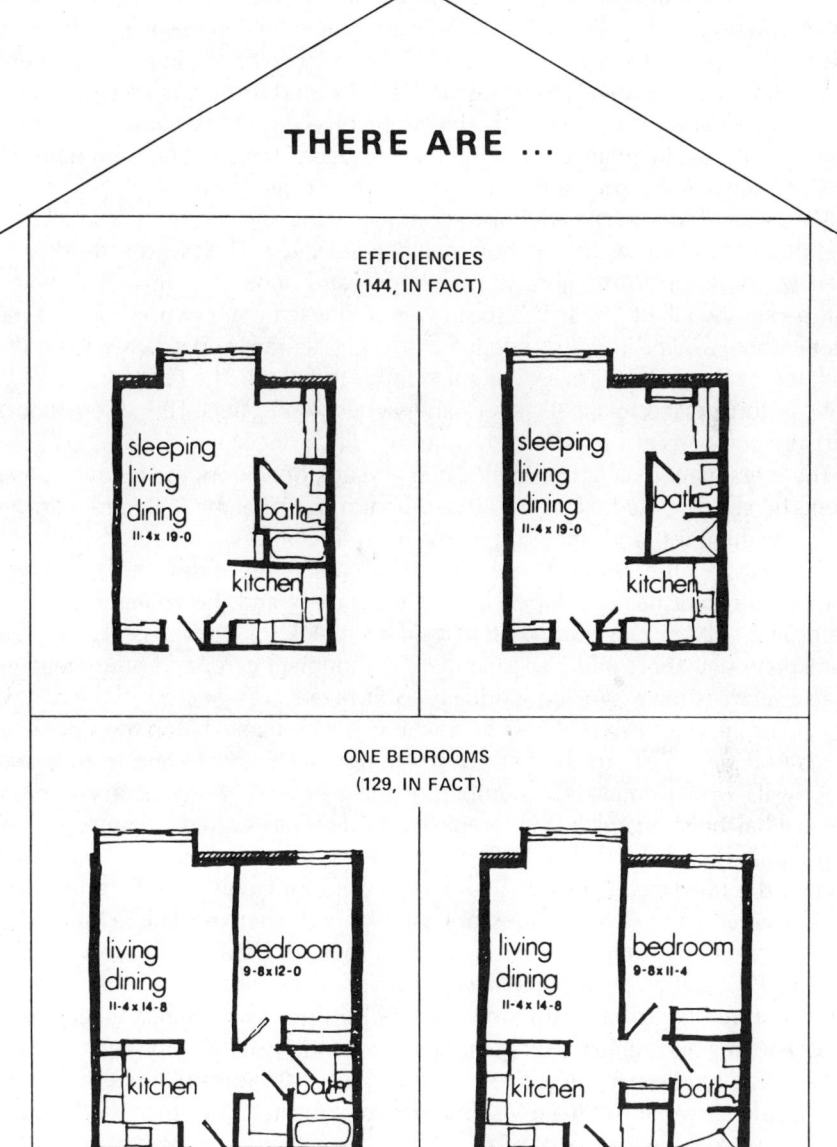

THERE ARE ...

EFFICIENCIES
(144, IN FACT)

ONE BEDROOMS
(129, IN FACT)

B

The resident manager, Mrs. Sandi Davenport, who uses crutches because of a childhood bout with poliomyelitis, has an apartment behind the office. Her enthusiasm and energy are typical of the efficiency and spirit of the project. There is a close link with Goodwill Industries, which is located several miles away. Lufburrow, the administrator of both, is deeply involved in the workings of Independence Hall and his wife is the building manager. Their strong commitment is solving many of the problems and moving the project forward.

The second floor of the administration building is reached by two small elevators that entail long waits for the wheelchaired. Nevertheless, the residents do manage to get up to the library, the chapel, and another room which was revamped in the fall of 1974. The room was an unused crafts/workshop and party kitchen until a blind resident opened a small restaurant and grocery store there with the backing of the Texas Commission for the Blind. The residents agree that it is "a good place to meet" over sandwiches and coffee. The little restaurant partially compensates for the lack of group dining facilities.

The rental pattern is noteworthy. After a year's operation, the following apartments had been rented: 18 of the 20 two-bedrooms; all of the 128 one-bedrooms, with a waiting list; and only 102 of the 144 efficiencies.

One-third of the residents are age 62 or older; the oldest is 91. "A good community spirit has developed among the elderly and the younger disabled," according to Mrs. Davenport. "If a resident is sick for a week or 10 days, the immediate neighbors and I will handle the shopping, care, and housekeeping."

The services have evolved gradually to fit needs. The first bus, which lacked a ramp or lift, has been replaced by a van with a hydraulic lift on the side; it runs all day taking people to the nearby shopping center and to and from work at Goodwill, which employs a number of the residents. A resident community council has been organized. A paraplegic resident has started a wheelchair sales and repair shop in the project. Some residents have planted ferns and flowers around the buildings. A picnic area and an outdoor game area for shuffleboard have been added. Extensive landscaping is planned. There is a link to hospital and medical services through ties to Goodwill's program. There is a grocery shopping service. Though there was originally no plan for attendant service, after six quadriplegics rented adjacent apartments and set up their own attendant service and housekeeping and dining arrangements, Independence Hall took over those attendant and food services (see Free Lives, Inc., Ch. 10). Some of the residents who are eligible for Medicare have Visiting Nurses come in to give them bathing care, if prescribed by their doctors.

The second floor apartments are reached by two elevators and by two sets of long ramps that double back and forth so that the incline is gentle enough for easy, though lengthy wheeling.

The kitchens have ample space underneath the shallow sinks for wheelchair use; low shelving; a conventional under-the-burner oven that is too low (some wheelchaired have added small countertop ovens and used the oven for storage; front stove controls; and an excellent refrigerator, though it lacks automatic defrosting and has a small freezer portion. The kitchens lack two of the usual special features: a pull-out board with cut-outs for mixing bowls and an adjustable height kitchen sink and work space. They have dishwashers and disposals, however. The bathrooms have drive-in showers and support bars on the walls, but the toilets are too low for easy use from a wheelchair.

Other special features include raised apartment numbers as an aid for the blind (two residents are blind), an emergency button in each apartment to alert the main office but no intercom to save steps, and a coin-operated laundry.

Financial eligibility is determined through verification from social security, employers, and other sources. The rents range $80–$187.74, and all include utilities, draperies, stove, carpets, dishwasher, and refrigerator. If 25% of a tenant's income is between the high and low rates, the 25% figure is the rent which is paid. If 25% of the income is over the high rate, only a credit check is required. If 25% is under the low rate, a committee determines eligibility. The program is subsidized rent, not rent supplement.

Dean Phillips, President and Chief Executive Officer of Goodwill Industries of America described the project as one of the mistakes from which knowledge and experience has been acquired. "After it was built, we were surprised to learn that all handicapped people didn't want to live in it. They didn't want to live only with other handicapped people. They wanted to live in a community. When we build again, we'll spread out into smaller units in communities."

CREATIVE LIVING

Address: 445 West Eighth Avenue, Columbus, Ohio 43210
Sponsor: Creative Living, Inc.
Date Opened: October, 1974
Number of Units: Total 18: All 1-BR
Cost: $333,100
For: All severely disabled
HUD Program: FHA Section 236
Architect: Charles M. Frank, assisted by Richard Eschliman and Associates, consulting architects

Creative Living is of particular interest as an example of a small residential unit where attendants are shared that was created by mobilizing a community to work with severely disabled individuals to solve environmental barriers (Fig. 13–12). Of further interest is the fact that the founders retained the original concept of no more than 20 residents and did not change from providing intermediate, rather than permanent, living arrangements. The project involved participation by severely disabled individuals, a university medical rehabilitation center, church groups, service clubs, lawyers, architects, professional consultants, FHA and HUD, and a well-balanced Board of Trustees and Women's Service Board.

The 18-unit apartment complex, with special facilities and 24-hour assistance for its severely disabled tenants, was opened in October, 1974, after nearly 6 years of planning by its nonprofit organization. During all these years the catalyst was Ernest W. Johnson, MD, Chairman of the Department of Physical Medicine at Ohio State University Hospitals, who worked closely with the project's archi-

Fig. 13–12. Creative Living apartment complex. **A.** The front doors of the apartments are under cover and open onto the grassy courtyard. **B.** The back doors of the apartments open onto a small patio.

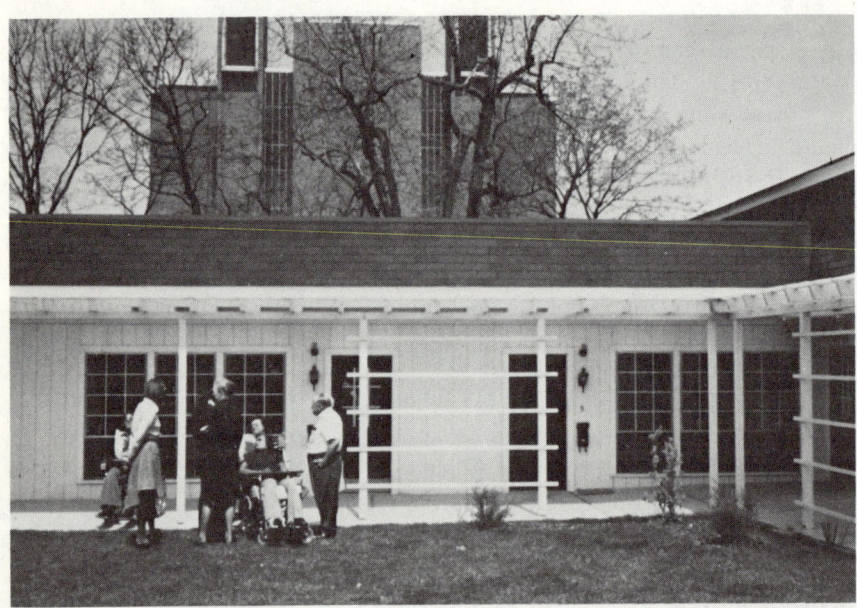

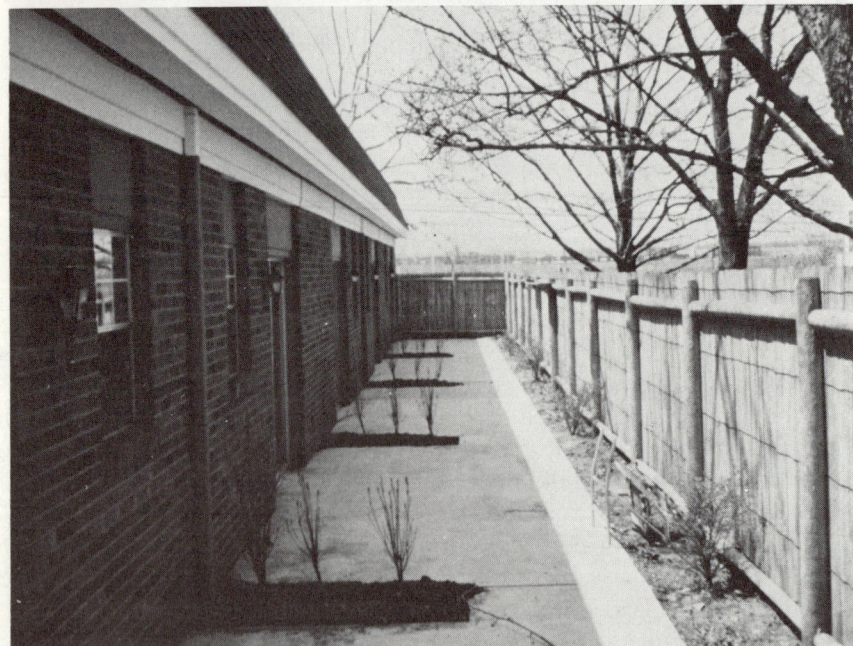

tect, Charles M. Frank, and its lawyer, Edward Whipps. Working along with them have been two quadriplegics, Richard N. Maxwell and Jack R. Dacre. Maxwell, an ex-Marine and C4-5 quad, was injured in a football game at OSU in the fall of 1963, rehabilitated at OSU Hospitals, graduated in 1969, and employed as Nursing Workshop Coordinator at Dodd Hall, the university's rehabilitation center. Dacre, a graduate of Otterbein College and an employee of the Ohio Department of Health, had spent 9 years in nursing homes or Dodd Hall.

In May, 1970, Creative Living, Inc., contracted with a Cincinnati-based consulting agency, Community Development Associates, Inc., to carry out a preliminary feasibility study to identify the probable market, facility costs and components, funding sources, and financial program. The cost of the study, $2800, was met through donations, the major amount from the Multiple Sclerosis Society. Questionnaires were sent to 153 disabled persons, aged 18–40. Of the 35 completed and returned, 29 (18%) indicated interest in an adaptive living facility.

The average age of the 29 interested respondents was 23; the average educational attainment was 12 years; there were 21 males; 21 were unemployed; and their disabilities included 12 quadriplegia, 3 partial quadriplegia, 6 paraplegia, and 1 each multiple sclerosis, cerebral palsy, hemiplegia, and birth injury.

By the fall of 1971, the site was determined when the Battelle Memorial Institute leased land adjacent to the OSU campus and within easy reach of Dodd Hall to Creative Living, with a 5-year contribution by Battelle of land rent. The 25-year lease is renewable by mutual agreement with the possibility of a further contribution by Battelle, depending on the success of the project. In May of the following year, rezoning and a zoning variance for the site were approved by the Columbus City Council.

COMMUNITY INVOLVEMENT AND FUND RAISING

The group gathered momentum and coherence, gradually expanding its actively working Board of Trustees to reach the community and build wide support. Creative Living (CL) was chosen as the official and perpetuating project of The Ohio Federation of Women's Clubs (OFWC), an 18,000 member organization to which more than 500 clubs belong; this action permitted CL to apply for financial and service support as well as support for legislation to assist the disabled in Ohio. Meanwhile, an annual membership drive was started and radio and TV publicity and local press coverage were successfully generated.

After only 2 years, by July, 1974, the OFWC had raised a total of $10,700, chiefly by collecting S & H, Top Value and Buckeye stamps; this money was used to purchase furniture for the lounge and community living area. In addition, they collected Betty Crocker coupons and exchanged them for the equipment needed in the kitchen. Individual clubs donated a washer and dryer and stereo equipment. The Altrusa Club of Columbus donated furnishings for some of the apartments. A living gift was presented by the Columbus Council of Garden Clubs of Ohio: the provision and maintenance of plants in the complex. Everett & Jennings donated $15,000 to make the film of a quadriplegic's life, starring Jack Dacre, titled *Still Life*. Substantial donations were received from the Columbus Foundation, the First Community Church Foundation, the Upper Arlington Rotary Club, the Women's Service Board (formerly Creative Living's Auxiliary), the Nationwide Foundation, the Columbus Alumnae of Delta Delta Delta Sorority, and the Franklin County Chapter of the Multiple Sclerosis Society.

FEDERAL ASSISTANCE

By the fourth year, a preliminary feasibility study had been made, nonprofit status secured, funds raised for interim operating expenses, and a site leased. CL then began a 2-year struggle to obtain federal assistance; CL's patient and determined efforts demonstrate that the way is not easy and that it requires the assistance of experts.

In February, 1972, Dr. Ernest W. Johnson, medical advisor, Charles M. Frank, President, and Paul Savage, Finance Chairman, went to the Regional V offices of the Social Rehabilitation Services in Chicago to discuss federal subsidies. In late summer of the same year, CL retained Sisson–Stern Co., a construction, regional packager, and contracting firm, to help obtain a Federal Housing Administration (FHA) commitment for an insured loan so that a construction mortgage could then be sought through a bank or other lending institution.

On January 5, 1973, a preliminary feasibility letter for a federally guaranteed mortgage was issued. Rejoicing was brief, however, for on February 28 CL received a letter withdrawing this feasibility letter. Further, it received word that the application must be reprocessed. During the 3-month delay, CL began to investigate financing from a private mortgage brokerage firm. At last, during the month of August a new conditional commitment was issued by the FHA which assured CL of an insured mortgage, of a reasonable amount, to cover the facility, as well as a major interest subsidy and supplemental rental funds for qualified tenants. However, it was February 4, 1974, before FHA closed the deal that resulted in a government insured mortgage of $333,100 over 40 years. This section 236 interest–subsidy program also provides $3703/year as rental supplement for qualified tenants.

THE APARTMENT COMPLEX

The facility is located in an area of older apartment houses, adjacent to the OSU campus. The one-story totally accessible complex is built around an open grassy courtyard, totally enclosed by three buildings and a high wooden fence; the spacious common lounge has a woodburning fireplace, TV, stereo, library area, and an adjacent small party kitchen. Off the hall are the offices of the staff assistant and the resident manager. The former has an intercom call board and a view of most of the apartment doors. Situated in convenient locations are covered vehicle loading areas and laundry facilities; a large parking lot for residents and their guests is located across the street.

Each apartment has a living room, bedroom, bath, and kitchenette; five of the units are larger than the others. Curtains, kitchen appliances, and an electric hospital bed are furnished with the apartment; the rest of the furnishings are supplied by the residents.

The bathrooms are enormous with wide doorways and accordion doors. The shower areas are a corner that can be curtained off; sinks and toilets are all of wheelchair height, and there are ample grab bars. The small electric kitchens were not designed for anyone in a wheelchair because it was incorrectly assumed that quadriplegics could not do any cooking and all the cooking would be done by attendants or relatives. However, several of the residents who are quadriplegic can do some cooking. For them, the oven is impossibly high, since it is placed in the upper cabinets. The drop-down kitchen table and work area are permanently set at a height that is too low for some wheelchair arms; they should have been made adjustable in height.

All doors are wide, and the light switches and thermostats are easily reachable from a wheelchair. The intercom is activated by a pressure pad connected by a cord to a panel by the bed. Residents whose hands are too weak to operate the pressure pad put it on the floor and run over it with their electric wheelchairs (the cord should be longer); one of the residents had hers redesigned to operate with less pressure. Each living unit is protected from fire and smoke by an alarm system and an automatic sprinkler system. Individual gas-fired forced air units provide heat in winter and cooling in summer.

RESIDENT SELECTION

The Screening Committee, composed of two doctors, two quadriplegics, and three trustees, worked out a philosophy of resident selection. Applicants must be in need of some personal care, either employed or enrolled in an institution of higher learning or in a vocational training program, and at least 18 years old. There is no defined maximum age, but if an individual no longer fits into the CL way of life, he will be counseled into a more appropriate residential facility. The committee concentrates on those aged 20–30 who want to be independent. The applicant must also be motivated to improve his situation, be able to direct or participate in self-care, have a desire to be part of the facility, and comprehend the implications of his disability. Finally, the applicant's family must be evaluated to determine finances and degree of support within the family environment. Each resident is subject to a semiannual evaluation by a committee of his peers. The admissions procedure consists of four stages: 1) collection of personal information, 2) investigation of medical and social background, 3) personal interview, 4) 6-month trial period.

RESIDENTS

The year 1974 was kaleidoscopic for Creative Living: ground was broken on February 22; eight residents moved in on September 22; and an open house, attended by more than 400 persons, was held on October 6. Of the eight first residents, four were employed and four were students. By mid-1975, there are 14 residents—11 traumatic quadriplegics and 3 poliomyelitis quadriplegics; 4 females, 10 males; the majority are in their 20s. One resident is working as a social worker in a cancer research project at University Hospitals; another, a lawyer from out of state, is studying to pass the Ohio bar examinations; another is working as a nursing workshop coordinator; another is a representative of the Ohio Department of Health in Dodd Hall; while another, an artist, paints with a brush held between his teeth (Fig. 13–13). Half are students at Ohio State; their fields are diverse: education, horticulture, social work, production management, business administration, social sciences education, and nursing home administration.

New residents are added very gradually because of the double problem of arranging financial aid and of meeting the criteria for residency. In some instances, an applicant's desire to move in has spurred him to make arrangements for a job or a training course.

RENT AND LIVING EXPENSES

The average total living expenses amount to about $400/month. For those whose income is limited to Supplemental Security Income, the amount of additional money needed averages about $250 monthly. Originally, CL had planned to meet an annual deficit of $3000 per resident. Fortuitously, additional government funds reduced the amount to $500–$700.

Fig. 13–13. Bobby Spencer, one of the quadriplegic residents, is a skilled mouthstick painter.

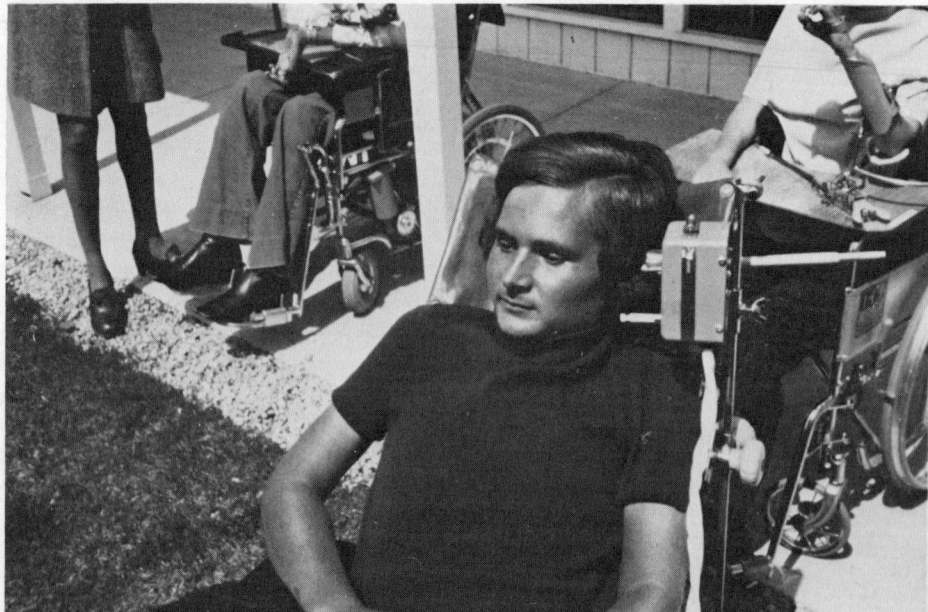

A typical student resident receives from the Bureau of Vocational Rehabilitation: tuition, books, rent (paid directly to CL), $25 for transportation, and $100 for food. Those in job training receive half-salary until ready for full employment. Most of their living expenses, excluding medicines and clothing, are paid entirely by the Bureau of Vocational Rehabilitation.

All utilities are included in the monthly rent of $124 (the rent supplement is $3703 annually). The rent does not include additional charges of $2 for the use of laundry facilities and $38 for the staff assistant service (this figure would have been about $112 if a special grant from the state had not been received).

ASSISTED LIVING FUND

A fund was established for the purpose of offering temporary financial aid to the residents. Funds advanced by CL are to be repaid when the individual attains an employment which will permit him to repay a portion or all of the sums advanced. As of April, 1975, the fund amounted to $51,000. The estimated needs for the first 12 months of operation are approximately $30,000.

STAFF

The resident manager, Gene Prichard, who has been disabled by respiratory poliomyelitis quadriplegia since 1940, is finishing up her undergraduate work at OSU and planning to earn a Master's in counseling and guidance (Fig. 13–14). An extraordinarily expert mouthstick typist, she has been a staff writer for several publications for the disabled as well as an active member of a number of organizations of the disabled. She is an excellent choice as manager—intelligent, perceptive, warm, and firm.

Staff Assistants (SAs) work in three 8-hour shifts. One is always on duty to provide emergency aid and nominal assistance (a drink of water, putting on or removing wraps, getting things off a shelf, personal hygiene needs, opening a door, or lifting into bed). In addition, they shovel snow, sweep the laundry room, and dust the common area. They are paid $3.10/hour, with more on holidays. There are three full-time SAs (5 days/week), three part-time (2 days/week) and two backup people. All but three are students, and all are trained in catheter changing and other necessary care.

Personal Service Attendants (PSAs) are also mostly students. All of them receive a 1-week intensive course at Dodd Hall under the supervision of Dr. Johnson to prepare them to handle all phases of quadness. Each resident is responsible for the hiring and paying of his or her own PSA, who gets the resident up and dressed in the morning and to bed at night, as well as doing light cleaning, laundry, shopping, and preparing some meals. Most of the residents require about 2 hours of assistance.

The Ohio Bureau of Vocational Rehabilitation has assigned a coordination or liaison counselor for all the CL residents to work out job possibilities and solve the complexities of support while in training or studying.

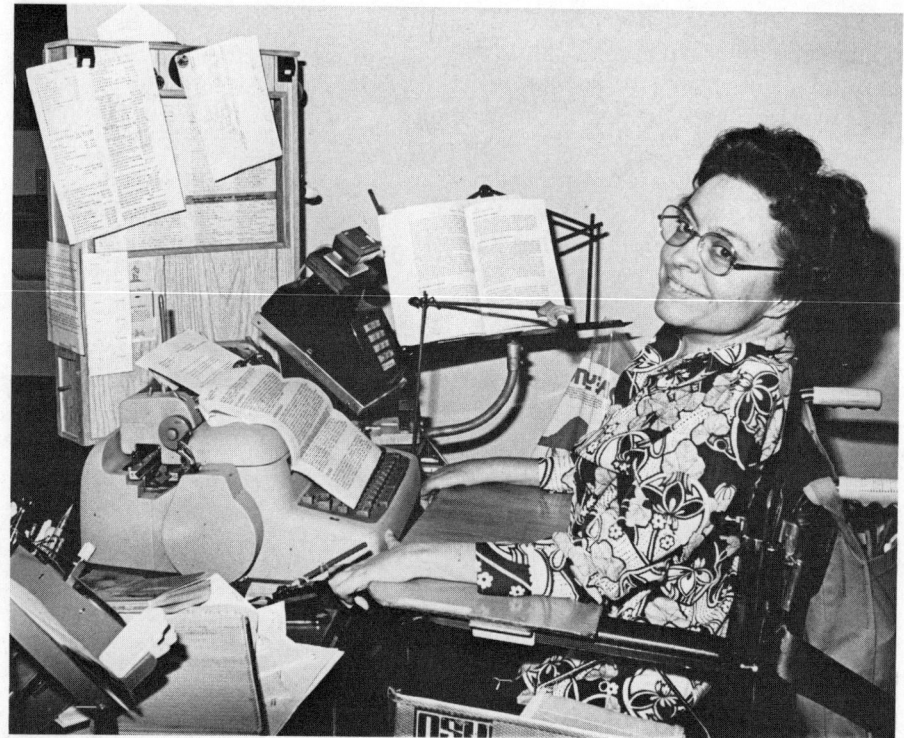

Fig. 13–14. The resident manager of Creative Living, Imogene Prichard, is an honor student at Ohio State University, an artist, a writer, and an extraordinarily expert mouthstick typist. (Photograph by Darry Dusbiber)

MEALS

Meals are a problem! Theoretically, the residents are welcome to eat in the Dodd Hall cafeteria about a block away. Actually, it is too far, there is too much traffic to cross, and it is too unpleasant to make the trip in winter. The residents often phone for deliveries of pizzas or submarine sandwiches at odd hours. Then, those who have to be fed run into the problems of job descriptions. The SAs do not have feeding on their job lists. Catering was explored and found to be too expensive. Besides, both catering and meals on wheels would run into the feeding problem.

Some residents are teaming up to share meals cooked in each other's apartments by one or the other's PSA, family, or friends. Perhaps, some sort of organized cooperative dining will be worked out using the party kitchen through the volunteers which CL is now recruiting. It is apparent that residents need more help at times than SAs and PSAs can or do provide. The whole CL program is so new that it has not had time to develop fully. It would seem that a resident couple might be the solution. The husband could work elsewhere and do maintenance/repair in off hours; the wife could prepare at least one communal meal a day and be available for the motherly things of life that are unlabeled and indescribable.

TRANSPORTATION

Thanks to a grant obtained from the Rehabilitation Services Commission (RSC) of Ohio, CL was able to purchase a 1974 Chevrolet van which had been specially adapted. Money was allocated to CL on a 4:1 basis, which meant that for each $1 CL appropriated the RSC appropriated $4. There are three drivers on call, or a friend, relative, or PSA may drive. The gasoline, insurance, and maintenance are paid by CL. The drivers are paid $2.75/hour if the van is used for personal errands or pleasure; there is no charge if it is used for school or work. OSU has a campus van with a ramp that can be used for attending classes; however, it stops operating at 5 P.M.

WHAT NEXT?

The problem looms of how to afford Creative Living after completing college or training and thus becoming ineligible for vocational rehabilitation support, but not yet earning enough to cover all the costs.

Bibliography

ADVENTURE IN A WHEELCHAIR. By Ida Daly, 1973, Seattle Handicapped Center, Seattle, Washington. $3.50.

THE HIGHLAND HEIGHTS EXPERIMENT. By Sylvia Sherwood, PhD, David S. Greer, MD, 1973, U.S. Government Printing Office. $1.25.

HUD-Assisted Housing for the Handicapped. By Morton Leeds, HUD CHALLENGE, Vol. VI, No. 3, pages 2–5, March, 1975.

A Living Environment for the Physically Disabled. By Dorothy A. Jeffrey, OTR, REHABILITATION LITERATURE, Vol. 34, pages 98–103, April, 1973.

A Public Housing Project for Physically Disabled Persons. By Ida Daly, ARCHIVES OF PHYSICAL MEDICINE AND REHABILITATION, Vol. 8, pages 387–388, 1971.

VISTULA MANOR DEMONSTRATION HOUSING FOR THE PHYSICALLY DISABLED. By Leon A. Pastalan, PhD, 1969, National Technical Information Service, Springfield, Virginia. $3.

"The way to a free and independent life is not to be well cared for. The way is to let the disabled be trained to take care of himself."

—Dr. Sven-Olof Brattgård, Sweden

14
Projects in the United States that Faded or Failed

From the mid-1950s to the mid-1970s more specialized housing projects for the physically disabled failed to materialize than succeeded. Now it seems as well, for many of the planners were entrapped by the prevalent "edifice complex" and concentrated their energies on a building for 100 or more disabled persons that would have segregated the disabled rather than integrated them into their communities.

Careful analysis of the unsuccessful project brings to light the basic problems: Appropriate housing at an affordable rent with supportive services is difficult to obtain because of the lack of choices, the lack of income, the lack of subsidized attendant care, the lack of accessible housing, the lack of adaptable housing, the lack of accessible transportation, and the lack of guidance from local, state, and federal agencies. Though some of the difficulties are being alleviated by current legislation and a more understanding climate, failures in the past emphasize the need to broaden the current changes.

TOO FEW—TOO MANY; TOO LITTLE—TOO MUCH

Most of the specialized housing projects that failed to materialize fall into patterns. One of the most common was the banding together of a few severely disabled persons to try to work out living arrangements with attendant care. As soon as the small group approached any professional in the housing field, whether governmental or private, they ran into the edifice complex. They were advised that they must plan in large numbers to make a project feasible and that, with such low incomes, the only route was public housing.

IRON LUNG POLIOS & MULTIPLEGICS, INC.

One of the small groups that was almost catapulted into planning a full-scale housing project was Iron Lung Polios & Multiplegics, Inc. Back in the mid-1960s, three members of the organization in Ohio, Susan Armbrecht, Mickie McGraw, and Donna McGwinn, all quadriplegic and dependent upon respirators part or full time, started with the idea of a small home with shared attendant care to be located in Chagrin Falls, a suburb of Cleveland.

Quickly, the number moved to 10–12 residents because friends who were disabled wanted to join them. "No. No. Uneconomical for so few," said the experts. "There should be 25–30." "No. No," said more experts, "that is not an economical number; you cannot 'mortgage out' with less than 100." "No. No," said some disabled, "if you have too few, you will have personality clashes; if there are enough people, everyone can find friends." "No. No," said other disabled, "if you have too many, it will just be another institution." So went the seesaw.

One of the "expert experts" who became interested in the then very novel idea of housing for the disabled with supportive services was a staff member of Urban America, Inc. This organization with the support of the Ford Foundation provided technical assistance and professional counsel to nonprofit sponsors of housing for the disadvantaged. The "expert expert" brought the proposed ILPM project to the attention of Robert C. Weaver, Secretary of HUD, and Philip N. Brownstein, Commissioner of FHA, and arranged for a small grant from Urban America to ILPM to determine the market by conducting a survey of the housing needs of the disabled *Rehabilitation Gazette* readers in Ohio.

In April, 1966, a questionnaire was sent to 383 severely disabled *Rehabilitation Gazette* readers in Ohio. A total of 217 questionnaires was returned (57%). Most of the respondents were "when-and-ifers" ("When and if my parents die, I shall need a residence"). An immediate need for housing with supportive services was indicated by 26 respondents (7%). Their average age was 38 years; average monthly income was $114.58; an average of 2.8 hours/day of attendant care was required; 20 needed a one-bedroom apartment, 3 required a two-bedroom apartment, and 3 required a three-bedroom apartment.

Urban America concluded that while most of the 217 who completed the questionnaire expressed a definite interest in specialized housing accommodations and anticipated that they would need it at some future date, the preponderant majority were in housing accommodations that were reasonably adequate at that time. Consequently, Urban America, Inc., did not encourage the development of a plan for two reasons: 1) it was doubtful a market could be validated for a project of sufficient size to make it feasible (75 units would have been the smallest number that could be considered), and 2) the staff required to provide the personal supportive service would present enormous financial and management requirements for which there were no existing tax-supported or philanthropic sources.

Though discouraged, the group tried private sources of funding; then, after careful consideration of the alternatives, the financial problems, and the status of similar projects, the group decided that the primary need was freedom—freedom of choice of where to live and how to live—that no single large facility could provide.

CHRISTOPHER FOUNDERS, INC.

One of the most surprising "fade-aways" was the project of Christopher Founders, Inc., a nonprofit organization composed of nondisabled persons whose goal was a residence for quadriplegics in Grand Rapids, Michigan. The residence, which actually resembled a large nursing home, would have had 4 private rooms and 56 semiprivate rooms, each with an adjoining living room, storage area, and a shared half-bath. There would have been a speaker-phone, nurse call system, treatment room, occupational and physical therapy rooms, living room with party kitchenette, dining room, barber and beauty shop, and additional storage area. The aim was "to develop a social setting for quadriplegics."

A survey of the quadriplegics in Michigan was made by sending questionnaires to organizations in Michigan, to the *Rehabilitation Gazette* in Ohio, and to the National Foundation—March of Dimes' central office asking that they forward the questionnaires to all quadriplegics known to them in Michigan. Responses were received from 225 persons: 105 (47%) were interested in residing in the home, 52 (23%) were not interested, and 68 (30%) were undecided. It was estimated 300–350 quadriplegics had been reached.

In 1967 architectural designs were completed, a site was chosen, construction details were completed, and preliminary staffing and service requirements were drawn up. With 33,000 sq ft, the total costs were estimated at about $1 million, plus land costs.

Planned as a licensed nursing home, financial support for the operation would have to come primarily from Medical Assistance under Title XIX and the social security incomes of the residents. Construction would be financed through Hill–Burton participation, donations from foundations and, if necessary, an FHA-insured mortgage. For a year everything ran smoothly. Then, in late 1967, the big obstacle: instead of the top rate of $16/day on which the plans all had been made, a cost of $17.50/day was found to be necessary. A commitment was sought from the Michigan Social Welfare Agency to permit the increased cost and allow Christopher Founders either to subsidize the amount or to bill the residents for the extra amount.

Finally, the directors gave up. The state would pay $16/day under Medicaid and absolutely no more. The actual costs finally came to $26/day. One of the directors reported that the state's regulations made everything as difficult as possible; the per diem grant would have had to be renewed every 90 days and persons would almost have to be terminally ill to get the $16. The director said that the project could not be feasible until there was either a national health plan or increased Medicaid; meanwhile, the board might buy some land and build a house for four or five quadriplegics and just start learning.

"ONE STOP" COMPLEX IN ROCHESTER, NEW YORK

During the summer of 1972, representatives of 15 rehabilitation, state, and local agencies initiated plans for a complex on 40 acres of surplus land near the Rochester State Hospital medical–surgical building. The centralized complex was planned to serve Monroe County's elderly, physically and emotionally disabled, and retarded citizens over the age of 16. The project was expected to accommodate more than 1000 residents as well as provide health and other services for hundreds of others living in the community.

The basic concept was to provide living accommodations for those who could not get by alone in the community and to have a variety of accommodations so that an individual could progress from one stage of independence to another as needs changed. As the plans were crystallizing, members of an organization of 300 disabled individuals known as Handicapped Independence through Housing, Education, Recreation, Employment, Inc. (HI HERE) adamantly opposed the inclusion of the physically disabled in the complex, which was planned for 400 elderly and 400 disabled or retarded persons. The organization termed the planning a ghettoizing approach that violated the rights of the disabled to live where they wanted without unreasonable or unnecessary restrictions; further, the organization criticized the professional agencies for not including the disabled in the planning.

There developed a petition battle between two groups of disabled individuals that appeared blow-by-blow in the newspapers. Members of the Cerebral Palsy Association, another group of disabled individuals, gathered 1500 signatures in favor of the complex. On the other hand, HI HERE gathered 9000 signatures opposing the project, plus the support of five city councilmen and five county legislators. For nearly a month, the battle raged. The Mayor of Rochester sided first with HI HERE, then with the complex planners.

As a result of the dissension, the complex was abandoned by the area planning council. Over the next few years, a task force was formed to develop a community-wide approach to rehabilitation issues. Over the years, too, other plans evolved. The leaders of HI HERE solved their own housing problems through marriage and sharing accommodations; United Cerebral Palsy and the Association for the Retarded have taken over several floors of housing for the elderly and set up apartment living arrangements for their disabled clients. The Multiple Sclerosis Society, which had been one of the principal organizers of the original plan, is looking into an offer to build several houses, distributed throughout the community, for small groups of people who need some form of assistance with daily living activities.

HOSPITALITY HOME, INC.

From 1961 to 1975, two determined disabled individuals, Ira J. Inman and Mabel Nebies, battled for a 150-unit apartment for members of their national social club, Indoor Sports Club. They fought from one site in Southern California to another, through lost options because of delays in Washington, through a promotor who confiscated funds, through a rejection by would-be neighbors as "undesirables," through inflated prices, for 14 years that would have tested Job.

After it was all over and the project was declared unfeasible, Inman wrote,

What we have been through, and this includes Jack A. Falkenberg, consultant, Ralph Flewelling, architect, and Miss Nebies and I, is not just frustration and agony, but hellfire. Personally, I have been a part of more than 100 sessions with Indoor Sports—just keeping the spark and hope alive—meetings with architects, building contractors, and, of course, the City of Hemet. I have driven thousands of miles, spent countless dollars for gasoline and other driving costs, meals, motels, and even booze. I have written literally hundreds of letters, worn myself and my patient wife to frizzles, spent sleepless nights, worn holes in my spinal cord injury tender bottom, argued and pleaded with people all the way from Indoor Sports to HUD and FHA officials to Senators and Congressmen. . . . I have made trips to Washington, D.C., and made miles of wheelchair tracks through the nation's capital, through HUD and FHA offices, all miles apart, and up and down the miles and miles of the hallways of House and Senate Office Buildings . . . Now I take consolation in the fact that I have done my utmost for a cause that I feel is worthy of it all.

LOSS OF A LEADER

Another pattern in the 1960s was that of a utopian plan created by one dynamic disabled individual who was unhappily institutionalized and wanted to escape to a one-piece housing, work, and social center. When that strong personality either found satisfying living arrangements, changed interests, or died, the plan faded away. It is interesting that most of these plans would have been for the disabled only and were not directed toward integrating the disabled within the community. This, of course, may be because many of these plans were made before integration was considered vital or maybe because the cocoon of institutionalization would naturally foster plans for life under one roof to avoid having to cope with transportation and the community.

The most dramatic example is the 20-year experience of New Horizons, Inc. The founder of New Horizons, a dream of a family home community for severely disabled persons, was the late Joan Herman, who was disabled by respiratory poliomyelitis quadriplegia and used a portable chestpiece respirator and an iron lung. She had been disabled by poliomyelitis in 1946, just after graduating from Concord Academy, when she was planning to enter Wellesley College. Before coming to New Britain Memorial Hospital, an enlightened chronic disease hospital, she had suffered the frustrations and limitations of a hospital for the aged.

At Memorial Hospital she found other young disabled persons who had lived in similar isolated situations. They joined together in May, 1955, to form New Horizons, Inc., and to work for more productive and meaningful futures by establishing a hospital residence with a homelike environment. They spent more than a decade planning to establish a workshop, community residence, gift shop, auditorium, chapel, swimming pool, school, and recreation facilities. They hoped that their plan could be made possible through federal legislation, state welfare, and family support as well as income from individual and group work.

Joan Herman was a brilliant and appealing leader. She set up a well-rounded board of directors, lined up a crew of volunteers, and solicited the support of such eminent personages as Dr. Howard A. Rusk, Dr. Jonas E. Salk, Mrs. Chester Bowles, and Dr. Roy Menninger. The board members and volunteers organized a series of fund-raising activities and solicitations that amounted to enough to purchase 23 acres of land and to build two pavilions and a hard-surfaced road, picnic area, and wheelchair paths. An incredible amount of volunteer energy went into the strawberry festivals, raffles, benefits, and the newsletter that recounted all the doings. All the work culminated in the symbolic burning of the $30,000 mortgage on the 23 acres of land on October 5, 1969.

Meanwhile, the dynamic Joan had found a more absorbing interest. In October,

1968, she sent a mimeographed letter to her friends explaining that she had become a Seventh-Day Adventist and her concepts of service to physically handicapped individuals had broadened. In August 1969, she left for a vacation at the Wildwood Hospital and Sanitarium, a medical missionary training center run by the Seventh-Day Adventists in Wildwood, Georgia. The holiday became a permanent move, for life with the New Horizons group had become incompatible with her new beliefs.

After Joan left, the momentum of her dream continued until the pavilions and the picnic area were completed. For a few years, life was settled in the attractive new wing of the New Britain Memorial Hospital (see New Horizons Wing, Ch. 11). The pavilions, shared with individuals and groups in the community, and transportation by means of a van and a bus made the residents a part of community life. Now, however, the dream has taken the form of a nursing home residence (see New Horizons, Inc., ch. 11).

In the mid-1960s, a number of similar situations involving individual leaders occurred around the country with other groups of disabled. A few examples are

1. A cooperative home for disabled persons who needed attendant care was intensely promoted by a young woman who was residing in a veterans hospital in Florida. When family circumstances permitted her to move into an apartment, the plan faded.
2. Two quadriplegics planned a self-sustaining vocational activity residence center for severely disabled individuals. The housing authority in Miami promised its cooperation if support could be secured from public and private health and welfare agencies. When one of the gentlemen died, the project evaporated.
3. In 1961, a young man, disabled by arthritis, planned a village in Arizona that would provide residential and vocational facilities for 16 disabled and 6 non-disabled persons and would become self-supporting. Plans included a telephone-answering service as well as bookkeeping, secretarial, and addressing and mailing services. The project faded away when the young man died.
4. In Philadelphia, a group of disabled persons, the American Society for the Physically Handicapped, led by a young woman disabled by arthritis, worked toward a housing project for the disabled. She made such waves about housing needs that HEW awarded a grant to the University of Pennsylvania School of Medicine to do a comprehensive study of the housing needs in Philadelphia. Though the project faded when she moved away, her work as a catalyst resulted in one of the most perceptive feasibility studies in the field. Titled, *The Physically Disabled and Housing*, it is summarized in Philadelphia Housing Studies, Chapter 16.

UNSUCCESSFUL COMMERCIAL VENTURES

Still another pattern for failure involves commercial ventures by nondisabled persons to attract disabled individuals to their care centers or condominiums. The usual procedure is to send press releases or advertise in the several nationwide publications beamed to the disabled and hope that customers respond. Replies were so scarce that the projects failed to materialize. Was it the method? Or was it because all were planned for independent disabled rather than for the dependent disabled who required some attendant care?

Between the years 1968 and 1971, attractive brochures with scale drawings advertised planned condominiums which would have been located in Seminole, Florida, and would have ranged from $15,500 for a one-bedroom and one-bath apartment to $24,500 for a three-bedroom and two-bath apartment. One-story apartments and a ramped swimming pool were planned. The site was near shopping, churches, bowling alley, and schools. Because of a poor response, no bank was interested. Finally, the units were offered for rent at $160/month. There was still no response and the project withered away.

In May, 1974, five accessible apartment buildings were planned to face the bay in Matlacha, Florida. Completely furnished, the rents were set at $200/month for one-bedroom apartments and $250 for two-bedroom apartments. The loan did not go through and the project was abandoned.

A development company in Mountain View, California, fanfared its plans to build a 52-unit complex meeting 702 grant requirements. It would have had a swimming pool, recreation area, exercise room, and a resident nurse. When only six replies were received in response to the ads and news stories, the project was abandoned.

PROJECTS THAT FAILED

OVERBROOK HALL, THE CLASSIC FAILURE

No account of the development of housing for the disabled in the United States would be complete without the oft-repeated story of Overbrook Hall. Briefly, the Philadelphia affiliate of the United Cerebral Palsy Association (UCP) started working on the project in 1951. To determine the need, questionnaires were sent to all families known to have a cerebral palsied member and conferences were held with the medical advisors and all the community agencies that provided services to the cerebral palsied (CPs).

Instead of taking the CPs that most needed the facility, those with severe involvement who required custodial care, it was decided to be cautious and take the mildly to moderately involved, aged 18–45 years, who could handle their own needs. The building that was selected was well-located, well-constructed, and contained a small elevator.

The elevator was symbolic of more complications. Before the residents moved in, it was impossible to get rulings on health and safety requirements because it did not fit into any existing category of residences or nursing homes subject to public supervision. After the project was in operation, the elevator had to be removed because it was approved for a private dwelling but not for an institution; there were constant inspections by the fire, health, and safety departments, and many expensive alterations had to be made.

In May, 1955, Overbrook Hall was opened with two young adult CPs. Residents were accepted on both a short- and long-term basis, and fees were established at $40/week. Most residents were supported by public assistance; others were employed at small salaries. The staff consisted of an administrator, a cook, two maids, and a maintenance man.

Occupancy was a constant problem, for though there were accommodations for 20, the building was never fully occupied during its 7½ years of operation. In fact, there were never more than 12 persons living there at one time. From May, 1955, to December, 1962, there were 60 residents (34 males and 26 females) ranging from those with no formal schooling to two college graduates. The average length of stay was 6–8 weeks. Many of the parents who had indicated acute need did not use the residence; they wanted it as insurance for the future but preferred to remain with present arrangements, no matter how unsuitable they might seem. Unsuccessful efforts were made to find residents outside the Philadelphia area and to use the space for respite care. During the summer of 1959, an experiment was made with 8 nonambulatory young men and women, between the ages of 16 and 30, who required attendant care. Living and dining rooms were converted into dormitories, and three practical nurses were hired. After 6 weeks, it was obvious that this was impractical in the present facilities. In addition, locating the residents for the experiment was difficult.

When studies showed that the direct cost of the program for the mildly to moderately involved CPs was about $1000 per resident per year it was decided to consider closing or discontinuing. The costs of altering the building to accommodate five to eight severely disabled persons were beyond the capabilities of UCP, and the residence was closed in December, 1962.

In its final report, the board of directors made several significant statements: 1) parents tend to keep their cerebral palsied children at home until a family crisis makes it impossible; therefore, supportive services in their homes and communities are vitally important; 2) parents have great anxiety about who will take care of their children eventually, and they need to be kept informed about alternatives; 3) long-term care of CPs will be most needed for the physically disabled retarded; 4) the provision of long-term care is a public responsibility; and 5) if a pilot residential project fails, there may be painful and perhaps harmful adjustments for some of the residents.

There were some optimistic results, however. It was felt that Overbrook Hall had functioned as an interlude of growth for some residents who made better adjustments after having learned a greater degree of self-sufficiency away from their families. According to the final report, "the establishment of such residences on a tax-supported basis might well yield gratifying results in salvaging mildly to moderately involved cerebral palsied adults from a lifetime of institution placement."

The experience spurred the Philadelphia UCP affiliate to take another look at long-term care. Its staff visited every public and private institution in the area and compiled a directory, explored foster homes, established liaison with other agencies for additional home services, and worked with them to explore the possibility of apartments in public housing projects for CPs.

MOTEL 66

From 1965 to 1971, Motel 66, a small motel which had been by-passed by a freeway, provided room and board for $150/month, plus $25 for attendant care, to 30 disabled residents from around the country. The staff consisted of a cook, an attendant, a waitress, and two maids. The motel was owned and operated by a retired couple who kept the expenses nominal by working along with the staff, taking night calls, and planning meals and entertainment. Until it closed because of the owner's death, it was the means for many disabled individuals to discover their potential for independent living—a working example of the value of a transitional facility.

"The abuses of institutions will be remedied not through new institutional programs, additional facility improvements, or better training and staff development, but through the active creation and promotion of open, integrated settings in local communities."

—Center on Human Policy

15
Alternatives for the Developmentally Disabled

In the last decade, the idea of deinstitutionalizing persons who are mentally retarded has swept Europe and North America like a tidal wave, creating a new spirit of optimism and a new vocabulary. Countless persons who had been indiscriminately categorized as "mentally retarded" and assigned to a life of custodial blankness have been moved out into the community into small familylike living arrangements. There, when they have adequate community services and positive direction, they have had a chance to learn the skills of independent living and to begin a transition to apartments of their own, employment in the community, and a normal chance to be happy and productive.

On the other hand, for others the pendulum has swung too quickly and too far. Without a comprehensive system of community backup services coordinated by a central agency, they have merely been moved from the isolation of a big institution to the isolation of a little group home institution, surrounded by unfriendly neighbors and out of touch with the community's facilities.

The new vocabulary has positive connotations and includes "citizen advocacy," "normalization," and "developmentally disabled." "Retarded children" are now "retarded citizens;" "crippled" are handicapped, disabled, or impaired; and people who are "patients" are actually called people, persons, individuals, residents, or clients. All of these concepts are relevant to the whole field of human service.

Legislation has implemented the new principles; among the first laws was the 1967 Swedish Code of Statutes which had far-reaching provisions and services for the mentally retarded. Developmental disabilities legislation in the United States was first effected in 1970. Successive laws have clarified the definitions and specified services, though the definition is still the subject of extensive Congressional debate. The 1973 extension of the Developmental Disabilities Services and Facilities Construction Act of 1970 (P.L. 91–517) defines developmental disability as "a disability attributable to mental retardation, cerebral palsy, epilepsy, or another neurological condition of an individual (including autism) found by the Secretary to be closely related to that required for mentally retarded individuals, which disability originates before such individual attains age 18, which has continued or can be expected to continue indefinitely, and which constitutes a substantial handicap to such individual."

Most of the projects listed on the following pages owe their existence to

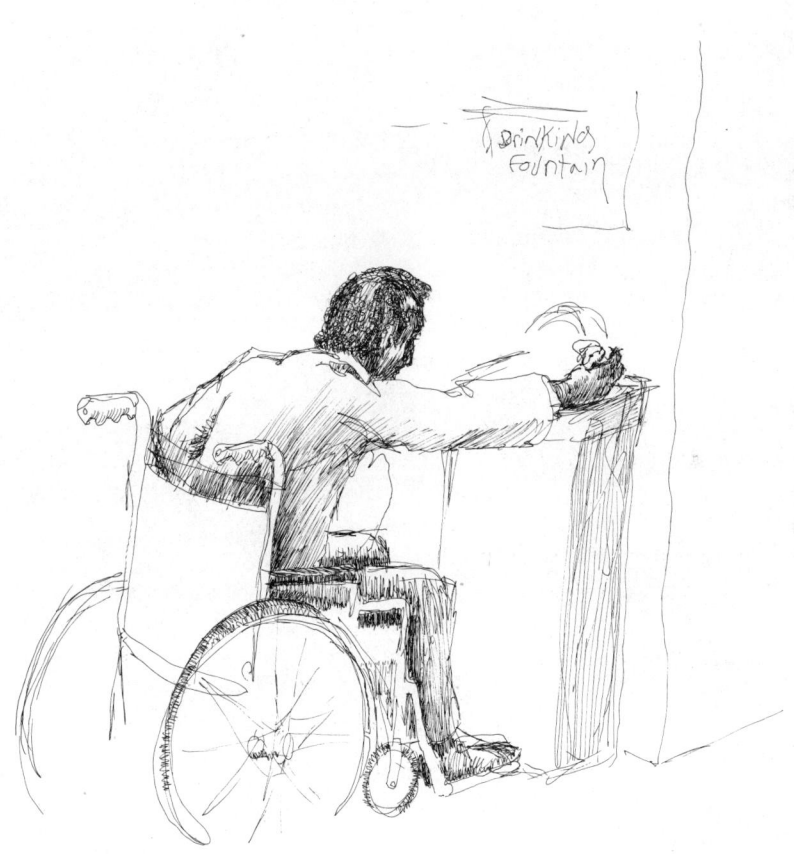

developmental disabilities legislation, which covers a wide range of services: mental health, special education, vocational rehabilitation, social services, health and medical services, special living arrangements, sheltered employment, recreation, protective services and other sociolegal services, information, referral, follow-along services, and transportation. Financing is on a federal/state sharing basis. Each state shares in the available federal funds according to the state's population, wealth, and need.

In addition, those concerned with developmental disabilities have been panning for gold in the Rehabilitation Act of 1973 (P.L. 93–112), Social Services Amendments (see Social Services Amendments of 1974: P.L. 93–647, ch. 7), and the Housing and Community Development Act of 1974 (P.L. 93–383). Under the latter, government funds may be applied to removing architectural barriers in existing facilities, as well as to developing facilities.

The developmental disabilities legislation has resulted in a central office in every state to deal with the problems of the developmentally disabled. In addition, in the more populous states there are also regional centers which act as clearinghouses to direct families to services—diagnostic, educational, psychiatric, legal, vocational, and medical. The centers do not operate major treatment programs but evaluate the needs of the disabled and their families, plan treatment programs, and arrange for treatments by state or private agencies, sometimes using their own funds, sometimes directing the families to other sources of aid.

Since the term, developmental disabilities is not universal, some of the agencies carry the label of a specific handicapping condition which is their primary concern. Parents would be advised to contact their local chapter of the Association for Retarded Citizens or of the United Cerebral Palsy Association and ask for advice and guidance. The agencies can assist with such important matters as determining the disabled individual's financial eligibility for Supplemental Security Income (SSI), which can mean a lifetime income from Social Security. Another area of vital concern is guardianship planning, including estate planning so that it does not jeopardize SSI. The agencies have relevant booklets and can suggest an attorney with experience in the field of estate planning for the disabled.

The excitement behind many projects is the fact that they were created by the intensity of individuals, often a mother who wants to benefit her adult child and others like him. It is encouraging to feel the power of one person with an idea, to see, for example, the dozens of group homes in Michigan because of one mother's dedicated work.

From experience and publications an optimum living arrangement evolves: it is a home or apartment, located near transportation, shopping, and community facilities; it has been decorated in a homelike way; each resident has his or her own room with individualized furnishings; there are no more than eight residents; a perceptive and understanding director has full authority, private quarters, and ample respite time; the neighbors have cooperated in the zoning changes and are involved in the project; the sponsoring organization provides a complete umbrella of supportive services; and the residents have opportunities to work, to attend school and church, to have hobbies, to enjoy social life and recreation.

STATE INSTITUTIONS

When deinstitutionalization was first legislated, it held the immediate promise of better care in centers close to the patient's family. However, of the more than 2000 centers planned after the passage of the Mental Retardation and Community Health Centers Construction Act of 1963, less than 500 had been built by 1975. Moreover, many patients have been discharged to nursing homes so inappropriate that some states are declaring moratoriums on further deinstitutionalization until satisfactory alternatives are available.

In spite of the developmental disabilities legislation, many developmentally disabled persons still reside in state institutions and need humanizing services. There will always be the necessity, of course, for some sort of institution for those who need lifetime support because of profound retardation or medical disabilities and for those who need a protective environment because of behavior problems such as delinquency, hyperactivity, or self-destructiveness. Both financing and watchdogging programs can be utilized to improve existing services and programs. The Hospital Improvement Projects and Hospital In-Training Programs provide federally financed assistance, and the Joint Commission for Accreditation of Hospitals has developed accreditation procedures to raise the standards of care.

State departments of mental health, voluntary agencies, and parents' organizations have effected significant improvements in the services and attitudes of existing institutions, both through in-service training and scholarships for institutional personnel and through physical improvements to the facilities. Further, voluntary agencies and parents have created many service programs: model home units within institutions so that residents can learn homemaking, including cooking, cleaning, and washing; grooming programs; social events such as dances, music, singing, and dramatics; transportation for the residents into the community and for the parents to visit the residents; continuing supervision and follow-up; and community education and involvement.

A unique and flexible system of partitions was used in New York State by the director of the developmental disabilities bureau to redo wards, buildings, and dormitories that accommodated more than 1000 patients in state institutions. Funds in the form of federal hospital improvement (HIP) grants were used to purchase modular partitions made by the InterRoyal Corporation, 1 Park Avenue, New York, New York 10016. The partitions can be varied to meet new program requirements without expensive changes to existing heating, lighting, and ventilation systems (Fig. 15–1).

NURSING HOMES

Before SSI, Developmental Disabilities Acts, and similar legislation there was the excuse of economic necessity for placement of young individuals and groups in nursing homes; alternative accommodations with supportive services were not feasible. It was relatively simple to place a young disabled person in a nursing home for the elderly, although such expensive services were not needed, and have the whole placement paid by Medicaid or Medicare.

Fig. 15–1. A. The 68 inch partitions, made by InterRoyal, have been used to break large wards and dayroom areas into colorful smaller living quarters and lounge rooms. **B.** The partitions include modular wardrobe furniture, consisting of a closet, exposed shelving, and lockable drawers, for each individual.

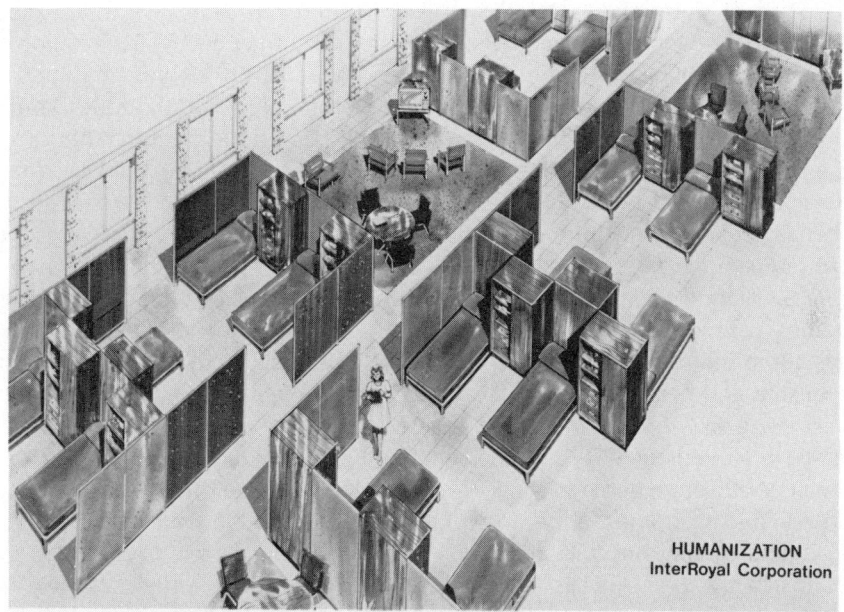

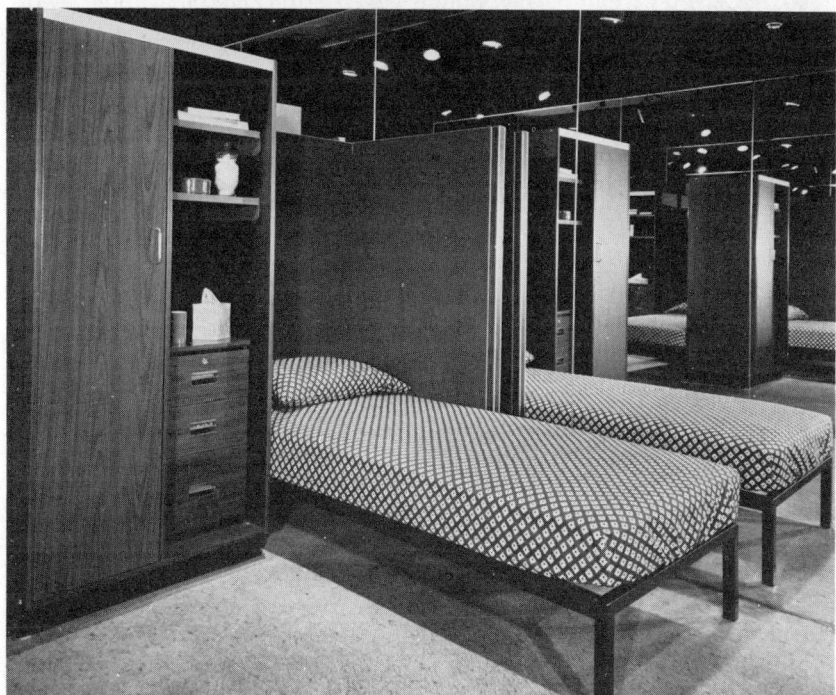

If there were any doubts about the suitability of nursing homes for young disabled, they would be quite dispelled by reading two recent publications. *Tender Loving Greed* by Mary Adelaide Mendelson, is based on her 10 years of study of the inner workings of the nursing home "industry." She visited 200 establishments in 21 states and found "scant evidence or even hearsay of truly excellent facilities." She found evidence of indifference to human needs, exploitation, and financial manipulations that make nursing homes a highly lucrative business. Her indictment includes these allegations: the government, which supports two-thirds of the one million people in nursing homes, is charged for drugs that never reach the patients; medical services are not delivered; equipment that is not needed and never used is installed to qualify for Medicare; money is stolen from patients; legal shenanigans, kickback arrangements, pyramiding mortgages, secret investments are rampant.

Mrs. Mendelson points out that an annual $3.5 billion pours into nursing homes, yet more money does not produce better care; she feels that the solution lies not in more money or more regulations, but in better use of the money now available and better enforcement of the present regulations.

Nursing Home Care in the United States: Failure in Public Policy was published in November, 1974, by the Senate's Subcommittee on Long-Term Care of the Special Committee on Aging. This report, based on a 15-year study of conditions in nursing homes, is the story of neglect by the 23,000 nursing homes in the treatment of the one million patients and neglect in the enforcement of basic standards by state officials and HEW. "Millions of older Americans who have already received care in nursing homes have not received maximum help," the report states. The report recognizes that many nursing homes provide quality nursing care, occupational and recreational therapy, and good medical services but "such homes are in a minority."

Following are some of the committee's uncheery findings: 82 is the average age of nursing home patients; average nursing home charges are $600/month; of the 815,000 registered nurses in the U.S., only 56,235 work in nursing homes; from 80%–90% of nursing home care is administered by orderlies.

Three of the committee's recommendations could also be quite relevant to young disabled: 1) health care should be provided in the home—thus helping more people and saving taxpayers' dollars; 2) financial assistance should be given to the children of the elderly so they can care for their parents in their own homes; and 3) gaps in Medicare coverage should be filled by the government.

The California study of the residential care needs of the severely disabled stated, "Despite the apparent logic of having severely disabled living together in a nursing home setup, this arrangement is demoralizing to the individuals, since the nursing home program is structured around old, dying people. . . . The disabled group feels as if they have been 'left for dead.' Not one disabled person living in a nursing home that was interviewed was happy."

In view of these indictments of some nursing homes, all sponsoring agencies who make or suggest a nursing home placement must do their own local investigating to be sure they are using one of the good ones, and they must maintain a hovering, watchdogging attitude as well as offer a range of supportive services, while seeking alternative youth-oriented arrangements.

INTERMEDIATE CARE FACILITIES

Planning a facility for multiply disabled persons who need supervision and assistance with daily living—custodial, but not medical or skilled care—can be a frustrating experience. In many states there is still no precise slot in the regulations for a residence geared to developmental programs for young, healthy disabled people.

Federal regulations governing intermediate care facility (ICF) services were issued by HEW in early 1974, and financial assistance to both eligible individuals and ICFs was authorized under the Medicaid program (Title XIX of the Social Security Act). The regulations established institutional and residential standards to which ICFs must conform in order to receive federal financial aid.

ECHOING HILLS RESIDENCE CENTER

Echoing Hills Residence Center, Warsaw, Ohio 43844, is an intermediate care nursing home which was constructed primarily for 20 cerebral palsied individuals in need of custodial care. In operation for 2 years, it has 20 regular and 2 day care residents whose ages range 18–50 and whose disabilities are primarily due to cerebral palsy; 14 are in wheelchairs. The per diem charge is $18.50; most of the residents are covered by Title XIX Medicaid. The programs range from continuing education at nearby colleges to working towards high school equivalency. A 20 passenger bus with a hydraulic lift takes the residents into town to church, shops, beauty parlors, and schools. Echoing Hills also provides a residential camp for persons with cerebral palsy.

THE PHOENIX RESIDENCE

After 3 years of work, the executive director of the Phoenix Residence, 1443 Stanford Avenue, St. Paul, Minnesota 55105 who is also the mother of a cerebral palsied son, Mrs. Margaret M. Ludden, has received a 1-year planning grant (ending December 31, 1975) from the Minnesota Developmental Disabilities Program to plan a facility for 48 multiply disabled adults. The program would be designed for residents' total developmental needs—physical, psychologic, and social. Programming has been approved, and provisional licensure as a Supervised Living Facility issued by the State Health Department. The facility would meet the requirements of the federal regulations for an Intermediate Care Facility/MR.

The site, on the river bluff, is Housing Redevelopment Authority land which is located near day activity centers as well as sheltered workshops. The facility will comprise 4 units of 12 persons each in 6 double bedrooms; each unit will have its own living and dining rooms and kitchen. A county-wide survey resulted in 93 potential residents over age 18, who are in state institutions, geriatric nursing homes, or other inhibiting settings. All are mentally retarded and/or otherwise developmentally disabled by cerebral palsy, seizure problems, or neurologic disorders. There is no continuum of services (except medical) after age 18 for people with these disabilities.

The board members are convinced that the levels of intelligence of the potential residents are undetermined because of inappropriate methods of testing and suppressive life situations; they anticipate significant development of intellectual and social potential in a homelike setting with services that maximize their abilities. Community and voluntary agencies and universities have been consulted in planning the programs, which will include a range of daytime activities, transportation to sheltered workshops, vocational, religious, and educational facilities, recreation, counseling, family involvement, audiology and speech therapy, dental and dietary services, a full-time registered nurse, medical, legal, and psychologic services, and physical and occupational therapy.

FOSTER HOMES FOR ADULTS

One of the first studies attuned to independent living was made by the New York Service for the Orthopedically Handicapped over the period 1961–1966 with a grant from HEW's Vocational Rehabilitation Administration. The study, published in 1966, had as its basic objective "to test the feasibility of a foster home program as an alternative to unnecessary inpatient care of adults with orthopedic disability." Two groups of adults, totaling 78, who appeared to be in need of some type of residential setting were selected for the study. One group had lived in various institutions for 15–28 years; the other was living in unsatisfactory situations in the community. The residents were given a weekend trial visit in the foster home before final placement was made and before any necessary physical modifications of the house were made. The social worker was always available to the resident or the family. The foster families received $175/month, then $200/month; the sponsoring agency paid $50, and the Department of Welfare paid the balance. When the residents were employed, they paid whatever they could afford. About one-third of the residents were working during the first 6 months, either in sheltered workshops or in the community; the longer they stayed in the community, the more likely they were to be employed. Though some found adjustment difficult, for many it was a major step from institutional life to relatively independent community living. The project demonstrated that disabled people, "with proper preparation and counseling, can live in the community as useful citizens, at a cost to the community far below that of hospital maintenance."

HOPE HAVEN WORK TRAINING CENTER

Hope Haven Work Training Center, Rock Valley, Iowa 51247, provides comprehensive rehabilitation, evaluation, training, and work programs to adults who are physically or mentally disabled, emotionally disturbed, or behaviorally or socially maladjusted. Living orientation is accomplished in a variety of settings, progressing from a model apartment for teaching independent living skills, to living in homes, foster homes, or supervised apartments within the community, and finally to independent functioning within the community. A 45-min slide presentation of the programs and services is available upon request.

VILLAGES

CAMPHILL VILLAGE

Camphill Village, Chrysler Pond Road, Copake, New York 12516, is part of the Camphill Movement which has schools and other working communities in many countries. The Copake village is a self-contained rural community that is home for about 100 mentally retarded adults and many staff members with their families. In a family atmosphere, the residents are provided training and work in farming, homemaking, and productive skills. Craft workshops and gift shops, as well as a mail order business in handwoven fabrics and handmade toys fill their lives. (The free catalog is charming!)

FIRCREST HALFWAY HOUSES

When Fircrest Halfway Houses (c/o Fircrest School, 1523 15th Street, N.E., Seattle, Washington 98155) were completed in 1969, they were first in the field

Fig. 15–2. Fircrest Halfway Houses in Seattle, Washington. **A.** The architect, Arnold G. Gangnes, was given an award by the national office of United Cerebral Palsy Associations, Inc., for his design. **B.** Site plan. **C.** Main floor plan. (Plans and photograph supplied by AG Gangnes, Architect)

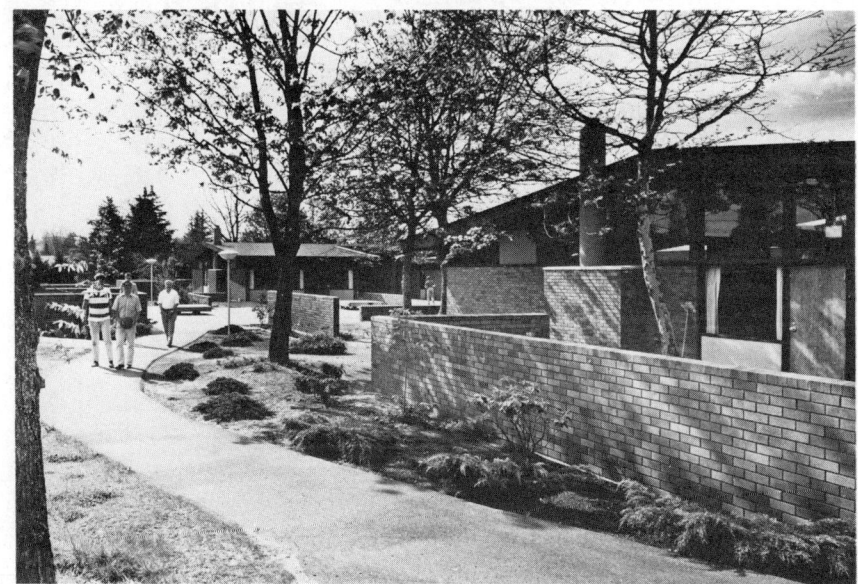

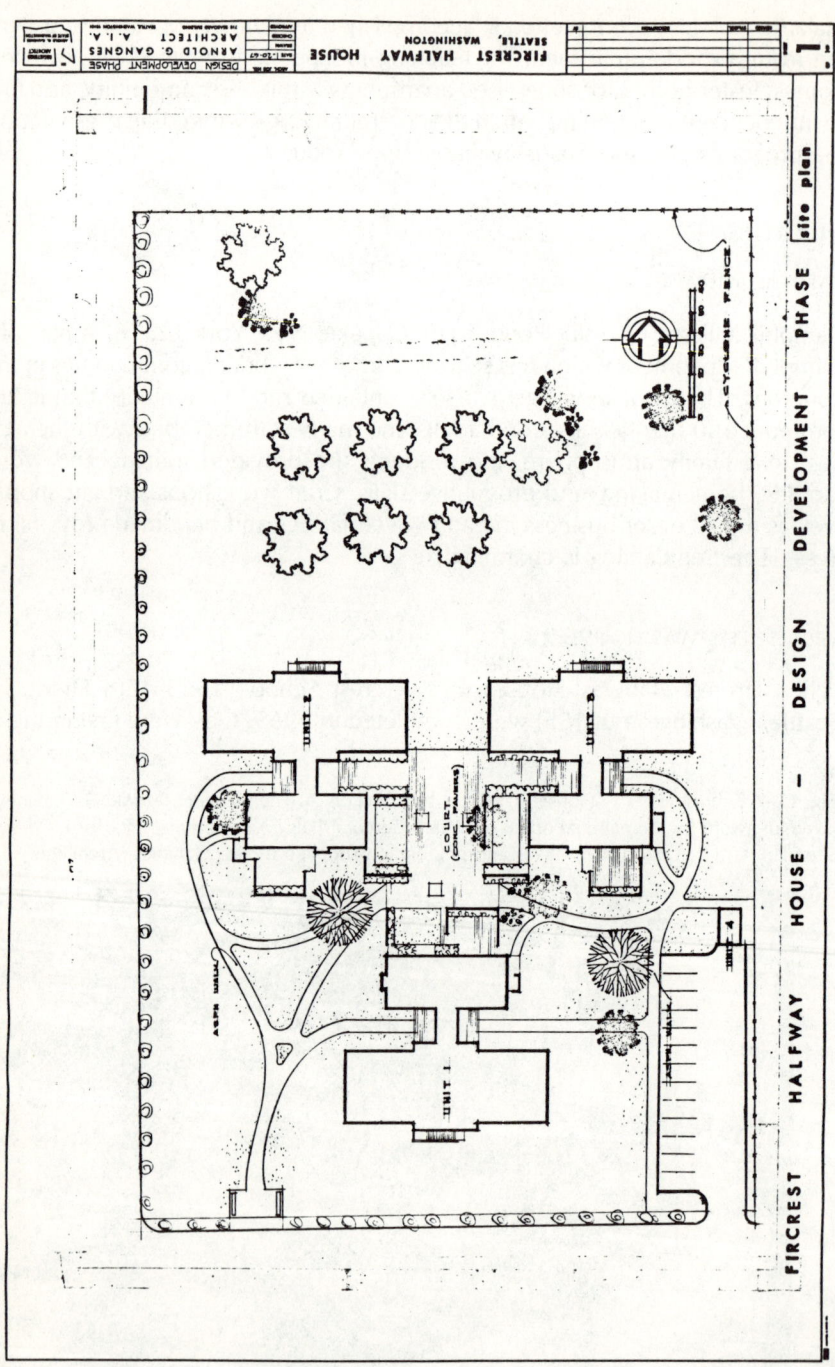

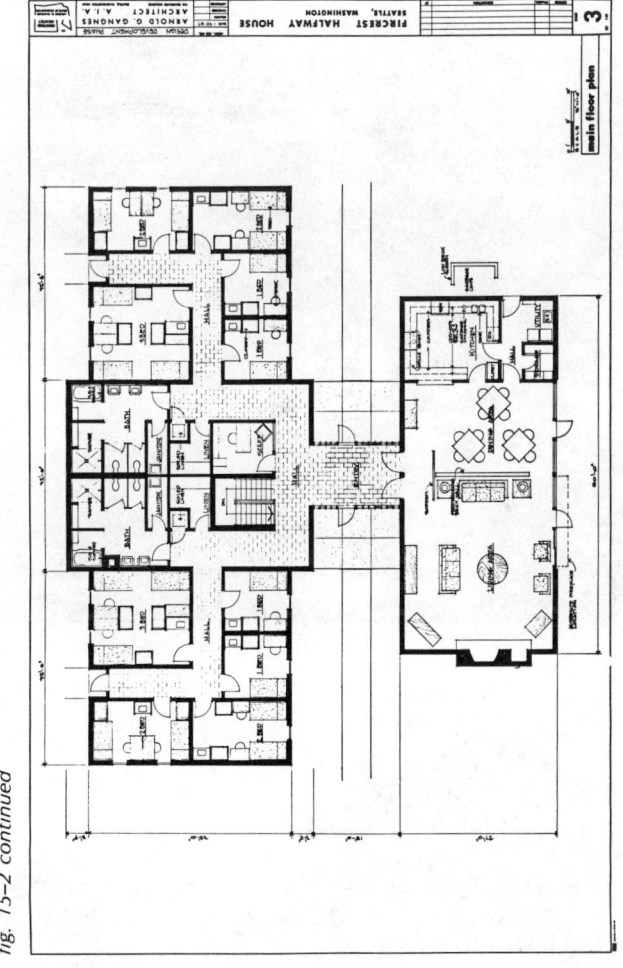

fig. 15-2 continued

Fig. 15–3. A. Handicap Village in Clear Lake, Iowa, a community of 152 mentally and physically disabled individuals who require special help and supervision in daily activities. **B.** A cottage unit. The central building contains a dining/living room, laundry, and kitchen; each of the wing buildings contains eight single bedrooms and a large bathroom. **C.** This homelike arrangement provides individual bedrooms, each with an emergency exit directly outdoors; the two cottage complexes, one for men and the other for women, have their own small living rooms and bathrooms with both tubs and showers. (Photographs courtesy of Dwayne L. Harris, Director of Development, Handicap Village)

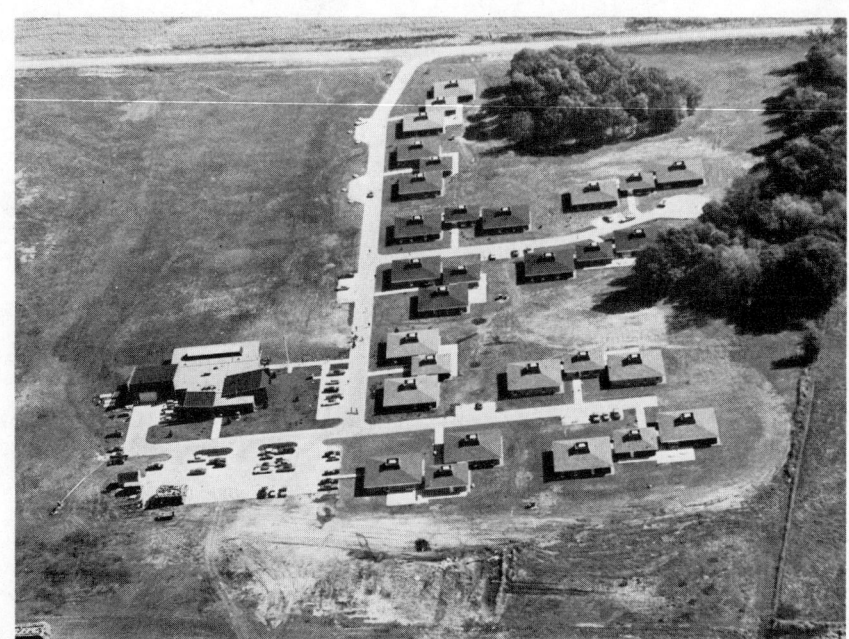

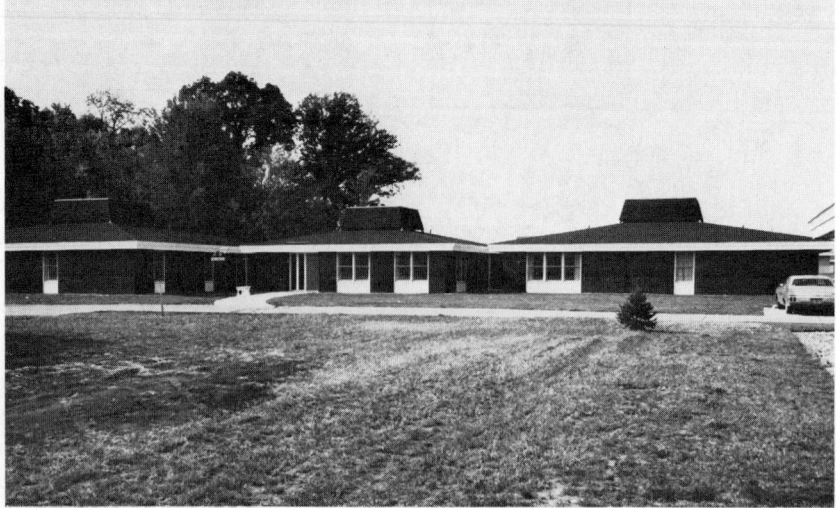

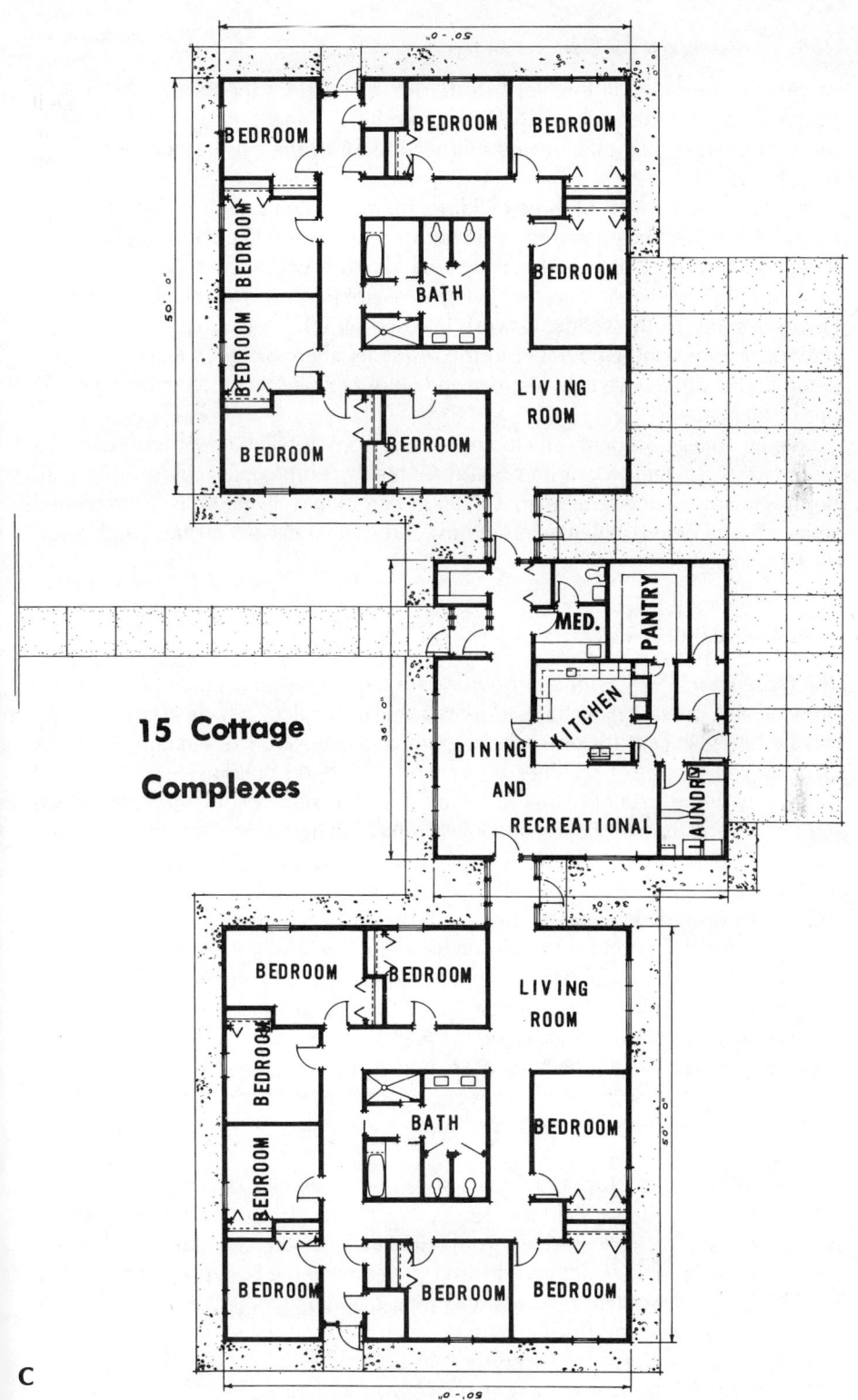

15 Cottage Complexes

of mental retardation in the Northwest. The mandate for the project, because it evolved from a state appropriation for more institutional beds, was that it serve 54 residents and that it be located on the grounds of the existing state institution (Fig. 15–2).

The complex consists of three buildings for 18 residents each, with 9 residents to a wing in one-, two-, and three-bedroom arrangements. Each building functions independently; each has its own living area, dining room, kitchen, outdoor dining patio, and lawn. The sleeping and living areas are purposely made quite separate because many of the residents work in low skill jobs with irregular hours. To provide stimulus and enjoyment to the residents, there are such luxuries as carpeted floors, decorative light fixtures, and landscaping. The project cost $10,300 per resident space.

Live-in college students, including many from foreign countries, work 15 hours/week for their room and board. A nearby community college offers in-house classes for the tenants that include community living skills, a graduated series of enrichment activities programs, and special classes for deaf and blind-deaf tenants.

HANDICAP VILLAGE

The December, 1973, issue of *The Rotarian* has a glowing account of the development and operation of this almost $2 million project which was built with private funds, except for one federal grant of $119,591. The director, Rotarian D. S. Boyer, who uses crutches because of childhood poliomyelitis, raised the monies, with the help of fellow Rotarians and the entire local community, from individuals and through Rotary auctions, Lions Club barbecues, Kiwanis concerts, church suppers, and youth marches.

Handicap Village, P.O. Box 148, Clear Lake, Iowa 50428, is geared to serve those who have gone as far as they can in other programs and who need more individualized opportunities to live and be useful (Fig. 15–3). Persons 16 and over having mental or physical disabilities that require special help and supervision in daily activities and living care are eligible. An approximate 50–50 ratio between the mentally and physically disabled is usually maintained; the mentally disabled provide the physical strength to push wheelchairs and do chores, while the physically disabled with mental capacity provide adult supervision. The present population consists of 152 residents. Their average age is 26–36; the oldest are in their 60s.

The staff for the 152 residents consists of 140 members. During the day, the ratio of staff to residents is at least 1:8; from 5 P.M. to 10 P.M., approximately 25 high school students are on duty; from midnight to 8 A.M. one staff member per cottage of 16 residents is up and dressed to help with the bathroom or whatever is needed. Two registered nurses and four community service staff schedule doctor appointments and shopping trips into the community. About 300 volunteers are available for various services.

The row of cottages resembles an attractive subdivision, with 10 large homes of stained wood. Each cottage consists of three contiguous units: a central unit that is 36' square and contains a dining/living room, laundry, kitchen, pantry, and medical room; with wings on either side that are 50' square and contain eight single individual bedrooms, a living room, and a bathroom; one wing is for men and the other for women; each cottage is limited to four residents in wheelchairs in order to share around the assistance needed with dressing, bathing, or mobility.

The main activities building contains a crafts room, ceramics activity room, classroom, music room, and offices, as well as a large "mall" with a skylight ceiling and an artificial green grass floor. A gymnasium, swimming pool, more activity rooms and an administration area are planned.

Utilizing behavior modification techniques, an incentive plan of rewards for activity participation provides spending money. Residents help with the menu planning (each cottage creates its own menus), grocery shopping, meal preparation, serving, and dishwashing, as well as making beds and doing the yard and home activities. Days are spent in the activity areas and in the classroom. The Handicap Village General Store, on the main highway, is an outlet for handicrafts and rummage sale items.

According to Boyer, a pattern of adjustment has evolved with experience. One of the primary problems is that too many of the disabled have not been given the chance to fail, the opportunity to learn by failure, because they have been overprotected by their families and their teachers. The Village practice is to refrain from doing anything for the residents that they can do themselves. The other major problem, inability to get along in a group, is often solved by moving residents from one cottage to another until they find the right milieu and realize that they must learn to live with themselves before they can accept and help others.

The overall cost per resident is approximately $550/month. Donations make up a portion of cost where subsidy is necessary. Most of the residents are on SSI or some form of social security program; in addition, the Village has a purchase of service agreement with the Iowa Department of Social Services involving a 75% reimbursement for custodial services over and above domiciliary care. County residents are eligible for day care services, home living, and functional educational allowances.

Integration within the nearby communities is part of the Village's positive plan. Residents go to town to the beauty shop or to the barber, they help buy groceries at three different stores, and the churches take the residents to whichever church they choose.

MOUNT OLIVET ROLLING ACRES

Mount Olivet Rolling Acres, Route 1, Box 576, Excelsior, Minnesota 55331, emphasizes training, learning, and living in a homelike setting. The home has accommodations for 66 mentally retarded persons. The facility consists of three houses and a central building with classrooms, activity area, dining room, kitchen and laundry facilities, and administrative offices. Each house has 22 residents, with 11 bedrooms, snack kitchens, a recreation room, and a large living room. The younger residents attend classes, and the older residents are taught to do jobs for industry, such as simple assembling and packaging procedures. Located on 23 acres of land bordering a small lake, the center offers recreational activities such as swimming, camping, boating, skating, and biking. Every opportunity is taken to integrate the residents into community life in nearby towns.

OPPORTUNITY VILLAGE, INC.

At the present time, Opportunity Village, Inc., R.D. #4, S.R. 741, Lebanon, Ohio 45036, is a community of 20 developmentally disabled adults falling into the areas of borderline, mildly, and moderately handicapped. In existence for only a few years, it is now using Otterbein Home's former nursing care building and actively planning for its future "village," which will include cottage living units, vocational training, and a retail complex. The retail complex is the intriguing part of the future plan; it will consist of a small amusement park with a children's petting zoo, a restaurant, a bakery, a greenhouse, a hayride, a pet store, a screen processing operation, and a country store.

RAINBOW VILLAGE

The St. Louis Association for Retarded Children (ARC) is constructing Rainbow Village, 1240 Dautel Lane, Creve Coeur, Missouri 63141, on an attractive piece of land in the midst of a suburb in three stages. The first stage, the Family Service Center, was opened in May, 1975. The Center is open to developmentally disabled individuals, regardless of age. It is available on a planned or an emergency basis 24-hours/day, 7 days/week. It can be used as a respite care facility for extended vacations or for a day or a few hours. The $350,000 structure includes seven double bedrooms, bathrooms, a living room, dining room, office, laundry, kitchen, basement recreation area, and two apartments for houseparents. The building is decorated in warm and happy colors and filled with living plants; the bedrooms are large and varied in decor.

The center is staffed with two couples who are resident houseparents and other paid staff, under the supervision of a social worker/registered nurse. Fees are based on the family's ability to pay; no individual will be denied services because of inability to pay. A van is available to take residents to workshops or school.

Two of the rooms are being used by Richard I. Goldbaum, PhD, the executive director of St. Louis ARC, 6372 Clayton Road, St. Louis, Missouri 63117, for a pilot project created with the Division of Mental Health for training and employing retarded adult women. In groups of four, they are being taken out of institutions and put through training programs to teach them to work as domestics in motels and private homes. They work during the week and return to the village over the weekends. They are taught to take care of themselves in a community, to handle money, to shop and to use public transportation. At the end of a year, they will move into apartments by themselves, and another group will be trained.

In the second stage, a community training and recreation center which will include classrooms, swimming pool, and gymnasium will be constructed. The third stage will involve residential housing consisting of seven separate houses, each designed for eight persons, with four double bedrooms, living area, dining area, kitchen, and laundry, under the supervision of resident houseparents. The final stage will be community living arrangements for those capable of living independently under the umbrella of the services of the complex.

ANNANDALE VILLAGE

Annandale Village, P.O. Box 7, Suwanee, Georgia 30174, is located on 120 wooded acres around a 15-acre lake, 30 miles northeast of Atlanta. The founder is an Atlanta physician, Maxwell Berry, parent of a mentally handicapped daughter. Training and education are geared to the needs of each individual resident. Outdoor work projects include gardening, forestry, and animal husbandry; indoor activities center around woodworking projects, arts and crafts, domestic arts, clerical work, and individual and group counseling sessions. Camping, fishing, horseback riding, boating, and sailing are all available. A personal interview with family and prospective applicant is required. The basic minimum fee is $600/month.

LAMBS FARM

Lambs Farm, Route 176 and Interstate 94, Libertyville, Illinois 60048, has been operated for more than a dozen years by the team of a former teacher and a former part-time bus driver for a school for the retarded. The team, Mrs. Corinne Owen and Robert Terese, bought the 50-acre farm with the help of millionaire W. Clement Stone; they employ 65 retarded adults. A variety of projects on the farm have developed and prospered: a pet shop, a bakery, a silk-screening shop, a gift shop, Heritage House, the Market, and a tearoom. Their dream is to build an entire community where young retarded adults can work and live and enjoy a happy family life.

GROUP HOMES

As a result of deinstitutionalization policies and new sources of income for individuals through social security, plus attendant care (chore service) allowances in some states, group homes are proliferating under many different auspices. Their growth is so mushroomlike that to find out what is happening it is necessary to maintain contact with each state's developmental disability organization as well as local chapters of concerned voluntary agencies.

The two examples detailed here typify the extremes of group homes—1) a comprehensive program by the state housing authority with the whole orchestra of relevant federal programs and 2) the brick by brick creation of a small home by a handful of parents with the wholehearted support of their local community.

Group Homes: One Alternative, a 38-page booklet by Robert Goodfellow, should be required reading for planners of group homes. Published in 1974 by the Center on Human Policy of Syracuse University, it may be ordered from the Human Policy Press, P.O. Box 126, Syracuse, New York 13210 for only 50¢. The booklet outlines the steps necessary to create a group home, emphasizing the necessity of having financial backing before starting (group homes cost about $6000 per person per year to operate), cautioning against grouping several homes in one section of town rather than placing them in different parts of the community, and detailing ways of guarding against resistance by the community and zoning problems. A check list to rate normalization warns against having more than eight residents—the size of a large family, using disability labels such as mentally retarded, having unhomelike names such as "Angels Rest," or using a home that is ayptical of the community. It asks such pertinent questions as whether residents have some power in making decisions that affect their lives, whether they have friends in the community, and if they enjoy "the dignity of risk."

MICHIGAN HOUSING AUTHORITY PROGRAM OF COMMUNITY CENTERS

Through a series of fortuitous happenstances, Mrs. Mary I. Wagner, the mother of a retarded son, was the catalyst for a statewide program by the Michigan State Housing Development Authority to establish group homes for adults who are mentally retarded (Fig. 15-4). Through equally fortuitous happenstances, a favorable social climate in Michigan has resulted in more small community-based homes for persons who are mentally retarded than in any other state. This climate has been fostered by cooperation between agencies and the creative utilization of such programs as HUD's Section 236, the Developmental Disabilities Act, Medicaid, and Aid to the Disabled.

In 1968, Mrs. Mary I. Wagner and a group of other concerned parents and professional persons formed a nonprofit corporation to cope with the problem of undeveloped capabilities and the lack of support services and social life for young adults who had successfully completed special education programs. The corporation, Community Living Centers, Inc., spent a year wrestling with zoning problems and the state's rules and regulations. Then they found a nursing home to rent and moved in 14 people; next they rented the house next door and had eight boys move in there with a teacher and a cerebral palsied housemother who is wheelchaired. They found that after people left home, they matured and did not need as much supervision. By the next May, they had started a home in Pontiac Township, about 20 miles away; then they found a 12-bedroom convent which they modernized and made homelike; and the following December they acquired a fifth house. In May, 1974, they went into a 2-year pilot project with emotionally disturbed retarded children who had been in institutions and who needed behavior modification to prepare them for foster home placement.

The activities of the residents of all the homes are programmed to use community resources to the maximum through YMCA and the churches. The residents

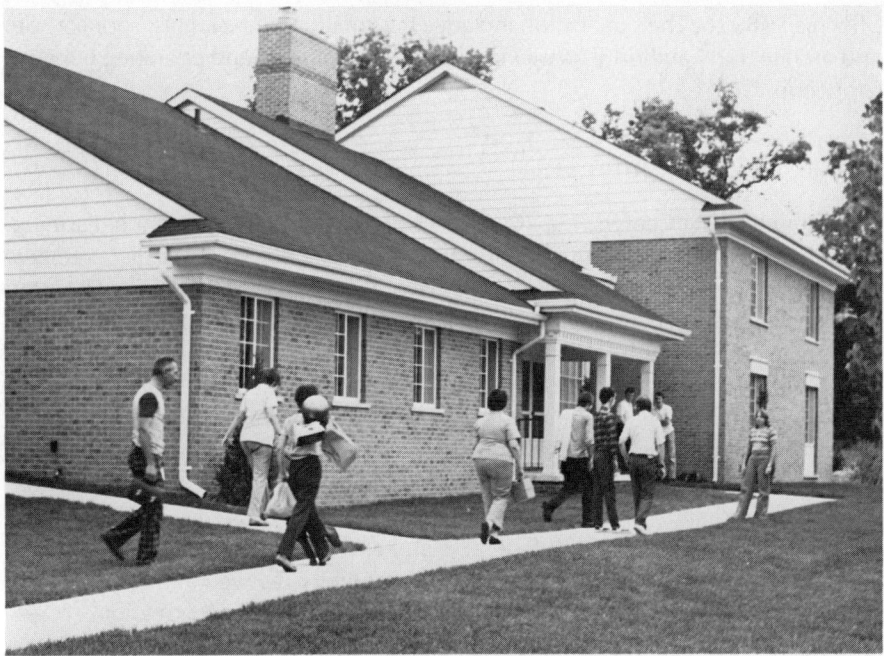

Fig. 15–4. Community living centers for the developmentally disabled are financed through the Michigan State Housing Development Authority. (Photograph supplied by Harold Mondol, Housing supervisor for Michigan State Housing Development Authority)

make their own beds, cook breakfast and lunch, set the table, and help with the housework. Dinner is a family meal for all. Each of the houses has a 15 passenger van which takes them back and forth to work and on shopping and recreation trips.

In 1970, one of the board members who was an architect and a builder happened to be in a meeting with the executive director of the Michigan State Housing Development Authority, and he asked if FHA Section 236 money could be used for the retarded. The executive director happened to be the father of a retarded son and became very interested in the project. He went to the Governor, who went to the Secretary of HUD, who happened to have a grandchild who was retarded.

So, the corporation started to work with HUD in 1970. After 3 years of work between the Housing Development Authority, State Department of Social Services (DSS), Department of Mental Health, and all the nonprofit agencies that have connections with the Housing Authority, the corporation began building a residence in 1973 and moved into it in 1974. Within a matter of months, 24 other nonprofit agencies had started building homes under the program.

For a detailed booklet on the program, request the *MR Housing Program—Guidelines—February, 1974* from the Housing Development Officer, Michigan State Housing Development Authority, 900 Commerce Center Building, Lansing,

Michigan 48926. The publication includes information on residents, sponsor, site and architecture, authority financing, supportive services, and operating budgets. (Appendix C)

COMMUNITY LIVING CENTERS, INC.

Community Living Centers, Inc. (CLC), 33229–31 Grand River Avenue, Farmington, Michigan 48024 has an administrative staff which consists of the executive director, Mrs. Mary I. Wagner, two social workers, and a secretary. The CLC staff provides vocational counseling, social and recreational programming, and general work planning for each resident.

CLC services are available to any retardate over the age of 18 who can benefit from the program. He or she must be able to care for his or her own personal being and possessions and also be able to work in the community, the training center, or in a sheltered workshop. IQ ratio is unimportant if the adult is functioning, benefiting, and contributing to his surroundings.

The staff works closely with federal, state, and county social agencies to provide vocational training and work in the community, as well as to insure good working relationships between employer and employee. Transportation, recreational and social activities, and medical care are provided. Each new resident is referred to the Division of Vocational Rehabilitation for evaluation before being assigned to a training program in a sheltered workshop.

The CLC homes are financed by a combination of federal (SSI) and state (DSS) sources that total $10 per person per diem. Any monies earned by the residents are deducted from monthly subsistence checks. Many of the residents have found employment in the community as janitors, dishwashers, or hospital aides and require only a minimum of financial assistance. A few are entirely self-supporting and do not depend on any aid.

COHOPE!

COHOPE! Community of Hope, Inc., Keezletown, Virginia 22832, is a privately financed nonprofit home that has a quiet feeling of warmth and enrichment. Geared to the needs of five wheelchaired cerebral palsied young adults with alert minds, the home was first planned in 1960; the building was started on donated land in 1969; and the first resident moved in during May, 1972.

The volunteer board of directors raises all the construction and operating monies, without federal or state grants or even a mortgage; presently, the board is launching a drive to add a wing to the present building. It will consist of an exercise room, rest rooms, storage rooms, and a laundry. Long-range plans include another residence building to take care of those on the waiting list.

Since most of the residents and the four day care students have received little or no schooling, the programs concentrate on education, utilizing the Reader's Digest Adult Reading Program, the Cyclo-teacher machine, and educational TV programs. The day education programs are directed by a full-time teacher and a second teacher who works 3 days/week and 1 weekend day. In addition, COHOPE! serves as a field training opportunity for the social services classes of a nearby community college and for senior student nurses from the local hospital.

The staff consists of two housemothers who work 4 days on and 4 days off, a housekeeper and an assistant housekeeper, an evening aide to the housemother, a cook who prepares the noon meal, an LPN who works part-time to do the night bedding down and the morning getting up, an office manager/bookkeeper, and a 2-day/week typist.

Costs per week average $1000. Income from the five residents averages $300/week (there is no set fee, each resident or parent pays as income permits). The board struggles to raise the difference. S&H Green Stamps and other trading stamps help pay for needed items as do several Wishing Wells located in six places in the state.

MARLBOROUGH HOUSE

Marlborough House, 1118 South Laclede Station Road, St. Louis, Missouri 63119, is sponsored by United Cerebral Palsy Association of Greater St. Louis, 8645 Old Bonhomme Road, St. Louis, Missouri 63132. The home, used for residential training and crisis and respite care, has a maximum time limit of 1 month's stay; cost per diem is $12. UCPA raised the $65,000 which covered the cost of the large old house and all alterations and furnishings. The largest house in its middle-class neighborhood, it had been vacant for 5 years because the owner was unable to have it zoned for commercial use; consequently, the neighborhood welcomed its use as a home again and zoning was no problem. Two rooms on the second floor are used by the resident houseparents, who do all the cooking and direct the activities, along with an advocate and case worker from the UCPA's staff. The first floor contains a living room, two big baths, two large bedrooms (three beds for girls, four beds for boys), a huge L-shaped recreation room that doubles as a dining room, and a kitchen. Safety regulations were fulfilled by having all doors open out, exit signs, ramps (the majority are wheelchaired), two water heaters (one for laundry, one with a low setting for residents), smoke detectors in every room (cost: $2000), and by having the whole house rewired.

HOSTELS AND HOSTEL/APARTMENTS

The lines of distinction between hostels, group homes, and apartments are blurred. Hostels will be used here to describe only those facilities that are labelled hostels.

NEW YORK STATE HOSTELS

Hostels are being developed at the rate of about 20 a year by the New York Department of Mental Hygiene, which contracts with a sponsoring local nonprofit agency for the operation of a facility and pays up to 50% of the net operating costs. In addition, it provides funds for furnishing and equipping the facility. Though hostel legislation allows for new construction or purchase of facilities, most recent hostels have been set up under a leasing arrangement. Rent paid by the sponsoring agency may be included in the operating expenses of the program. Facilities range from part of a floor of a modern high-rise complex in Rochester to a former convent building in Schenectady. Most are designed for about 10 or 12 people. A directory of 46 hostels, dated October, 1974, is available from the Hostel Programmer, Department of Mental Hygiene, 44 Holland Avenue, Albany, New York 12229.

TANYA TOWERS HOSTEL APARTMENTS

Tanya Towers Hostel Apartments, 620 East 13 Street, New York, New York 10003, are sponsored by United Cerebral Palsy of New York City (UCP of NYC), 122 East 23rd Street, New York, New York 10010. In October, 1973, UCP of NYC leased 13 apartments on one floor of a ten-story apartment facility which had been built especially for the elderly and deaf. The apartments, with fully equipped kitchen, terrace, air conditioners, and low tubs and grab bars were decorated and furnished (all with the same plastic furniture, alas) by UCP. The complex, in a slum area, zoned for urban renewal, includes a large community room, spacious enclosed and secure landscaped outdoor sitting area, and laundry room.

The apartments are arranged to have space for 16 multiply or developmentally disabled adults, two temporary accommodations for respite care, an apartment for a live-in home assistant, and one for a common dining room.

The staff consists of a hostel director, a full-time sleep-in home assistant, a relief assistant for weekends, a part-time counselor who works with UCP of NYC, and a part-time bookkeeper and secretary. The staff can be expanded on a daily or hourly basis if needs increase.

The residents, in the upper ranges of retardation, are selected by an Admissions Committee because of their potential to develop self-care skills and eventually move into their own apartments. It is anticipated that 60% will use the apartments as a transition to more independent living and 40% will reside there permanently.

All residents must participate in a program outside of the residence every day. Most of them use the UCP of NYC bus and attend recreational, therapeutic, or educational programs at the UCP center. A number of the residents are taking a course in communication for the deaf so they can use it with the other residents of the building. Most of the hostel residents mingle with the other tenants in the community rooms and laundry and participate in the tenants' council.

Through a complicated arrangement of matching amounts with the New York State Department of Mental Hygiene, under the Congregate Shelter B rate, each resident receives $375/month which is turned over to UPC of NYC for the operating costs (food, rents, salaries, equipment, maintenance, laundry, and transportation). UCP of NYC reimburses the residents with $33 for spending money. Some residents also have social security checks, and others have earnings from the sheltered workshop; thus all have reasonable amounts of spending money unless they are on SSI only.

In addition to the 16 apartments, UCP of NYC has rented several other apartments in Tanya Towers for disabled married couples who participate in their programs and has helped them to secure allowances for whatever is needed in the way of full- or part-time housekeeping services.

In order to establish a residential facility in each of the four boroughs it serves, UCP of NYC plans to open a similar hostel in the Bronx in 1976 which will accommodate between 15 and 20 disabled adults. In Staten Island, it has made arrangements with a commercial nursing home, Hyland Manor, to accommodate 20 moderately disabled persons. Meanwhile, work continues on the Brooklyn Campus, a complex that was started in 1970 and that will eventually serve more than 500 children and adults.

ELMER LUX HOSTEL

The Elmer Lux Hostel is sponsored by the United Cerebral Palsy Association of Western New York, 119 Halbert Street, Buffalo, New York 14214. Opened in 1973 with spaces for 18 residents, the hostel is planned for residents who stay for 1 year of intensive services, 6 months of less intensive services, respite care up to 30 days, or occasionally overnight. The majority of all the residents in the first years came directly from institutions or had been institutionalized at some time. The age range is 18–40.

The first year's report contained an interesting observation on the financial problems of the first year: "In budget terms, 18 residents were supposed to 'roll in' and the hostel would be filled. It simply doesn't work this way. The group process only starts as people are introduced slowly. The facility itself takes time to become a home and not just a building. Supportive services cannot be overtaxed all at once, but developed and changed over a targeted period of time." By the end of the first year, there was a waiting list. The facility has an approved rate of $350/month. All benefit checks (SSA, SSI, VA, etc.) name the resident as payee; he then pays for his own monthly room and board.

EXCEPTIONAL PERSONS, INC.

Exceptional Persons, Inc., P.O. Box 690, Waterloo, Iowa 50704, operates two hostels with supervision and training for young physically or mentally disabled adults who are in a vocational adjustment training program or are on job placement; in addition, it has recently opened a group home for severely retarded who will need lifetime protective services.

The first home, provided by the First Presbyterian Church of Cedar Falls, Iowa, began in May, 1969, and accommodates 9 men; the second, provided by the Nazareth Lutheran Church of Cedar Falls, began in May, 1974, and accommodates 12 women. Houseparents live in the homes on a 24-hour/day basis and are supervised by Exceptional Persons, Inc. Costs for care at the hostels are borne by the resident, Goodwill Industries of Northeast Iowa, Iowa Division of Rehabilitation, Education and Services, the county of legal settlement, parents, or a combination of individuals and agencies. A singular follow-up advocacy program after the residents leave the hostels provides regular and systematic contact for as long as necessary to help assure a good adjustment to independent living.

APARTMENTS AND GROUP HOME/APARTMENTS

The gradations of independence through utilizing existing apartments with varying degrees of supportive services were pioneered by the Spastic Children's Foundation (SCF) for their young adults (see The Spastic Children's Foundation, Ch. 8). The SCF system is the most comprehensive and functional in the country, the most adaptable to all levels of mental or physical disabilities. A number of apartment-based projects are relevant to planners of living arrangements for the developmentally disabled (see Ch. 10, Apartment Living Arrangements); the following are geared specifically to those with developmental disabilities.

YOUNG ADULT INSTITUTE RESIDENCE

Young Adult Institute Residence, 4–21 27th Avenue, Astoria, New York 11102, is located in the Goodwill Terrace apartment building, which was specifically built for the disabled. The group apartments are managed and financed by the State Department of Mental Hygiene. The program, which has been in existence for 5 years, was started by Professor Thomas Robert Ames of Manhattan College. The basic charge per month covers maintenance, salaries for counseling and management services, rent, utilities, laundry, and food (all the food in the program's store is free). The 33 residents, both men and women, range in age 21–43. The residents work in sheltered workshops or in competitive employment as messengers or cleaners.

Living in these apartments is the middle stage of development towards independent living. After living at an adjustment center where they learned traveling on public transportation, budgeting, and self-direction in day or evening programs, the residents progress to satellite apartments, which may be located wherever they choose to live, and they are independent except for continuing counseling service that is available as needed. A number of the residents have married and moved out to these satellite apartments. The management and the residents' organization raise monies for parties and extra expenses by bingo games and other group activities.

CONVERTED SHOPPING CENTER APARTMENTS

The UCP of Franklin County, 2144 Alger Road, Columbus, Ohio 43227, rented some by-passed shopping center space and converted it into a service center. In addition to UCP, the Volunteers of America has offices there, and there are 300 apartments adjacent. UCP has taken over 12 of the apartments for an assisted living program. Before an individual can move into an apartment, he or she must attend a home management course and must be carefully evaluated so that any adaptive equipment which might be needed can be installed. A couple lives on the premises to serve as houseparents to the residents. Each individual is responsible for his own rent and is engaged in some form of work activity.

In addition to the apartment project, UCP has evolved a system of supplying services for which it has a contract with the county welfare department, funded by Title IV funds. The services include adult day care, foster care, chore service, transportation, and health care (OT, PT, or doctor). Payment is worked on a unit of service basis, with a module of $6.18 for every unit. Thus, 45 min of chore service, or 45 min of OT time, or a morning of adult day care each equal one unit of service.

DEVELOPING OPPORTUNITIES IN INDIVIDUAL RESPONSIBILITY (DOIR)

DOIR (Adult Program Director, United Cerebral Palsy Association of Pittsburgh, House Building, 4 Smithfield Street, Pittsburgh, Pennsylvania 15222) is a supportive service program which sparkles with originality and exemplifies the importance of working with a wide range of community forces. Shortly after a federal grant had been received in July, 1974 for the purpose of developing opportunities for growth in independence, contacts were made with the Pittsburgh Housing Authority (PHA) and with public and private agencies concerned with service to the developmentally disabled.

To solve the money problem, the project planners "nailed down two funding sources to be blended into a concerted funding stream." The project was divided into staff and hardware and included 11 workers of varying responsibility, three adapted vans, consultant services, and rent for an ancillary office. This portion, funded under Title XX of the Social Security Act, is a 75/25% matched program; its budget totals $90,000 with the $22,000 match provided by the Alleghany County Mental Health/Mental Retardation (MH/MR) Program.

According to Allen Condeluci, Adult Program Director,

The hardware portion includes furnishings and adaptations for 15 apartments and office equipment. This portion of the program is funded under the Developmental Disabilities Discretionary Fund and is an 80/20% match. This budget totals $61,000 and the $11,000 match is provided by UCPA of Pittsburgh in kind, and MH/MR in Allegheny County.
The total program budget is $150,000 and the per diem rate is $13.50/day.
The beauty of this program, however, is not the per diem. Rather the beauty is that it is normalizing for the residents involved. The apartments selected are scattered throughout West Gate Village, a private housing development, funded under Section 236. Since the local housing authority has long-term leases on 60 units within this 260-unit development, they will function as rentor. Our residents are eligible for a 75% reduction as dictated under Section 8. In dollars and cents this means that the resident on SSI ($181/month in Pennsylvania) pays $30/month for rent and utilities. The resident signs his own rental agreement, pays his own rent, buys and prepares (sometimes with assistance) his own food and runs his own life. It is normalization in action.

In order to be admitted, individuals must be physically and developmentally disabled, have the mental and physical potential for independent living, and be able to transfer onto a toilet, tub, or stairway lift. The residents are selected on a 50–50 basis, half coming from the community and half from state-funded institutions. Residents are selected by an admission committee comprised of representatives of UCPA, County Mental Health and Mental Retardation, appropriate Base Service Units, and officials from community institutions. Potential residents from the institutions spend a "break-in" period at Hamarville Rehabilitation Center to be oriented to independent activities of daily living. Each resident is involved in some day programming, either at a therapeutic activity center, a sheltered workshop, or gainful employment.

Explained Candeluci,

Under DOIR three essential elements are married together, enabling the exceptional resident to be "on his own." These three elements are the meat and potatoes of independent living. They are

1. Provision of a counselor/advocate. This worker is concerned with investigating existing community resources necessary to support and insure independence in living. The counselor will also act as a caseworker, catalyst, advocate in procuring services and negotiating the overall human service network on the resident's behalf.
2. Provision of transportation service. It is not enough to place the developmentally disabled adult in the community; architectural barriers and problems in transportation must be considered. With this in mind, the program calls for the purchase of a van capable of transporting eight residents.
3. Purchasing of adaptive equipment. The Developmental Disabilities grant provides approximately $750 to be used for any adaptive device considered essential to independent living. This includes grab bars, ramps, stairway lift, raising and lowering cabinets, and adapting wheelchairs. In addition, furnishings are funded under the DD grant. However, the adults in the program will select their own furnishings to match their taste.

As of early 1976, 27 residents had been assisted in a variety of settings, including 6 placed in high rise apartments and 6 at West Gate. Initially, we assisted two cerebral palsied residents to move in with an able-bodied volunteer. Since he owns the home and lives there, he is able to provide the needed physical assistance for a fee. Since both residents are SSI recipients, they qualify for Allegheny County Institutional District Adult Service Supplement. The MH/MR catchment area was able to provide homemaker service 1 day/week. With DOIR grant money we were able to "adapt" the home and provide some transportation. Food stamps were procured for the SSI residents who qualified and the white identification medical card, available to SSI recipients, assisted in costly medical needs.

This is but one example of how we have used the DOIR approach in setting up two residents. Obviously there is no "pat" system in dealing with a disability as diverse as cerebral palsy. The options are as great and creative as the worker and clients involved.

We are convinced that this is the soundest way to normalization. These residents, who under different circumstances would be placed in an intermediate care facility or nursing home, now have the option of living in the community in various adapted apartments on their own.

Bibliography

United States Bibliography

Architecture, By Arnold G. Gangnes A.I.A. Reprinted from MENTAL RETARDATION, Grune & Stratton, Inc., 1970. Available from National Association for Retarded Citizens, 2709 Avenue E East, P.O. Box 6109, Arlington, Texas 76011. 28 pages. 1973. 50¢. A review of the history and developments of architecture and design for the mentally retarded, the 28-page booklet illustrates examples in Europe and the U.S. The theme of the article is "If you wouldn't design it for your own home and family, don't design it for the retarded."

DIRECTORY OF FACILITIES FOR THE LEARNING-DISABLED AND HANDICAPPED. By Careth Ellingson and James Cass. Harper & Row, 1972. $6.95. A 624-page encyclopedic soft cover book that includes analytic descriptions and comparative data of diagnostic facilities in the United States and Canada. An invaluable guide to diagnostic services, it includes clearcut information on each facility to enable parents as well as professional persons to make well-informed decisions.

FUNCTIONAL AIDS FOR THE MULTIPLY HANDICAPPED. By Isabel P. Robinault, PhD. Harper & Row, Publishers, Inc., Medical Department, 2350 Virginia Avenue, Hagerstown, Maryland 21740. 1973. $10. This 233-page resource book was prepared under the auspices of the United Cerebral Palsy Associations, Inc. The emphasis is on practical, specific information such as what to use, where to purchase it, or how to make it. While the book concentrates on individuals who are cerebral palsied, many of the ideas are applicable to all sorts of other disabilities. A valuable source of information for professionals and planners of residential facilities, the book can be a form of group therapy for parents of cerebral palsied children.

GROUP HOMES: ONE ALTERNATIVE. By Robert Goodfellow. Human Policy Press, P.O. Box 126, Syracuse, New York 13210. 50¢.

Hostel Apartments. By E. Younker. In PROCEEDINGS OF A CONFERENCE ON HOUSING ALTERNATIVES FOR HANDICAPPED ADULTS. New York City, April, 1974.

HOW TO ORGANIZE AN EFFECTIVE PARENT GROUP & MOVE BUREAUCRACIES. By Charlotte Des Jardines. 1971 Co-ordinating Council for Handicapped Children, 407 South Dearborn, Room 950, Chicago, Illinois 60615. $1.50. The publication urges parents to assert themselves, to stop feeling insignificant and apologetic for asking a bureaucrat to do the job for which their taxes are paying him, stop begging, stop being patient, stop accepting excuses, stop being afraid of offending bureaucracies, and be persistent and use mass action.

INDEPENDENT LIVING—A STUDY OF THE REHABILITATION OF PHYSICALLY HANDICAPPED LIVING IN FOSTER HOMES. By H. E. Young. New York, New York Service for the Orthopedically Handicapped, October, 1966.

MANAGING RESIDENTIAL FACILITIES FOR THE DEVELOPMENTALLY DISABLED. By R. C. Scheerenberger. Charles C Thomas, Springfield, Illinois 62717. 281 pages. 1975. $16.50. Primary attention is given to philosophy, personnel, organization, leadership, planning, and organized labor.

MR Housing Program—Guidelines—February, 1974. Free from Housing Development Officer, Michigan State Housing Development Authority, 900 Commerce Center Building, Lansing, Michigan 48926.

NEW ENVIRONMENTS FOR RETARDED PEOPLE. By Arnold G. Gangnes, AIA. Superintendent of Documents, U.S. Government Printing Office. 1975. $1.15. During the 4th World Congress on Mental Retardation in Montreal, Canada, October 1972, the Architectural Planning Committee of the International League of Societies for the Mentally Retarded displayed photographs and architectural details of projects all over the world. The 42 most outstanding of these projects are presented by the PCMR in this handsome booklet that includes the photographs and floor plans.

NEW NEIGHBORS. THE RETARDED CITIZEN IN QUEST OF A HOME. U.S. Government Printing Office, Washington, D.C. 20402. #4000–00310. 1974. $2.10. Fourteen contributors discuss philosophical and practical aspects of the retarded citizen's need for a home in the community.

NURSING HOME CARE IN THE UNITED STATES: FAILURE IN PUBLIC POLICY. By the Subcommittee on Long-Term Care of the Special Committee on Aging, United States Senate; U.S. Government Printing Office, Washington, D.C. 20402. $1.85.

OPERATING MANUAL FOR RESIDENTIAL SERVICES PERSONNEL. By Joanne F. Holland and Robert F. Rubeck. Nisonger Center for Mental Retardation and Developmental Disabilities, the Ohio State University, Columbus, Ohio. 142 pages. 1974. $4. The collection of articles deals with practical problems.

THE ORIGIN AND NATURE OF INSTITUTIONAL MODELS. By Wolf Wolfensberger. Human Policy Press, P.O. Box 126, Syracuse, New York 13210. $2.

PEOPLE LIVE IN HOUSES: PROFILES OF COMMUNITY RESIDENCES FOR RETARDED CHILDREN AND ADULTS. Stock Number 1700–00143. Order from Superintendent of Documents, U.S. Government Printing Office, Washington, D.C. 20402. $1.50.

RESIDENTIAL CARE NEEDS: A REPORT TO THE CALIFORNIA STATE LEGISLATURE. By California Department of Public Health, Bureau of Chronic Diseases, California, 1969.

SEXUAL RIGHTS FOR THE PEOPLE . . . WHO HAPPEN TO BE HANDICAPPED. By Sol Gordon. Human Policy Press, P.O. Box 126, Syracuse, New York 13210. 50¢.

STANDARDS FOR RESIDENTIAL FACILITIES FOR THE MENTALLY RETARDED. The Accreditation Council for Facilities for the Mentally Retarded, 875 North Michigan Avenue, Chicago, Illinois 60611. May, 1971. $3.50.

TENDER LOVING GREED. By Mary Adelaide Mendelson. New York, Alfred A. Knopf, 1974.

With a Little Help from My Friends. By Elliott McCleary. THE ROTARIAN. Vol. 123, No. 6, pages 24–27, 47–50, December, 1973.

ZONING FOR FAMILY AND GROUP CARE FACILITIES. By Daniel Lauber and Frank S. Bangs, Jr. American Society of Planning Officials, 1313 East 60th Street, Chicago, Illinois 60637. 1974. $6. This 30-page booklet is an excellent summary of the zoning problems related to the development of community-based facilities for the disabled as well as the mentally ill, drug users, and public offenders. It is a very helpful source of information on public attitudes toward group care facilities, current zoning treatment, court decisions, and recommended zoning treatment.

UNITED STATES SOURCES OF INFORMATION

The Center on Human Policy, Division of Special Education and Rehabilitation, Syracuse University, 216 Ostrom Avenue, Syracuse, New York 13210. An advocacy program, sponsored by the Social and Rehabilitation Service of HEW, the center operates two model group homes, sponsors the Parents Information Group and the Central New York Parents Action Group, and provides legal advocates to parents. The legal group has effected significant policy shifts through negotiations with institutions, school districts, and other service agencies. Its advocacy material includes booklets, slide shows, manuals, and handbooks. Free list available from Human Policy Press, P.O. Box 127, Syracuse, New York 13210.

EXCEPTIONAL CHILDREN. Published 8 times a year by The Council for Exceptional Children, 1920 Association Drive, Reston, Virginia 22091. $12.50/year.

THE EXCEPTIONAL PARENT, P.O. Box 964, Manchester, New Hampshire 03105. Six issues per year, $10/year.

Kennedy Center, 4695 Main Street, Bridgeport, Connecticut 06606. Request list of monographs.

National Association of Private Residential Facilities for the Mentally Retarded, 6269 Leesburg Pike, Suite B-5, Falls Church, Virginia 22044. This is a nonprofit educational corporation organized in 1970 by leaders of private residential care facilities to maintain high quality services and share information and problems. The aim is to assure the quality of life for the developmentally disabled in "out-of-home" living situations—residential facilities, community-based living units, hostels, foster homes, and any form of residential service delivered by nongovernmental agents. Active membership costs $20/year; associate, $5/year. Membership includes a newsletter and a wide range of services and information, a good investment for planners as well as operators of facilities. *The Directory of Members,* $5, includes the name, address, administrator, phone, and licensed capacity of 403 facilities in 35 states; it is an invaluable source of information on what is actually in existence in the field of residences for the developmentally disabled.

THE RIGHT TO CHOOSE. ACHIEVING RESIDENTIAL ALTERNATIVES IN THE COMMUNITY. National Association for Retarded Citizens, P.O. Box 6109, 2709 Avenue E East, Arlington, Texas

76011. 1973. $1.25. Attractively presented and clearly outlined, the 80-page handbook is an excellent guide to developing appropriate services in a logical step-by-step process. Among the topics covered are comparison of costs for lifetime services, defining the need, writing the proposal, getting help, source of funding, restrictive codes, mechanics of administration, selecting residents, operating the program, and evaluating the program. It has an excellent bibliography and glossary.

Though the guide is beamed toward those who are mentally retarded, it would be useful to anyone planning residential services for any age or disability. In addition, a helpful set of booklets, titled *Residential Programming for Mentally Retarded Persons,* costs $1.50. Ask for a list of the association's other publications.

New York Department of Mental Hygiene, 44 Holland Avenue, Albany, New York 12229, publishes a free biweekly tabloid newsletter, *Mental Hygiene News.*

Ohio Department of Mental Health and Mental Retardation, Residential Licensure Section, Room E-104, 2929 Kenny Road, Columbus, Ohio 43221. A list of Ohio single family homes, intermediate care facilities, and group homes is available on request.

Ohio Developmental Disabilities (ODD), Inc., Suite 212, 2238 South Hamilton Road, Columbus, Ohio 43227. Organized in November, 1972, this nonprofit voluntary organization is made up of the Epilepsy Association of Ohio, Ohio Association for Retarded Citizens, and United Cerebral Palsy of Ohio. None of the ODD programs fall under the state's service delivery system, yet each one works cooperatively with the state system to achieve maximum effectiveness. ODD was organized to plan, coordinate, and implement programs of statewide significance for developmentally disabled citizens.

To date, all funds have been provided by the Ohio Developmental Disabilities Planning and Advisory Council. However, private funds are being solicited for additional activities. Presently, three programs are being administered by ODD: 1) District Citizens Committees, which are the local resource for the development of citizen response to federal, state, and local planning; 2) State Personal Advocacy Office, which coordinates private advocacy programs; and 3) Residential Services Program, which has concentrated on documentation of the need and published *Guidelines for the Establishment of a Group Home, Resource Guide—Services for Persons with a Developmental Disability,* and *Community Living for Ohio's Developmentally Disabled Citizens.*

In addition, ODD publishes a free quarterly, *Community Living News,* and its community support team provides consultation to local individuals and agencies in the planning and development of residential services as well as assistance with legislation, funding, licensing, zoning, and expertise in the areas of staff and programming.

Of special interest are the published proceedings of ODD's Residential Services Seminar II, *Residential Options for Ohioans with a Developmental Disability.* The seminar's recommendations would be helpful to others concerned with these common problems: residential models and programs, manpower resources and training, zoning, licensing, and public relations and funding.

The President's Committee on Employment of the Handicapped, Washington, D.C. 20210. Ask to be on their free mailing list for *Performance* and request *Abroad in the Land: Legal Strategies to Effectuate the Rights of the Physically Disabled."*

The President's Committee on Mental Retardation (PCMR), Regional Office Building #3, Room 2614, 7th and D streets, S.W., Washington, D.C. 20201. Request a list of their publications and ask to be on their regular mailing list. Specifically request *Changing Patterns in Residential Services for the Mentally Retarded,* by Wolf Wolfensberger et al. and *Silent Minority.*

CITIZEN ADVOCACY FOR THE HANDICAPPED, IMPAIRED, AND DISADVANTAGED: AN OVERVIEW. Prepared by Wolf Wolfensberger for PCMR. Superintendent of Documents, U.S. Government Printing Office, Washington, D.C. 20402. 1972. $1. The 59-page booklet outlines a program for private citizens to act as advocates. It points out that the disabled are at times harmed by the very services designed to protect them.

Note: PCMR has launched a comprehensive study of the building codes and zoning ordinances which frequently serve as major impediments to the establishment of group living arrangements for the disabled. Examples are requested from those who have experienced problems.

Telephone aids for teaching the mentally retarded to use a telephone include a 29-page teacher's guide to learning concepts, suggested games, flipchart, flash cards, and teletrainer. For information, contact local telephone company.

United Cerebral Palsy Associations, Inc., Governmental Activities Office, Chester Arthur Building, 425 "Eye" Street, N.W., Washington, D.C. 20001. In the early 1970s Elsie D. Helsel, PhD, became UCPA's Washington representative to work for legislation for the disabled. To share legislative information with UCPA's 300 state and local affiliates, she created an extraordinarily informative newsletter, *Word from Washington*. It is a treasure! It is also free. Each monthly issue summarizes the current legislation relevant to the disabled, giving precise details on its possibilities, and lists new publications, reports, and studies. Of special value is the 200 page looseleaf ORIENTATION RESOURCE NOTEBOOK ON GOVERNMENTAL ACTIVITIES published in April, 1976 and available for $12.

United Cerebral Palsy Associations, Inc. 66 East 34th Street, New York, New York 10016. Request their list of publications. The range of subject matter covers every phase of long-term care; most of the pamphlets or reprints will be sent free of charge or for a small fee. Among the most helpful are NO PLACE LIKE HOME, $2.25, HANDBOOK ON TRANSPORTATION, $1, and HOUSING FOR DISABLED PERSONS, an annotated bibliography prepared by Hofstra University, free.

Canada

The National Housing Act in 1973 empowered the federal housing agency, Central Mortgage and Housing Corporation (CMHC), to make 100% loans for new construction, as well as for purchase and improvement of existing buildings, for dormitory or hostel accommodations for the mentally retarded. In addition, "start-up funds," not exceeding $10,000 are available to assist a nonprofit group in preparing a loan application to CMHC. The Canadian Association for the Mentally Retarded (CAMR), a federation of associates in every province, is creating small homelike living units for the mentally retarded of all ages scattered throughout communities. CAMR has been buying or leasing existing facilities rather than constructing new homes and has been working to have unrealistic building and fire regulations reviewed and revised.

The Canadian Association for Mentally Retarded sponsors the National Institute on Mental Retardation which is headquartered at Kinsmen NIMR Building, York University Campus, 4700 Keele Street, Downsview (Toronto), Ontario M3J 1P3, Canada. NIMR is preparing a manual on residences which will include reports from all 350 local Associations for the Mentally Retarded concerning the growth of residential facilities, staffing patterns, and financing. CAMR publishes a delightfully informative quarterly, *Mental Retardation/Déficience Mentale*. It is a bargain at $2/year in Canada as well as foreign countries.

THE PRINCIPLE OF NORMALIZATION IN HUMAN SERVICES. By Wolf Wolfensberger. NIMR. 1972. $8.50 in Canada, $9.50 outside Canada. Dr. Wolfensberger of Syracuse University was a visiting scholar with the Institute in the early 1970s, and NIMR has published his two best-known books. One is this 258-page book which traces the term *normalization* from its origin in 1969 in Denmark to its development in Sweden.

CITIZEN ADVOCACY AND PROTECTIVE SERVICES FOR THE IMPAIRED AND HANDICAPPED. By Wolf Wolfensberger and Helen Zauha. NIMR. 1973. $7.50 in Canada, $8.50 outside Canada. This 278-page book promotes citizen advocacy as one of the means of effecting integration and normalization. The volunteer efforts of a competent, mature citizen based on a one-to-one relationship can work wonders. The book discusses the disabled person's legal rights and presents a sensitive collection of subjective reactions and feelings by disabled individuals. A comprehensive outline of the history of protective services by Elsie D. Helsel, PhD, includes the major types of protective services—guardianship, adoptive parenthood, conservatorship, and trusts.

Request the NIMR list of publications; there are some excellent books, booklets, and reprints at small prices. A few examples:

Apartment Living. By W. Wolfensberger. #H77. 25 pages. 1971. 50¢.

A Selective Overview of the Work of Jean Vanier and the Movement of L'Arche. By W. Wolfensberger. #H90. 22 pages. 1973. $1.50 abroad.

Help Yourself to Food. By the Ontario Association for the Mentally Retarded. #H86. 59 pages. 1972. $2. A simple illustrated cookbook for use by the retarded.

Lifelong Homes for the Adult Mentally Retarded. By J. Vanier. Reprint DM/MR. #H80. April, 1969. Psychology of adult retarded and philosophy of care evolved at L'Arche, France. 10¢

Residences for Retarded in Canada. By CAMR. List of public and private facilities. Reprint DM/MR. April, 1971. 10¢

Residential Care for the Mentally Handicapped. Conclusions of the International League of Societies for the Mentally Handicapped Symposium in Frankfurt, September, 1969. 31 pages. $1.

Great Britain

Centre on Environment for the Handicapped, 24 Nutford Place, London W1H 6AN. List of publications available on request.

Designing for Mentally Handicapped People. Residential Care. Full conference text. 1971. 40 pence (80¢).

The Use of Normal Housing by Mentally Handicapped People. By Sandra Francklin. 1973. 85 pence ($1.70).

Improving Existing Hospital Buildings for Long-Stay Residents. (CEH Design Guide 1). By Jean Symons. 1973. 60 pence ($1.20).

Training Centres for Mentally Handicapped People. By Sandra Francklin. Reprint from BUILT ENVIRONMENT, October, 1973. 15 pence (30¢).

Trends in the Design of Residential Accommodation for Mentally Handicapped People. By George Miles. Reprint from BEACON, Spring 1974. 15 pence (30¢).

Hostel for Mentally Handicapped Adults. Halstead, Nether Priors, Essex; William Apps, County Architect, Essex County Council. 1974. 15 pence (30¢).

Campaign for the Mentally Handicapped (CMH), 96 Portland Place, London W1N 4EX. Founded in 1971, this group seeks more widespread use of ordinary housing for the mentally handicapped. "The use of ordinary housing will mean considerable reduction in building costs. . . . but any money that can be saved must be channelled into stronger administration, better domiciliary services, and more staff."

Future Services for the Mentally Handicapped. 1971. 15 pence (30¢).

Even Better Service for the Mentally Handicapped. 1972. 50 pence ($1).

Two Years After the White Paper. The paper lists points of action if true community care is to become a reality. 1973. 35 pence (70¢).

Homes for Mentally Handicapped People. By Sandra Francklin. Aimed at architects, this paper describes the design and adaptation of small group housing. 1974. 25 pence (50¢).

Integration or Segregation? The Choice in Practise. 1974. 25 pence (50¢).

CMH pioneered conferences involving mentally handicapped people:

Our Life. Report on the first conference in Britain for mentally handicapped people. 1972. 50 pence ($1).

Listen. Report of the follow-up conference. 1973. 50 pence ($1).

A Workshop on Participation. 1973. 50 pence ($1).

The Spastics Society, 12 Park Crescent, London W1N 4QE. The Society's free list of publications covers the range of concern and care for spastics. The latest helpful publication, *Aids for the Handicapped,* is available for 50 pence ($1) plus 10 pence (20¢) postage. The *Spastic News,* a lively and informative monthly in tabloid form, would be an addition to all cerebral palsy chapters. An annual subscription costs 60 pence ($1.20).

"Until we construct and remodel buildings to make them completely accessible to and usable by the physically handicapped, a large number of persons will be denied full independence and participation in our society. . . . I have confidence in the ability of our architects to provide the essential and artistic means if they are so directed."

—Peter Lassen, AIA JOURNAL, "Buildings for All to Use."

16
Statistics, Legislation, Standards, Codes, and Studies

DEFINITIONS

The definitions that relate to ability to live with or without the assistance of another human being for some or all essential functions are the most meaningful in terms of planning for housing and services needed. Definitions of the disabled can only be vague descriptions, however, because most people are not static in their disability. They are constantly acquiring more skills through experience or equipment, coasting in a remission, losing ability because of a progressive disease, or slowing down because of the normal processes of aging.

Following is a selection of definitions:

U.S. DEPARTMENT OF HOUSING AND URBAN DEVELOPMENT (HUD)

"A handicapped person is one who has a physical impairment which a) is expected to be of long, continued, and indefinite duration; b) substantially impedes his ability to live independently; and c) is of such a nature that such ability can be improved by more suitable housing conditions."

SOCIAL SECURITY ACT

"A disabled person is unable to engage in any substantial gainful activity by reason of any medically determinable physical or mental impairment which can be expected to last for a continuous period of not less than 12 months."

REHABILITATION ACT OF 1973

"A severe handicap is a disability which requires multiple services over an extended period of time and results from amputation, blindness, cancer, cerebral palsy, cystic fibrosis, deafness, heart disease, hemiplegia, mental retardation, mental illness, multiple sclerosis, muscular dystrophy, neurologic disorders (including stroke and epilepsy), paraplegia, quadriplegia and other spinal conditions, renal failure, respiratory or pulmonary dysfunction, and any other disability specified by the Secretary of HEW."

CONFERENCE OF THE CANADIAN REHABILITATION COUNCIL FOR THE DISABLED

"A disabled person is a human being who through disease, illness, congenital condition or traumatic experience, is impaired in functioning in one or more areas of daily living. This functional impairment causes unusual and undue dependency on one or more other human beings and/or mechanical devices."

HANDICAPPED AND IMPAIRED IN GREAT BRITAIN. PART I

"Disabled—the loss or reduction of functional ability"

"Impairment—lacking part or all of a limb, or having a defective limb, organ, or mechanism"

"Handicap—the disadvantage caused by disability"

STATISTICS

The numbers of the elderly in the U.S. are countable: there are now more than 20 million people who are 65 years of age or older, representing nearly 10% of the population. The numbers of the disabled are not so precisely countable and the range of estimates is wide. The data of government agencies—National Center for Health Statistics, Rehabilitation Services Administration, Social Security Administration, U.S. Census Bureau, U. S. Office of Education, and the Veterans Administration—and the Mershon Center of Ohio State University do not yield information that can be precisely related to planning housing.

In 1974–1975 four authoritative agencies used the government data to reach similar conclusions as to the number of people whose mobility is limited by environmental barriers. HUD's October 1975 Interim Report of its work on the new ANSI standard concludes that the target population for barrier-free design— the entire elderly population plus the younger disabled population—totals 32,030,000 people or 16% of the U.S. population. The National Center for a Barrier Free Environment estimates "that one out of ten persons has limited mobility due to a temporary or a permanent physical disability." The President's Committee on Employment of the Handicapped concludes from the figures of the 1970 Census that one out of every eleven adult Americans is disabled. The first report of the Architectural and Transportation Barriers Compliance Board states that "approximately 22 million or 10% of the entire population in the United States have physical impairments which restrict them from normal daily activities."

Fortunately, more precise data on the spinal cord injured are becoming available so that eventually they can be used to pinpoint the need for centers and transitional housing. Presently, unpublished data from a 1971 Health Interview Survey of the National Center for Health Statistics, HEW, show an estimated 102,000 paraplegics (of all ages) and 51,000 quadriplegics. The incidence rate is 0.5/1000 for paraplegics and 0.3/1000 for quadriplegics.

The National Institute of Neurological and Communicable Diseases and Stroke of the NIH is sponsoring a study of the incidence of head and spinal injury in the U.S. The study is being made by Research Triangle Institute, P.O. Box 12194,

Research Triangle Park, North Carolina 27709. The 26-month study will be completed in December 1976.

The first mandatory registry for spinal cord injuries in the U.S. was legislated in Florida in June, 1975. For information, contact Wendy F. Leader, Project Director, Central Registry, 1309 Winewood Boulevard, Tallahassee, Florida 32301.

A National Spinal Cord Injury Registry has been initiated by the Medical University of South Carolina. A biannual newletter reports the results of the studies. For details contact Thomas B. Ducker, MD, Principal Investigator, Spinal Cord Injury Registry, Division of Neurological Surgery, Medical University of South Carolina, 80 Barre Street, Charleston, South Carolina 29401.

ARCHITECTURAL BARRIERS LEGISLATION

The construction and criteria standards pioneered by the Veterans Administration in the 1950s were used as the basic ingredient for the *American Standard Specifications for Making Buildings Accessible to, and Usable by, the Physically Handicapped* (ANSI A117.1–1961). These ANSI specifications, approved in 1961, were the product of 3 years of work and research under the leadership of the National Society for Crippled Children and Adults, the President's Committee on Employment of the Handicapped, Committee A-117 of the American Standards Association, the American Institute of Architects (AIA), and about 75 associations, societies, and agencies. Among the individual leaders of the study were Leon Chatelain, Jr., a Washington, D.C. architect, and Professor Timothy Nugent, whose adaptations at the University of Illinois were used in the research.

NATIONAL COMMISSION ON ARCHITECTURAL BARRIERS

In 1965, under P. L. 89–333, a National Commission on Architectural Barriers was established to evaluate the nationwide problem of architectural barriers. The Commission's comprehensive 54-page report, *Design for All Americans,* is available from the U.S. Government Printing Office for 50¢. In addition to the report, the Commission arranged for cost studies by the National League of Cities, which found the increased cost of making three new buildings accessible (a civic center, a city hall, and a hotel) to be less than one-tenth of 1%; the League also computed the extra costs of making seven hypothetical buildings barrier-free to be less than one-half of 1%.

ARCHITECTURAL BARRIERS ACT OF 1968

P. L. 90–480, amended by the Act of March 5, 1970 (P.L. 91–205), was designed to implement the recommendations of the National Commission on Architectural Barriers. The 1968 Act provides that buildings constructed, altered, leased, or financed in whole or in part by federal funds be designed so as to be accessible to the disabled. All types of buildings, except residential and certain military structures, are covered by the Act, including the Washington, D.C. area transit system.

STATES' BARRIERS LEGISLATION

In 1961, the first federal grant was given to the Minnesota Society for Crippled Children and Adults to provide statistical data on the extent of architectural barriers in four communities. In 1963, Minnesota and North Carolina became the first of the states to enact barrier-free legislation at the state level. Since then, almost every state has enacted some form of legislation, though the laws of many states are so hampered by restrictive clauses or lacking in enforcement mechanisms that they are mere tokens.

William B. Hopkins, Director of Public Affairs of the Minnesota Society for Crippled Children and Adults, Inc., spearheaded the adopting of the 1971 legislation to expand accessibility requirements to all buildings except single and two-family residential buildings and farm buildings. In addition, he helped make Minneapolis the first American city with a curb-ramping program; between 1968 and 1974, Minneapolis installed approximately 9000 curb ramps.

IOWA STUDY OF CONFORMANCE

To test the effectiveness of P.L. 90–480, Edward H. Noakes, AIA, Chairman of the Committee on Barrier-Free Design of the President's Committee on Employment of the Handicapped, initiated a study of conformance to ANSI standards of 34 buildings that had been constructed in Iowa with federal funds. The report, *Accessibility: the Law and the Reality,* concludes that the majority of the projects were not fully accessible and that there was a lack of understanding of the problems of the disabled.

NATIONAL POLICY STATEMENT

As of May, 1974, a Task Force, convened at the initiative of the AIA, agreed upon the following National Policy Statement:

In the United States today it is estimated that one out of ten persons has limited mobility due to a temporary or permanent physical handicap. Improved medical techniques provide some mobility where it was not possible in the past, and an expanding population of older persons is increasing this number every year. Yet, in general, the physical environment of our Nation's communities continues to be designed to accommodate the able-bodied, thereby increasing the isolation and dependence of disabled persons. To break this pattern requires a national commitment.

Therefore, it shall be national policy to recognize the inherent right of all citizens, regardless of their physical disability, to the full development of their economic, social, and personal potential, through the free use of the man-made environment.

The adoption and implementation of this policy requires the mobilization of the resources of the private and public sectors to integrate handicapped people into their communities.

REHABILITATION ACT OF 1973 (P. L. 93–112)

The Rehabilitation Act has tremendous potential for those with the most severe disabilities and for the elimination of barriers for all disabled.

Sections 501 and 503

The Affirmative Action programs required for the employment of disabled employees by firms contracting with the government may include the provision of barrier-free work areas.

Section 502

The Architectural and Transportation Barriers Compliance Board insures that certain buildings financed with federal funds are accessible, investigates alternative approaches to accessibility, and determines what measures are being taken by government and private agencies to eliminate barriers. Among the initial staff members is the long-time champion against barriers, Mrs. Kathaleen C. Arneson of the Rehabilitation Services Administration. Three of the staff members are wheelchaired: James S. Jeffers, Peter Lassen, and Larry Kirk. In March, 1975, Jeffers was named Executive Director of the Board. Infractions regarding compliance should be reported directly to the Architectural and Transportation Compliance Board, Room 1004, Switzer Building, 330 C Street, S.W., Washington, D.C. 20201.

Section 504

Section 504 deals with nondiscrimination under federal grants. Regulations may require accessible college campuses wherever federal scholarships or federal research funds are used.

HOUSING AND COMMUNITY DEVELOPMENT ACT OF 1974 (P. L. 93–383)

The Act includes provisions which focus specifically on the disabled. Under the Section 231 mortgage insurance program nonprofit or profit motivated groups and public agencies may sponsor the construction or rehabilitation of specially designed rental housing for the elderly or handicapped. The program provides for insured loans at 8½ percent interest, plus ½ of one percent mortgage insurance premium.

Section 202 construction loans are available to nonprofit or cooperative sponsors of housing specially designed for the handicapped, participating in the Section 8 Housing Assistance Payments Program, which replaces Section 23, (see Leased Housing under Section 8, Ch. 10).

Clarifying information is contained in the report of a seminar on the implementation of the Act as it impacts on the disabled. The report, *Proceedings: A Seminar on Housing for the Disabled: A Local Perspective,* is available without charge from Housing Council of Niagara Frontier, 238 Main Street, Buffalo, New York 14202.

STANDARDS

During the summer of 1974 HUD awarded $256,000 to Edward Steinfeld, School of Architecture, Syracuse University for a 2-year study to update and expand the 1961 standard. This standard of the American National Standards Institute (ANSI) applied principally to public buildings. The new standard is a performance standard emphasizing the concept of adaptability. It includes dwelling units and related exterior spaces and will have a great impact on the design of housing and the environment. The new standard will be submitted to ANSI for adoption and to HUD for inclusion in the Minimum Property Standards.

In October 1975, HUD published the results of the first year's work, *Interim Report: Barrier-Free Access to the Man-Made Environment—A Review of Current Literature*. The theme of the study is indicated:

The civil rights of disabled people are slowly but surely being guaranteed through legislation and court action. Although people with disabilities are not yet included in civil rights legislation, there is a trend in other legislation to mandate antidiscriminatory guarantees similar to those that racial minorities, women and the aged have received regarding employment, use of places of public accommodation, housing, etc. The right of access to the built environment is firmly established in existing civil rights legislation, although it is not specifically directed to access by disabled people. Specific policies need to be created that implement total accessibility for disabled people to all community support systems. This will insure that one group of people is not unwillingly segregated from full participation in normal community life.

The interim report covers the demography of disabled people, standards and codes review, review of human factors research, spatial behavior of disabled people, building products review, and performance criteria. It concludes, "The individual can make adaptations to a poorly fitting environment but successful adaptations can often be made more appropriately and effectively through design. . . . For a relatively low cost existing environments can be modified to allow people with disabilities to interact competently in them."

ACCOMMODATIONS FOR THE PHYSICALLY HANDICAPPED, VA CONSTRUCTION STANDARD CD-28 (OCTOBER 15, 1973). Order from Office of Construction, Veterans Administration, 810 Vermont Avenue, N.W., Washington, D.C. 20420. This standard is very wheelchair-oriented. The VA requires conformance to these supplementary standards as well as to ANSI. Details are periodically reviewed and updated.

BUILDING CODES

NATIONAL BUILDING CODES

Most of the larger government units in the United States subscribe to one of the major national building codes. Generally, the codes are remedial regulations that are directed toward stability and sturdiness of construction, fire safety, and health and sanitation. Within the last few years, all 3 "general interest" model codes—Building Officials and Code Administrators (BOCA), International Conference of Building Officials (ICBO), and Southern Building Code Congress (SBCC) —have added requirements to meet the needs of the disabled. The 1975 edition of BOCA, for instance, includes a number of provisions for wheelchair accessibility in public buildings. In addition, 1 in every 25 residential units in residential hotel buildings and residential multifamily buildings must be made accessible to the disabled, and they must be proportionately distributed throughout all types of units.

A list of the building codes and standards publications is available from James R. Dowling, Director, Codes and Regulations Center, American Institute of Architects, 1735 New York Avenue, N.W., Washington, D.C. 20006.

Though inclusion of accessibility features in the codes is a big step forward, it is only the beginning. Local communities are permitted to delete sections before adoption, so the inclusion of these provisions does not ensure that they will be adopted in each town. It is the responsibility of local organizations and individuals representing the disabled to influence their communities.

STATE BUILDING CODE: NORTH CAROLINA

The North Carolina Building Code, one of the most comprehensive and effective building codes in the United States, is presented in an attractively illustrated book, *An Illustrated Handbook of the Handicapped Section of the North Carolina State Building Code* published in 1974. It was financed by the Governor's Study Committee. Ronald L. Mace, the architect who created the book and its illustrations, is wheelchaired himself; his illustrations cover every phase of the building code relating to public and residential buildings; also included are wheelchair specifications and relevant legislation.

The details listed in the public building section are covered in the 1961 ANSI standards, but they seem more meaningful with the Mace touch of clarity. Suggestions for privately owned residential projects include elevations and floor plans derived from specifications for kitchens and bathrooms.

The book may be ordered from the North Carolina Department of Insurance, P. O. Box 26387, Raleigh, North Carolina 27611. Price: $1.50.

Legislation on Rights and Tax Credits

North Carolina has passed legislation requiring that 5% of the total number, or at least one toilet room in publicly owned projects or privately owned hotels, motels, schools, and institutional residential projects conform to the minimum accessibility requirements cited. Residential units for the disabled must be distributed equally in a project; they may not be segregated. Statutes also establish curb ramp standards and the rights of the disabled to the use of public conveyances, public places, and guide dogs.

Tax credits are allowed in North Carolina for removal of architectural barriers. In determining state net income, the entire cost of renovation to an existing building or facility to make the toilets and entrances accessible can be deducted. A credit of $550 against income tax is allowed to corporate or resident owners of multifamily rental units for each dwelling unit that is constructed to conform to the building code standards for handicapped living units.

Minimum Residential Construction Suggestions

Based on guidelines from HUD, the following suggestions are made for one of every ten units of privately owned residential projects intended to be sold primarily to North Carolina's physically disabled and/or elderly:

1. Level throughout the unit
2. Kitchens constructed or adjustable to the following
     34 in. high work surfaces
   * Cabinet toe space: 6 in. deep, 84 in. high
     Range with front controls; oven housing top not over 52 in.
     Controls for vents and lights mounted on countertop
     Open space under sink: 30 in. wide, 29 in. high
     Sink: 5 in. deep, lever faucets
     Wall cabinets: adjustable shelves, bottom 16 in. above work areas
   * Turning area: 5 ft clear space between walls or cabinets
     Hot water: insulated exposed lines or maximum temperature set at 120°F
   * Refrigerators: frost-free or self-defrosting, freezer at top
     Under counter clear knee space: 30 in. wide, 24 in. deep; height: 29 in. underneath, 30 in. to countertop
   * Doors: 32 in. clear opening, operable by single effort; swing out or slide
3. Closets with adjustable shelves (4 ft 2 in. to 5 ft 4 in. above floor) and adjustable poles (4 ft to 5 ft 6 in. above floor)
4. Bathrooms, constructed or adjustable to the following
   * Doors swing out or slide, 32 in. clear space
     Clear floor space: 5 ft × 5 ft between cabinets or walls
     Stainless steel handrails on each side wall: 33 in. high; 54 in. long; bear 250-lb load; 1-½ in. clear space between rail and wall
     Lavatories: top 2 ft 10 in. from floor; front 22 in. from wall; 5 in. deep; single lever controls
     Hot water: insulate exposed lines or set at 120°F
     Showers: minimum 3 ft 4 in. × 4 ft 6 in. clear inside; no curbs; seat hinged to wall 19 in. above floor; single lever controls 40 in. high
   * Mirror and one shelf no higher than 40 in. from floor
     Medicine cabinets: adjustable shelves; top no higher than 6 ft
     Toe space of cabinets, same as kitchen
5. Window sill heights 30 in. from floor, except in kitchen and bathroom
6. Electrical wall outlets: minimum, 16 in. from floor, except special outlets in kitchen and bathroom

Minimum Residential Construction Requirements

Privately owned residential projects with more than ten individual residential units shall have 5%, or a minimum of one unit, meet the requirements for exterior accessibility. Doors shall be on one level or accessible by ramps (1 in 12, 8.33%) or elevators.

Kitchens shall meet only the requirements listed which have an asterisk(*). Bathrooms shall also meet only those requirements which have an asterisk*, plus the following: 6 ft between walls except at tub wall and if 5 ft × 5 ft clear floor space is not available, a wall-hung lavatory must be used.

STATE BUILDING CODE: MASSACHUSETTS

The legislation of Massachusetts relating to barriers is unique because its Architectural Barriers Board writes and enforces its own regulations for new buildings and trains local inspectors. The legislation has been developed under the leadership of another wheelchaired architect, Robert J. Lynch, AIA. It provides for accessibility in an unusually broad range of privately financed buildings that are open and used by the public. Further, it provides that at least 5% of the units in hotels, motels, and apartments with 20 or more units must be accessible and usable by the disabled.

CITY CODE: NEW YORK CITY

The New York City Building Code as it relates to accessibility of public buildings is analyzed in a delightfully illustrated booklet, *Barrier-Free Design, Accessibility for the Handicapped.* The authors, Phyllis L. Tica and Julius A. Shaw of the Graduate School and University Center of the City University of New York, have created a helpful 31-page booklet. Copies may be ordered from Educational Resources Information Center, EDRS, P.O. Box 190, Arlington, Virginia 22210.

CITY CODE: CHICAGO

HANDICAPPED CODE AMENDMENTS TO THE MUNICIPAL CODE OF CHICAGO discusses the strong amendments, adopted in 1973, which are included in the Structural Section of the Building Code. Order from Index Publishing Corporation, 308 West Randolph Street, Chicago, Illinois 60606. $4.20.

SURVEYS AND STUDIES

A few of the most significant surveys and studies are presented here in detail because of their comprehensiveness and their recommendations and conclusions.

TWO CALIFORNIA STUDIES OF RESIDENTIAL CARE NEEDS

NEED FOR RESIDENTIAL CARE OF SEVERELY HANDICAPPED CHILDREN AND ADULTS OF NORMAL MENTALITY. Final Report of the Senate Fact-finding

Committee on Labor and Welfare. Published by the California Senate in 1965.

In response to complaints about the lack of residential care services by parents, voluntary agencies, and disabled individuals and groups of disabled individuals, the California Senate Fact-Finding Committee conducted a statewide study of the residential needs of mentally normal severely disabled persons. A total of 4000 questionnaires were distributed by United Cerebral Palsy Association affiliates throughout the state and in Southern California by the Crippled Children's Society of Los Angeles. The majority of the 326 returned questionnaires were from individuals aged 15–19, living with their parents, and disabled by cerebral palsy.

As a result of this study, in 1965 the legislature authorized a 4-year pilot project to determine the needs for residential care services. The project expenses were estimated at $100,000 for the first year, $175,000 in the second year, $175,000 in the third year, and $100,000 in the fourth and final year.

RESIDENTIAL CARE NEEDS. HANDICAPPED PERSONS PILOT PROJECT. A Report to the California State Legislature. January, 1969. State of California, Department of Public Health, 2151 Berkeley Way, Berkeley, California 94704.

In this study, the term residential care was used in the broad sense, embracing all types of services and living arrangements for individuals who are severely disabled. Specifically, it was not used to denote special institutions, but included a flexible range of housing situations and a determination of which care services were essential and appropriate for the individual disabled person's well-being.

Two locations were chosen for the study: Sacramento County and the City of Long Beach. The two local project staffs consisted of a medical social worker, public health nurse, and a clerk. Working with local agencies, the staff selected 115 severely disabled persons who represented the entire gamut of severe physical disabilities, age, living situations, and backgrounds.

To determine the extent of the need for residential care services in California the number of severely physically handicapped persons of normal mentality was estimated by a count of all severely handicapped persons under 65 years of age known to be living in Sacramento County on a given day. Information was gathered through 100 voluntary, health, and welfare agencies, as well as public schools, physicians, and nursing and boarding homes. Based on these data in California in July, 1968, there were approximately 9600 severely physically disabled persons of normal mentality in need of residential care services. The Sacramento data indicated that two-thirds were over 20 years of age.

The two staff teams worked closely with their disabled persons, exploring every avenue of community resources and agencies, analyzing and alleviating or correcting, where possible, their needs for attendant care, information services, personal and family counseling services, equipment, employment, education, vocational training and counseling, medical supervision, nursing, recreation, and transportation. The teams had funds available to take care of immediate needs, such as installing ramps, instructing the family in the use of equipment, hiring a tutor, furnishing a hydraulic lift, finding a suitable apartment, installing an additional toilet, making a loan to purchase an electric typewriter, teaching self-care and grooming, purchasing furniture, paying for all or part of attendant care services, and arranging for dental and medical care.

The study found that, of the estimated 10,000 Californians under 65 who were severely disabled and in need of residential care services, probably no more than 2000 had critical needs not being met at any one time. It was also found that

1. The range and degree of needs and dependence on others make the physically disabled a distinct group for which the combination of existing assistance programs is inadequate.
2. No one agency meets their multiple, complex, and varying needs.
3. Architectural, transportation, and attitudinal barriers block the piecing together of services.
4. The individuals have alert, active minds, normal ambitions, normal emotional needs and reactions, normal abilities for creativity, and normal desires for mental stimulation, occupation, recreation, and community life.
5. For all of them the range of activities is restricted because no one has found a way to bring services into the residence.
6. Most disabled persons can and do live independently in the community and express a strong desire to continue doing so. More could and would live at home if there were better and easier means of providing occasional respite for the family or emergency substitute care.

The study group made the following recommendations:

1. Establish a state program to see that adequate services are provided locally to care for the comprehensive needs of the severely physically handicapped of normal mentality, drawing upon all available government, voluntary, and private resources in the community
2. Establish local supervisory teams composed of a nurse and a social worker to determine the individual's needs, to find sources of necessary services, and to see that they are coordinated, delivered, and changed as needed
3. Provide for the temporary shelter and residential care of those disabled persons who ordinarily live at home
4. Provide funds to modify dwellings and repair or purchase equipment necessary to maintain a disabled person in his own home or to preserve the integrity of his family
5. Provide case management and ongoing residential care service by a health-oriented community agency, such as a coordinated home care or other agency
6. Emphasize preventive care
7. Provide reasonable attendant type care, as needed, to be given by adequately trained and supervised nonprofessional personnel
8. Seek flexibility in interpretation of regulations governing federal, state, and local programs for this group
9. Develop and utilize the talents and abilities of the disabled
10. Develop protectorship services and accept the responsibility for the provision of care when no one else is able to do this

A state residential care program, according to the study, would average $83.33/month per person, compared to $766/month for care in a special institution. Care in regular institutions would average $511/month: a) $165/month for boarding homes, b) $426/month for extended care facilities, and c) $1800/month for hospital care.

If the recommended residential care services were available, the vast majority of the disabled would be able to live in their own homes, where they prefer to live, and generally fare better; they would receive as wide a range of services and as satisfactory care in the home as in an institution. The provision of temporary or respite care would make it possible for some disabled now living in institutions to return to their homes. For a few others, special housing, such as a protective facility, may be necessary. The longer special housing can be avoided, however, the happier and more independent the person, and the more economical his care.

MASSACHUSETTS HOUSING STUDIES

HOUSING NEEDS OF THE HANDICAPPED. A study conducted by the Massachusetts Association of Paraplegics, Inc. in cooperation with the Massachusetts Council of Organizations of the Handicapped. Published in 1970.

The Massachusetts Association of Paraplegics, Inc. (MAP), under the leadership of Elmer Bartels, a quadriplegic, is one of the most outstanding groups of disabled in the United States. As a cohesive group, MAP has tackled the problems of the disabled through cooperation with local community agencies. Although in the mid-1960s MAP approached the housing problem with the belief that a single large facility would solve the problem, it was soon realized that the way to solve the problem was not through a single facility but through legislation, information, and services that include transportation, equipment, minor adaptations, and attendant care. Subsequently, MAP and the Massachusetts Council of Organizations of the Handicapped effected legislation that provides a minimum of 5% barrier-free housing within all state-aided projects for the elderly built after January, 1970; it has watchdogged housing that was built with federal funds to be sure that it conformed to the requirement of 10% barrier-free units; and it has set up a functional service within the Boston Housing Authority to provide services, information, and equipment.

This study was based on two surveys made in 1965 and 1966. The projections beyond the actual numbers seem a little tinged with the preconception that a large housing facility was needed, but the results are interesting because many of the areas covered are unique.

The first study, in 1965–1966, surveyed the 250 MAP members with the following results: 59% felt their own living facilities were adequate; 60% would have been interested in moving to some kind of halfway housing. In the second study, in the autumn of 1966, questionnaires were sent to more than 3000 disabled persons, including 400 MAP members as well as the Massachusetts members of the Paralyzed Veterans of America (PVA). The summary results are based on 951 responses.

The general characteristics of the sample were as follows: 53% were single, 28% were high school graduates, 25% had some college, 52% were unemployed, 49% used a wheelchair, 29% used crutches, and 27% used leg braces. Disabilities included poliomyelitis (26%), cerebral palsy (17%), paraplegia (16%), quadriplegia (9%). More than half were not interested in moving to another part of the state if special housing were provided near an educational or vocational training facility. Age distribution was: 21–29 (22%), 30–39 (19%), 40–49 (22%), 50–59 (16%), 60–64 (4%). Assistance was needed: 19% needed an attendant; 18% needed a housekeeper; 6%, a visiting nurse; and 4%, meal delivery service. The range of ability to pay was $40–$160/month, with the majority able to pay less than $100.

There was no clear preference as to type of facility wanted: 32% wanted regular apartments and 34% preferred their own homes; 61% wanted a 50–50 disabled and nondisabled tenant population, 7% wanted 100% disabled, 5% wanted disabled and elderly, 14% wanted 80% disabled and 20% nondisabled. Several design features were suggested: 13% wanted common dining facilities, 12% wanted employment in the building, 10% wanted shopping within the building; 11% wanted recreation within the building. Special features mentioned included special kitchen features (8%), special bathroom facilities (4%), garage within building (7%); 1%–5% wanted elevators, ramps, railings at stairs, wide doors, physical therapy, and emergency call system.

The group involved in this study is unusual in that it is younger than a typical cross section of the disabled, whose numbers increase with age. This is probably explained by the relative youth of both the MAP and PVA membership. Another interesting point is that, although 49% used a wheelchair, only 4% wanted special bathroom facilities, and only 3% wanted wider doors.

Recommendations that were made as a result of the study were

1. Low rent or subsidized apartments with services
2. Units for disabled within public housing
3. Tax incentives for private contractors to build accessible homes
4. Low cost program to assist the disabled to become homeowners
5. Establishment of a housing council to define priorities and develop legislative and social programs

HELPING ALL THE HANDICAPPED. Prepared by the Massachusetts Vocational Rehabilitation Planning Commission.

The Commission, established to study the existing and future needs of the disabled throughout Massachusetts made the following recommendations through its housing committee:

1. Require integration, no architectural barriers, and supportive services
2. Establish a state housing supervisor, an area advisory committee, and an area coordinator
3. Change public housing restrictions to make occupancy easier for a larger number of disabled individuals
4. Build all new public housing units that have elevators so that they are barrier-free; those without elevators should have first floor barrier-free apartments.

ADAPTIVE HOUSING FOR THE HANDICAPPED. By Paul L. Fishman. A feasibility study carried out under the direction of Hermann H. Field, FAIA, in the Long-Range Planning Department of the Tufts–New England Medical Center. Published in 1971, the study was financed through a grant provided by the Medical Rehabilitation Research and Training Center, Tufts University School of Medicine.

When a site for sheltered or adaptive housing near Tufts–New England Medical Center seemed possible through urban renewal activities, a grant was secured for a 1-year study. The study involved a proposal for a 100-unit facility geared to younger independent disabled persons alone or in small families. The proposal was soon altered to include 100 units of adaptive housing and 100 units for the elderly, plus a small attendant care facility for those disabled who could not live independently. The units for the elderly were added to go along with existing programs. The attendant care facility was soon eliminated because of 1) disagreement about the degree of skill necessary to care for spinal cord injured and 2) uncertainty as to how such a level of care would be managed with existing state laws.

Although the project was abandoned, the study is a valuable analysis of the housing problem, including a review of existing projects and studies, as well as public housing legislation and programs, methods of sponsorship, and minimum accessibility details.

The study recommended that

1. Revolving funds be made available for nonprofit groups to sponsor adaptive housing.
2. Units of adaptive housing be produced as part of ordinary housing.
3. Barrier-free design in family housing be encouraged by HUD.
4. Medical centers sponsor projects combining housing plus limited health care services for transient and permanent residents.
5. A central resource system—agency, bureau, person, or group—be established to monitor housing activities, both public and private.

Fishman concluded that the only way architectural barriers can be uniformly eliminated from all structures is through modifications of local building codes, and the most promising course to barrier-free housing seems to lie in development of housing suitable for the disabled but available to all. Fishman echoed the thoughts of Marie McGuire Thompson, formerly of HUD, "I believe the whole area of resident care and activity needs a separate entity set up, an incorporated body able to take the responsibility and assume the risks, if any; also free to buy and maintain equipment, establish relationships with facilities and services in the community."

There are two major problems with nursing homes: 1) they are designed for care of elderly persons who are chronically ill or convalescent and 2) they are staffed to provide more expensive care than is required by most young disabled persons.

Housing Alternatives for Individuals with Spinal Cord Injury. By Frederick A. Fay. Reprinted from SELECTED RESEARCH TOPICS IN SPINAL CORD INJURY REHABILITATION. A collaborative Rehabilitation Services Administration and Training Centers Task Force Project, July, 1975.

Order from Frederick A. Fay, PhD, Director of Research, Rehabilitation Research & Training Center, Tufts University, 185 Harrison Avenue, Boston, Massachusetts 02111.

The author, a quadriplegic, earned his PhD at the University of Illinois in educational psychology. He has a private practice and serves as a consultant in nursing and rehabilitation care facilities in Boston. He suggests two alternative solutions to housing the spinal cord injured. Solution A is total accessibility. "Nearly every paraplegic and many quadriplegics can live in virtually any housing alternative that is accessible to them—from log cabin to penthouse. Generally, these persons prefer to be totally integrated into their community. . . . It seems obvious that the ultimate goal in changing our housing must be a barrier-free environment that is totally accessible to all."

Solution B involves group residences.

Three distinct groups appear to benefit by some sort of group residence (hostel, halfway house, motel, dormitory, clustered housing, congregate housing, commune, etc.). First, many high level quadriplegics (C2–C4) may require skilled nursing as well as housekeeping and attendant care, and have found sharing the costs, rent, maintenance and help with other quads to be quite economical. Second, many paraplegics and quadriplegics who benefit by the "peer therapy" of the SCI center, but who no longer need the costly support services, have found great benefit in transitional halfway houses that bridge the gap between hospital dependency and community self-sufficiency. Third, there are a small minority of persons with SCI who simply prefer life in a community of disabled individuals or feel that a specialized facility is better than no facility.

PHILADELPHIA HOUSING STUDIES

THE PHYSICALLY DISABLED AND HOUSING. A PHILADELPHIA STUDY. By D. B. Columbus and W. J. Erdman. Final Report Planning Grant VRA-DRF-PD-28-6. HEW.1968. Survey of Disabled Persons Reveals Housing Choices. By D. B. Columbus and M. L. Fogel. JOURNAL OF REHABILITATION, March–April, 1971.

As a result of the zeal of the president of the American Society for the Physically Handicapped for a housing project, the University of Pennsylvania School of Medicine obtained a research grant from HEW to study the housing needs of the disabled living in the Philadelphia area. A questionnaire was mailed to 385 persons with stabilized medical conditions who had been patients of the leading hospitals in Philadelphia. The 93 (29%) returned forms represented numerous disabilities. Only one-third of the respondents were interested in moving into special housing.

Because of the low completion rate of questionnaires, an interviewing system was added. Eventually, 455 people had either filled out the questionnaire or been interviewed. Of these, there were 236 males and 219 females; the mean age was

51; the majority (219) were married and living in their own homes; only 47 lived alone; and 279 needed some type of attendant care for their daily routines.

Most preferred to live in housing which was designed mainly for the nondisabled but which would accommodate a few disabled persons. In other words, they wanted the same housing available to all others, but made architecturally accessible. All adult age groups rejected a facility designed to accommodate only disabled persons. Two-thirds of the total group preferred to remain in their present living arrangements where family members could assist them with daily needs.

In the total group, only a small percentage (9%) had been disabled since birth. Since the mean average age was 51 and the average length of time since onset of disability was 15 years, many were middle–aged by the time they were disabled and had already established their own living patterns.

The authors concluded

There was the realization that as in all housing there should be a wide variety of good, well-designed choices available to the disabled of all economic levels because no single facility in a city would fulfill all of the requirements for all of the disabled.

. . . and unless a percentage of the federally sponsored and also privately financed housing units are designed to be accessible to the disabled, their housing problems will remain unsolved.

Successful rehabilitation is inextricably intertwined with the environment in which the disabled live.

Housing for the Disabled: II. Characteristics of those Willing to Move to Specially Designed Facilities. PERCEPTUAL AND MOTOR SKILLS Vol. 32, pages 212–214, 1971.

This follow-up study of the one-third (134) in the earlier Philadelphia studies who wanted to move to a special facility was also supported by a grant from HEW. In contrasting those willing to move and those who preferred not to move, differences and similarities of the two groups emerged.

On the average, the would-be movers were more likely to be city apartment dwellers, single, male, users of wheelchairs or braces, and to have a lower income than the nonmovers. Further, there were more young people in the group, and they were more accepting of housing for the disabled only but less accepting of integration of the elderly.

The authors conclude that, based on this survey, the housing needs of those willing to move would consist of low to moderate cost units with kitchens and bathrooms designed to accommodate those who use wheelchairs and braces. Further, since 194 (43%) required two or more bedrooms for family members who would take care of their basic daily needs, "it is illogical to plan housing for the disabled without considering family members or other personnel who could fulfill these duties."

One of the positive results of the study was making the Philadelphia Housing Authority more aware of the needs of the disabled for low income housing and for information on the housing rights granted to them by the 1964 and 1965 legislation that made housing available to them in public housing projects for the elderly.

NEW YORK STATE HOUSING STUDY

RESIDENTIAL NEEDS OF SEVERELY PHYSICALLY HANDICAPPED NON-RETARDED CHILDREN AND YOUNG ADULTS IN NEW YORK STATE. By Joseph Fenton, EdD, with the assistance of Robert E. Ayers. Rehabilitation Monograph No. 46. New York University, Institute of Rehabilitation Medicine. 1972.

Dr. Fenton presents the results of his 1969 survey in a comprehensive 188-page analysis. His method of distributing the questionnaires insured unusually wide coverage: over 10,000 questionnaires were distributed by professional staff members of more than 100 public and voluntary agencies. After eliminating those from individuals over the age limit of 55 or mentally retarded, the reports of 2575 severely physically disabled persons in need of long-term residential facilities were accepted and analyzed.

It was found that the number of disabled increased with age, thus the largest group was aged 40–55; 30% required attendant care, but the rest were quite independent or needed only occasional assistance; 88% lived in their own homes, foster homes, or relative's homes which were considered inappropriate; 12% lived in institutions such as nursing homes, hospitals, or infirmaries. The great majority were disabled by cerebral palsy (20%), muscular dystrophy, multiple sclerosis, spinal cord injury, arthritis, and poliomyelitis.

One of the most interesting tables was that listing the reasons those living at home needed residential facilities: 820 (39%)—family physically unable to maintain demands for adequate care; 355 (16.9%)—inadequate services available in community; 228 (10.8%)—parents or spouse aged; 188 (8.9%)—to relieve members of family for other obligations.

Particularly depressing was the study of 500 proprietary nursing homes in upstate New York which cared for 57 patients under the age of 50 in an environment without challenge or recreation. Almost equally depressing was the study of 58 disabled persons under age 55 at the Goldwater Memorial Hospital Public Home Infirmary, 82% of whom were between ages 21 and 39 years, disabled primarily by poliomyelitis and cerebral palsy; functionally, 10 were relatively independent and 34 were dependent.

Dr. Fenton concluded

"Suitable" public, voluntary agency or private long-term residential facilities are virtually nonexistent in New York State for severely physically handicapped children and adults of "normal" intellect. If, however, these same disabled individuals were mentally retarded, mentally ill, juvenile delinquents, criminals or criminally insane as well, they would be eligible to benefit from a "residential" program operated by one of the Departments of the State of New York.

Dr. Fenton made 18 specific recommendations, many of which are relevant to other states and communities. Following are the highlights:

1. The planning and administering of a residential program for the disabled should be delegated to a single state agency.
2. Regional committees should be designated to coordinate programs on the community level.
3. For those who require some assistance, group living residential facilities should

be located throughout the state; the facilities should be available for respite care.
4. For those disabled persons who can live alone, individual housing facilities, apartments, private homes or motel type facilities should be constructed; they should be centrally located and have subsidized rent and transportation.
5. For those who wish to remain in their own homes, state funds should be available for home services including recreation, counseling, and family aides; funds should also be available to make adaptations to the homes.
6. HEW should be urged to incorporate federal–state cost sharing provisions to encourage a nationwide residential facility program.

Of special significance are the services that were reported as "needed but not receiving." In the order of most often reported to the least: recreation, vocational evaluation and counseling, social services, transportation, occupational therapy, friendly visitors, psychologic services, physical therapy, schooling, attendant care, homemaker services, home care program, speech and hearing therapy, physical follow-up, medical evaluation, public health nursing, general hospital care, and an assortment of miscellaneous services.

BRITISH ANALYSIS OF COSTS OF CARE OF DISABLED

CARE WITH DIGNITY. AN ANALYSIS OF COSTS OF CARE FOR THE DISABLED. Report by the Economist Intelligence Unit. Revised edition. National Fund for Research into Crippling Diseases, Vincent House, 1 Springfield Road, Horsham, Sussex RH12 2PN, England. January 1974. £3.

The study compared the costs of caring for disabled people at home with a range of domiciliary services (£16–£30/week), in a specialized residence such as a home for spastics (£18–£35/week) in a chronic hospital (£25–£30/week), and in an acute hospital (£100/week). Thus, it is typically around £10/week cheaper at home than in long-stay hospitals or residential homes.

A fascinating assortment of facts came out of this study.

Only 10% of the disabled are under age 50.

Sickness, disability, and old age account for the public expenditure of nearly £6 billion, 13% of the Gross National Product and 28% of the total public expenditure.

Most of the expenditures are on institutions. No machinery exists whereby savings in institutional costs through effective community care can be transferred to the community care services.

The population of the severely disabled will rise at the rate of 2%/year.

Local authority and voluntary homes accommodate 8300 disabled individuals under 65, most of whom are over 50. The Cheshire Homes, the largest of the voluntary groups, have spaces for 1500 disabled. With the Spastics Society and other voluntary agencies 5000 people are accommodated.

All one-bedroom council flats should be built with grab bars in the bathroom, waist-level electrical fittings, and bannisters or handrails.

Existing waiting lists are a poor guide to potential demand. People are reluctant to move to different surroundings, even to much more suitable accommodations.

"A satisfactory housing situation for the disabled will not be achieved unless a wide choice is available."

The study includes two proposals for improvement: 1) a group of financial institutions aimed at catering to the needs of the disabled—a housing association, house agency, finance house, and a building society and 2) a "boarding out" project for "fostering" adult disabled at a salary large enough to attract competent housewives. The author cites the Danish plan of paying families to take care of their disabled and the Belgian centuries-old tradition of caring for disabled people, especially the mentally retarded within the community. One in six Belgian families cares for a disabled person and, since World War II, has been paid by the state.

The study revealed the abysmal ignorance about useful devices or equipment on the part of the disabled as well as professional personnel. In addition to the displays in London run by the Disabled Living Foundation, the Spastics Society, and the Central Council for the Disabled, the suggestion is made for a country-wide mobile display service. The aim would be reach the disabled, their doctors and nurses, their relatives and neighbors. Specially equipped and staffed vans or caravans would tour the country with self-contained exhibitions.

Alternative suggestions include: 1) secure space in one or more of the major department stores which have country-wide branches and mount displays of devices that could travel from store to store and 2) make systematic presentations on educational TV and radio programs covering various phases of living with disabilities.

Bibliography

THE AMERICAN PEOPLE, By E. J. Kahn, Jr., Baltimore, Penguin Books, Inc. 1975.

Chronic Conditions and Limitations of Activity and Mobility United States—July 1965—June 1967. Series 10. No. 61. National Center for Health Statistics, Public Health Service, U.S. Department of Health, Education, and Welfare, January, 1971.

Chronic Conditions Causing Activity Limitation. Series 10. No. 51, National Center for Health Statistics, Public Health Service, U.S. Department of Health, Education, and Welfare, 1969.

Current Estimates From the Health Interview Survey United States—1972. Series 10. Number 85, National Center for Health Statistics, U.S. Department of Health, Education, and Welfare, 1973.

Design for All Americans. A Report of the National Commission on Architectural Barriers to Rehabilitation of the Handicapped. Washington, D.C., U.S. Government Printing Office. 1967.

Disability in the United States. A Compendium of Data on Prevalance and Programs, edited by Lawrence E. Riley and Saad Z. Nagi. Columbus, Ohio, The Ohio State University, 1970.

An Epidemiology of Adulthood Disability in the United states, by Saad Z. Nagi. Mershon Center, Columbus, Ohio, The Ohio State University, 1975.

Findings of the 1970 APTD Study. Part I. Demographic and Program Characteristics. Washington, D.C., U.S. Department of Health, Education, and Welfare. September 1972.

Findings of the 1970 APTD Study. Part II. Financial Circumstances. Washington, D.C., U.S. Department of Health, Education, and Welfare. December 1972.

The Goal Is: Mobility! Environmental and Transportation Barriers Encountered by the Disabled, by Ruth Lauder; Washington, D.C., U.S. Department of Health, Education, and Welfare. 1969.

Limitation of Activity Due to Chronic Conditions, U.S. 1969 and 1970, National Center for Health Statistics, U.S. Department of Health, Education, and Welfare. Series 10. No. 80. April 1973.

One in Eleven Handicapped Adults in America. A Survey Based on 1970 Census Data, by the President's Committee on Employment of the Handicapped. Washington, D.C. 1975.

Proceedings: A Seminar on Housing for the Disabled: A Local Perspective. Housing Council of Niagara Frontier, Buffalo, New York 1975.

"Selected Facts and Figures About the Disabled and the Disadvantaged," National Citizens Conference on Rehabilitation of the Disabled and the Disadvantaged. Washington, D.C. Department of Health, Education, and Welfare, June 1969.

Social Security Survey of the Disabled: 1966; Reports No. 2, 3, 6. by Lawrence D. Haber; Social Security Administration, U.S. Department of Health, Education, and Welfare, 1968–1969.

"Spinal Cord Injury. Hope Through Research." Public Health Service Publication No. 1747. Health Information Series No. 143. Prepared by the Information Office, National Institute of Neurological Diseases and Stroke, National Institute of Health. Washington, D.C. U.S. Government Printing Office, Reprinted 1970.

"Studies in Housing for the Handicapped." by Charles Gueli and Deborah Greenstein; *HUD Challenge,* Vol. VI, No. 3, pages 22–25, March, 1975.

"To Help the Physically Handicapped," in "Looking Ahead;" *HUD Challenge,* Vol. 5, No. 7, page 1, July, 1974.

Travel Barriers. Transportation Needs of the Handicapped, prepared by Abt Associates, Inc. for U.S. Department of Transportation. Washington, D.C. August 1969.

Use of Special Aids, United States 1969 (Series 10, No. 78), National Center for Health Statistics, U.S. Department of Health, Education, and Welfare. December 1972.

United States Census Summary 1–715. Detailed Characteristics. Table 220 "Characteristics of the Noninstitutional Population 16 to 64 Years Old With Work Disability: 1960."

"It is amazing how much the cause of the disabled is being pushed, first by the disabled themselves, and secondly by the general public. The days when only the specialized agencies were involved in pushing for change have hopefully disappeared."

—*Pierre Gariepy, Alberta Division Canadian Paraplegic Association*

17
Canada

HEALTH SERVICES

The administration of health services in Canada is a direct responsibility of the provincial governments, which may delegate certain functions to local or municipal governments. The federal government does not itself operate a medical care insurance plan; the Medical Care and the Hospital Insurance and Diagnostic Service Programs, which cover over 99% of the population (about 22.5 million), achieve a national health program through a series of interlocking provincial plans.

Any resident of Canada, whether a citizen or not, employed or unemployed, is eligible for the insurable benefits of the health insurance programs. The Canadian programs are financed on a current basis through taxation, premium payments, or modest utilization fees.

The Hospital Insurance and Diagnostic Service Program covers inpatient care (including drugs and diagnostic tests) and outpatient services that vary from province to province. The Medical Care Program covers all required services by medical practitioners.

SOCIAL SECURITY SYSTEMS

FINANCIAL ASSISTANCE FOR THE DISABLED

The Canada and Quebec Pension Plans cover those with a severe disability who have made contributions to the plan for a minimum of 5 years.

Through the Canada Assistance Plan, the federal government and the provincial governments share the costs of assistance to disabled persons in need. The provinces determine the eligibility, decide on the amount, and provide the assistance, which may include prostheses, medical appliances, costs of transportation for medical treatment, and the costs of care in special homes for the disabled, elderly, and others with special needs.

Financial assistance also varies widely. For instance, in Ontario, there became effective in January 1975 a minimum guaranteed income of $2750 for all disabled over age 18 and all aged over the age of 65, while British Columbia guarantees an income of $213.85 to a single disabled person and $427.70 to a married couple.

Workmen's Compensation recipients receive wheelchairs, appliances, minor home renovations, hand controls, and drugs. Their compensation is based on

75% of their most recent earnings and an allowance for an attendant, wife, or other family member.

VOCATIONAL REHABILITATION OF DISABLED PERSONS (VRDP)

The federal government and the provinces share the costs of vocational rehabilitation services, such as counseling, assessment, services of restoration and training, employment placement, maintenance allowances, transportation, tools, books, and attendant care, as well as staff and administrative costs. Such programs vary from province to province and depend on local interpretation of need. Provinces may or may not pay for hand controls, ramps, hydraulic lifts, or power-driven wheelchairs.

NATIONAL REGISTRY

There is no national registry of disabled persons in Canada, although several different types of reporting systems and registries have been established for purposes of research, prevention, or treatment. Since 1966, the Department of National Health and Welfare has operated a surveillance and monitoring system for congenital anomalies with the participation of British Columbia, Alberta, Manitoba, New Brunswick, and Ontario. The British Columbia Registry of Handicapped Children and Adults is considered one of the best registers in Canada.

CENTRAL MORTGAGE AND HOUSING CORPORATION (CMHC)

In many ways, the approaches of the United States' HUD and Canada's CMHC to the problems of housing the elderly and the disabled are quite similar. Both have developed rent subsidies; both are working on proportions of disabled persons in housing for the elderly; both are working toward integration of all types of persons in all types of housing and toward the provision of supportive services.

Regulations for access to public buildings are contained in the Supplement No. 5 to the National Building Code, *Building Standards for the Handicapped,* but they are effective only when the document is adopted as a municipal bylaw.

RECOMMENDATIONS FOR THE FUTURE

NATIONAL CONFERENCE OF THE PHYSICALLY DISABLED

The Canadian Rehabilitation Council for the Disabled (CRCD) is a national federation of the voluntary organizations concerned with and committed to helping the physically disabled. Its quarterly publication, *Rehabilitation Digest,* covers the entire spectrum of disabilities and is an excellent source of information on the activities of the voluntary organizations throughout Canada.

One of the Council's outstanding contributions to the welfare of the disabled is the National Conference of the Physically Disabled which it convened November 4–7, 1973 in Toronto. Working in seminar sessions, the 150 participants explored common problems in the areas of education, financial security, recreation and culture, social responsibility, transportation, and housing. Their recommendations and resolutions concern the problems faced by all disabled persons everywhere. The housing recommendations include: design 10% of all units in new multiple housing projects for the disabled; allow remodeling for the disabled to be tax deductible; and incorporate courses on the needs of the disabled in schools of architecture. The resolutions are printed in full in the Fall/Winter 1973–1974 issue of *Rehabilitation Digest,* which can be ordered from CRCD, Suite 2110, One Yonge Street, Toronto, Ontario M5E 1E8. 75¢.

TORONTO TASK FORCE

"This City is for all its citizens no matter how palsied their step or frail their grasp," stated Mayor David Crombie in his inaugural address on January 3, 1973. Shortly thereafter he initiated a Task Force to study the problems of the disabled and elderly and invited all concerned to participate. The Task Force's recommendations are presented in a 100-page report written by Pamela Cluff and Jane Staub, Toronto. *The Mayor's Task Force Report Re Disabled and Elderly.*

The report, available from City Hall, City of Toronto, covers services, leisure and recreation, employment and income, transportation, education, and housing. Some of the housing recommendations are of special interest: fund an information center to assist those looking for suitable accommodation; make special provisions for the development of small group homes in areas zoned for single family homes; and furnish consultation services and financial assistance for home repairs to the elderly and disabled.

SOCIAL PLANNING AND REVIEW COUNCIL OF BRITISH COLUMBIA

The need for change through public awareness and action by government and private agencies is the strong recommendation contained in the working paper, *Housing for the Handicapped,* presented by a committee of the Panel for Guidance of Handicapped of the Social Planning and Review Council (SPARC) of British Columbia in March, 1973, and available from SPARC at 2210 West 12th Avenue, Vancouver V6K 2N6, British Columbia. The Committee on Housing for the Handicapped was composed of representatives from the fields of health, welfare, rehabilitation, architecture, and voluntary agencies concerned with the disabled.

One of the most noteworthy of the recommendations is that specially designed rental hostels (residences with shared laundry facilities, communal dining and recreation rooms, usually with housekeepers) be integrated into the planning of low income housing developments to accommodate those who are unable to live independently and that capital support for these buildings be provided by the Federal Government under the National Housing Act (1954 Section 15).

The report summarized the existing facilities for the dependent disabled—those individuals who require a lesser degree of care than provided at nursing home level and yet who need some degree of assistance with self-care: 1) private homes; 2) licensed boarding homes, costing a minimum of $150–$174/month; 3) licensed boarding-home care, costing $200/month, with some supervision (perhaps the most desirable but also the scarcest); 4) nursing homes and private hospitals, costing a minimum of $358/month; 5) general hospitals, costing $45–$65/day; 6) extended care facilities, costing $15–$20/day (patient pays $1/day); 7) rehabilitation centers, costing up to $50/day (patient pays $1/day).

HANDICAPPED HOUSING SOCIETY OF ALBERTA

In a fascinating evolution, disabled individuals and groups in Alberta coordinated their efforts into one cohesive organization, the Action Group of the Disabled, 10325—83rd Avenue, Edmonton, Alberta. With the aid of a 5-month federal grant under Local Initiative Program, a team of ten disabled persons began its activities in 1972 by compiling a registry of the physically disabled in Edmonton and by gathering data to establish their needs.

REGISTRY AND LIFESTYLE RESEARCH

The registry was prepared by arranging for the various agencies serving the disabled to mail questionnaires to their clients. In addition to the name of the individual, the questionnaire requested information on the age, sex, medical diagnosis, disability, and educational and employment status. Of the 3387 questionnaires sent out, 730 were completed and returned.

In the second phase of the project, in-depth personal interviews were conducted with a sample population of 40 persons selected from the registry. During the same study, another survey, specifically oriented to young and middle-aged disabled persons living in institutions, was taken. These 23 individuals expressed great dissatisfaction with their living accommodations: they had no privacy, no responsibilities, and little recreation; they wanted individual bedrooms, a homelike atmosphere, and more normal lifestyles. The fascinating report of these studies, *Research on the Life-Styles of the Physically Disabled,* should be required reading for planners of any type of group housing. It can be ordered from Alberta Committee of Action Groups of the Disabled, #4, 10015—82 Avenue, Edmonton T6E 1Z2, Alberta.

HOUSING *CHARETTE*

The philosophy of the Society is that those affected by decisions should be allowed to participate in the process leading up to them as well as in the actual making of them. To engender this philosophy, a 5-day housing *charette,* financed by a $10,000 grant from the provincial government, was held in April, 1973. The charette is basically an intensive process of community planning aimed at community change and allowing citizens to participate in creative decision-making processes. Primarily, the charette participants—65 disabled persons—indicated a need for change in the process by which the decisions which determine their future are made. Three basic recommendations evolved:

1. It must be a fundamental criterion that all future housing for the disabled be based on a) maximized independence for the disabled and b) optimized integration of the disabled into the community.
2. All future housing for the disabled must include the disabled in its programming, design, construction, and management. This shall also apply to all programs other than housing.
3. A program of public and special education relative to the disabled should be developed to provide an information exchange between the disabled and the public-at-large. This program will be designed and operated by the disabled with financial subsidy from the provincial government.

The final report, *Handicapped Housing Charette,* is available from the Handicapped Housing Society of Alberta. It recommends that a housing complex which includes a broad spectrum of services be designed and managed by residents with varying degrees of physical disabilities. Other recommendations include more comprehensive home services, a guaranteed income, and accessible transportation.

Housing Master Plan

To continue the momentum developed at the charette, the Housing Society initiated a Tri-Level Governmental Committee on Housing for the Handicapped, which consisted of persons from all three levels of government and members of the Housing Society. The committee for funding agreed to fund a program study to produce a master plan on a housing complex for the physically disabled.

The total program study, covering research on disabled housing, identification of financial resources, land search, costs analysis, and determination of the best methods of implementing the project, is documented in the Society's comprehensive report titled, *Access: Housing.* Of particular interest are the drawings and plans of the central city location by Thorkelsson Architects and the tabulation of the results of the very extensive questionnaire used in the survey of 81 potential residents. This report which should also be required reading for all who are planning housing and services for the disabled, is available from the Handicapped Housing Society of Alberta.

The specific recommendations of the potential residents include: a location in normal residential settings near commercial, cultural, and recreational facilities; a ratio of no more than 50% disabled; a mix of incomes; a staff to provide a scheduled number of hours of assistance in daily living; a few hotellike temporary quarters; a maximum use of neighborhood recreation facilities; a choice of dining services; and intensive occupational therapy for all new residents to prepare them for independent living.

The research team wholeheartedly recommends the charette format for future endeavors. Those who reside in the complexes will be housed in accommodations which they helped to initiate, plan, and design. It is they who determined the size, location, integration, services, and administration.

Future plans of the Society include developing the proposed housing complex, providing for some units in all future city public housing developments, developing architectural plans for single dwelling units, and acting in an advisory capacity for groups of individuals that are developing units.

SERVICE ORGANIZATIONS

CANADIAN PARAPLEGIC ASSOCIATION

The Canadian Paraplegic Association, 520 Sutherland Drive, Toronto M4G 3V9, Ontario, operates the world's largest comprehensive system of rehabilitation services for the spinal cord injured. Significantly, the managing director, G. K. Langford, the executive directors of its divisions in the provinces, and the majority of the members of the National Board of Directors and the regional Boards of Management are themselves wheelchaired by spinal cord injuries.

Directing the Association's efforts toward a satisfying and fulfilling restoration of the spinal cord injured to the community, its counselors begin working, under medical guidance, with newly disabled paraplegics and quadriplegics as early as is feasible. They continue their guidance and supervision in the hospital, at home, and in every stage of adjustment.

The Association supplies and maintains equipment; it provides counseling, employment guidance, legal aid and information services, vocational training, educational supervision, direct financial aid and loans, and assistance with housing and home care services, including attendant care. It owns and operates the new 106-bed Lyndhurst Hospital that specializes in the treatment and rehabilitation of the spinal cord injured in Ontario. It acts as an advocate for the spinal cord injured at all levels of government and with the community. National news relating to spinal cord injury are reported in its excellent quarterly, *The Caliper,* which has a subscription rate of $2/year.

Operating under a federal government charter granted in 1945, the Association is headquartered in Toronto at the Lyndhurst Hospital. Each of its seven divisions —Atlantic (Nova Scotia and Prince Edward Island), New Brunswick, Quebec, Manitoba, Saskatchewan, Alberta, and British Columbia—has its own Board of Management. Funding of the association varies from province to province, but consists generally of provincial and municipal government grants, as well as corporate and private donations, plus fees for services rendered to provincial and other agencies. Some divisions utilize the United Way fund-raising.

LOCAL INITIATIVES PROGRAM

While the Local Initiatives Program (LIP) is not managed by the disabled, nor specifically geared to them, it has been of great value to tens of thousands of unemployed and underemployed disabled and nondisabled persons. With a minimum of red tape, unemployed individuals as well as groups and local organizations have applied directly to the federal government for grants to establish programs for employing persons who are unemployed or on welfare in useful local activities. The only restrictions are that the products may not be sold commercially and that any project involving the local government must be discussed with the local authorities. The only criteria for employment on a project are unemployment and a willingness to work for a maximum of $100/week.

Efficiency has been high and direct costs and failures low. The products include specialized toys for blind and disabled children, and the projects include day care centers, low income housing rehabilitation projects, information centers for disabled and immigrants, transportation and delivery services for elderly and disabled, rural and urban clean-up and pollution control, and senior citizen "handyman" teams. The projects cover the whole range of Canadian territory, from urban centers to Indian reservations and remote fishing villages. Many of the programs have continued and become self-supporting; many of the individuals have become permanently employed.

INFORMATION SERVICE FOR THE DISABLED IN ALBERTA

In 1972, some of the disabled persons who had worked on the Action Group of the Disabled Research Team received an LIP extension to set up an information service, Social Services for the Disabled. The chief concern expressed by the disabled when they had been interviewed for the original report was that they were not aware of what services were available to them. The areas covered by Social Services for the Disabled include housing, employment placement, and information on financial assistance through the social security systems. A "hand-in-hand" type of assistance was established, a service that welcomes persons who are disabled into the office to discuss their problems with the staff members, who are also disabled.

Social Services for the Disabled concentrates its efforts on helping the disabled seek and attain proper employment. The organization contacted all three levels of government so that it could refer prospective candidates to the proper channels for employment. To establish initial contacts in the business community, a letter was sent to 935 businesses in Edmonton to encourage them to hire persons who are disabled. Further services include medical and legal information and home services, such as homemaker service.

HANDICAPPED RESOURCE CENTRE IN BRITISH COLUMBIA

The Handicapped Resource Centre, Suite 101—8185 Main Street, Vancouver, V5X 3L5, British Columbia, was created and funded with the cooperation of a number of agencies: the British Columbia Division of the Canadian Paraplegic Association, the Urban Design Centre, Company of Young Canadians, Opportunity for Youth Program, and United Community Services. Known initially as the Vancouver Resource Centre for the Disabled, the agency is primarily concerned with locating suitable housing services, and equipment for the disabled. By the end of its first year, the agency had grown into an effective and independent organization which employed nine disabled members of the Canadian Paraplegic Association, under the leadership of Les Watson, Executive Director.

According to the December 1, 1974, *Progress Report to the Provincial Government,* the Centre dealt with 496 clients and made 292 placements in the period from January 1, 1974, to November 30, 1974. In April, 1974, the Vancouver Resource Society for the Physically Disabled set up a committee to develop alternative lifestyles for people who require some daily personal care but who do not wish to live in institutions or at home with relatives. The results of the committee's work are the following projects.

Group Home, 885 West 46th Avenue, Vancouver, British Columbia

In April, using the offices of the Handicapped Resource Centre as a base, the committee hired a coordinator to establish a group home for the physically disabled. Start-up funds for this purpose were received from Central Mortgage and Housing Corporation. Application forms were sent to institutions, hospitals, rehabilitation centers, social workers, and disabled individuals. Applicants were screened and interviewed to determine level of interest and the amount of attendant care required. Of the 75 applicants, one was chosen as the core member; this person chose the second; the two of them chose the third, and a fourth, until the group was formed.

The Handicapped Resource Centre leased a suitable house, made financial arrangements with the Department of Human Resources, and began remodeling. This involved a ramp around one side of the house from the back door, an enclosed elevator from the basement to the first floor, and alterations to the bathrooms. Furniture was donated or purchased. Two live-in attendants were hired, and the residents moved in on August 1, 1974.

Group Home, 5434 Manson Street, Vancouver, British Columbia

The lease agreement for this residence was signed by the Vancouver Resource Society for the Physically Disabled. The Handicapped Resource Centre assumed responsibility for the renovations and finding the four tenants. Arrangements were made through the Division of Health, Care and Aging to subsidize the tenants so those who were on assistance programs could afford to live there. The Division also obtained "special needs" money to purchase household furnishings such as a dryer, refrigerator, linen, and dishes. Two of the four tenants moved in while the renovations were in progress and participated in the planning of the ramps, handrails, and other adaptations.

Proposed Group Homes

The Handicapped Resource Centre has been asked to assist in planning housing, in Kitsilano, for four children from Sunnyhill Hospital and for four or five young deaf adults attending the Western Institute for the Deaf.

Community Involvement

The Handicapped Resource Centre worked with the Vancouver Parks Board to create a summer program of crafts, picnics, bus tours, and a Thursday evening "coffee shop." In addition, a production group composed of physically disabled individuals was formed to plan and produce programs on the new community-based FM radio station. The programs will air the needs of the disabled as well as introduce outstanding people in the disabled community. While the production crew learns radio skills, the advisory group is raising money for the 1-hour/week show. The remaining monies will be raised from agencies which want to have programs made about their organizations; other revenue will be obtained through the sale of programs to other radio networks.

QUEBEC STUDY OF INTEGRATED HOUSING

In August 1974, the Quebec Division of the Canadian Paraplegic Association received a grant from the Department of National Health and Welfare to study integrated housing. The objectives of the 3-year study are 1) to find conventional housing in dispersed locations and make it accessible for 30 quadriplegics and 2) to coordinate arrangements for community services and home care which will enable them to live as independently as possible. Both the director, Ghislain Cayouette, and the coordinator, Patricia Konecny, an architect, are paraplegics. They hope to create a program that can be implemented nationwide.

HUDAC'S MODEL HOME FOR WHEELCHAIR LIVING

The Housing and Urban Development Association of Canada (HUDAC), the voice of Canada's housing industry, has designed and constructed a model home through a committee, HUDAC—Greater Vancouver, with the cooperation of the British Columbia Division of the Canadian Paraplegic Association and the Central Mortgage and Housing Corporation. The house was designed to demonstrate that a house for the wheelchaired could be constructed at a reasonable cost. The main objective was to dispel the fears expressed by builders that housing for the disabled involves many extra expenses, looks institutional, and would be unsatisfactory for the general public. The committee first set up the criteria for the design and then made the actual working drawings of the house. As the design criteria process evolved, it became evident that the changes and improvements required to make the house more convenient for a person in a wheelchair were not of a major nature. In fact, the end product is a home which will be more convenient for everyone, disabled or not (Fig. 17-1).

The final design for the model home called for a three-bedroom house with 1500 sq ft of space and a two-car carport. It is located at 12736 Campbell Place, Surrey, British Columbia, in the Glen Robertson West Subdivision. Designed for a homemaker in a wheelchair, the plan requires only 75 sq ft of additional space in the slightly wider halls, roomier bathrooms, and in the 5 ft diameter turning radius for a wheelchair. Most of the special features are in the design of the

Fig. 17–1. HUDAC Home for Independent Living. (Photograph courtesy of G.K. Langford, Managing Director of the Canadian Paraplegic Association)

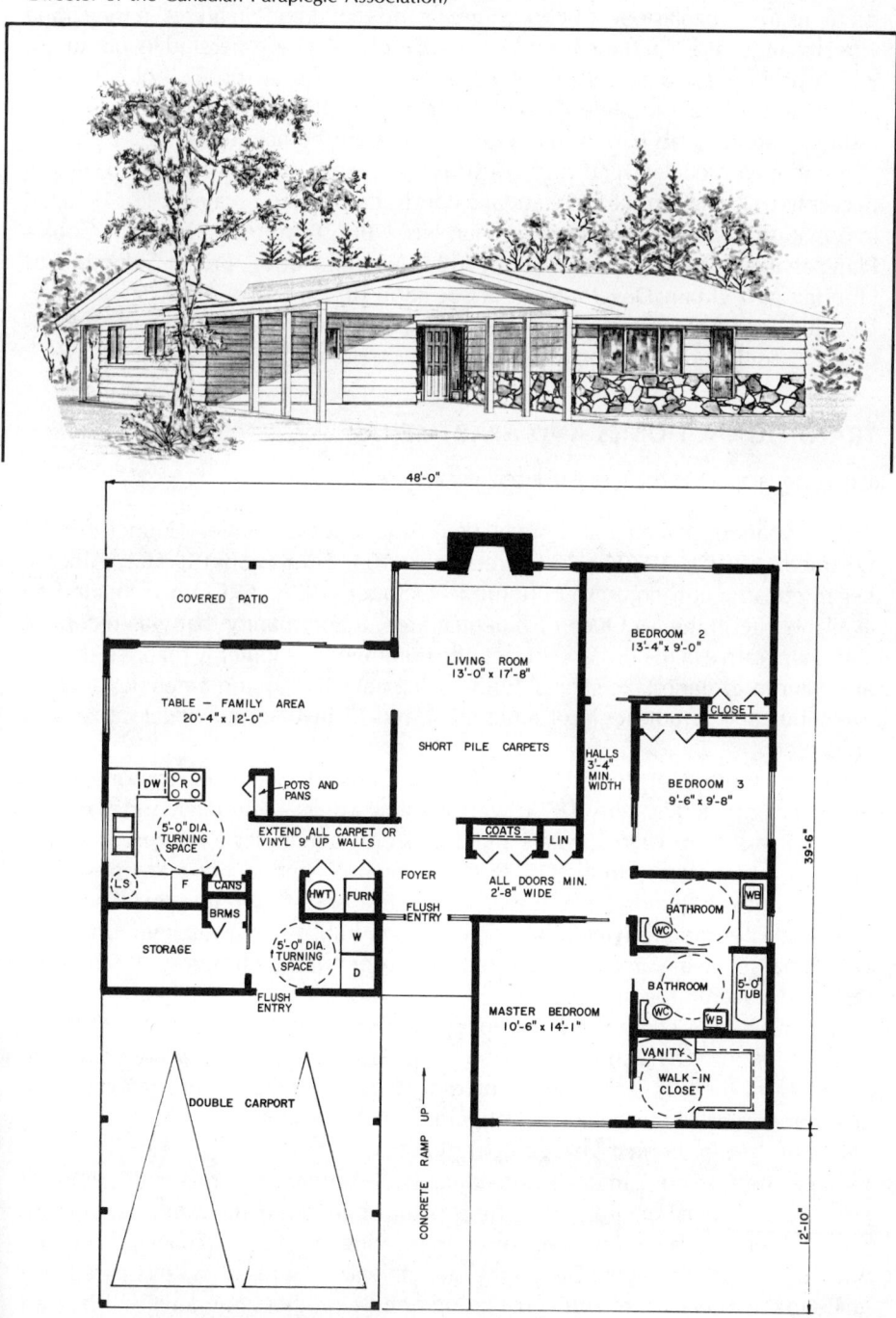

bathrooms and the kitchens and are not readily apparent. Most of them conform to the criteria of the Central Mortgage and Housing Corporation and cost little or no more than regular construction. One of the few unique features is the Crane wheelchair lavatory in the master bathroom with solenoid-operated lever faucets which provide six different preset water temperatures at the flick of a switch. Adequate backing is provided in both bathrooms so that the future purchaser can install whatever grab bars or lifting aids that might be needed.

A complete detailed record of construction costs was maintained and, where necessary, alternate prices of standard construction were obtained. For detailed information, request a brochure on Plan No. NB-228 from the designer, Cook's Plan Service & Drafting Ltd., 13659—108th Avenue, Surrey, British Columbia, or Housing and Urban Development Association of Canada, Greater Vancouver. Detailed accounts are included in the Spring, 1975 issues of the Canadian Paraplegic Association's *Caliper* and the British Columbia Division's *Paragraphic*.

TRANSITIONAL HOMES AND APARTMENTS

THE ELVES HOUSE—GROUP HOME PILOT PROJECT #1

After 3 years of planning and organizing, Alberta Rehabilitation Council for the Disabled (ARCD), 10201—104 Street, No. 504, Edmonton T5J 1B2, Alberta, began construction on a group home in October, 1974. ARCD had located an available site in the McQueen residential area, a community that was receptive and cooperative in the project. In fact, the community voluntarily rezoned the site and offered to undertake special fund-raising activities to add amenities such as a minibus and remote control equipment and to involve individual citizens as volunteers.

Group Home Pilot Project #1, 143 Street and 107 Avenue, Edmonton, Alberta, was opened in June, 1975, with 9 young adults—4 women and 5 men—ranging in age from 18 to 35 years and disabled by quadriplegia (4), cerebral palsy (4), and rheumatoid arthritis (1). Planned for both permanent and transitional living in a family atmosphere, the residence is a one-story frame dwelling, with nine single bedrooms, living room, dining room, hobby room, kitchen, tub room, wheelchair cleaning area, storage area, staff room and bathrooms, attached garage and covered loading dock.

Each resident is charged $3/day for room and board. In addition, the Government of Alberta, Division of Services for the Handicapped, has approved a grant to ARCD for the first year of operation of up to $21 per diem. Applications to the government for ongoing operational grants will be submitted on the basis of the actual budget in the first year of operation.

Since there is no Canadian precedent for a staffing pattern for this type of physical and social environment, the provincial government, with related community agencies, is underwriting and participating in a staff training and orientation course. Over a 4-year period the staffing will be studied and evaluated as a guide to the operation of additional group homes in other communities. The staff of 9 young people had an intensive two-week training course at Alberta College.

The staff members work in 3 shifts at the home. Six are personal care attendants, 1 staff supervisor, a cook, and a housekeeper. The residents are involved in every facet of running the home.

PARAPLEGIC LODGE

In the early 1960s, the British Columbia Division of the Canadian Paraplegic Association began promoting the concept of a hostel house to assist paraplegics and quadriplegics over the difficult transition period following discharge from the G.F. Strong Rehabilitation Centre. It was estimated that two distinctly different types of housing were needed: 1) a hostel halfway house for limited stays immediately after individuals have left the rehabilitation center but before they are ready to go into the community, while arrangements are being worked out for job placement, transportation, vocational training, and education; 2) a permanent residence with individual rooms and common dining facilities where there would be a limited amount of assistance available. There was doubt as to whether it would be best to concentrate on one dwelling or "scatter the money into several different buildings where there would be others besides paraplegics and quadriplegics."

The National Office of the Canadian Paraplegic Association guaranteed the initial $30,000 required to purchase land for a hostel. In 1970 a piece of land with a spectacular view of the North Shore Mountains was acquired at 3655 Clarke Drive in the City of Vancouver. Since it was located in a residential section, it was necessary to have it rezoned. Meanwhile, the Division gained assistance in the managing and operating of the hostel when the Lions Club of South Vancouver agreed to form a new society, Lions Paraplegic Lodge Society. Total costs were initially set at $359,000. In the final analysis, total costs were in excess of $400,-000 (land, $70,000; furnishings, $40,000; building, $270,000; landscaping, taxes, etc., $20,000).

The Lodge's first tenant moved in on December 10, 1972, 11 years after the B.C. Division had started to work on a hostel project. The unique complex of treated cedar consists of three houses triangularly built around a sun court and connected by outside covered walkways (Fig. 17–2). The facility is designed to accommodate 24 paraplegics and quadriplegics. It has been averaging about 18 paraplegics and 6 quadriplegics.

Two of the three houses contain six apartments each. The apartments consist of a living room, bedroom, and patio with a private entrance. In addition, each house has a shared kitchen and a laundry. The third, the main house, contains six apartments for double occupancy by quadriplegics, which are designed to be shared by a spouse, a parent, or a paraplegic to provide the necessary assistance with daily living activities. The main house also contains a large lounge for the use of all residents and a kitchen with facilities for up to ten quadriplegics. The caretaker's suite is subtly located on the second floor of the main building, emphasizing that he is the caretaker of the building, not of the residents.

The architects, Barry Downs and Dick Archambault, and their entire staff

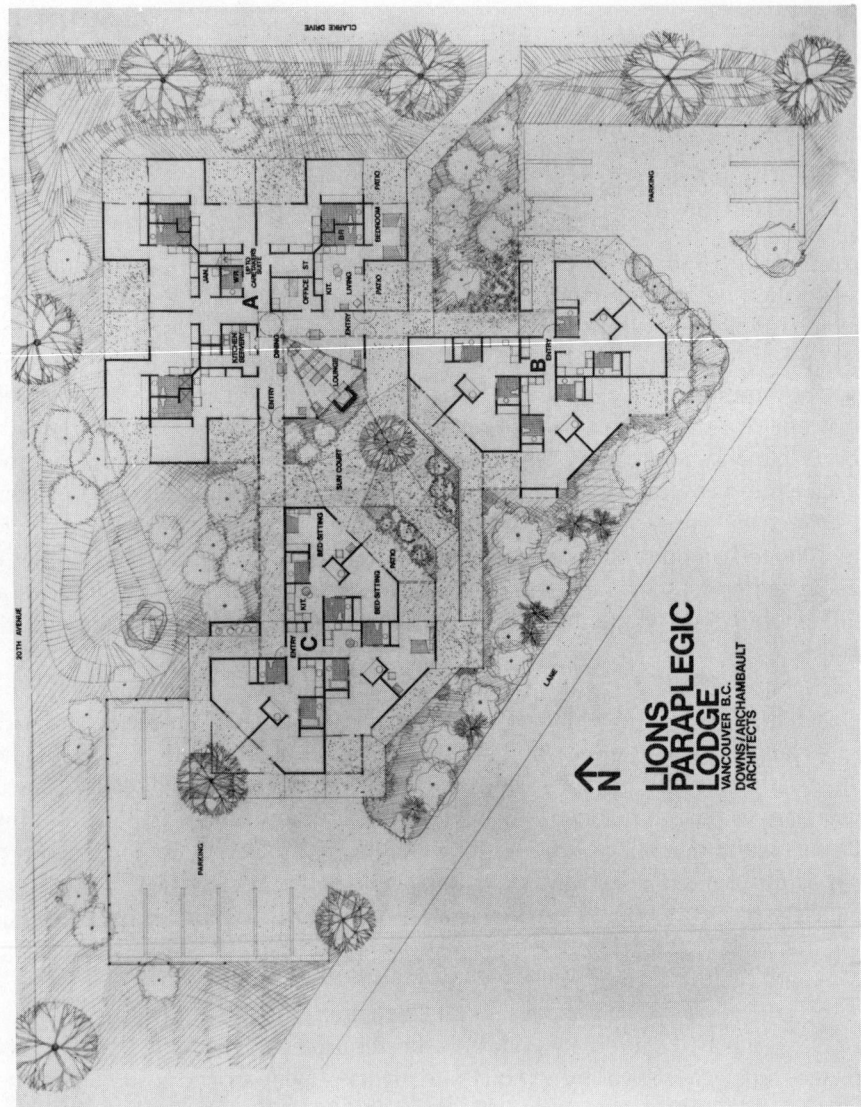

Fig. 17-2. A. The British Columbia Division of the Canadian Paraplegic Association was the prime mover in the construction of the Paraplegic Lodge. **B.** General view of the units. **C.** The central lounge area looks out on the inner court. **D.** The furniture is simple and movable. **E.** Double occupancy unit. (Canadian Architect 2, 1974; John Fulker, photographer)

fig. 17-2 continued

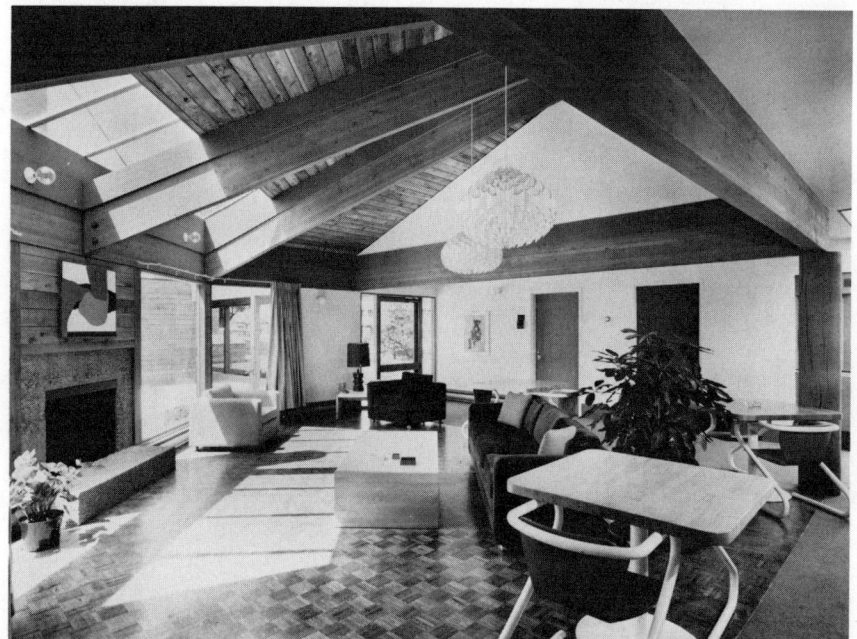

B

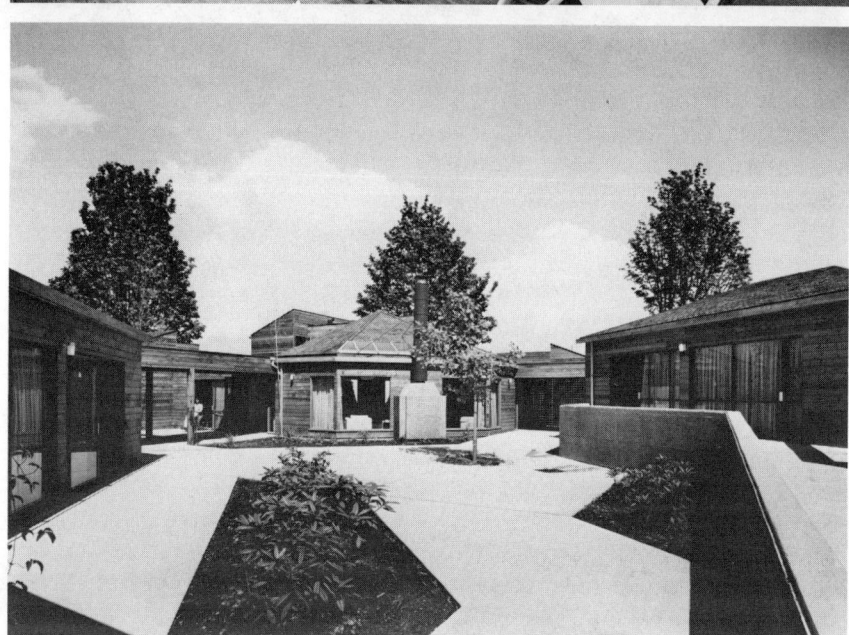

C

fig. 17-2 continued

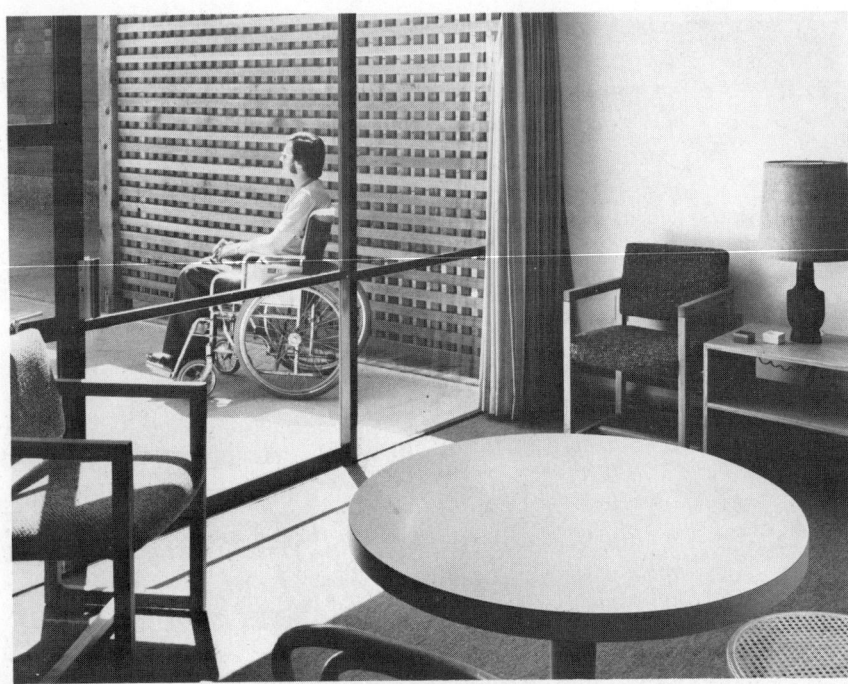

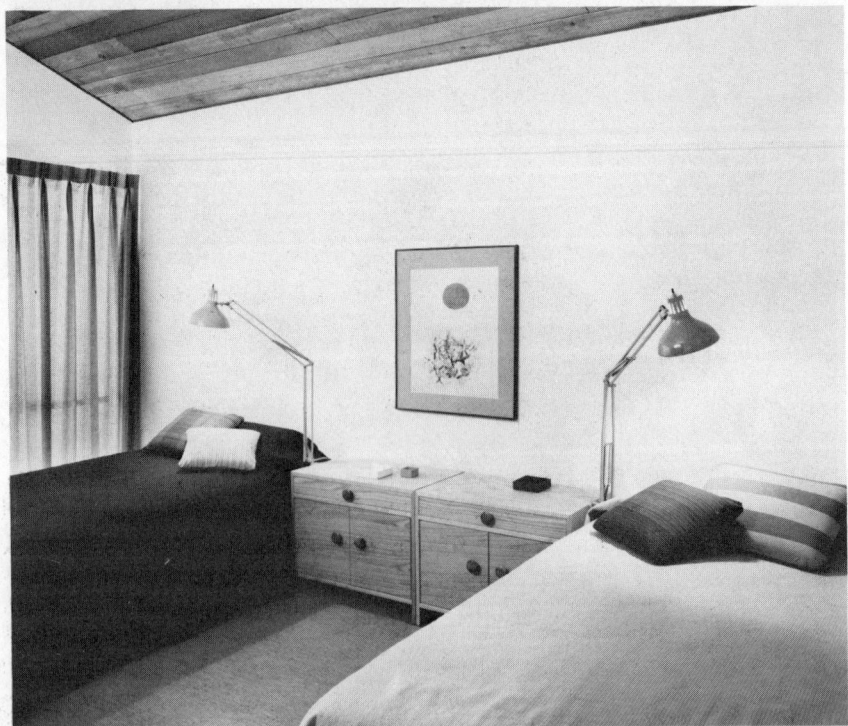

borrowed wheelchairs and used them in their daily activities around their office to gain an appreciation of problems such as the location of light switches, the widths of doors, and the arrangements of kitchens and bathrooms. As a result, the entire complex is designed for wheelchair living. The architects rejected a system of height-adjustable bathroom and kitchen fixtures and used standard equipment such as ranges with front controls and single-handled lever faucets, because they believed the residents should not live in a temporary Utopia but be prepared to cope with normal housing and equipment.

The lodge has only three rules: 1) a suite is to be treated as if it were the tenant's own home; 2) tenants are responsible for keeping and leaving their suites as they found them; 3) tenants may not behave in a manner that disturbs other tenants. The reaction of the tenants has been so favorable that many are reluctant to leave.

According to the 1973 Annual Report, the Lodge is financially sound and out of debt except for the mortgage. The tenants pay sufficient rent to make it self-supporting: completely furnished, a single accommodation is $165/month, and a double is $125/month per person. The tenants have widely varying economic backgrounds: some are on welfare, some receive Workmen's Compensation or veterans' payments, some receive insurance disability, and others pay their own way. The Department of Human Resources subsidizes part of the rent for persons on disability pension; depending on need, this may reach approximately 60% of the rent.

The staff consists of two persons, a manager and a manageress. They work 7 days/week unless they wish to bring in substitutes to replace them on weekends.

Doug Mowat, executive director of the Canadian Paraplegic Association, emphasizes that the Lodge is a transitional residence for temporary, short-term accommodation. In a fascinating article in *The Canadian Architect,* he describes it as "a place to live from the time the patient leaves the rehabilitation centre until he has totally accepted his disability, made the social adjustment to his new way of life and obtained further education—all leading to job placement, personal independence, and self-sufficiency." He feels that the key reasons for the success of the project are the design and the central location—close to shopping, transportation, education, and entertainment.

WHEELCHAIR HOUSING CENTRE, TEN TEN SINCLAIR

The 7 years of planning by the Canadian Paraplegic Association (CPA) that went into the Wheelchair Housing Centre, Kingsbury and Sinclair, West Kildonan, Winnipeg, Manitoba, started in November 1967 with an analysis of the housing and special accommodation needs of 245 paraplegics on the active files at the CPA office. Of this total, 121 (49%) were in need of more suitable accommodation or would need other arrangements in the near future; the average person in the files was aged 40, single, relatively independent physically, unemployed, on welfare, and living with parents.

The CPA drew up plans for a residential facility and selected a site within wheeling distance of the Garden City Shopping Center, a recreation park, and a community club; the site is located on a bus line and near a direct route to downtown. The most important reason for selecting this site, however, was its nearness to the Luther Home for the elderly which had demonstrated a special interest in and understanding of its residents, including a number of young quadriplegics. The Luther Home offered to manage the wheelchair housing centre.

Ground was broken in July 1974 after 2 years of careful planning and close liaison between CPA and the Board of the Luther Home. The 2-year scrutiny included approval of the planning by the Manitoba Housing and Renewal Corporation (MHRC), of the funding by the Central Mortgage and Housing Corporation, of the rezoning by the Community Committee, and of the program and operation by the Care Services Branch of the Department of Health and Social Development.

The structure consists of 75 individual suites distributed over two floors. Each suite contains 500 sq ft and consists of a living room, kitchen, bathroom, and bedroom, as well as ample storage space. To avoid concentrating a large number of severely disabled persons in one area, there are only 25 quadriplegic units. The other 25 wheelchair suites are for tenants who are personally independent, such as paraplegics, but who can benefit from a variety of shared services and developmental programs. The remaining 25 suites are for nondisabled tenants, "from all walks of life, chosen for their interest and ability to associate with their wheelchair neighbors." Some are university students and retired couples or others who qualify for MHRC housing. The residents moved in between July and December 1975.

A Special Consultant has been hired to assist the more severely disabled tenants develop maximum physical independence through aids and appliances and other supportive systems. The aim of the project is to provide the disabled tenants with the training and experience that will eventually enable them to move into their own apartments or homes within the community with assistance from visiting home care orderlies and homemakers if required.

POINT PLEASANT LODGE

Opened in December, 1974, Point Pleasant Lodge, Halifax, Nova Scotia, provides temporary accommodation for persons with a variety of disabilities. It is used by those who are attending hospitals as outpatients or are involved in rehabilitation programs. It contains 55 single hostel units (12 of which are designed for wheelchair users) and 52 double units.

LONG-TERM RESIDENTIAL FACILITIES

BATTIN–FIELDING MEMORIAL HOUSING

Plans for this housing complex in Saanich began in 1966 with a $100,000 donation by Mrs. Elsie Fielding. It was completed 7 years and 1½ million dollars later, under the aegis of the Victoria and Vancouver Island Multiple Sclerosis Society, Suite 408, 723 Fort Street, Victoria V8W 1H1, British Columbia.

Fig. 17–3. Battin-Fielding Memorial Housing. **A.** The Victoria and Vancouver Island Multiple Sclerosis Society sponsored this 60-unit project. **B.** The two upper floors are planned for senior citizens; the two lower floors can be reached by ramps. (Williams DJ: Victoria is location of centre for disabled, MS Canada 1(4): 4–5, 1974)

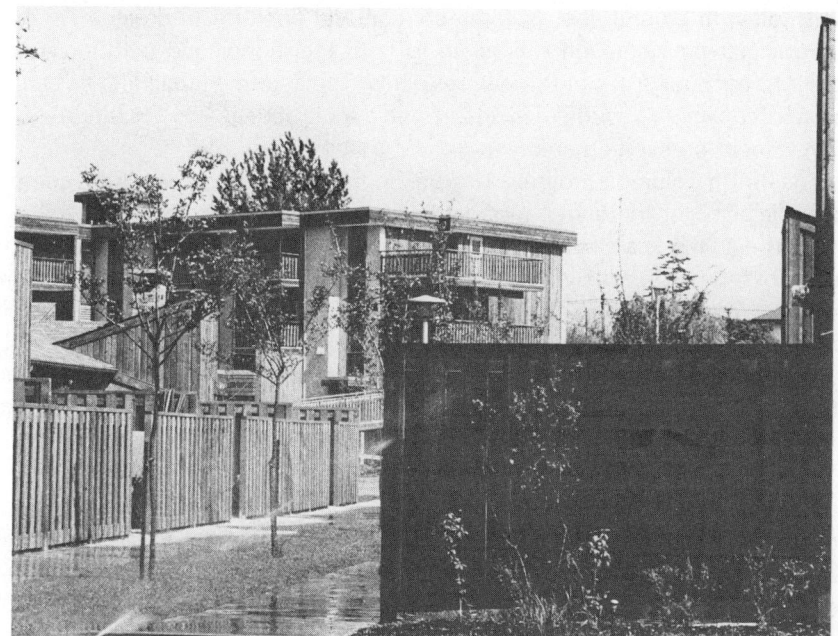

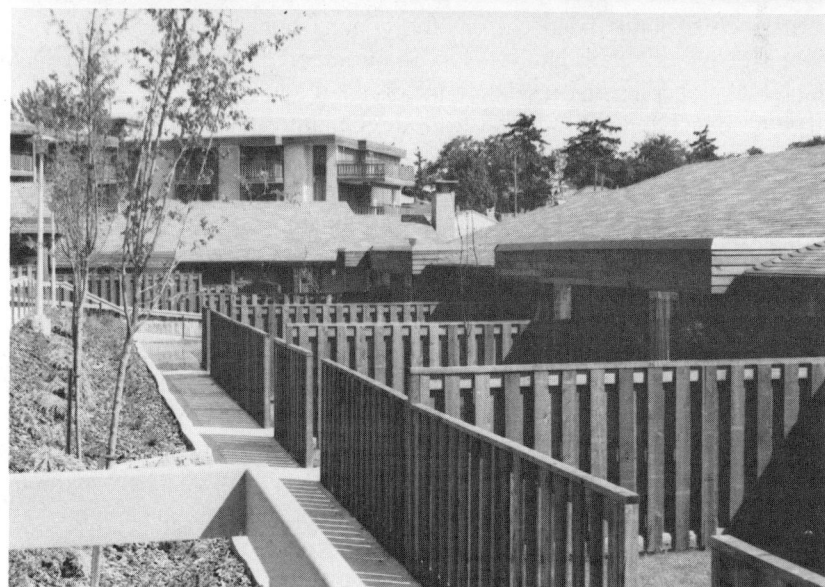

This handsome multilevel project was designed as an integrated development for disabled persons and their families and senior citizens. The four-story apartment building contains 12 one-bedroom units and 48 bachelor units (Fig. 17-3). The townhouse clusters consist of 4 three-bedroom units and 15 two bedroom units, all with ground floor accommodation and open beam design.

Particular consideration was given to both the indoor and outdoor areas in order to encourage visiting among residents. The apartment building has a common balcony with a southern exposure and a social lounge which includes a small refreshment preparation area.

The British Columbia Housing Management Commission operates the complex, and eligibility for the complex is based primarily on need.

The next step is an Activity Centre to be built in the heart of the complex at a cost of more than a million dollars. The center will contain medical examination rooms, workshops and activity rooms, a library, classrooms, rest areas, and a cafeteria. It will be used by clients from many community agencies: visiting nurses, meals on wheels, physiotherapy and occupational therapy, assessment of the disabled, transportation, recreation, and education.

BELLWOODS PARK HOUSE

In 1965, the City of Toronto deeded to the Adult Cerebral Palsy Institute of Metropolitan Toronto property that was located in the west central section close to transportation, recreational, educational, religious, and shopping facilities. The Ontario Government gave a capital grant of $5000 per bed. The Institute raised the balance of funds needed from the general public and in February 1967 opened Bellwoods Park House, 300 Shaw Street, Toronto M6J 2X2, Ontario which was Canada's first residence for disabled adults.

The residence receives support from the Ontario Ministry of Community and Social Services. Out of a monthly pension of $238.77, a resident pays $165.77/month for his room and board. The government provides a per diem subsidy of $11 for residential care and $17 for extended care. The per diem cost at Bellwoods Park House is $13.24 per resident. The ratio of staff to residents is 1:2.

A descriptive brochure emphasizes that Bellwoods Park House is a home "in every sense of the word, providing a room of one's own, a place of one's own, a life of one's own." Although preference is given to cerebral palsied men and women, others are admitted. The residence presently accommodates 61 single adults, (42 women and 19 men) whose average age is 35. About 80% are cerebral palsied. In order to be admitted, a person must be over 18 years of age, mentally competent, and physically able to look after himself with a minimum of assistance. Persons with a progressive disease are excluded.

The residence has attracted the active involvement of 40 volunteers and 33 community service organizations. The Board of Education provides teachers at the residence as well as correspondence courses. The Toronto Public Library Board established a core library at the residence and sends a librarian once a week to distribute books and stimulate interest in reading. Residents attend bowling and swimming programs, go on shopping trips, and attend theaters. Contact with the immediate community has been mainly through the churches.

Residents are encouraged to do as much as they can for themselves and to assist in light housekeeping duties. Twenty-three of the residents act as receptionists in the office, operate the elevators, and assist in general maintenance. For these services, a small remuneration is given to augment the "comfort allowance." Nineteen residents attend the Corbrook Sheltered Workshop for disabled adults, and three are enrolled in secondary schools.

The residents are represented on the Administrator's Advisory Committee by nine of their number who are elected annually. In this way viewpoints, complaints, and suggestions of the residents and the administrator are discussed. Matters that concern policy are referred to a liaison committee which is made up of representatives from the Residents' Council and the Board of Trustees.

A touch of irony: during the years of fund raising, the need for a residence for adults was often dramatized with life stories. The most frequent story told was that of an intelligent and compassionate cerebral palsied gentleman in his 50s who had lived in a hospital for some 20 years while directing a service to shut-ins. When Bellwoods Park House was completed and the gentleman was invited to move in, he declined. The residents seemed too young for him, and he preferred to stay in his own familiar surroundings.

PARTICIPATION HOUSE

A project of the Cerebral Palsy Parent Council of Toronto, Participation House, P.O. Box 264, Markham L3P 3J7, Ontario, opened in November 1972 about 20 miles from Toronto. It offers permanent accommodation to 38 severely disabled individuals, respite care for 6 during vacations or emergencies, and recreational, workshop, and activity programs for 75 daytime participants.

The complex, designed with wind-swept roofs and hexagonal rooms, consists of administration quarters, a ramped water therapy/swimming pool, a large greenhouse, and six bungalows. Each bungalow simulates a family home unit for six persons. The six single rooms can be converted into three double rooms through the use of sliding walls. In addition, each bungalow contains a living room, dining room, and three bathrooms.

Admission to Participation House is open to young adults 18 years of age and over with severe multiple disabilities. The residents must be capable of participating in, and benefiting from, the programs offered. Accommodations are available to any resident of Ontario, with priority given to nearby residents. All admissions are made on a 3-month probation basis. Programs offered include workshop, recreational activities, and therapeutic schedules.

MAISON LUCIE BRUNEAU

Since Maison Lucie Bruneau, 2222 East Laurier, Montreal H2H 1C4, Quebec was founded in 1969, it has been the only place in Quebec with accommodations for quadriplegics. All disabilities are represented among the 80 residents and the outpatients, and their ages range 18–50. In most instances, the $9.65 cost per diem is paid by the government of Quebec. Two persons share a room. The five-story facility includes a communal dining room, a number of workshops, and home care services.

CHESHIRE HOME FOUNDATION—CANADA INC.

The transplantation and mutation of Cheshire Homes from England to Canada is significant because 20 years of experience in England are being utilized and efforts are being made to avoid repeating the mistakes of the past. For instance, the numbers of residents are small compared to the early English homes, the locations are "in the heart of things" rather than in the country, most of the rooms are single rather than multiple, and the residents are taking an active part in planning social activities.

The Cheshire Home Foundation, headquartered in London, sent Mrs. Pamela Farrell to Canada in 1970 to explore the possibility of stimulating development of homes for the disabled. Encouraged by the enthusiasm expressed by disabled young adults and their parents, it was decided to establish a home in Toronto. Subsequently, the Cheshire Home Foundation, 11 Lowther Avenue, Toronto M5R 1C5, received a Charter under the Charitable Institutions Act in June 1971 to set up homes throughout the province.

The following suggestions for developing Cheshire Homes are detailed in a seven-page "Manifesto:"

Men and women aged 18–50 years are eligible for entry. Having entered, residents may stay for the rest of their lives, if they so desire. They must be physically disabled and require assistance with the activities of living, they must be in a reasonably static physical state or have an only slowly progressive condition. (Most frequent disabilities are cerebral palsy, spina bifida, spinal cord injury, muscular dystrophy, multiple sclerosis, and Friedreich's ataxia.) Potential residents must be mentally alert and able to contribute to the familylike atmosphere. Residence is available to those of any race, religion, creed, or social status, whether or not they are financially able to pay.

The way of life is as close to normal living as possible; residents are free to come and go. Bedrooms accommodate one or two people; meals are communal. Work facilities or opportunities are arranged where possible (perhaps a workshop room with printing press, duplicating machine, and carpentry tools). Social activities are organized by residents. There is involvement with the outside community and volunteers. The homes are as fully self-governing as possible, although they are administered by a committee which may employ a director.

Residents may continue under the supervision of their own previous medical specialists; arrangements should be made with local practitioners for routine examinations and for a system of medical coverage.

The site should be centrally located, near public facilities. The building may be a big old townhouse, a custom-built home, units incorporated into a public housing project, a hostel type building with some units for disabled plus necessary services, satellite units related to a central facility, or apartment units within an apartment complex for nondisabled persons.

Tentatively, there should be accommodations for 5 to 25 persons, an administrator's permanent live-in suite, several sitting rooms, dining room, craft room, activities spaces, library, and a kitchen large enough to allow disabled residents to participate in meal preparation. In addition, there might be garden and recreation areas, physiotherapy services, and laundry facilities.

McLEOD HOUSE

McLeod House, 11 Lowther Avenue, Toronto M5R 1C5, Ontario is the first Cheshire Home in North America (Fig. 17–4). Opened on June 21, 1972, it is in half of a three-story Victorian residence in the midtown Annex district, near theaters, museums, libraries, art galleries, parks, restaurants, and other community resources. A number of structural changes were necessary, including the installation of an elevator and ramps, as well as shelving and storage facilities. The original cost of the house was $68,000; the cost of the remodeling has been about $30,000.

Fig. 17–4. McLeod House, the first Cheshire Home in North America, was opened in 1972. (The ramped side of the building is McLeod House.)

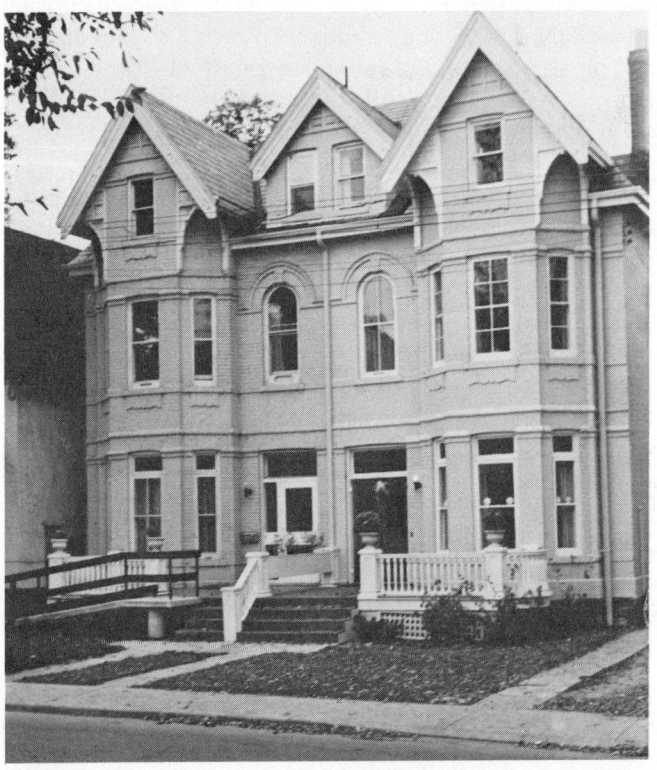

Zoning regulations restricted accommodation to five residents, and fire regulations required that any resident should, in the event of an emergency, be able to get down stairs unaided. The layout of the first floor, with living/dining room and kitchen, is that of any family home. On the second floor, there are three bedrooms, one single and the others shared; one room has been set aside as a quiet study area.

By the end of January, 1973, McLeod House had its full complement of five residents: three male and two female, aged 18–30 years, with disabilities ranging from osteogenesis imperfecta to an unknown tropical disease, and an educational range from Grade 7 to a Bachelor of Science.

All residents were admitted initially for a probationary period of 1–2 months, after which each left for a short while in order to make a final decision. The Admissions Committee feels that this admissions procedure, by which all new applicants became well acquainted with existing residents before moving in, eliminated most problems of adjustment and ensured a high degree of compatibility.

The paid staff of one full-time administrator and one part-time domestic helper is augmented by a small core of volunteer workers, including two university students studying nursing and social work who help in the evenings and on weekends. Individual volunteers help with decorating, shopping, cooking, outings, typing, and grooming. Groups lend their support in fund raising and arranging social activities.

The amount of money from the Provincial Government fluctuates according to the number of people living at the house and the operational costs incurred. The Government subsidy is 80% of operational costs to a maximum of $11 daily for each resident on assistance (*i.e.,* a disability pension). The resident's portion of the per diem cost is $5.50, which is deducted automatically from the pension each month. A full-paying resident pays the total per diem rate.

Housekeeping is a responsibility shared by staff, residents, and volunteers. Menus are planned by the residents 1 week in advance, and a shopping list is prepared for the volunteer who makes a weekly trip to the local supermarket. The preparation of meals is also a cooperative affair.

Medical services are provided by the St. George Health Centre. Services have included frequent home visits by doctors and nurses as well as a monthly sanitary inspection in compliance with regulations of the Charitable Institutions Act.

The operation of the project depends on a successful working relationship with three branches of the Ontario Ministry of Community and Social Services: 1) Family Benefits advises the residents on personal financial matters and provides information on financial assistance available to the disabled; 2) Vocational Rehabilitation Services provides educational counseling and career information; 3) Homes for the Aged Branch provides a consultant to develop a system of documentation in such areas as fire regulations, medical services, dietary services, and financial records. The Branch has been interested primarily in senior citizens and only recently recognized that an adult group home fills the particular emotional and social needs of young physically disabled adults.

HASTINGS–PRINCE EDWARD CHESHIRE HOME

The Hastings–Prince Edward Home, 246 John Street, Belleville K8N 3G1, Ontario is the second Cheshire Home in Canada; it opened in March, 1974, with two young men and one young woman in their early 20s. After 9 months of operation, there were six residents, ranging 21–41 years of age, with disabilities ranging from cerebral palsy and spina bifida to quadriplegia.

The residence is a large Victorian house that has been renovated to include lower countertops, countertop stove, grab bars in the bathrooms, and an extension to house the elevator. It is located in the downtown area, near all facilities, including the library, arena, and shopping. The director, Mrs. Irené Sansom, strives for a cooperative living environment with each one helping with the running of the Home. Involvement and interest of the community have been keen; service clubs have been generous with donations; high school students have been used for extra coaching in basic academic skills; and community college students have been used in field placements.

Most of the residents participate in the activities of a social group for the physically disabled that include wheelchair basketball, bowling, and swimming. Since the Home is located next to a secondary school, some of the residents are taking night school courses in painting, jewelry making, or gourmet cooking. One of the male residents works as a night clerk at a nearby motel; another works 1 day/week at a florist shop making wreaths and arrangements.

CLARENDON HOUSE CHESHIRE HOME

As of December, 1974, the steering committee (c/o Mrs. Jane Staub, Ontario Children's Centre, 350 Rumsey Road, Toronto 17, Ontario) had signed a 10-year lease for five apartments on the second floor of Clarendon House, a new apartment building in central Toronto. Eventually, the apartments will provide units for 10–12 tenants, offering them physical care, meal preparation, and housekeeping. The committee decided to start with five tenants in order to gain more extensive knowledge of the needs for support services, the types of housing wanted, and the extent and form of training required for the care staff. When they have acquired experience in the physical care of the first five tenants, they will select the remaining five to seven tenants with the help of the first tenants.

CHESHIRE HOMES OF YORK, INC.

Under the chairmanship of Dr. John Whittaker of Ontario Crippled Children's Centre, the steering committee (c/o Miss M. A. Wickham, Secretary, 74 Sherwood Avenue, Toronto M4P 2A7, Ontario) has defined its plans to build a residence in north Metropolitan Toronto for 15 young disabled adults who require supportive but not nursing care, who are unable to live independently, and who are aged 18–40 on admission.

DURHAM REGION CHESHIRE HOME

After a year of fund raising the steering committee of the Arts Resource Centre, Civic Administration Complex, 50 Centre Street South, Oshawa L1H 3Z7, Ontario, located a five-unit apartment building available in the center of Oshawa. Approval for a capital loan was received in November, 1974, from Central Mortgage and Housing Corporation. An elevator and a ramp were constructed and other minor renovations made to accommodate 10–12 physically disabled residents and 2 staff members.

A brief from the admissions committee recommends that admissions be regulated over a period of time; opening with two residents, adding the rest over a period of 6–12 months in order to lessen initial adjustment problems. Further, it recommends that the staff be employed about 4–6 weeks before the opening date. Three types of residents are recommended for admission: two or three severely disabled, such as quadriplegics, who require extensive care but are independent in moving about in motorized wheelchairs; two or three moderately disabled, such as hemiplegics or paraplegics who have maximal use of one or more limbs; and two or three residents with other disabilities (blindness, deafness, or loss of one limb).

Since the admissions committee is trying to provide a normal home, it feels there is no need for structured programming of activities, although there will be access to craft and art materials, books, games, and a hobby/work area. Routines should be established by the residents. The Residential Council will meet on a regular basis, involve all residents and a staff representative, have a formal committee structure, have the authority to make decisions governing in-house structure and functioning, coordinate services such as volunteers, and request outside consultation if necessary.

It is recommended that four staff members provide the services needed: a live-in supervisory couple to handle housekeeping duties (including preparing and serving one meal a day), maintain house and grounds, deal with minor repairs, and assist the residents (including transference, turning in bed, recreation, shopping expeditions, and helping when they prepare their own meals); a live-in assistant supervisor; and a bookkeeper–typist who will not live in.

ASHBY HOUSE GROUP

The Board of Directors (c/o Mrs. Mira Ashby, Social Service Department, Toronto M5G 1L7, Ontario) decided to fill the need for a residence for persons specifically suffering from brain damage, usually as the result of motorcycle and auto accidents. The residents will be ambulant males, between the ages of 17 and 35, whose medical treatment has been completed. The residence will be in a reasonably central location, zoned for nonresidential use. It will have accommodation for six to eight residents and two live-in staff members. Meals will be prepared on the premises. An application for a start-up grant has been made to Central Mortgage and Housing Corporation.

SASKATOON CHESHIRE HOME

On land donated by the City of Saskatoon and with financial backing of the Kiwanis Club of Saskatoon, the first unit of the Saskatoon Cheshire Home, 314 Lake Crescent, Saskatoon, Saskatchewan, was started in October, 1974. With accommodation for eight severely disabled adults and an attached suite for houseparents, it is the first of four units in a condominium type of building development which will ultimately house 30–40 disabled persons. Initially, the Victorian Order of Nurses will provide nursing care on a visiting basis.

The Cheshire Homes in Canada are fascinating. They demonstrate the need for flexibility and show the advantages of a central organization. Most importantly, they show how the steering committees reflect the needs of different communities. In the preceding examples of homes, for instance, there are wide variations. The types of residents and the numbers (4–40) all are different, yet overall purposes and financial arrangements are similar.

MISCELLANEOUS LOW RENTAL HOUSING

The following examples of low rental housing in Alberta, Manitoba, New Brunswick, and Nova Scotia typify the trends in housing through local housing authorities. All these examples are cited by officers of the Canadian Paraplegic Association.

ALBERTA

Executive Director Pierre Gariepy reports, "Generally, the climate for disabled people is good: the provincial government has made help to the disabled one of its priorities; the city of Edmonton has ramped downtown intersections, is putting up excellent special low income housing, and is working on improvements in the transportation system."

MANITOBA

Executive Director A. T. Mann reports that a number of wheelchair units have been made available through the Manitoba Housing and Renewal developments. However, existing regulations still preclude applications by wheelchair tenants below 45 in projects for the elderly, and most of the facilities for the wheelchaired are "bachelor" type units rather than family type units. Increasingly, commercial apartments have made modifications such as small ramps or wider doorways.

NEW BRUNSWICK

Executive Director B. G. Hallam sketches the programs available in New Brunswick.

Our provincial government provides a Disability Allowance of $199/month and will allow extra monies for orderly and attendant care by nonfamily members. Many of our clients live at home with their families with this income. The New Brunswick Housing Corporation provides wheelchair-accessible units within its low rentals and senior citizen complexes and makes special low interest loans available for our paraplegics and quadriplegics to renovate their homes for wheelchair use.

New Brunswick is a very rural area. In fact, there is no central urban area in the province, but rather three major cities, no one of which exceeds 100,000. Two-thirds of our clients live in rural areas and their opportunities for employment are extremely limited. We are studying the possibility of establishing a small paraplegic lodge. We think this might encourage some of our rural clients to live in the city and find employment.

We conduct quite an aggressive campaign both publicly and privately for the removal of architectural barriers. So far this has resulted in a bylaw in Fredericton requiring public buildings to be accessible, and several private apartment owners have erected buildings with level entrances.

NOVA SCOTIA

Resettlement Officer Lynn B. Stow summarizes the progress made during the last year:

1. City housing. The Halifax Housing Authority has made provisions for the wheelchaired in two low rental projects. Ahearn Manor, Gottingen Street, Halifax, has six well-designed wheelchair units. (Unfortunately, they are all on the ground floor and not dispersed throughout the building as suggested by the Canadian Paraplegic Association.) Westwood Towers, 6701 Chisholm Avenue, Halifax, is designed with wide doors in all the apartments and a ramped front entrance.
2. Senior citizens housing. The Housing Commission is beginning to include wheelchair units.
3. Private developments. A new high-rise apartment building contains at least two units designed for wheelchairs. The owners of the apartment building, Park Victoria on South Park Street, will widen the bathroom doors if a wheelchair occupant wishes to rent a unit.
4. Senior citizen center. The proposed Northwood Centre, a special care residence and day care for the elderly center, is planning to provide several levels of care to senior citizens, with good provision made for those who are wheelchaired: self-contained apartments, home care, supervisory care (homemakers, meals, laundry), limited personal care (help in daily activities, dressing, bathing), and intensive personal care (continuous nursing).

Bibliography

ACCESS: HOUSING. Handicapped Housing Society of Alberta, 1973.

"Cheshire Homes Foundation—Canada Inc.—A Manifesto." 1973.

Design for the Wheelchair Tenant. By D. L. Mowat. CANADIAN ARCHITECT, Vol. 19, No. 2, page 22. February, 1974.

HANDICAPPED HOUSING CHARETTE. Handicapped Housing Society of Alberta, 1973.

HOUSING FOR THE HANDICAPPED. A Working Paper. Prepared by the Panel for Guidance of Handicapped, Social Planning and Review Council of British Columbia, 1973.

Lodge for Paraplegics, Vancouver. By Downs/Archambault: CANADIAN ARCHITECT, Vol. 19, No. 2, pages 20–22. February, 1974.

Published by the Minister of National Health and Welfare, Queen's Printer for Canada, Ottawa:

THE CANADA ASSITANCE PLAN. Cat. No. H76–1873. 1974.

DISABILITY BENEFITS. Cat.No. H76–870. 1970.

WORKING PAPER ON SOCIAL SECURITY IN CANADA. (DOCUMENT DE TRAVAIL SUR LA SÉCURITÉ SOCIALE AU CANADA). 2nd edition. April 18, 1973.

HEALTH SERVICES IN CANADA.

THE FEDERAL MEDICAL CARE PROGRAM. Questions and Answers. 1974.

REVIEW OF HEALTH SERVICES IN CANADA. 1974.

SOCIAL SECURITY IN CANADA. (la Sécurité sociale au Canada). Cat. No. H13–1/20. 1974.

REPORT ON RESEARCH ON THE LIFE-STYLES OF THE PHYSICALLY DISABLED. The Action Group of the Disabled Research Team, Edmonton, Alberta, 1972.

"Resident Care in Canada." By Douglas G. Seaton. Paper presented to the Conference on International Rehabilitation Patterns for the Multi-handicapped. New York City, 1971.

Victoria is Location of Centre for Disabled. By D. J. Williams. MS CANADA, Vol. 1, No. 4, pages 4–5. Winter, 1974.

"It is nothing short of a national scandal and a terrible indictment of modern society that we should even be discussing the integration of the disabled. They should never have been segregated."

—James Loring, Director, the Spastics Society

18
International Experiences

GREAT BRITAIN

Housing for the disabled and elderly in Great Britain is changing and complex. It is changing, as is housing around the world, because of the growing spirit of independence of disabled and elderly individuals. It is changing from custodial residential care in country mansions supported largely by voluntary organizations to adapted or "mobility" housing within ordinary housing projects, with the addition of resident caretakers, and to adaptations to existing housing, with the addition of supportive services brought into the home.

It is complex because it is provided, not by the central government, but by various combinations of local district councils, county councils, and voluntary and other organizations. Thus housing is subject to the state of local finances and to the decisions of local officials and local and national voluntary organizations.

The three basic types of special accommodation for the disabled are: 1) Residential care is a communal living arrangement that includes room, board, and personal care, provided either by voluntary organizations or county councils; 2) Individual self-contained units which may be owned or rented are provided by district councils, new town corporations, voluntary housing associations, private individuals, and organizations; many of these units are sheltered housing, with a resident warden on call for emergencies; 3) Chronic sick units provided by Regional Health Authorities furnish constant nursing care.

RESIDENTIAL CARE

Two voluntary organizations—The Cheshire Foundation for the Sick and the Spastic Society—pioneered residential care in Great Britain beginning in the early 1950s. For the next 20 years, both had periods of phenomenal expansion, purchasing and converting large country mansions into homes and work centers for the disabled, developing strong regional branches, and maintaining training centers for the staff members. By the early 1970s, when both reached a peak of establishing residential centers along the same set patterns, they began to develop alternatives to meet the changing times and the changing needs of their residents. Unfortunately, because of the general recession of the mid-1970s, many of the creative ideas for alternatives to institutional living remain in the planning stage.

The Cheshire Homes

The Cheshire Homes, started by Group Captain Leonard Cheshire in 1948, number more than 100 homes, about half of them in Britain and the rest in South America, Africa, Canada, India, Europe, and the Middle East. There are about 2000 residents in the homes in Britain and 1262 residents overseas. A central Trust, known as The Cheshire Foundation Homes for the Sick, 5, Market Mews, London W1Y 8HP, England, a registered charity, presides over all the homes in the United Kingdom. It owns all the properties and acts as a guarantor to the public that the individual homes are run in conformity with the aims of the Foundation.

Each home is autonomously run by a Management Committee of volunteers drawn from the local community. The committee decides all matters of policy, admits residents, appoints staff, and raises money. The larger homes have a resident warden in charge, but most of them are run by a matron or nursing sister with a permanent staff of trained and semitrained nurses and other housekeeping help. Special training in residential care is available to staff members. This includes a 1–1½ year course, covering both theoretical instruction and in-service training.

The majority of the homes have a policy of admitting only the younger disabled, between the ages of 18 and 40, who have a long prognosis. Married couples, the aged, and the mentally retarded are not usually included, but have a few homes for their own separate groups. The homes average about 40 residents, both men and women, and have a balanced selection of disabilities.

The operating costs of the Homes have been kept relatively low through services performed by volunteers and the residents. Thus, in England, the average cost per diem is £5, ($10) compared with £10–£15 ($20–30) in a National Health Service Hospital with chronic sick facilities. Residents pay none, part, or all of their costs. Depending upon their ability to pay, they are sponsored by local authorities or various service clubs or associations.

In addition to its residential homes, the Foundation has recently developed more integrated adaptations:

1. "Bread-winner" bungalows on the grounds of several existing homes for couples, one of whom is disabled and who may spend the day in the home.
2. A four-bed nursing wing and a day center in connection with Tulse Hill, a complex of 40 houses and apartments built by the Greater London Council for families with a disabled member.
3. Ground floor apartments for four disabled students at Oxford who require personal assistance.

The Spastics Society

Since The Spastics Society, 12 Park Crescent, London W1N 4EQ, England, was founded in 1952, it has established over 160 facilities for the cerebral palsied and helped over 25,000 individuals. The Society's role has changed drastically during its 22 years, evolving from isolated custodial care to integrated independent living facilities. It is sensitive to the humanity and individuality of the cerebral palsied, due in large part to its dynamic director, James Loring, who has created innovations such as a traveling exhibit of aids demonstrated by an occupational therapist, toy libraries, weekend conferences of disabled persons and staff members, accommodations for severely disabled married couples, special facilities for disabled students, and a training college for staff and voluntary workers.

The Royal Hospital and Home for Incurables

Located on 24 acres, the Royal Hospital and Home for Incurables, (West Hill, Putney, London SW15 3SW, England,) has residents from all over the United Kingdom and abroad. It is said that under its roof are more people disabled by multiple sclerosis than under any other roof in the world—more than one-third of the 221 residents have MS. It is a voluntary hospital, founded in 1854 to provide a home with medical and nursing care for those who need long-term care.

The Marie Foster Home

(Barnet General Hospital, Wellhouse Lane, Barnet, Hertfordshire EN5 3DJ, England.) The Barnet and District Branch of the Multiple Sclerosis Society of Great Britain and Northern Ireland worked for 14 years to raise funds to build the Marie Foster Home which provides accommodation for 30 disabled individuals in ten single rooms, four two-bed rooms, and two six-bed dormitories.

In addition to this home, the Multiple Sclerosis Society has a full-time short-stay holiday home in Scotland, another in the West of England, and another in Sevenoaks.

Charities Digest

The Family Welfare Association's annual guide contains a classified list of all charities in the United Kingdom, the best source of listings of voluntary organizations which operate residential facilities. The 1975 edition is available from Family Welfare Association, 603–503 Kingsland Road, Dalston, London E8, England; or Butterworth, 2265 Midland Avenue, Scarborough M1P 4S1, Ontario, Canada. Butterworth's price is $9.65 plus 30¢ postage.

SELF-CONTAINED HOUSING

To provide for the disabled and elderly who do not need the nursing care of residential homes but need some daily help, the local authorities have developed a program of sheltered housing with resident wardens. The warden looks after the heating and cleaning, as well as answering emergency calls that may involve calling the doctor, helping with personal care and shopping, some occasional cooking, or household work. The housing authority normally builds these projects and pays for their operating expenses, and the welfare authority contributes to the warden's salary.

Fig. 18-1. Habinteg. **A.** The below counter storage units on castors have pull-out shelves with bowl cut-outs; the doors have D-handles and looped pulls. **B.** The kitchen counters can be adjusted in height between 2 feet 7 inches and 3 feet (787–914 mm). **C.** Toehold space under the tub leaves space for the base of a lift; the fold-away support by the toilet was imported from Scandinavia. (Photographs supplied by Roman Halter and Associates, Architects, courtesy of the Architects' Journal)

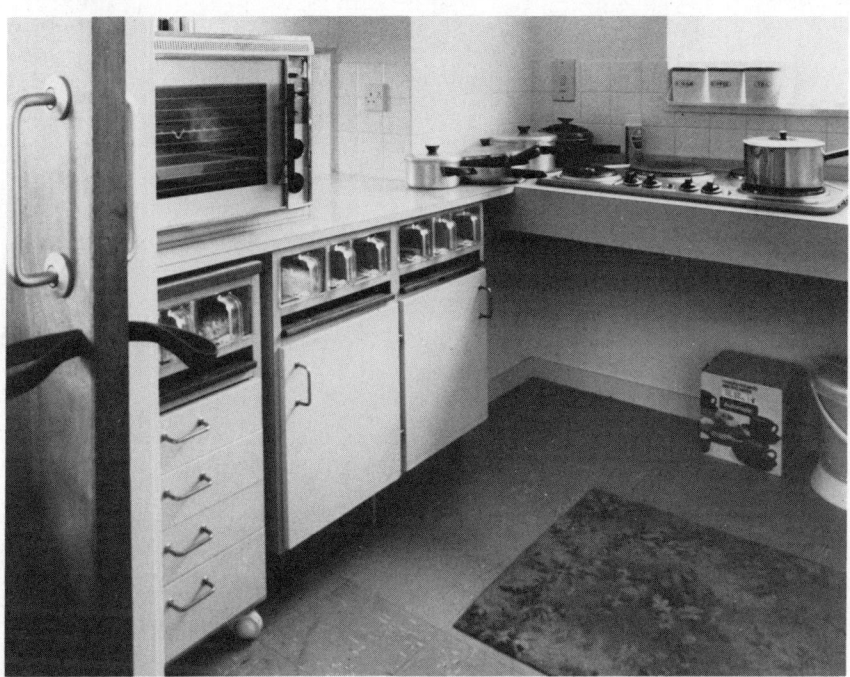

A

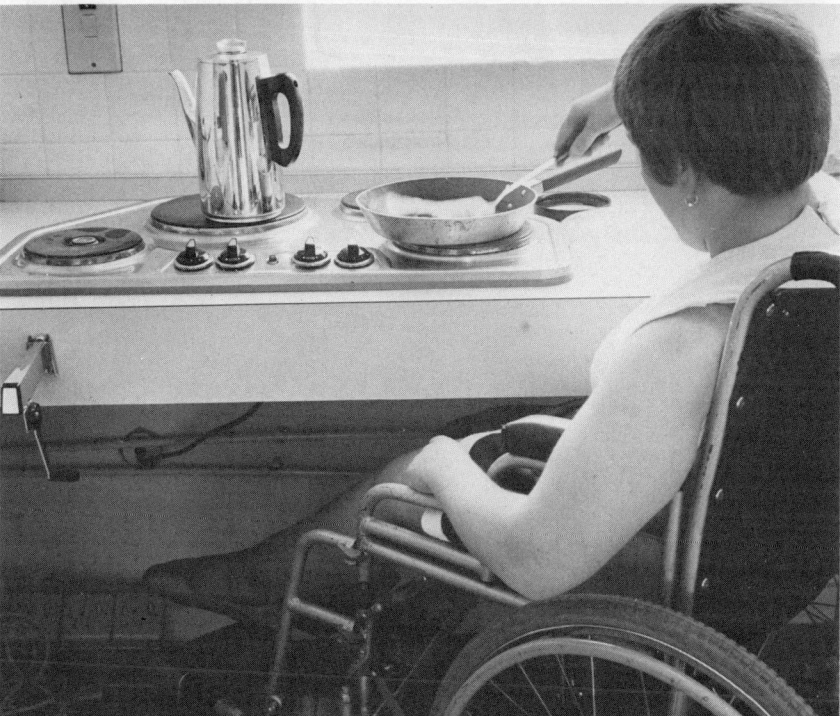

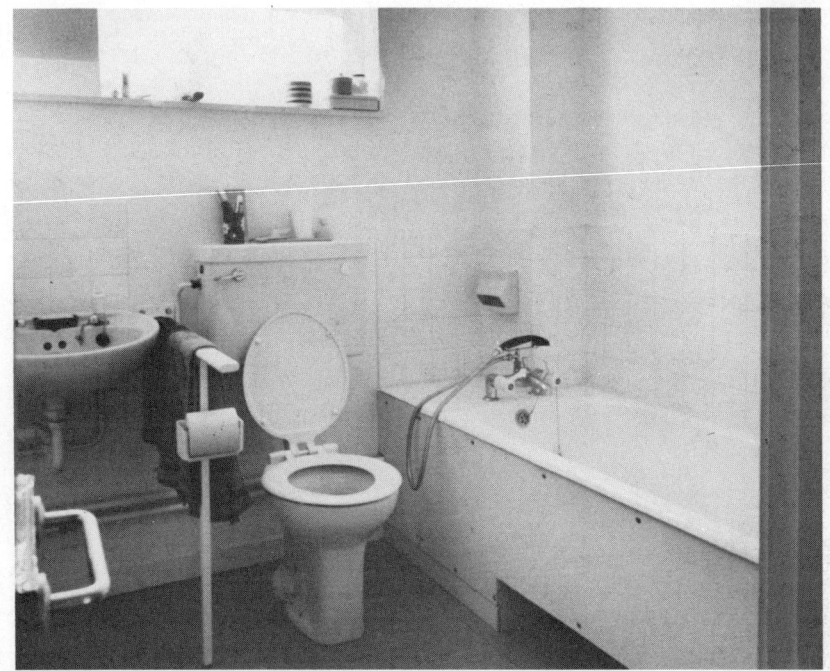

C

Habinteg

Habinteg at Moira Close in Haringey, North London, is the first project completed by the Habinteg Housing Association, 6 Duke's Mews, London, England (Fig. 18–1). Sponsored by the Spastics Society, it provides integrated housing for elderly and disabled individuals. Though the proportion of disabled is limited to a maximum of 25%, all the units have ramped entrances and wide doorways. A community assistant and his wife care for the needs of both disabled and nondisabled. The first Habinteg was so successful that 26 additional projects are planned throughout Great Britain.

Inskip St. Giles Housing Association

Disabled club members raised funds to build 25 special units, serviced by a warden, within a large housing development (Jolliffe House, 22 West Street, Poole, Dorset, England). Fifty percent of the taps on basins and kitchen sinks were converted to electrical operation.

John Groom's Association for the Disabled

Under its former name, John Groom's Crippleage, the Association, 10 Gloucester Drive, Finsbury Park, London N4 2LP, England, had been providing voluntary services since 1866. In the early 1970s, the Association began to provide specialized housing within ordinary projects. The first, Princess Crescent, 9 Princess Crescent, Finsbury Park, London N4, consists of 13 apartments. The kitchen cupboards on tracks were imported from the Swedish Fokus Society; even the refrigerator is adjustable in height; the toilet is cantilevered with space at either side for transference; the ground floor apartments have Clos o Mat toilets and showers; handrails are minimal and fitted as needed. The details are photographed in a booklet available from the Association for 25 pence.

The Thistle Foundation

The Thistle Foundation, Craigmillar, Edinburgh EH16 4EA, Scotland, was established in 1944 for veterans and their families; it was one of the first communities of self-contained houses with medical care and supportive services at hand. The community of 300 people comprises 97 houses, 6 bungalows, and a residential care hostel for 16 single men and women. Every house is connected by a covered passageway to the central clinic, physiotherapy and occupational therapy departments, gymnasium, swimming pool, and recreation hall. On the grounds there are fields for archery and other sports, a bowling green, and a games court. The Foundation maintains the houses but the residents are expected to furnish them and pay for their own living expenses, including heat and light. The houses are subsidized and the residents pay about one-seventh of the cost of comparable council houses.

The new hostel is linked in the same way as the houses to all the facilities by a covered way. Opened in 1971, the attractive home has 12 one-room suites (bed–sitters), each with its own shower room, and 2 double rooms, each with its own large bathroom.

In addition to the Thistle Foundation, a number of other Scottish voluntary organizations are operating or planning housing projects. For further information, contact the Scottish Information Service for the Disabled, Claremont House, 18/19 Claremont Crescent, Edinburgh EH7 3QD, Scotland.

PREFABRICATED HOUSING

Guildway Limited, Portsmouth Road, Guildford, Surrey, England, which is one of England's largest manufacturers of factory-made houses, has developed designs for local authorities to use in apartments and houses for elderly and disabled persons. The firm has designed units with standard items that are suitable for the wheelchaired and has made provisions to add special features as needed. The doors are 826 mm (32-½ in.) wide and the halls are extra wide. Electric sockets and light switches may be placed at any height. An open space may be created below the kitchen sink by eliminating a cupboard. In the bathroom, a shower basin may be provided instead of a tub; it may be fitted with grab bars, a pole, and a shower chair. The toilet may be raised to 432 mm (1 ft 5 in.) and grab bars attached to an adjacent wall. The garages and paths may be extra wide and the passageways covered. Guildway also makes special adaptations in homes for individuals.

YOUNGER CHRONIC SICK UNITS

In the late 1960s the Department of Health and Social Security initiated a crash program by the Regional Hospital Boards to get the younger chronic sick out of hospital geriatric wards. The amount of £5,000,000 was earmarked for building units to care for long-term patients aged 15–59. Most were to be built on hospital grounds and average about 25 patients per unit, some in single rooms but most in four-bed wards.

SPINAL CORD INJURIES FACILITIES

Sir Ludwig Guttmann, who pioneered the modern concept of comprehensive treatment and rehabilitation of the spinal cord injured, set up the Stoke Mandeville National Spinal Injuries Center in 1943 in anticipation of an increased number of spinal cord casualties during the Spring Offensive of 1944. In addition to Stoke Mandeville, which has facilities for about 225, Sir Ludwig set up seven other small spinal injuries units in the United Kingdom and influenced the creation of units in 24 other countries.

Though he emphatically recommends the establishment of a hostel and a sheltered workshop near every center for those who are unable to return to their homes, very few of the centers have them. He particularly recommends the hostel–workshop for the developing countries where it would be impossible for the spinal injured to return to their villages in the bush. For those who return to their homes, he urges that every center set up a follow-up service with regular home visits by medical and social work staff members.

Most of the residential facilities for paraplegics or quadriplegics maintain workshops or encourage work in the community. The Sir Ludwig Guttmann Hostel at Stoke Mandeville Hospital maintains facilities for 30 persons, mostly in single rooms, who are in need of long-term care. Lyme Green Hall in Cheshire and Kytes Estate in Hertfordshire were started for ex-servicemen of World War II and have special bungalows for those who live with their families. The Duchess of Gloucester House in the industrial area of outer London, has inexpensive wardlike accommodations for employed paraplegics numbering 70 men and 6 women.

The Spinal Injuries Association (SIA), 24 Nutford Place, London W1H 6AN, England, was officially inaugurated in February, 1974. The disabled men and women who formed SIA felt the need for communication and information on many aspects of the care of the spinal cord injured, such as provision of housing, hostels, holiday accommodation, emergency care, equipment and transport, research and investigation into employment and other problems. The aim of the SIA is to help identify and solve these problems.

RELEVANT LEGISLATION AND REPORTS

Chronically Sick and Disabled Persons Act of 1970

While Great Britain's disabled population has not created its own club type housing projects as have disabled groups in some other countries, it has been phenomenally successful in influencing both legislation and the creation of the position Minister for the Disabled which is now filled by the very effective Hon. Alfred Morris. The Chronically Sick and Disabled Persons Act, the culmination of a very effective publicity campaign mounted by an organization of the disabled, Disablement Income Group (DIG), made it mandatory for local authorities to provide a comprehensive service for disabled people, requiring them to: 1) find out the number of disabled people in their community and assess their individual and collective needs; 2) provide an effective information service; and 3) improve the range of their services.

DIG also runs a social work advisory service on financial matters for disabled who may wish to write for advice and publishes a quarterly, *Progress,* as well as informative pamphlets. DIG's excellent publication, *An ABC of Services and General Information for Disabled People,* costs 10 pence (20¢) or is free to disabled individuals. It can be obtained through DIG, Queen's House, 180/182A, Tottenham Court Road, London W1P OBD, England.

Department of the Environment Circular 74/74

In May, 1974, the Department of the Environment published a joint circular with the Welsh Office, *Housing for People who are Physically Handicapped,* to assist the local housing authorities to meet housing needs. It emphasized that housing for the disabled should be arranged in the community, not in hospitals or residential homes, that it is preferable to adapt existing homes rather than to rehouse people, that specially designed housing would be needed only by those who are totally dependent on wheelchairs for living or housework, and that mobility housing, with a few special features, would be suitable for many disabled people as well as nondisabled people and would quickly widen the choice of available housing.

Working Party on Housing for Disabled People

The Working Party on Housing for Disabled People, established by the Central Council for the Disabled under the chairmanship of Professor John Greve, has produced an Interim Report that specifically recommends establishing an agency to help disabled and elderly people find suitable accommodation to buy or to rent. Such an agency might encourage private house builders, social service departments, and housing associations to make provisions for disabled people within the private sector of housing.

Copies of the report may be obtained from the Central Council for the Disabled, 34 Eccleston Square, London SW1V 1PE, England, for 30 pence (60¢).

AUSTRALIA

Australian social welfare services are provided by the Australian Government, its seven state governments, voluntary agencies, and church organizations. The Australian Government Rehabilitation Service, with centers in all state capitals provides support for training as well as residential and day services for those assessed as capable of filling a definite occupation within 3 years of training. It also provides free care in public hospitals and other medical services to pensioners, subject to a means test. The Department of Social Security deals with social security, welfare, the health insurance fields, and social planning.

In 1963, the Australian Council for the Rehabilitation of the Disabled (ACROD) was established by more than 70 voluntary agencies and churches which had pioneered in providing employment and housing for the disabled, primarily through large sheltered workshops, some of which had adjacent residential facilities. In recent years, however, as the numbers of the severely disabled increased and the costs of care spiraled the government has subsidized capital building costs and initiated a maintenance subsidy.

In common with most of the world, Australia does not have a national registry of those who are disabled, has placed more emphasis on housing for the elderly than for the young disabled, has a means test unrelated to the needs of the severely disabled who require attendant care, and places more emphasis on institutionalization than on normalization. The development of hostels, of small group homes, and of adapted housing and services within the community has not kept pace with the needs of young, healthy disabled. On the other hand, in nearly every state individuals and groups of disabled have been the catalysts for the establishment of residential facilities and workshops.

NEW SOUTH WALES

The House With No Steps

(49 Blackbutts Road, Belrose 2085.) This network of residences, workshops, and training centers has evolved under the leadership of Lionel Watts, MBE, who is severely disabled by poliomyelitis. The network began modestly in 1962 with the founding of a sports and social club, the Wheelchair and Disabled Association. The first program involved securing transportation for disabled people from all over Sydney to attend the meetings of the club.

In 1964 a sheltered workshop was started, other sports clubs opened, and plans initiated for a residence. The next year the government donated 2½ acres of land for a residential/workshop complex.

In 1966 the vocational training unit was opened. In addition to employment in the two large workshops, the unit furnishes a variety of services: counseling; assessment; home visits; work placement; financial assistance; advice on equipment, community resources, and pension payments; transportation; and sports and social club activities.

In 1969, 20 Independent Living Units were opened (Fig. 18–2). Designed for individuals who can live without assistance, each unit contains two beds and built-in wardrobes, a kitchen preparation shelf which extends into the living room

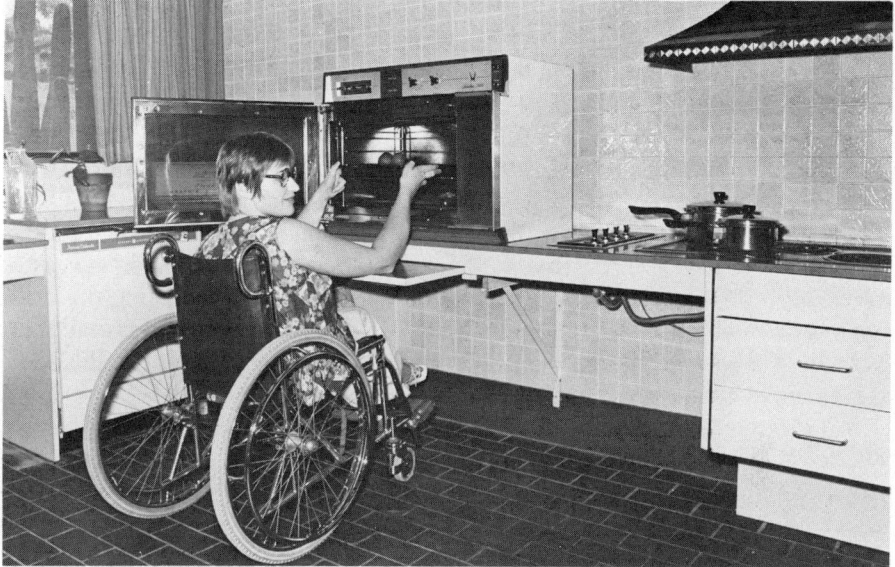

Fig. 18–2. Evelyn Moxey demonstrates the oven shelf in one of the 20 units in the House With No Steps at Belrose, Sydney.

as a buffet-dining table, and special bathroom and toilet facilities. Through a wall of glass, an outside, enclosed Japanese ornamental garden forms an integral part of the living area. The grounds are landscaped and accented with natural rocks and waterfalls.

In 1970, Lachlan House With No Steps Committee formed to raise funds in Forbes for a workshop and hostel complex. A training program was started for young quadriplegics in hospitals to teach them to use the telephone in industry, selling, market research, and answering services.

In 1971, Phoneability Enterprises formed to expand the use of the telephone in industry. Six quadriplegic men at headquarters use the phone to sell stationery, office equipment, swimming pool accessories, and advertising space. Other quadriplegics work from home using special phones provided by the Association. Additional communities started hostels and workshops. Additional assessment and training centers opened in two communities.

In 1972, Capricornia House With No Steps formed at Rockhampton as the regional center for the Queensland Central Coast. A special bus was purchased and a job training center for spinal cord injured persons opened.

In 1973, a center opened to train disabled young men and women in catering techniques, cooking, kitchen work, cleaning, and waitressing. First International House With No Steps was established in Manila. A car with hand controls was purchased and driving instruction courses started.

In 1974, another sheltered workshop opened and another bus was purchased. Holiday camps started to train employees in self-care and independent living. A canteen opened to provide hot or cold meals to the office and workshop staff.

Civilian Maimed and Limbless Association

Another complex of facilities in the Sydney area that includes workshops, transportation, and residential accommodations was started in 1954 by a disabled couple, the late Mr. and Mrs. H. Bedwin, MBE. Both were quadriplegic, Hugh because of polio and Hazel because of rheumatoid arthritis. The Civilian Maimed and Limbless Association (CMLA), 159 Princes Highway, St. Peters, 2044, an association of people who are disabled, has grown to a membership of some thousands with a network of six workshops in Sydney and Newcastle. Over 3000 disabled workers have entered the CMLA workshops; 250+ have gone to normal jobs, 400+ are still in the workshops, and there are practically none on the waiting list. Some of a fleet of 17 transport vehicles are driven by disabled persons.

In 1956 the association purchased for residential accommodations an historic old house in Dulwich Hill with large rooms and wide verandahs known as Gladstone Hall. A ramp and alterations allowed accommodation of six disabled boarders cared for by housekeeper/cooks.

Three-year lobbying work of the organization effected a law in 1963 granting a subsidy by the Government of $2 for every $1 raised by welfare organizations for the provision of accommodation for disabled persons working in sheltered workshops, provided the building costs do not exceed $4800 per new person. As a result, in 1966 Gladstone Hall was enlarged to accommodate 30 people, modernized to include a community kitchen, dining and sitting rooms, and matron's quarters.

The original aim was to create self-supporting workshops and hostels, have the workshop employees be able to earn, together with the invalid pension, the equivalent of the basic wage, and to employ only physically handicapped people of normal working age, 16–60. But pressures changed the policies to include those with mental handicaps and the elderly. At any one time, over 40 categories of physical disability are represented in the workshops, the most common source of disability is cerebral palsy, with epilepsy, polio, arthritis, and quadriplegia the next most common.

Significantly, the work force includes over 50% mentally retarded and mentally disturbed persons. The Association's quarterly publication, *Fortitude,* reports, "the mentally handicapped person can often supply the physical bridge for his physically handicapped fellow worker. The effect seems to be that a sense of importance is built up in the mentally handicapped person which has, in many cases, resulted in considerable development of previously latent potential." The Association reports that its policy of a piecework rate at the same earning rate as outside industry results in phenomenal developments in both physically and mentally disabled people, that the correlation between IQ and work capacity is very low, and that degree of motivation and interest are the most important factors. It also found that the borderline IQ level (about 70) is the most troublesome and that the 50 IQ level is the minimum that can be successfully mixed. Supervision costs are higher with the mentally retarded than with the physically disabled, but transport costs are higher with the physically disabled.

Social services and welfare work became increasingly important as the numbers of workers increased. Problems include placements in open industry, acute housing problems, pension difficulties, and making of aids for use in the workshop as well as at home. Advice is given on the installation of ramps, raising of chair heights, lifting devices, extension of tap handles, and other mechanical aids. Most of the work involves couselling and consulting, "Our counselling ability is gained from our own handicapped people and represents the total of their combined experience."

According to the organization's secretary, Ben Meads, during the 1970s the emphasis has turned more towards the operation of sheltered workshops and less towards living accommodations because much greater numbers of the disabled can be helped through employment than from an equivalent investment in housing.

The Spastic Centre of New South Wales

The Spastic Centre of New South Wales, Allambie Heights, Sydney 2100, operates a medical treatment unit and school for nearly 300 metropolitan children, transporting them to and from their homes daily; residential hostels for trainees and country children and young adults; a small school and treatment unit at Newcastle some 60 miles north of Sydney; a mother and babies training program for 300 very young cerebral palsied babies; and Centre Industries, an industrial training unit for severely disabled cerebral palsied persons.

The Centre is based on the principle that if the parents cannot pay with money for the years of treatment given to their children, they can pay with work. Mothers and fathers are each expected to volunteer for 1 day/month or provide a substitute worker. The system has many hidden benefits, such as a subtle form of group therapy as parents share problems with other parents while working together.

Centre Industries was established in 1961 with its single objective to provide training and employment for the most severely disabled cerebral palsied. Operating in the highly competitive telecommunications and electronics industry, its output for 1975 is expected to exceed $6,000,000. Presently employment stands at 260 disabled (of whom 222 are cerebral palsied) and 553 nondisabled workers. It provides real, not token, employment with the ultimate aim of placement in open industry. The trainees are paid at nondisabled piecework rates for their work. Payment is based strictly on production and includes a pension allowance from the Government.

Door-to-door transportation and mobility within the factory are vital. Thirty-eight buses pick up and return 370 children and adults daily, with a nominal transport charge of $1 weekly from all adult trainees.

The Centre has designed and produces, at a cost of $500, an inexpensive electric wheelchair with the controls and seat assembly suited to each individual's requirements; it may be controlled by a joystick or a push-button. The chair cuts the labor costs of pushers and adds freedom of action and excitement to work.

The Centre's Personal Independence Program has paid dividends in the resulting increase in self-confidence and independence in personal activities. For example, the program covers all aspects of a cerebral palsied girl's personal needs. Each girl is given highly individual training in the most suitable of nine foot–square cubicles containing assorted toilet adaptations and rails of different heights. The girls learn to cleanse, put on make-up, dress, and attend to toilet needs by themselves, with whatever gadgets and equipment are necessary. The program is directed and planned by a cerebral palsied trainee who has designed the necessary plumbing and other adaptations needed for the program. Though it may take years, most of the girls learn to take care of themselves so that they may go to work in other factories where there are no special facilities.

Cherrywood Village

In 1965 the State granted 90 acres of land to the Foundation for the Disabled for a residential and occupational complex for physically handicapped people. Cherrywood Village, located in Kingswood, a semirural area 35 miles west of Sydney, was planned to attract its able-bodied neighbors with sports and recreational areas as well as an occupational center, thus minimizing segregation and isolation.

The first unit, Cutler House, was dedicated in 1968. The hotel/motel type residence, built around a courtyard, consists of 40 self-contained units, each with its own shower and toilet facilities, sick bay, gymnasium, recreation area, workshop, and a heated swimming pool.

The Paraplegic and Quadriplegic Association of New South Wales

Founded in 1961, the Paraplegic and Quadriplegic Association of New South Wales, 833 King George's Road, South Hurstville 2221, fills a variety of the needs of its 810 members, of whom 714 are disabled. Current projects include developing a manual of equipment and services, researching and furnishing equipment, operating the workshop Paraquad Industries which specializes in gauge and instrument repairing, researching the possibilities for employment of quadriplegics, developing a quadriplegic driver-training vehicle, continuing its survey of all paraplegic and quadriplegics in New South Wales (the total number now surveyed stands at 760), acting as consultant on architectural barriers at motels and universities, participating in national and international sports, providing holiday accommodations, and planning hostel facilities. Further, with the help of local Rotary Clubs, the workshop has been enlarged and a wheelchair bus purchased.

Following their pilot project of adapting an existing bungalow for four or five self-sufficient paraplegics, the Association is planning a hostel for quadriplegics to be built in the vicinity of a large public hospital in Sydney, with national and state government assistance. The hostel, with a 40-bed capacity, will have rooms for one, two, and three persons and will have a sheltered workshop attached.

QUEENSLAND

Community Home Care Service

S. D. Tooth, Minister for Health, summarized the Queensland home care service for the elderly and disabled in a Department of Health booklet, *Community Home Care Service:*

This new service is based on the premise that it is possible for the elderly and the disabled to receive a competent, helpful, and sympathetic service within the comforting confines of their own homes and familiar surroundings. It is envisaged that this service will enable those in need to continue their lives in dignity and in the pride of self-sufficiency.

The service is based on the retention of the patient's own doctor as the key person in medical care and, at the same time, the provision of skilled help where it is needed in the domestic social work and public health nursing fields. The cooperation of voluntary and church-sponsored organizations is being actively encouraged. It is realized that only if all community-based groups work together will an effective service be developed.

Community Home Care Service provides free of charge or for a very minimum fee: nursing consultation in the patient's own home, investigation in social problems, advice on associated health problems, and regular domestic help in the home for as long as it is considered necessary by the Home Care Service.

Brisbane Spastics Centre

The Brisbane Spastics Centre provides education for 80 school children and nursery facilities for 30 children under school age. In addition, the center operates a residential home for 60 adults at New Farm, a suburb of Brisbane, and an outpatient treatment center for 200 children.

Paraplegic Welfare Association of Queensland

In 1974, the Paraplegic Welfare Association of Queensland, 93 Stafford Road, Kedron, Brisbane, bought land in the Brisbane suburb of Belmont. It is in the process of raising funds to build a hostel for its quadriplegic members.

SOUTH AUSTRALIA

Much of the information on housing facilities in South Australia was compiled with the assistance of D. J. Forward and Erich Krell. Miss Forward, a founder of the Phoenix Society and volunteer editor of its quarterly magazine, has been disabled by a hip disease since childhood. Mr. Krell, a high level quadriplegic, is a member of the International Association of Mouth and Foot Painting Artists.

The Phoenix Society, Inc.

The Phoenix Society, Inc., P.O. Box 112, Cowandilla 5033, established its sheltered workshop in 1958 for physically handicapped persons over 15 years of age. It provides employment and rehabilitation services for 220 workers, 56 of whom are mentally retarded. Transportation is provided for those too disabled to use public transport. Presently, the Society is trying to work out a hostel scheme by leasing or buying a large old house and putting a half dozen workers in it as an experiment.

Phoenix, a nonprofit organization, shares the monies produced from work contracts with its workers. The work opportunities vary widely to suit all types of disabilities: woodwork, spray painting, production line assembly, packaging, collating, bulk postage mailing services, subassembly work, general office work, and general gardening and ground maintenance.

A warmth and friendliness make Phoenix a special place for its workers. In 1974, 21 of its disabled workers received awards for continuous service of 10 or more years. Social and recreational activities are an important part of the work and include the annual picnic, Christmas parties, barbecues, concerts, specially designed "games evenings," and cricket matches.

Home for Incurables

The Home for Incurables, 103 Fisher Street, Fullarton 5063, provides a home for just over 400 people certified as having a chronic disease which is incurable and needing nursing care, excluding those with cancer, tuberculosis, epilepsy, blindness, or mental diseases of any kind. Residents pay fees according to their means, and every resident is left with some spending money. To meet the needs of the more than 400 on the waiting list, a new building is planned that would increase the number of residents to 800 and the staff from 240 to 450.

Mitchell Park Village

Mitchell Park Village, 33 Thirza Avenue, Mitchell Park, South Australia 5043, completed in 1967, consists of two courts, Orana and Coorinda, which comprise 26 apartments, family houses, and single units. Kitchens have sinks with space underneath, lowered cupboards, and eye-level ovens with doors which open sideways. Bathrooms have handrails, accessible wash basins, and showers large enough for wheelchairs. There are no steps and all doors are extra wide. The exteriors are attractive and bright, with gardens and lawns maintained by the Housing Trust.

Reactions of the disabled to Mitchell Park Village are mixed, ranging from enthusiasm to feeling that it is too segregated, too lacking in contact with the "real" world.

Paraplegic Association of South Australia

Situated within the Spinal Injuries Unit at Morris Government Hospital, the Paraplegic Association of South Australia, Folland Avenue, Northfield 5085, provides for the general welfare and care of the spinal cord injured, including physical training, transport to work or workshops, education, recreation, and domiciliary services. It also keeps in touch with former patients in the Northern Territory and maintains a branch at the large country town of Mt. Gambier where there is an independent sheltered workshop, Heritage. Those who have returned to their homes may receive the daily assistance of district nurses, meals on wheels, and other domiciliary services. The South Australian Housing Trust will adapt doorways and build ramps for some. Those without homes live at the hospital on a temporary basis or at the Home for Incurables; some attend sheltered workshops.

Small specialized residential centers for those with sensory disabilities include: the South Australian Blind Welfare Association, P.O. Box 1105, Adelaide 5001 which is planning a complex of 23 units for communal living by blind persons, both employable and elderly, adjacent to its new headquarters and the South Australian Adult Deaf Society, Inc., 262 South Terrace, Adelaide 5000 which provides a young peoples' hostel attached to the center for young deaf men and women mainly from the country.

Bedford Industries Vocational Rehabilitation Association, Inc.

Founded by the South Australia Tuberculosis Association, Inc., Bedford Industries, Goodwood Road, Panorama 5041, has evolved into an extensive sheltered workshop under the directorship of Kenneth T. Jenkins, chairman of the World Commission on Vocational Rehabilitation. The workshop provides a work-oriented setting in the manufacturing, marketing, and accounting fields. The activities include engineering, electronics, woodwork, textiles, book-binding, stationery, printing, painting, packaging, and subcontract. The more than 600 workers have a wide range of disabilities. Buses provide transport to and from work and lunch is served for a nominal fee. Social and recreational activities are organized by a Social Committee.

To provide accommodation for workers from the country, an attractive hostel was added in 1974 on a 9½ acre site of "bush land" near the workshops. The director describes it:

"Bal-yana" comprises 50 single motel type self-contained suites, each with its own private bathroom and bed-sitting room. Twelve of these suites have been specifically designed to accommodate severely physically handicapped occupants.

At present there is a communal dining room/lounge and residents are provided with breakfast and an evening meal on weekdays and three meals a day at weekends and on Public Holidays. In addition there is a small kitchen on each floor of the accommodation section where it is possible to prepare light meals when required. An additional sitting room for use as a reading room is provided. Shortly an additional 20 suites will be provided, and a recreation/games room, a television room and reading room will be added.

One of the conditions of entry is that the handicapped client must work, although not necessarily at Bedford Industries; in fact, some are employed in outside industry. It is intended that Bal-yana be a transition house for the majority of its residents, although some residents are likely to remain there for the rest of their working life.

Home Care Services

Meals on Wheels, Inc., 97 Fullerton Road, Kent Town 5067, provides home services for small charges to anyone with a doctor's certificate stating details of need: 1) A daily midday hot three-course meal is delivered from eighteen metropolitan kitchens and eight country and suburban kitchens; 2) Home Help Service provides laundry and/or house cleaning from once every other week to 3 hours/day; 3) Hair care service is given by voluntary trained hairdressers; 4) Befrienders are trained to visit and chat and do a few personal favors; 5) Standby Service is provided by visitors who give the family a few hours away from home; 6) A Heavy Cleaning team brings the home up to standard to enable Home Help to cope with regular cleaning; 7) Chiropody services include a mobile foot clinic and a visiting chiropodist.

Four metropolitan hospital centers provide free or for a nominal charge home nursing care, physiotherapy, social work, chiropody, occupational therapy, housekeeping and home help, sitters, linen and meal services, and the loan of appliances.

TASMANIA

Mary Guy, who is quadriplegic because of poliomyelitis, furnished the information on Tasmanian services. She is active in organizations of the disabled that are attacking architectural barriers and promoting a residential center.

"There is not a hostel, residence, or anything similar for the physically handicapped in this State. There are several hostels for retarded children, and one for retarded adults if they are employed at a sheltered workshop. If a physically handicapped adult does not have a family to care for him he must go to a government institution for the elderly, or a rest home for the elderly, or to a home in Perth (about 90 miles north of here) which is for the incurably ill.

"The Housing Department will give special consideration to a handicapped person who applies for a unit and over the past few years has helped many disabled people to live with reasonable independence. The Department will also help to design a house suitable for a disabled person and will adapt an existing house or unit of the Department if it is needed.

"Tasmania has a statewide Meals on Wheels Service for the elderly and disabled run by a voluntary group and subsidized by the State and Australian governments. A nominal fee is charged for the meals. In addition, the State subsidizes a housework service for light housekeeping for a small fee. Volunteers support a District Nursing Service which is available without charge; a similar service is run by the St. Vincent de Paul Society."

VICTORIA

Angus Mitchell House

The Angus Mitchell House, 61 Sutherland Road, Armadale, is a hostel built by the Victorian Society for Crippled Children and Adults, 524 Collins Street, Melbourne

C1). All facilities are specially geared for as independent a life as possible. Much of the equipment, such as hydraulic lifts, was donated by the Rotary Club of Melbourne. Admission is limited to those between the ages of 14 and 40. Most of the residents are country people in the metropolitan area for long- or short-term training or employment; they are charged according to their ability to pay and have a choice of companionship or privacy. During a typical year, between 50 and 60 men and women are provided with accommodation at various times, about 30 usually in permanent residence.

Hilltops Holiday Home

Another project of the Victorian Society for Crippled Children and Adults, Hilltops Holiday Home, Hoddle Street, Yarra Junction, is in the mountains and provides not only outings for children, but also weekend holidays for single adults and young people's groups, as well as for families with a member who is disabled. The home is operated year-round by an experienced, mostly volunteer staff.

Glen Waverly Rehabilitation Centre

Designed for 100 resident and 50 nonresident trainees, the Glen Waverly Rehabilitation Centre, Glen Waverly, Victoria, includes administration and medical buildings with facilities for five doctors, a clinical psychologist, social workers, speech therapists, and physiotherapists. The educational section has three large classrooms and study rooms, a library, and offices for counselors and tutors. The occupational therapy area has work areas for light trades, radio, and office procedures, as well as a model kitchen, bedroom, and bathroom where the skills of daily living are taught and practiced.

There are also workshops for woodwork, machine and sheet metal work, welding and process work. The work conditioning unit is conducted on strictly industrial lines, and the residents are employed on subcontract work under normal industrial conditions.

Other areas provide a dining room with cafeteria or waitress service; a canteen; a library; a theater for cinema, concerts, dances, and other entertainment; basketball and tennis courts; a small bowling green; and a farm area of approximately 2 acres for rural work. Staff accommodation comprises a residence for the manager and assistant manager as well as a self-contained flat for the matron and a four-bedroom flat for four nurses. Three motel type rooms are provided for parents and other visitors from country areas.

Residential sections house more than two-thirds of the residents at ground floor level. Lounge rooms, TV and writing rooms, toilets, bathrooms, and laundries are located near the bedrooms. The planning and location blend with existing and future private residences in the area.

Deva Hostel

Managed by the Victorian Society for Crippled Children and Adults, the "Deva" Hostel, 10 Acland Street, St. Kilda, is planned for severely disabled young men and women who, in a sheltered environment, are able to go out to work. There is a flat within one section of the hostel for women to try caring for themselves by doing their own marketing, housework, cooking, etc. The staff of the hostel is at hand if emergency assistance is needed.

WESTERN AUSTRALIA

A community welfare organization sponsored and supported by the general public, the Paraplegic Association, 184 Cambridge Street, Wembley, represents the approximately 336 quadriplegics and 240 paraplegics in Western Australia. Its workshop, Paraplegic Agencies, specializes in party hats, toys, decorations, handbags, mocassins, and cane and woodware manufactured by paraplegics.

In November, 1969 the Paraplegic Association opened the Quadriplegic Centre, Selby Street, Shenton Park, Perth, to assist quadriplegics in their return to the community. Located on a 5-acre block area adjoining the Royal Perth (Rehabilitation) Hospital, the Centre uses the hospital's kitchen and laundry facilities. It endeavors to provide a home environment, while offering special medical and nursing care as required, with a minimum of trained staff. The building comprises: a 30-bed "C" Class Hospital for the after-care of patients on completion of their acute treatment, as well as for those who live in unsuitable conditions in various parts of Western Australia; residential units for quadriplegics and paraplegics working in sheltered workshops or in private industry; and a sheltered workshop to provide employment and to study and assess the physical capacities of quadriplegics.

In addition to providing this residential care for a few cord injured individuals, the Association endeavors to assist many of them in their adjustment to life in their own homes. To supplement the skilled nursing care of the Silver Chain Nursing Service, a Home Nursing Advisory Service appoints a trained Nursing Sister to visit the homes of the Association members. The service includes regular follow-up after discharge, including information about home adaptations and equipment, and advice and assistance to the families.

Further, the Association is the voice of the spinal cord injured in "negotiations with governments and the general public, on pension anomalies, tax exemptions on motor cars, better group transport, provisions of surgical requirements, better wheelchairs, home visits, counseling and welfare."

NEW ZEALAND

Auckland Coordinating Council for the Disabled

The Auckland Coordinating Council for the Disabled, P.O. Box 1426, Auckland, formed in 1969 by the Rotary Club of Auckland, coordinates the activities of its member organizations. Present membership consists of 27 Full Member (voluntary) organizations and 36 Associate Member (statutory) organizations. The Council endeavors to avoid duplication of services, conducts surveys to provide accurate information to the government, and publishes a magazine, *Accord,* and sponsored a wheelchair guide to Auckland, *Access.*

The Council works with the government to make government accessible to the disabled, to build two "State House" demonstration houses, and to provide a realistic set of criteria for accessibility in housing. These criteria would not add to the cost, but would facilitate entry to all rooms in a house and make any extra modifications regarding toilets a simple procedure.

Disabled Re-Establishment League, Inc.

A government agency, the Disabled Re-Establishment League, Inc., P.O. Box 1426, Auckland, deals with vocational rehabilitation assessment and work experience. It is closely allied with the Coordinating Council. Staff members act as the liaison between the disabled person, employer, and the medical team, making recommendations concerning vocational rehabilitation and future employment; a regular follow-up plan is included in the service.

Laura Fergusson Trust for Disabled Persons, Inc.

The Laura Fergusson Trust, 244 Great South Road, Auckland 5, was established in 1967 to assist disabled persons in the solution of their residential problems. The Trust has built a home in Auckland with accommodation for 33 and is planning to build additional facilities in other areas.

Disabled Citizens' Society

In 1942, a paraplegic, Horace Cadogan, started a social club for other disabled persons. In March 1974, this Disabled Citizens' Society, P.O. Box 5062, Auckland 1, opened a complex that includes a new factory, office, cafeteria, boardroom, wheelchair workshop, administrative area, and reception facilities. The building is the first stage of a larger complex to include a hospital, gymnasium, swimming pool, and workshop.

The Disabled Citizens' Society has created a number of innovative ways of making money through its workshops: selling imported wheelchairs and aids; converting old newspapers into paper wool with a paper-shredding machine and selling the wool to manufacturers as a packing material; labeling honey pots for export to Japan; subcontract work (manufacture of cedar-wood cigar boxes, cleaning clock and electrical gauge faces); and repairing and servicing wheelchairs.

The Society maintains branches in Hamilton, New Plymouth, Dunedin, and Invercargill. It has purchased a holiday home, Sea-Side Camp, in Omana for members and their families. Regular indoor bowls and darts evenings are held at the center.

Civilian Maimed Association of New Zealand, Inc.

The Civilian Maimed Association, P.O. Box 8159, Auckland, has 14 centers throughout Auckland. Its training is geared not only to the rehabilitation of workers into normal employment but also to work for the general welfare of the homebound.

Home Services

The Extramural Hospital of the Auckland Hospital Board, 24 Mountain Road, Epsom 3, Auckland 3, provides nursing services and medical social workers as liaison between the hospital, the disabled person, and the home. Occupational therapy under the direction of a medical practitioner is available to elderly and disabled individuals in the home; it involves both modifying or adapting the home as well as the community and teaching the disabled persons and relatives how to gain the optimum level of independence. Also under the direction of a medical practitioner, a physiotherapist gives the disabled individual and his family exercise programs, information on equipment, and advice on overcoming architectural barriers. Two therapists advise families of children disabled by cerebral palsy on management and training in the home.

A pool of equipment for loan includes beds, cots, mattresses, crutches, commodes, frames, hand hoists, bed cradles, walking aids, and wheelchairs. In addition, dietetic advisory service, linen service at a small charge, wheelchair service, meals on wheels, chiropody services, and a mail order service of ileostomy, colostomy, and urinary appliances are provided. Household help is available for those who can be maintained at home with this assistance, as against requiring admission to a hospital. Day care services are being developed at most hospitals for elderly persons living at home.

ASIA

The crux of the problem in Asia is that there are too many people and too few services. Nevertheless, there is progress, and there are many dedicated professional people and growing numbers of disabled persons working to coordinate the needs of the disabled into their national frameworks.

Though there has been increasing recognition of the economy of and the need for integration of the disabled in education and employment, there has been almost nothing developed nationally in the way of residential facilities. The only homes are institutions for handicapped children, the aged, and the blind, often run by religious orders. There is some custodial care for veterans and those with leprosy and mental retardation. Long range plans for hostels for employed disabled workers are only at the discussion stage. The Cheshire Homes Foundation of England operates 19 homes in India, as well as homes in Hong Kong, Indonesia, Malaysia, Philippines, Singapore, Shri Lanka, and Thailand.

Fig. 18–3. A. Bamboo latrine with a raised doorway to make it harder for snakes and other vermin to get inside. **B.** Cutaway view of a Philippine family's bathing area. The waste water drains into a soak pit.

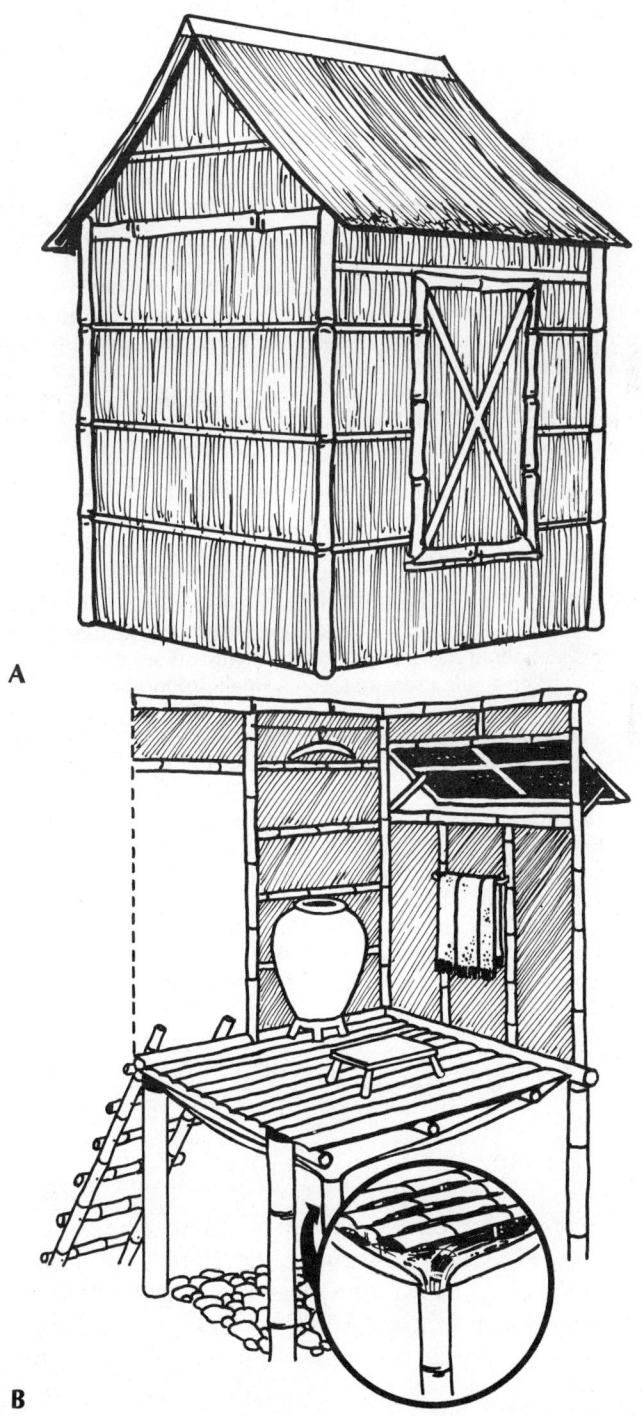

THE JOURNAL OF REHABILITATION IN ASIA

To keep abreast of developments in Asia, one must subscribe to *The Journal of Rehabilitation in Asia,* a gold mine of information. Its editor and founder, Mrs. Kamala V. Nimbkar, the doyenne of rehabilitation in Asia, was one of the 1972 Lasker Award winners for distinguished international service to the handicapped. Subscription to the quarterly journal is available for Rs. 12/- in India, $3.50 or equivalent in Canada, U.S.A., and other countries. Order from The Amerind, 15th Road, Khar, Bombay 400 052, India.

In the January 1975 issue of the *Journal,* Mrs. Nimbkar outlines the problems of wheelchairs and housing in Asia in an editorial titled, "Wheelchairs in Asia."

All the material one finds in Western rehabilitation journals, the books on the subject of wheelchairs with increasing improvements, gadgets, etc. raises the question—just when, where and how can we use wheelchairs in Asian countries. Here are some of the questions to ask ourselves in this matter. How many of the handicapped in India can afford a wheelchair? How many can all the Red Cross Branches, Rotary, Lions, and other service organizations supply? If the disabled do manage to secure one, will it be to their measurements, residual muscle strength, suitable for self-propulsion?

Mrs. Nimbkar adds that wheelchairs are useless in most of Asia—in the villages because of mud, soft sandy roads, or rocky lanes, in the cities because of deep gutters, rubbish, or uneven paving.

Let us consider the housing situation. Where in the village houses would you keep the wheelchair? Once in connection with a Paraplegia Project I visited a number of village homes of our clients and about the only place for a chair was suspension from the ceiling. In the cities there might be a little more space in a small proportion of the homes and the wheelchair could be a change from the bed or a chair. But why not put castors and a braking arrangement on an ordinary chair, much cheaper and more suitable.

One thing I might mention, in Malaysia in the forest and rural areas, houses are often built on stilts and those are very difficult for anyone with a disability to get in and out of as there are ladderlike steps and no way to use crutches, wheels or anything—and too high to have a ramp (Fig. 18–3). This must be true in parts of Africa also.

In Baroda a group has come up with what they call a "mini-wheel chair" which is really a platform on wheels with a number of improvements. Something similar has been developed in Vellore. These are certainly generally more useful and so why are they not being produced in quantity? I do not know the answer but my guess is that we still suffer from an inferiority complex and want to do what the West does and are imbued with the idea of being "up" and not down on the floor and yet all over Asia I venture to say that the majority of people live on the ground or floor.

So, let us think about this problem and perhaps one day the most suitable type of "wheelchair for Asia" will be found.

JAPAN SUN INDUSTRIES AND MODEL HOME, TETRA-ACE

Dr. Yutaka Nakamura, an orthopedic surgeon, is also the founder and director of Japan Sun Industries, Kamegawa, Beppu, Oita. During the 1964 Paralympic Games in Tokyo, Dr. Nakamura was struck by the fact that most of the contestants from out of the country were employed and lived in the community, whereas the Japanese competitors were patients in hospitals. As a result, he founded Japan Sun

International Experiences 357

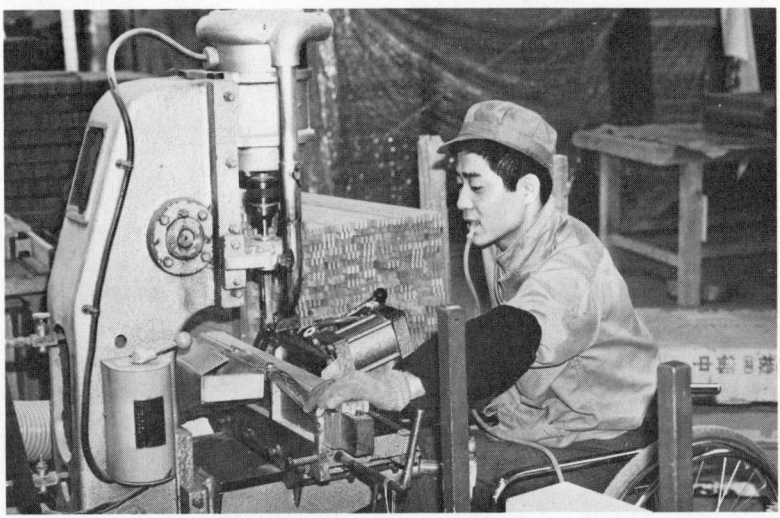

Fig. 18–4. A tetraplegic (quadriplegic) operates the lathe by sucking and blowing on the tube of the Possum switch. (Photograph courtesy of Dr. Yutaka Nakamura, Director of Japan Sun Industries)

Fig. 18–5. Moving lanes between floors make the entire building easily accessible. (Nakamura Y: Working Ability of the Paraplegics. Paraplegia 11(2): 182–193, 1973)

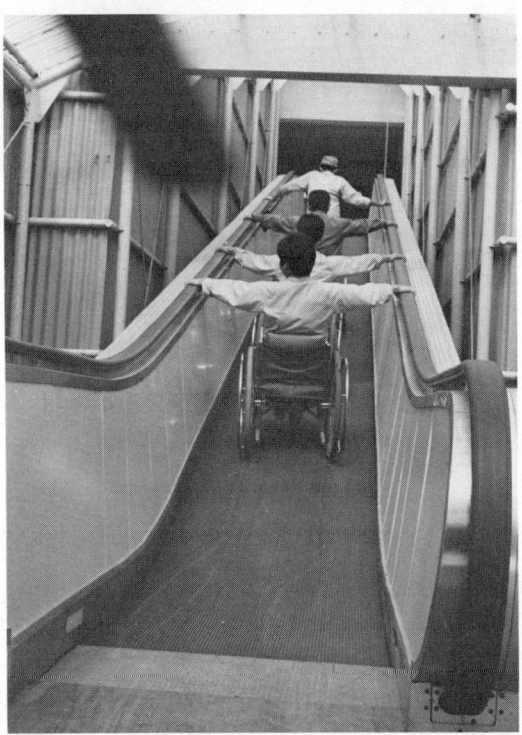

Fig. 18–6. A. Beds in the Tetra-Ace house may be moved up to the ceiling. **B.** Kitchen in Tetra-Ace. **C.** Specially designed bathroom. **D.** Typical Japanese toilet. **E.** Battery-powered wheelchair with lift; all the operations of the lift are triggered by whistle. **F.** Electrically powered wheelchair for use in Japanese style house with tatami mats. (Photographs courtesy of Dr. Yutaka Nakamura, Director of Japan Sun Industries)

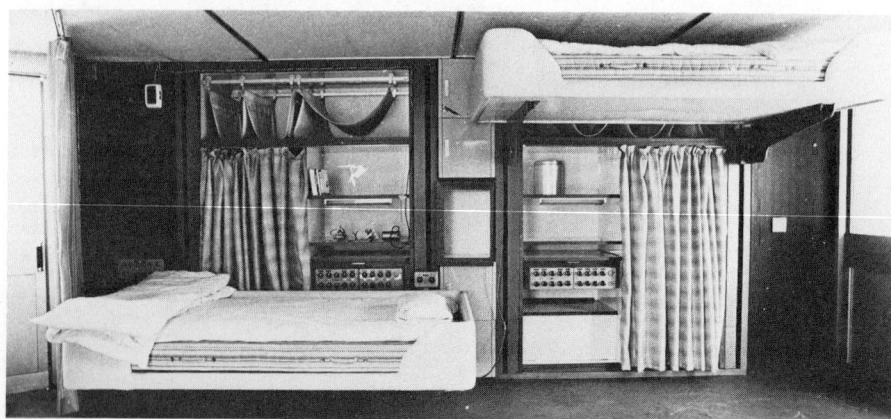

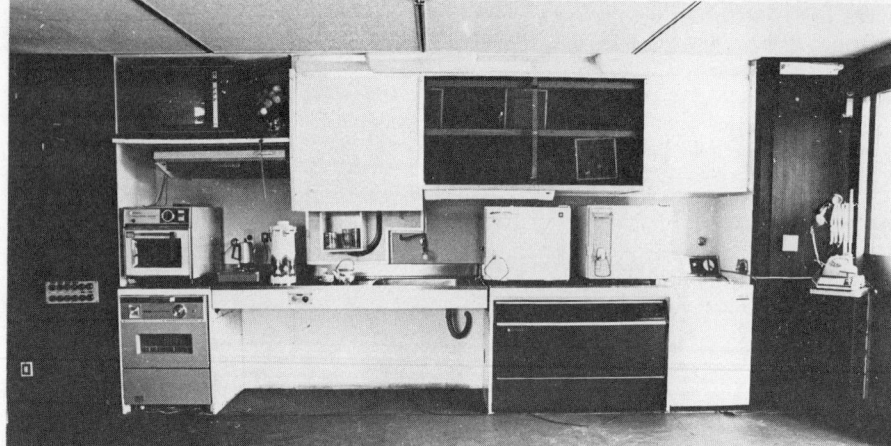

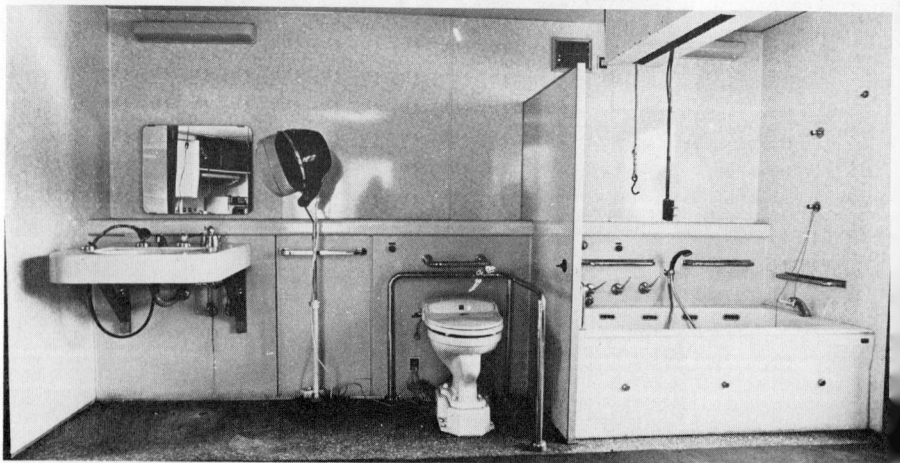

International Experiences   359

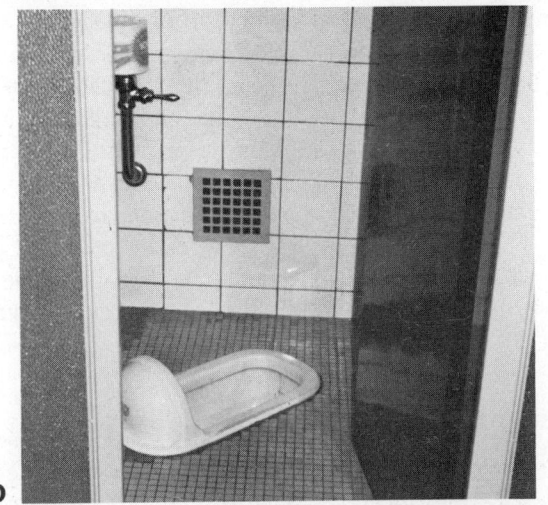

D

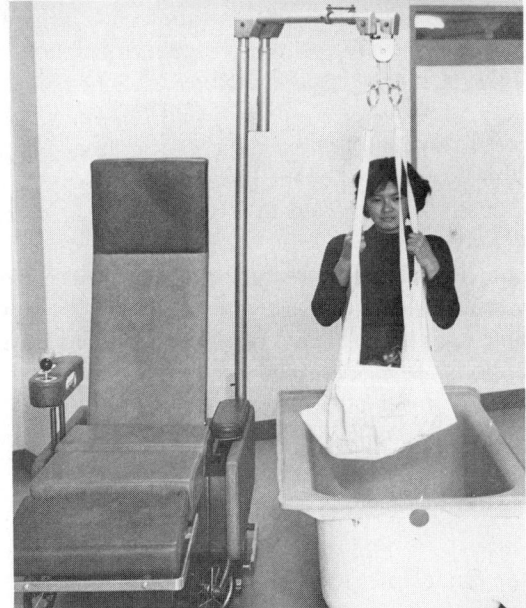

E

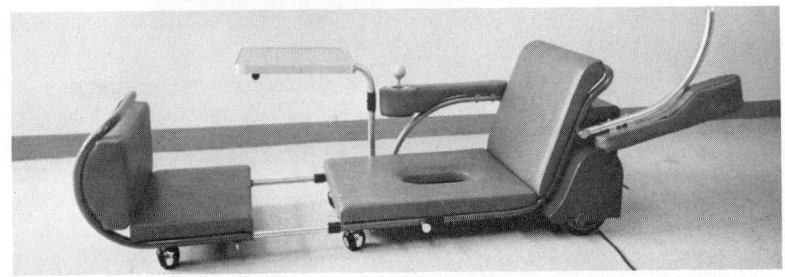

F

Industries the next year to give employment to paraplegics. It is now the largest factory in Beppu City, employing 345 disabled persons (40% in wheelchairs) and grossing about $4,000,000 annually. The complex consists of the main building, the Human Resources Institute, the International Training Institute, and Omron Taiyo Electronics Co.; the facilities include a gymnasium, swimming pool, hot spring bath, barber shop, and bank. The Omron Taiyo Electronics Company is owned and managed by the 50 wheelchaired persons who assemble electric parts.

Of the 345 disabled workers, 273 are male, 72 female; the disabilities include: spinal injury (64), cerebral palsy (123), polio (41), muscular dystrophy (9), amputee (15), deaf (15), and miscellaneous (78).

Dynamic Medical Rehabilitation

Scientific studies are made of each worker's physical measurements, muscular power, and reach; respiratory and circulatory functions are measured while working; and switches or levers of every machine are located where each worker can attain maximum efficiency with minimum fatigue. Adaptations include a Possum (breath-controlled) switch on a lathe and elbow switches on the rolling machine (Fig. 18–4).

Using the Cornell Medical Index, psychologic tests are administered immediately after the worker has been hired, after 2 months, and after 1 year. In the first tests, about 40% proved to have neurosis; in the third tests, about 28%.

To cut down on decubiti or pressure sores from prolonged sitting there are regular push-ups and massage to music in the morning, at noon, and in midafternoon. All the spinal cord injured have weekly inspections by a doctor and periodic urine tests. Sports are emphasized because it was found that active sports participants had much lower rates of absenteeism.

Throughout the factory independence is emphasized. For instance, there are moving lanes between floors (Fig. 18–5), the toilets are at a convenient height for transfer from a wheelchair, and there are automatic wheelchair washers.

Model House for Quadriplegics

A model house, Tetra-Ace, was created to demonstrate that quadriplegics can live by themselves with mechanical aids (Fig. 18–6). Ultra sound waves operate the elevating beds, doors, curtains, rotating shelf, toilet, telephone, and television. The electric wheelchair lowers to the level of the Japanese who sit on tatami mats rather than chairs.

FURTHER RESEARCH ON QUADRIPLEGIA

Dr. Masao Nagai, a C5–7 quadriplegic, who is in charge of the Psychiatric Department, National Rehabilitation Centre for Physically Impaired, reports the results of a 1974 study of Japanese traumatic quadriplegics on which he worked with the Hakone National Sanatorium. Questionnaires were sent to 32 university hospitals, 20 labor accident hospitals, 134 public and 92 private hospitals. Of 1606 myeloparalytics, tetraplegics number 640, the largest number ever counted in Japan. It was found that hand function and urologic disorders were still the main concerns. This study and other data suggested that the low rate of vocational rehabilitation in Japan was due to the unfavorable social environment, not to the lack of motivation. It was considered that the environment could be improved by changing the industrial structure, the sociopsycholgic attitude, and by improving communication and transportation. Further, 58% wanted nursing homes established and 42% wanted to have social surroundings improved for the homebound.

The Centre is developing unique aids to assist the severely disabled individual to live independently. Among the devices are an automatic human washer that consists of an upright enclosed tub with a sliding seat (Fig. 18–7). A similar enclosure functions as an automatic hair washer. An ingenious power feeder enables the user to eat and drink by himself by manipulating four head-operated switches (Fig. 18–8).

JAPAN ABILITIES, INC./JAPAN ABILITIES ASSOCIATION

In April, 1966, 200 disabled individuals met in Tokyo to form the Japan Abilities Association 17-3, 5- Chome Yayogi, Shibuya-Ku, Tokyo, Japan. Their rallying placard proclaimed, "I seek opportunity, not security."

Fig. 18–7. Automatic human washer with sliding seat; a selective switch controls shower, washing, and drying. (Photograph courtesy of Dr. Masao Nagai, Director of Psychiatric Department, National Rehabilitation Centre for Physically Impaired)

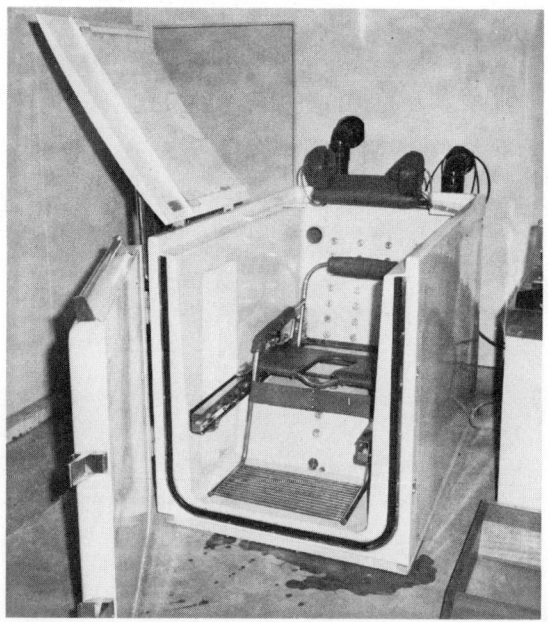

Fig. 18–8. A. Power feeder is operated by pushing buttons with the head. **B.** Power feeder. (Photograph courtesy of Dr. Masao Nagai, Director of Psychiatric Department, National Rehabilitation Centre for Physically Impaired)

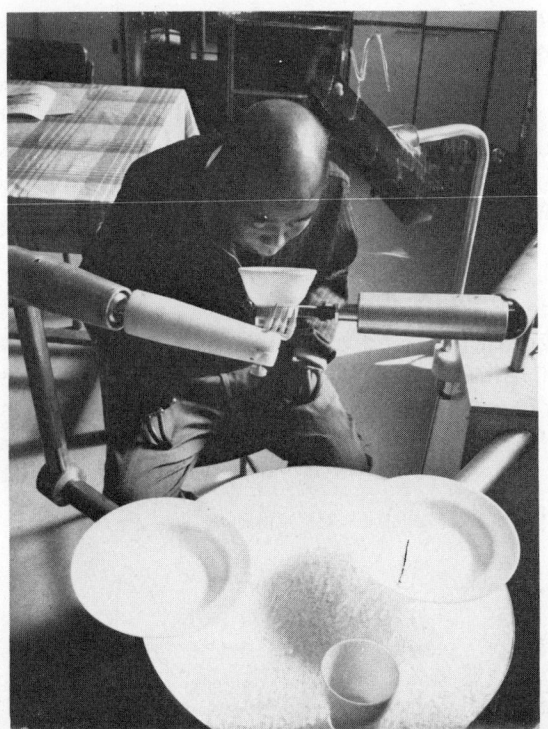

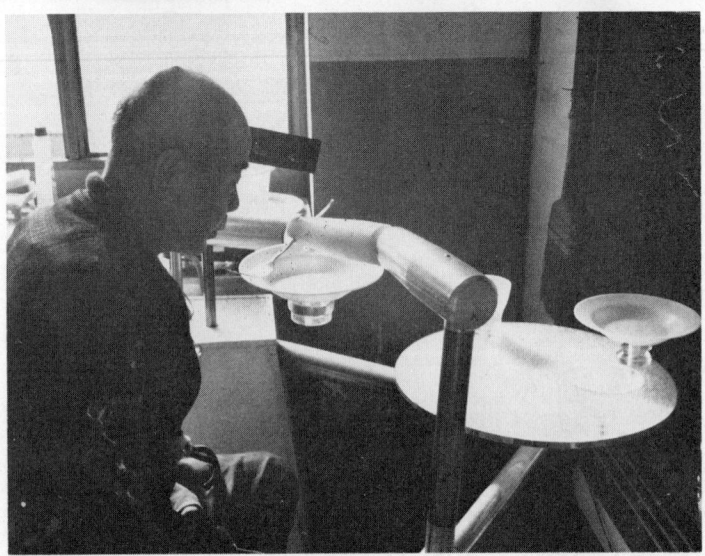

Two months later, Japan Abilities, Inc. was founded by Hiroyasu Itoh, who had been disabled by poliomyelitis since childhood. With the example of Henry Viscardi's Abilities, Inc., the support of the director of Tokyo Light Printeries Association, and a capital of a 1.5 million yen investment by 20 disabled individuals, the company started a printing business (Fig. 18–9). After a frustrating 3-year struggle, the company began to prosper and the sales have continued to increase year after year, now exceeding 100 million yen a year. The company competes with other Japanese corporations on the basis of price and quality. Without subsidy from any source, it has been showing a profit and expanding. About half of the company's employees are physically disabled.

The company subsequently launched an incinerator division to develop antipollution techniques, and with an affiliate, Abilities Data Service, Inc., has started a joint venture that is expanding and prospering.

In January, 1974, Japan Abilities, Inc. started a business of supplying training equipment and medical aids for the disabled and the elderly. In July of that year, its social and political organization, Japan Abilities Association, held the first exhibition of rehabilitation equipment for the disabled in Tokyo. The exhibition, which introduced about 200 items of equipment, was made possible through the cooperation of some 20 manufacturers and was surprisingly successful. The Association had expected about 100 visitors; over 3000 people visited the exhibition in 1 day. The exhibition marked the beginning of the Association's growth to more than 1000 members. It now publishes a bulletin with a circulation of about

Fig. 18–9. Photo-type setting machine operator at Japan Abilities, Inc. (Photograph courtesy of Hiroyasu Itoh, President of Japan Abilities, Inc.)

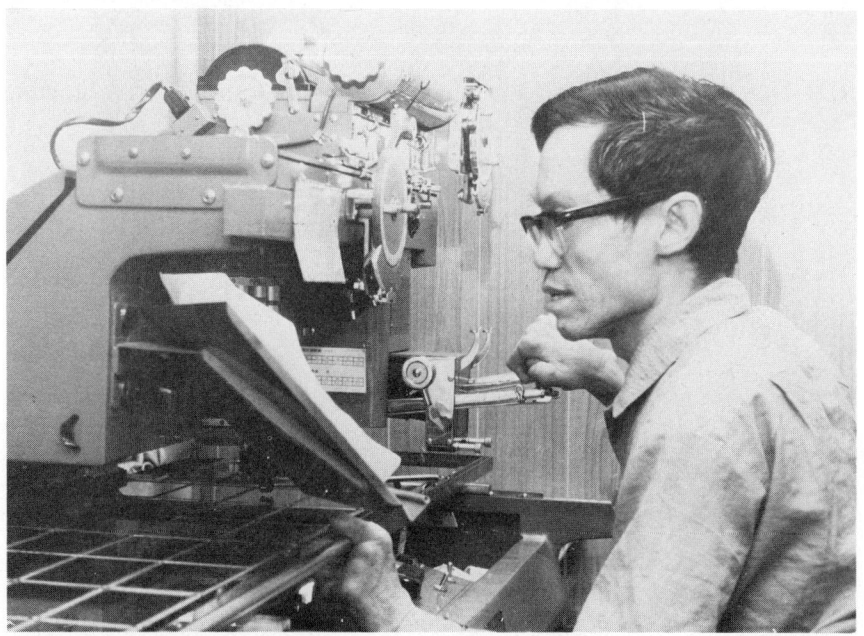

10,000, holds an annual national convention, conducts marriage and employment counseling, and has an arts and crafts club, a sports club, and a ham radio club (Figs. 18–10 and 18–11).

New Rehabilitation Equipment and Aids Division

The new rehabilitation equipment and aids division of the company is aimed at sales through the direct mail system to Japan's physically disabled and aged

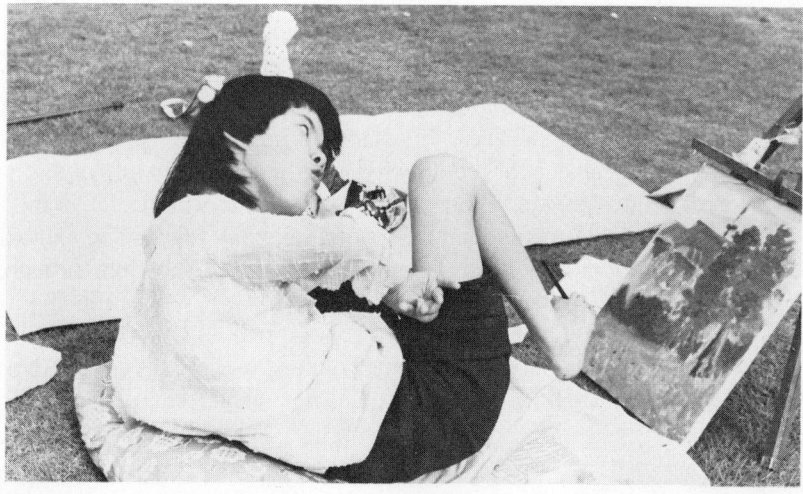

Fig. 18–10. Japan Abilities Association's art club training course. (Photograph courtesy of Hiroyasu Itoh, President of Japan Abilities, Inc.)

Fig. 18–11. A member of the Ham Club of Japan Abilities Association, the Sky Friend Club JRIZNH. (Photograph courtesy of Hiroyasu Itoh, President of Japan Abilities, Inc.)

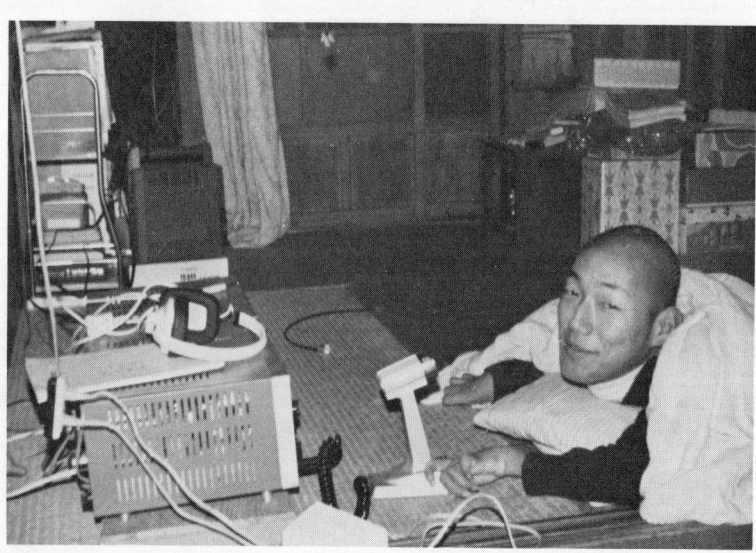

individuals as well as hospitals and welfare facilities. According to Itoh, there are about 3 million disabled people and 360,000 "helpless aged people" in Japan (population: 109 million). The direct marketing system enables the company to lower prices by 20%–50%. The items carried in the catalog include both manual and electric wheelchairs, bathtub lifts, and eating and other daily living aids. The manufacturers include British and Japanese companies. The target is 180 million yen in sales by distributing the catalog three times a year.

The company plans to set up a franchise chain of 500 service shops in key cities throughout Japan and to supply 5000 rehabilitation aids and equipment from domestic and foreign manufacturers at reasonable prices. The service shops will be located at convenient places, such as department stores, drugstores, drive-ins, bicycle shops, and medical instrument stores. The personnel in the shops will be disabled. The Japan Abilities Association will expand into communities from these shops.

On segregated housing, Itoh states,

We wish to sustain our own lives as independent citizens and workers. In other words, we wish the handicapped to be an active part of society. About half of our employees are handicapped; however, we treat all the employees without distinction with regard to work and salary. To associate the handicapped with the nonhandicapped in business is the purpose of Japan Abilities. The company does not provide the handicapped employees with special boarding houses because if they do not live in ordinary housing with nonhandicapped people and cannot go to the office, the company's policy does not make sense.

Abilities Data Service

One of its affiliates, the Abilities Data Service, Inc., is preparing a list of the physically disabled and helpless aged and of hospitals and social welfare institutions. Initially the list will include 100,000 names. The Japan Abilities Association will send direct mailings to all on the list, advising them to visit the nearest service shop and see the aids that interest them; in each area there will be people who can demonstrate how to use, repair, and maintain the products.

CZECHOSLOVAKIA

The first collective home for the disabled in Czechoslovakia was completed in 1973 as a result of a dozen years of work by a group of disabled individuals led by Jan Posker, who is disabled by muscular dystrophy. The 11-story facility, containing 100 apartments, is located in a complex that includes a 200-bed medical rehabilitation center, a swimming pool, an assembly hall, a 200-bed social care institute, apartments for health service personnel, restaurants and shops, a sheltered workshop for 200 disabled workers run by the Union of Invalids, and facilities for social activities and sports (Fig. 18–12). All the facilities of the complex are accessible, and personal assistance is available as needed. Further information is available from Vedoucí Strediska Pro Invalidy, 747 63 Hrabyne u Opavy, Czechoslovakia.

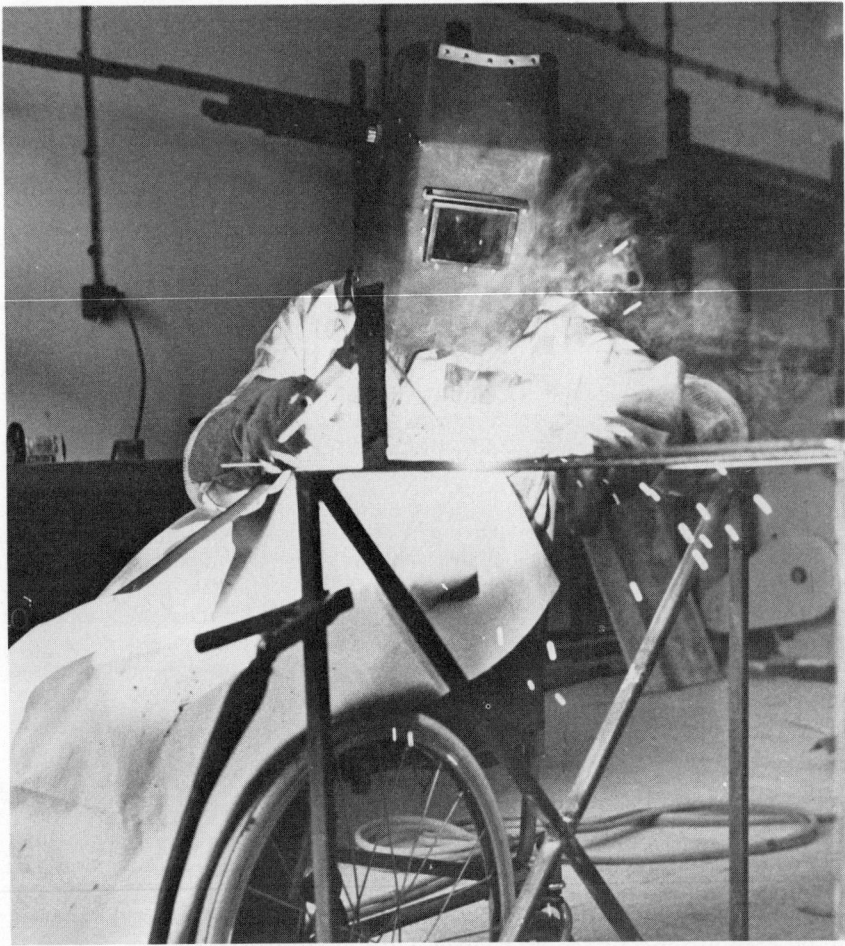

Fig. 18–12. Stanislav Lašák, a welder at the East Slovak Steel Works before a motorcycle accident 5 years ago, had been unemployed until he moved to the cooperative home. He is a welder again in the maintenance shop. (Krausová: Born Again, Czechoslovak Life 28(4): 22–23. Photograph by O. Karasek)

DENMARK

Many of the benefits and services now available to the disabled in Denmark were originally conceived by a private foundation, the Society and Home for the Disabled, which was founded in 1872. During the 1950s, the disabled organized the National Association of Disabled, now consisting of 22,000 disabled persons with 50 local branches. The Association carries out social advisory work and operates holiday and recreational activities, as well as sheltered work establishments. In addition, it initiated the Cripples' Building Society, 1 Hans Knudsens Plads, DK 2100 Copenhagen Ö Denmark, which built and operates 12 collective houses or other specially adapted apartment buildings and more than 100 single family houses all over the country (Fig. 18–13).

Fig. 18–13. A. The Danish National Association of Disabled built 100 of these adapted homes which it rents to disabled individuals and their families. **B.** Design for a wheelchair kitchen in a single family home. (Photographs courtesy of Preben Höybye-Mortensen, Society and Home for the Disabled)

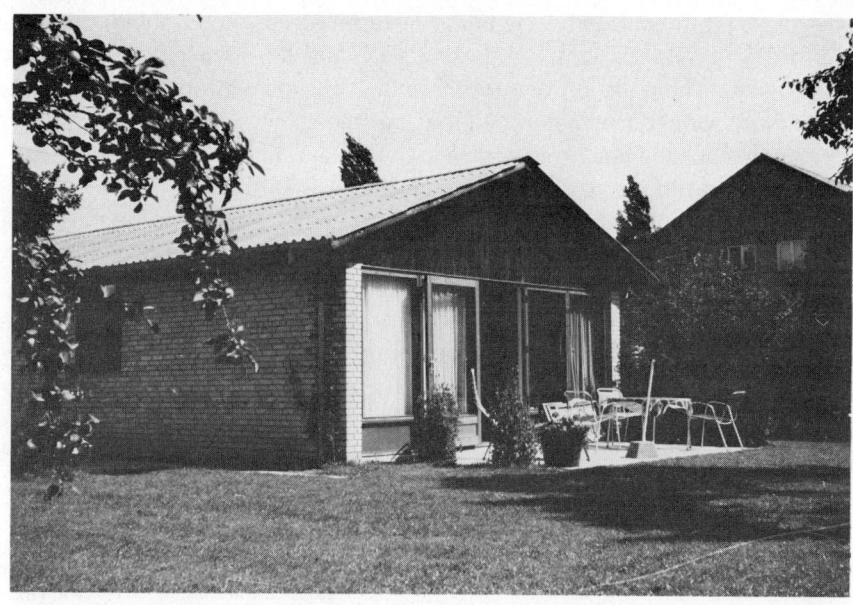

A

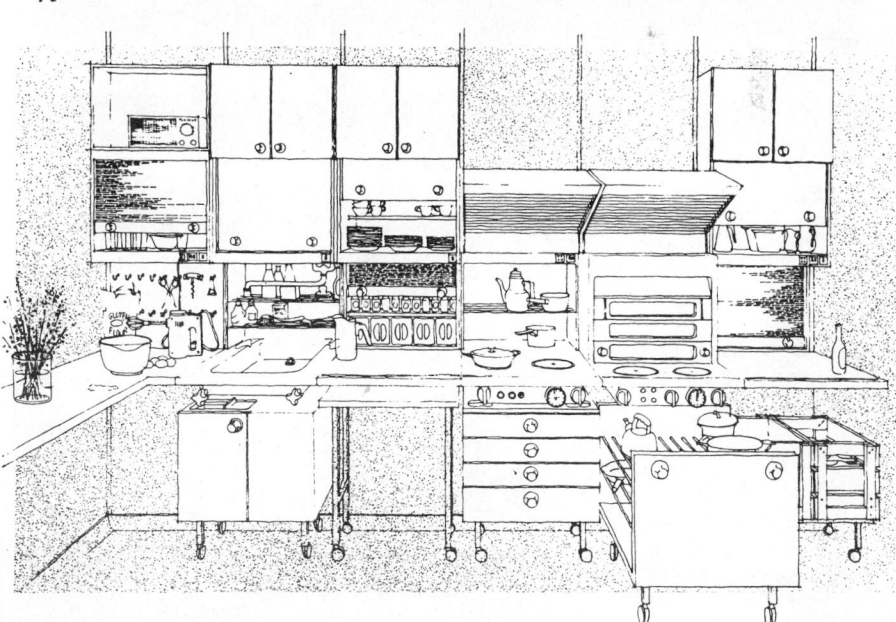

B

The collective house at Hans Knudsens Plads was the first of its kind in the world. Completed in 1959 at a cost of 15½ million Danish kroner, the building has 13 floors and 425 tenants. There are 170 apartments, all of which are adapted for the disabled, though only one-third are reserved for the disabled, one-third being for the orthopedic hospital nursing staff, and the remaining third for the general public. There are 60 one-room units, 31 with two rooms, and 70 with three or more rooms. The majority of the apartments have only a kitchenette for lighter meals since the tenants may dine in the restaurant on the premises or have dinner sent up from the restaurant kitchen (Fig. 18–14B).

There is a cleaning staff available to clean the apartments. The disabled who need attendant care for dressing, bathing, or toilet may phone for one of the 8 helpers that are paid by the government (Fig. 18–14). The staff totals 35 persons.

The 13th floor contains a nursing home for 15–17 poliomyelitis patients who require respiratory equipment. Single persons live in the nursing home; married persons live with their families during the day and sleep in the home at night or when their families are away. On the tenth floor are 26 single and double rooms for the use of disabled persons from the provinces while they are under treatment. In addition, 7 apartments accommodate 24 severely disabled young people who

Fig. 18–14. Bathroom at Hans Knudsens Plads with specially designed toilet and support bars that swing up to store on the wall. (Photograph courtesy of Preben Höybye-Mortensen, Society and Home for the Disabled)

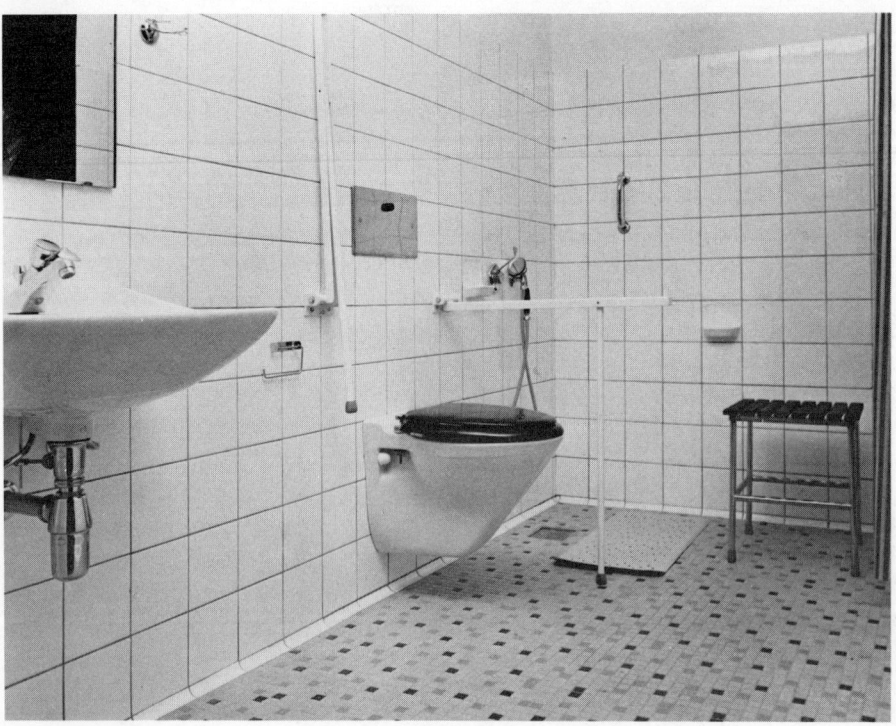

otherwise would have been in nursing homes. They are supervised by a male nurse.

In the collective houses and other blocks of apartments, only one-third are used by the disabled because it is considered desirable for disabled people to be integrated with the nondisabled. As an incentive to make adaptations for the disabled, the Ministry of Housing will cover the extra expenses of special equipment in collective houses. Public loans may be given for the adaptation or conversion of flats or houses to make them suitable for disabled persons.

Disability allowances are paid for those who cannot work or who are undergoing training, but a special grant is also paid to those who have serious medical disabilities and are employed. It is considered an incentive to work and a compensation for special expenses and trouble which the disabled person must encounter to keep his job.

An interesting experiment is the employing of a family member by the government to take care of a severely disabled relative. The relative is given some hospital training and then paid according to the financial needs of the family. This plan keeps the family together and saves public funds, since the cost of maintaining a patient in his own home is less by a third than the cost of maintaining him in a hospital; in addition, hospital beds and personnel are released for other purposes.

FEDERAL REPUBLIC OF GERMANY

This capsule of information is condensed from a very comprehensive survey of rehabilitation and residential facilities in West Germany which Marji Cappel prepared for the text. Because the survey far exceeded the space limitations it will be published in installments in the REHABILITATION GAZETTE. Wheelchaired and slightly ambulatory, Marji has been disabled by poliomyelitis since 1959. She is an artist and a poet; her husband is a professor.

Health insurance in Germany dates back to Prince Otto von Bismarck, who instituted social welfare legislation between 1881 and 1890. The present German government's policy is that it is far wiser and cheaper to pay for training an individual than to support him all his life by public funds. It has promised everyone the right to rehabilitation and integration into normal social life. Health insurance is obligatory for all employees. A 1971 law requires every business employing 16 or more persons to employ 6% disabled (at least 50% incapacitated) or pay a substantial fine. Sozialhilfe ("social help"), financed by social insurance fees and taxes, covers all necessary rehabilitation, equipment, and prosthetic devices.

Stiftung Rehabilitation, 69 Heidelberg 1, Postfach 101409, West Germany, is a huge government organization comprising many institutions. Among its concerns are social and professional education, medical and nursing care, psychologic and social therapy, sociology of education, rehabilitation counseling, vocational assessment and evaluation research. Its goals are to enable 80% of all disabled to be assimilated into normal social life by the early 1980s, to find a satisfying place in life for the other 20%, and to prevent disability. Stiftung is an excellent source for advice on architectural planning of buildings for the disabled.

Charitable religious organizations maintain the majority of the long-term residences and workshops for the disabled. Bethel, near Bielefeld, run by the Protestant State Church, was founded in 1867. It is a town in itself, with a population of 14,000, including 4000 disabled (epileptics, mentally ill or retarded, alcoholics, juvenile delinquents, migrant workers, elderly, and displaced). The Joseph's Association is part of Caritas, a charitable organization of the German State Catholic Church, which opened its first home for the disabled in 1864. It maintains 11 different establishments for disabled children and youth, 40% of whom have cerebral palsy.

Other significant organizations providing residential facilities: 1) Pfennigparade ("penny parade"), 8 Munich 40, Barlachstrasse 38, West Germany, concerns itself primarily with those disabled by poliomyelitis. It provides a 56-unit apartment house, a boarding home for students, an intensive care ward, and a computer programmer department. 2) Sozialhilfe, Selbsthilfe Koerperbehinderter e.V. (Social-Help, Self-Help for Physically Disabled), which was founded in 1955 by paraplegic Herr Eduard Knoll, includes 6000 other disabled members in 35 groups in different cities. The central establishment at Krautheim, 7109 Krautheim/Jagst, West Germany, contains living facilities with attendant services for 51 permanent residents and 30 guests. The organization has extensive plans for expansion. 3) Fokus-Deutschland, 2071 Hoisbuettel, Hamburger Str. 107a, West Germany, uses Swedish designs for special kitchen and bathroom installations in several hundred apartments designed for the disabled and interspersed among regular apartments. The installations are paid for by public funds, trade unions, insurance companies, or social offices. An interesting feature is that in the calculation of state support for rent for low income families, a disabled person counts as two.

A comprehensive book on the planning and construction of buildings for the disabled, both public and residential, was published by Deutsche Verlags-Anstalt in Stuttgart in 1974. Written by two of Germany's leading architects, Herbert Kuldschun and Erich Rossman, the book, *Planen und Bauen fuer Behinderte,* covers construction in Germany, Holland, Denmark, Sweden, and Switzerland. Copiously illustrated with photographs and floor plans, its only possible drawback is the fact that it is written in German.

FINLAND

The first philanthropic organizations at the turn of the century were the associations for the blind and deaf. Later, the associations to assist the disabled servicemen were formed. Eventually, all the organizations evolved into the Association of Disabled (Invalidiliitto r.y., Mannerheimintie 44, 00260 Helsinki 26, Finland). The Association is the nationwide central organization of the local associations of disabled persons. It safeguards the interests of the disabled in social planning and advises and guides individual disabled persons. It has developed rehabilitation hospitals, vocational training institutes, sheltered workshops, homebound work centers, holiday facilities, and residences.

FRANCE

A paraplegic, Joelle Hathaway of Pacific Grove, California, contacted the housing projects in France and translated their correspondence and brochures.

Groups of disabled individuals in France have been increasingly successful in establishing their own residential centers. Though in many instances only the first of a planned chain of residences with attendant care is in operation, the patterns are set, the models are functioning, and the future residences are on the drawing boards.

Guide de la France pour les Handicapés Physiques is a 382-page guide in French and English which is available from Comité National Français de Liaison pour la Réadaptation des Handicapés. A travel guide to Paris for the disabled, it includes accessible hotels, motels, homes, and apartments for vacation or year-round living.

Groupement des Intellectuels Handicapés Physiques, a dynamic group of young disabled students and professionals, recently opened its first residence for 25 at 8, Rue des Myosotis, 545 Vandoeuvre, Nancy, near the University of Nancy. The cost of accommodation is paid by a combination of Securité Sociale and l'Aide Sociale, with contributions from the residents' families, when possible. Transportation is furnished and meals are brought from the university restaurant.

The Club des Genêts, Boîte Postale 98, 79200 Parthenay, France, opened the first of a chain of residence clubs in 1972 (Fig. 18–15). The monthly dues include

Fig. 18–15. A. First residence of Club des Genêts. **B.** Eventually, such residences will cover all of France.

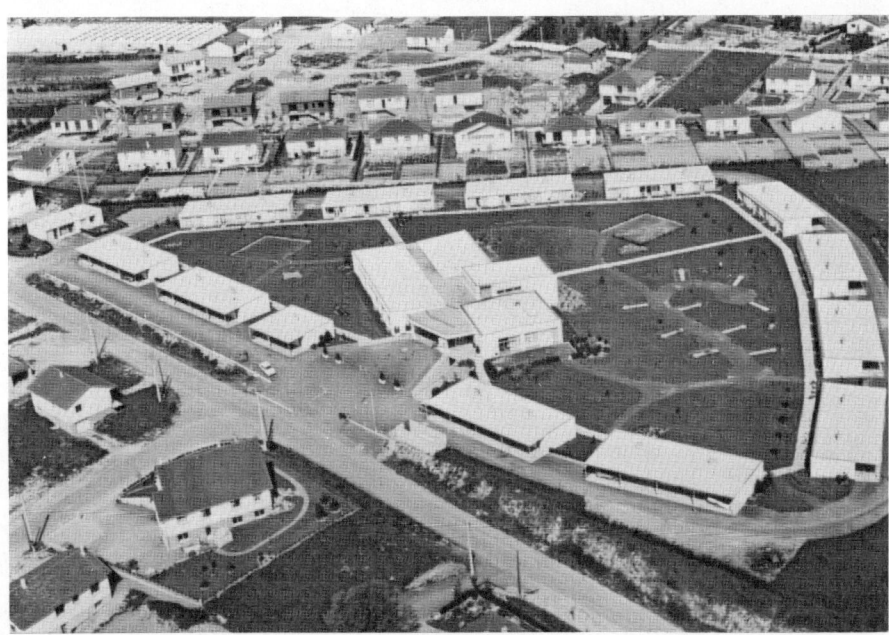

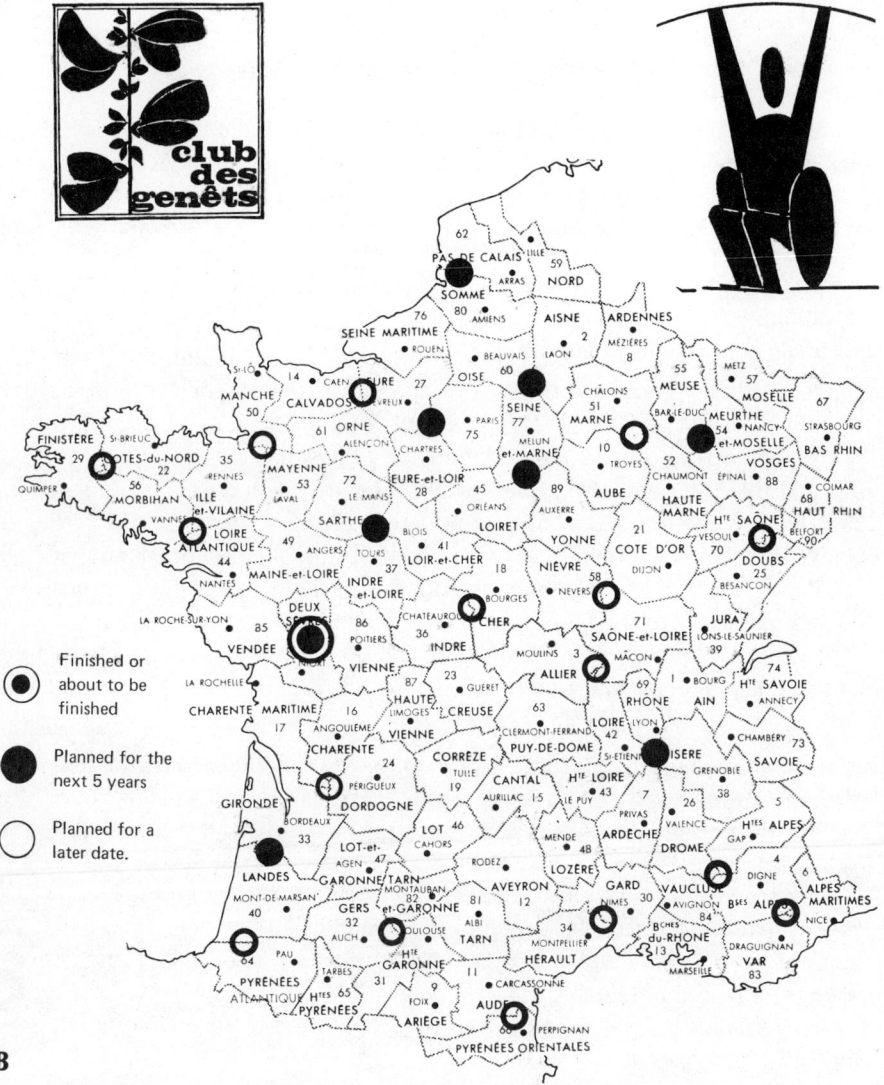

B

a furnished apartment, utilities, three meals a day, wine, and all services and leisure facilities of the club house.

Founded in 1933, Association des Paralysés de France, 27 Avenue Mozart, Paris 16, France, is composed of physically disabled individuals and parents of disabled children. It operates more than a dozen residences throughout France.

The following organizations concerned with housing for the disabled may be contacted for further information:

Association Française de Normalization, 23, rue Notre-Dame des Victoires, Paris 2, France.

Association pour le Logement des Grand Infirmes, 16 rue Hamelin, 75016 Paris, France.

Comité National Français de Liaison pour le Réadaptation des Handicapés, 38, Boulevard Raspail, 75007 Paris, France.

THE NETHERLANDS

The Netherlands Central Society for the Care of Disabled has acted as the central organizing body for rehabilitation activities since its founding in 1899. It has been concerned with rehabilitation and housing for many years, publishing one of the first studies of special adaptations, *Housing for the Disabled,* in 1960. Financial assistance is available for adapting homes or apartments to suit the individual's needs. Home service centers provide assistance (nursing care, home care, attendant care, laundry, and meals).

Het Dorp, Heijenoordseweg 150, Arnhem, Holland, is a village community of 400 severely disabled men and women which was developed by Dr. Arie Klapwijk, director of a rehabilitation center for children, and opened in 1966. Details are available in the booklet, in English, *Het Dorp: A Unique Experiment in Humanity* from Het Dorp. The village is located on a wooded and rolling 44-acre site at the edge of the residential area of Arnhem, a town of 300,000. To facilitate integration and employment the village comprises a shopping center, supermarket, post office, workshop, gasoline station, restaurant, barber shop, beauty parlor, and travel agency.

Each resident has his or her own self-contained apartment, individually furnished and equipped. Each group of ten apartments is a self-sufficient unit, with a laundry room, guest rooms, kitchenette, and a large living/dining room. The main meal is brought from the central kitchen. Nine of the apartments are assigned to the disabled, the tenth is for a staff attendant known as a "dogela." Most of the 200 dogelas live at Het Dorp, thus giving a more normal balance to the village. The cost per diem is about $18; those who can afford it pay their way; others are supported by the state and the Het Dorp Foundation. About half of the disabled villagers work in the sheltered workshop. Het Dorp may seem to be a ghetto, but it is an alternative to institutionalization and offers a well-designed setting for those who need and want its sheltered life.

SWEDEN

by ADOLF RATZKA

Adolf Ratzka has been quadriplegic and dependent on a respirator for sleeping because of poliomyelitis since he was 18. He was born in Czechoslovakia, grew up in Bavaria, and attended the University of California, Los Angeles. He is a doctoral candidate in urban economics from UCLA and has been doing his dissertation research in Stockholm since 1973.

Neutrality and nonintervention during both World Wars, industrialization, and 40 uninterrupted years of social-democratic administration have turned Sweden into a modern and wealthy nation. Considered by many a testing ground for new ideas in social planning, Sweden has received much attention and criticism.

The provision of public housing receives high priority by the government. About 90% of the total current construction is financed in part by government loans at below market terms. Eligible households are entitled to a housing allowance; the amount depends on family size, income, and housing costs. An annual income of some $10,000 might be considered average for full-time work. If this is the only income of a family of four, an additional $2500 in the form of the various allowances might be forthcoming. Yet taxes might amount to $4000. Taxation is rather progressive; on an income of $30,000 one might have to pay 87%.

Planning for housing the handicapped is done at the local, county, and central government level, usually by public agencies with well-defined tasks rather than by the handicapped. Most interesting to foreigners is probably the Handikappinstitutet, (address: Handikappinstitutet, Fack, 161 25 Bromma 1) which is the main public organ for generating research, developing new products, and disseminating information. Equipped with an electronics lab and an automotive workshop where cars are modified for para and quad drivers, the Institute houses periodic conferences and exhibitions on technical aids as well as an impressively comprehensive library and the Committee on Technical Aids, Housing, and Transportation (ICTA) of the International Society for Rehabilitation of the Disabled. The other main research center is Professor Brattgård's Institute for Research for the Handicapped at Gothenberg University.

Most municipalities have a Handikappråd (Council for the Handicapped) whose purpose is to coordinate planning efforts between the various city departments and to serve as a clearinghouse for information on new developments that might benefit the disabled population. These councils also exist at the county and the national level.

In Stockholm there is also the Handikappbyrån (Office of the Handicapped), a branch of the city administration that runs such programs as the Transportation Service for the Handicapped and the Housing Allowance for the Handicapped. The office also runs an information service concerning not only the various services the disabled are entitled to but also accessible places such as restaurants, theaters, shops, etc., in Stockholm and popular vacation spots.

Most of the handicapped are members of the two large organizations of the disabled. One is a coalition of all the special membership groups like the Association of Traffic and Polio Victims, the Association of the Blind, etc. The other organization consists of members with all types of mostly physical disabilities. These two organizations have a net of local chapters all over Sweden and well-established political connections. There has been much improvement in the situation of the disabled in Sweden–due in large part to the lobbying efforts of these organizations. But change comes slowly. The organizations are heavily bureaucratized, and a good deal of effort seems to go toward maintaining them. Other activities include keeping the membership informed about their rights, running vacation resorts, a citizen band radio club where an operator passes messages from disabled drivers on to third parties via telephone, and organizing social functions.

In dealing with the authorities the organizations rely exclusively on their board members. Their style is—typically for Sweden—cooperation, not confrontation. Younger, impatient members seem to get soon frustrated judging from the very few faces under 35 at the meetings. A refreshing contrast to these established organizations is the tiny Anti-Handikapp group with chapters mainly in Lund and Stockholm. Conditional to the integration of the disabled is a basic change in the structure of Swedish society which leads to political, economic, and social equalization. Toward this goal Anti-Handikapp is working through such activities as issuing a quarterly magazine, performing plays, arranging exhibits, and organizing handicapped youth.

In addition to the assistance programs for the general population, the handicapped are entitled to several other such services. In order to qualify for the following programs the nature and extent of the disability has to be certified by a medical doctor or rehabilitation specialist such as the district nurse or a physical therapist at the district hospital.

A disabled person with no or insufficient income from employment receives a $250 pension, just as a retired person does, plus an additional $65/month in recognition of the fact that a disabled person has generally higher costs of living. A disabled student, in addition to the $200/month study loan, is entitled to a $125/month pension.

A whole range of technical aids, including power wheelchairs, is provided free of charge regardless of income. To name just a few, the list of free items includes patient lifters, page turners, hearing aids, tape recorders, prosthetic devices, a whole array of household helps such as dishwashers and washing machines, etc., if the need is certified. A disabled person who is dependent upon an automobile for transportation in connection with work or education qualifies for financial help in purchasing and modifying the car. For those disabled persons who cannot or prefer not to drive their own car and cannot use public transportation, a special transportation service is provided in many communities.

Most cities have a Home Service (Hemtjänst), a branch of the city's Social Services Department, through which the aged and handicapped receive help in their daily living routine, *i.e.,* with shopping, cooking, cleaning, and personal hygiene. In an interview with the department, needs are assessed in terms of hours of help. This service is means tested, but low income persons receive it free. Most of the helpers are middle-aged neighborhood women who receive a base rate of $4.50/hour on week days and up to $6/hour for nights and weekends. Since $4.50 is close to the bottom of the wage rate, there is a chronic shortage of helpers in Stockholm.

In Stockholm the policy is to reduce total housing costs to the household to 12 to 20% of the gross income depending on family size. Conditions are certification of the disability and a functional housing unit. Amounts of up to $3750 and in some cases even more can be granted to adapt housing for a handicapped person. The grant, called Bostadsanpassningsbidrag (Housing Adaptation Grant) is not means tested. The sum can be applied to existing housing whether owner occupied or rented as well as to housing to be constructed. Depending on the individual's needs rooms can be added, walls moved, stairs ramped, tracks for patient lifts mounted to the ceiling, kitchen and bathroom equipment changed, etc. In the case of expensive modifications the authorities will investigate alternative solutions such as moving to another place. In general, however, the policy is to enable persons who become disabled to remain where they have been living if they so desire.

The so-called "interspersed housing units for the handicapped" (insprängda handikapplägenheter) may be in municipally owned or cooperative housing or built by other nonprofit construction firms. There are a few specially designed apartments in many of their large high-rise developments, but statistics on the number of such units are unavailable at this point. Their production is tied to new construction activity. With the present slump of the construction industry and 10,000 vacant apartments in Greater Stockholm, the number of such units for the handicapped is not likely to increase considerably in the near future.

Fig. 18–16. The Fokus apartment at Mölndal near Göteborg. **A.** The 48 square meter apartment is for one person. **B.** The 78 square meter apartment contains two rooms and a kitchen. **C.** The 96 square meter apartment with three rooms and a kitchen is planned for families. **D.** A Fokus kitchen assembly designed for use by a single person. All working areas can be adjusted in height. Telescopic plastic pipes and flexible hoses are used at the sink. **E.** The shower and the sink are interchangeable and may be raised or lowered. There are alarm buttons in every room. (Drawings and plans supplied by Dr. Sven-Olof Brattgård, The Folkus Society)

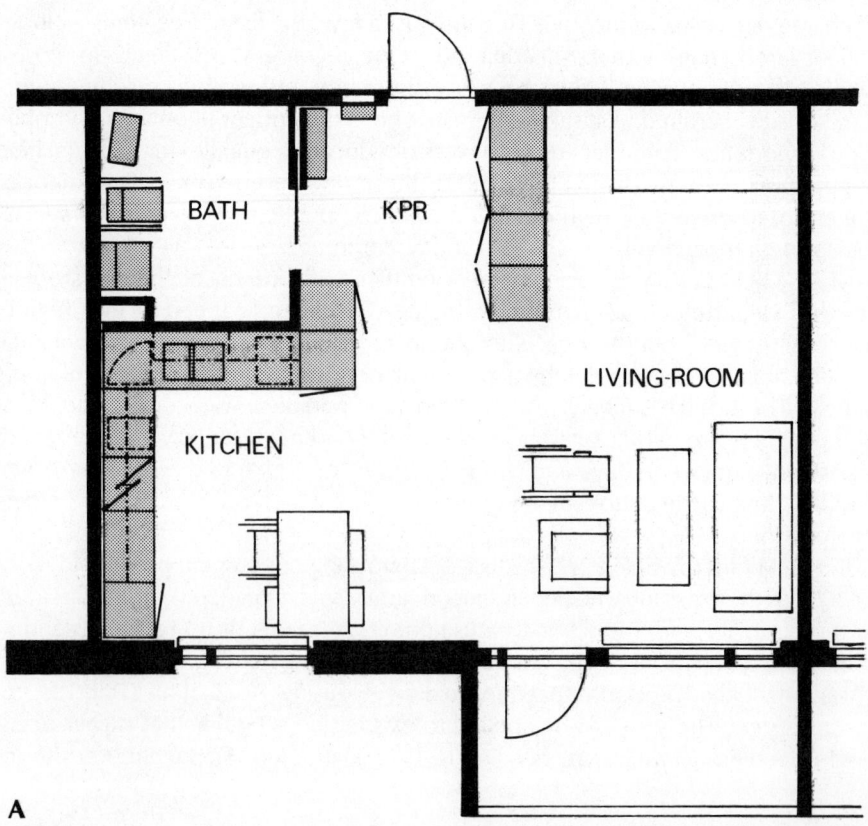

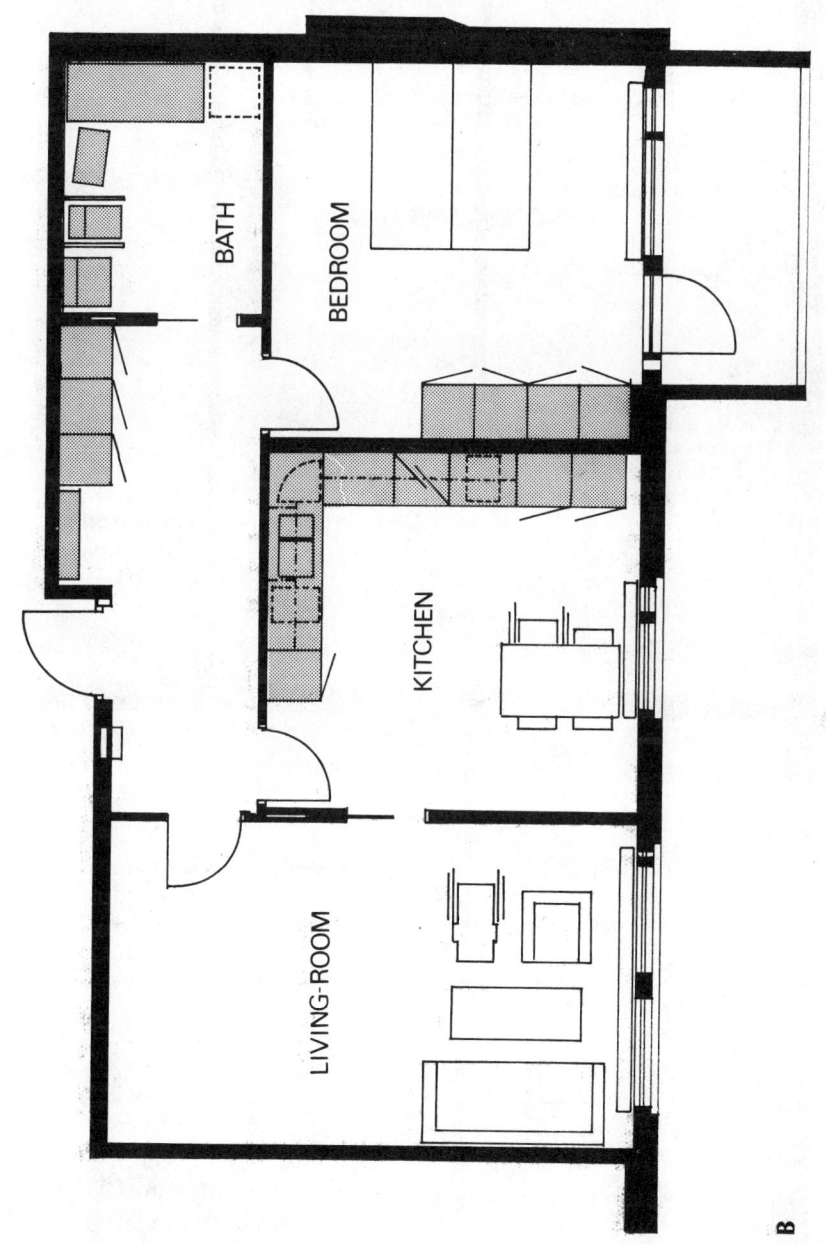

B

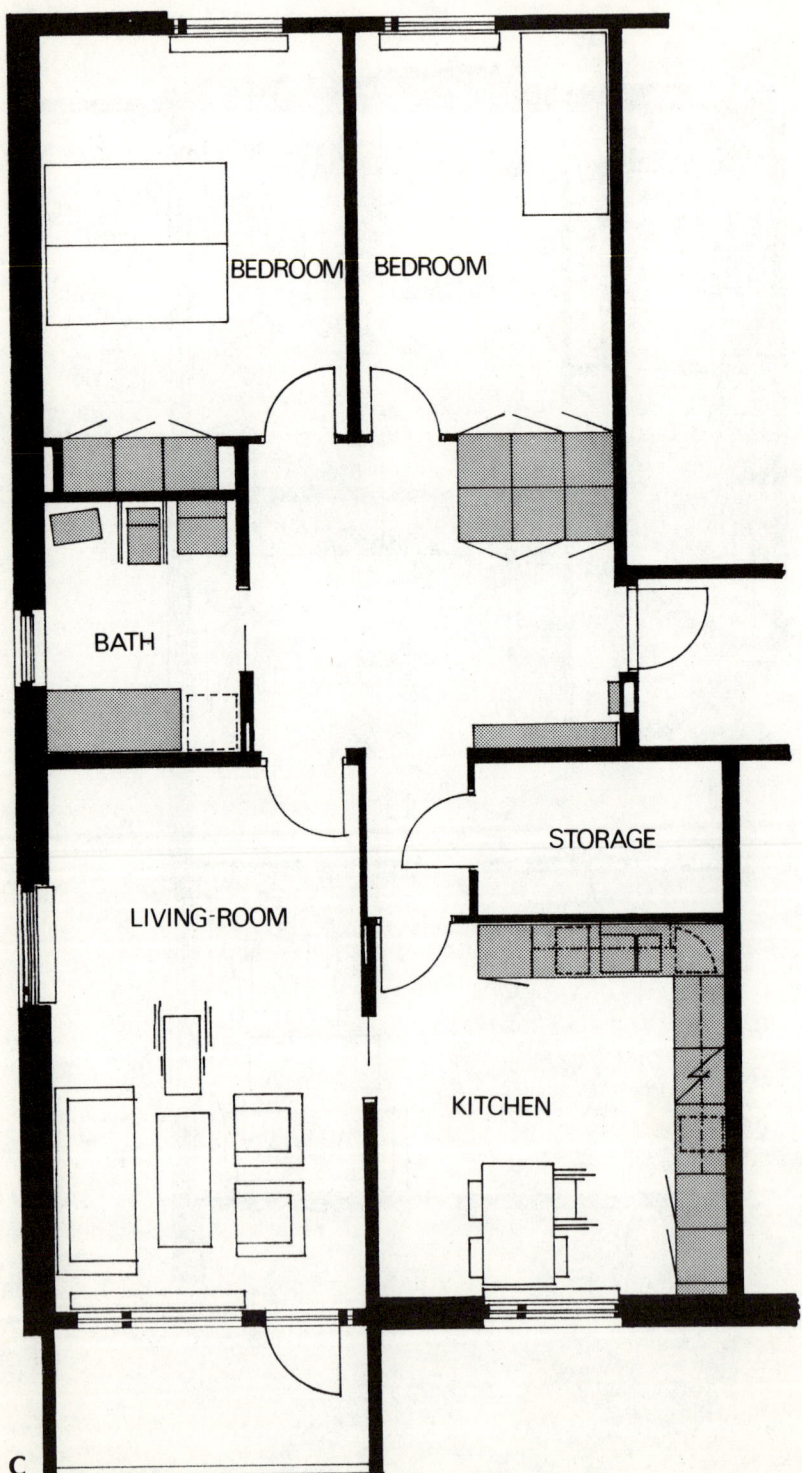

fig. 18–16 continued

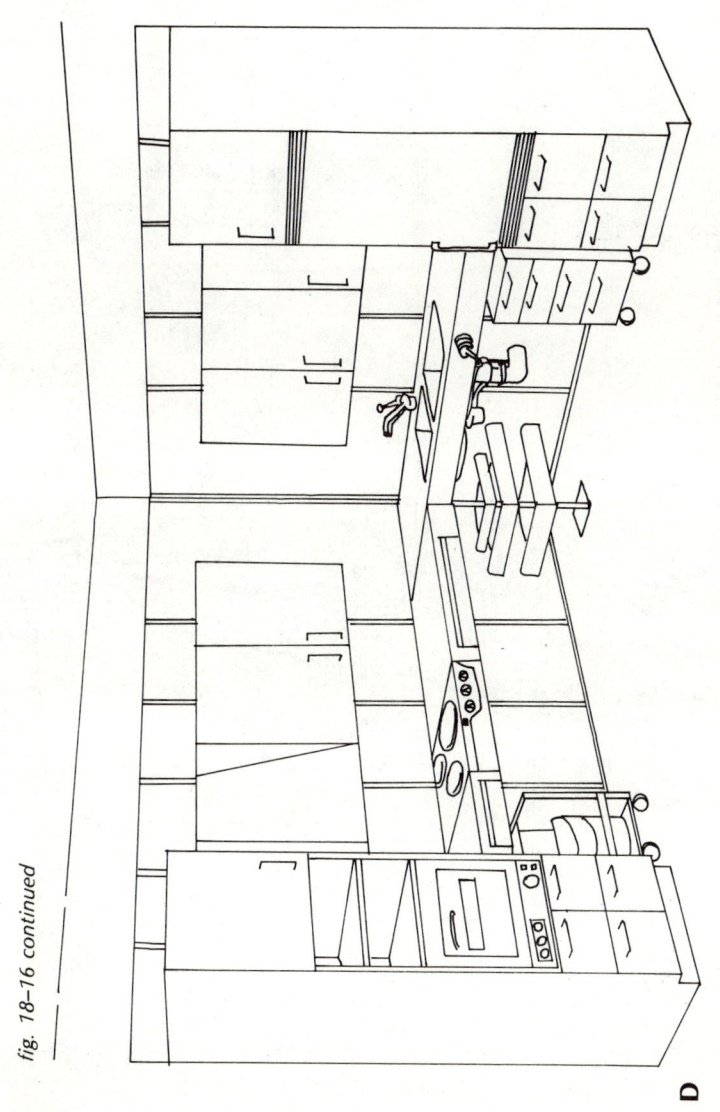

fig. 18–16 continued

D

fig. 18–16 continued

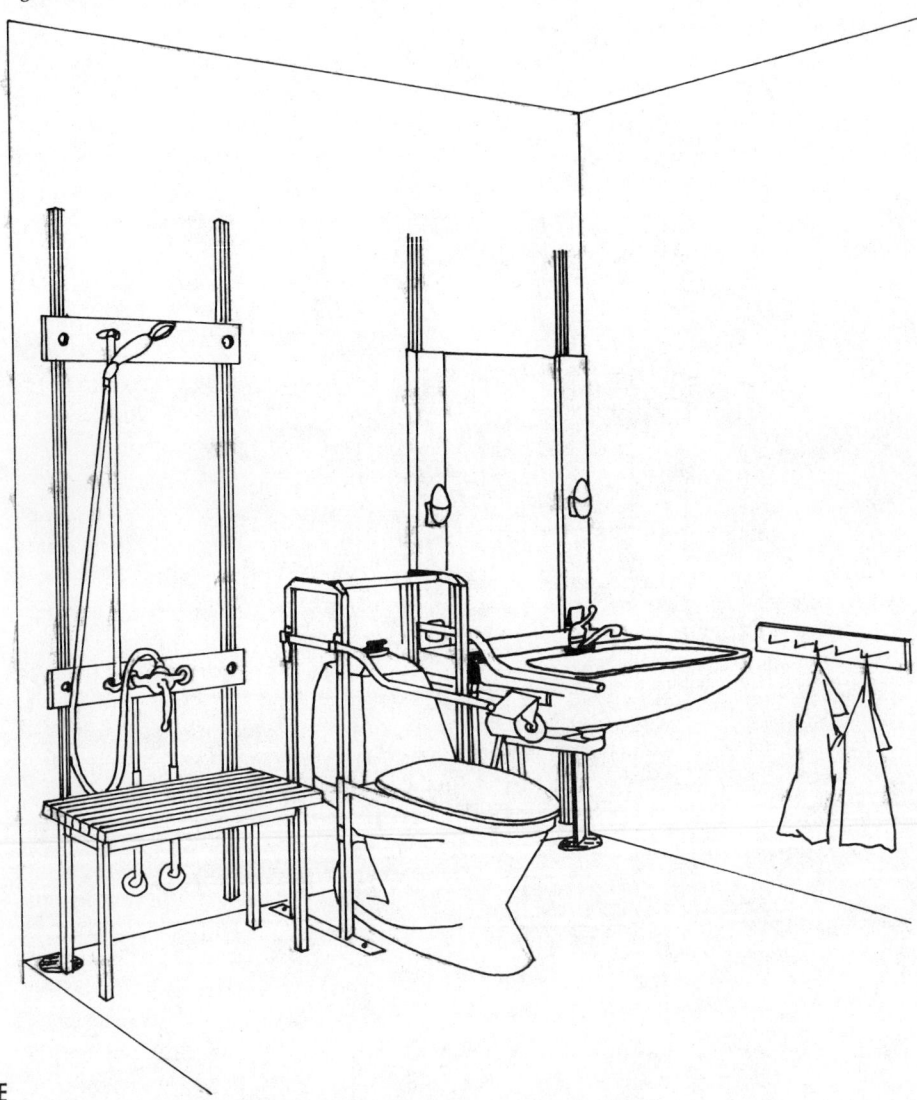

E

Another alternative for wheelchair living are the Service Houses (Service hus). The idea is derived from the Scandinavian and East European cooperative movement and is quite old: many households living in high density in a large building complex make it possible to provide services that are unavailable or too costly in terms of time and money to families living in, say, single family housing, services that are meant to free the individual from many chores, to enable him or her to participate in many group activities and to escape the isolation of the nuclear family.

There are 500–600 such Service House apartments in Sweden today. Of these,

260 were built by the now defunct Fokus Society, whose activities began in 1964. Fokus can be considered a pioneer in providing actual examples of housing integration. The society has been discontinued for lack of funds, but its concept is still valid (Fig. 18–16). Since other countries have become interested in the work of the Fokus Society, more detailed information is included in Appendix D.

There are not enough halfway houses where the young handicapped or recently disabled person can try independent living after institutionalization yet have a reliable backup system. Originally the Fokus apartments were planned for this purpose, but due to the very low turn-over, the Service Houses became permanent housing. After waiting a long time to get into a Service House, a resident is not likely to leave its convenience and security.

The question here is: What should be the long run goals of a housing policy for the handicapped? Most want complete housing integration, that is to be able to visit neighbors and friends, to stay overnight where one pleases, and to choose one's residence with the same degree of freedom as the general population. It seems clear that the concept of Service Houses and interspersed apartments, with their limited choice of locations, conflicts with this goal. To remedy the present shortage of housing and service facilities in the short run more Service Houses and interspersed units are needed. But to push these housing forms as long run solutions means to give up the goal of housing integration; the existence of Service Houses and interspersed units serves as an excuse on the part of society not to make all housing adaptable to wheelchair living.

The handicapped population in Sweden is probably materially speaking better off than in most other countries. In comparison to the general Swedish population, however, the disabled as a group are still underprivileged in terms of income, educational achievement and job opportunities, as government investigations have shown. Despite the efforts in the area of housing, service and transportation they are handicapped by severe restrictions in their mobility, choice of location, and lifestyle.

This is generally the danger with special solutions to the problems of the handicapped—"special" in the sense that some measure is aimed exclusively at the handicapped. An example is the Transportation Service for the Handicapped. It serves to segregate the handicapped from the general population and relieves the public transportation authorities from making all busses and subways accessible to everybody including those who are temporarily or permanently handicapped be it because of a cast, old age, pregnancy, a baby carriage, a wheelchair or because of blindness. Here another example of a "special" solution: The entrance to one of the new and accessible subway stations in Stockholm consists of perhaps 10 swing doors. One door in the middle, marked with the international symbol of access, is about 6" wider than the rest. Instead of simply making all doors 6" wider the architects remind us through the symbol

NORWAY

Details of the architecture and housing for the disabled in Norway may be obtained in the following publications in Norwegian:

BOLIGER FOR ALLE? (Freedom for All?). By Laila Nikolaisen and Marit Skiple. Oslo. Norges Vanfrelags. 120 pages. August, 1974. The publication describes architectural details of housing for the disabled, particularly adaptations to bathrooms and kitchens. It is available from Sosialforlaget A/S, Dopsgt. 7, Oslo 1, Norway, for kr. 17.50 ($3.15).

PROGRAMMERING OG LANLEGGING AV UTBYGGINGSOMRÅDER. By Marit Skipple. Oslo. Norges Vanførelag. 104 pages. October, 1974. This attractively illustrated report by architects and medical personnel summarizes the planning for integrating the disabled into housing programs.

SPAIN

Information on housing in Spain may be secured from Fraternidad Católica de Enfermos, Domicilio Social, Montserrat, 30, Madrid 8, Spain, an international organization of disabled individuals. The members of the more than 50 chapters in Spain hold monthly meetings in their centers, which are always open. Some have organized work projects, others serve wine and snacks to the general public; most have space for residential facilities for permanent and transient guests.

SWITZERLAND

Several projects involving small numbers of apartments for the disabled within normal apartment houses have been opened in Lancy and Geneva within the last few years. Details of these and more traditional facilities are contained in the book, *Institutions de Réadaption,* which has a section on apartments and homes, vacation homes, workshops, schools, and hospitals. Priced at 15 Swiss francs, it is available from Zentralsekretariat Pro Infirmis, Feldeggstrasse 71, Postfach 129, CH—8032 Zurich, Switzerland.

YUGOSLAVIA

The imaginative rehabilitation program of Yugoslavia, operating from 12 rehabilitation centers located throughout the country, is incorporated into the national health program. At present, 95% of the people who need rehabilitation are covered by national health insurance; the others pay for their own medical needs or are assisted by local governments.

As a result of the services of the centers, permanent institutional care is almost unknown in Yugoslavia. While a patient is in a center he is instructed in self-care, given vocational retraining, and his home is adapted to his needs. If the immediate family or relatives are unable to manage his care, foster homes are secured. Some centers send busloads of physiotherapists out each day to the homes of patients who cannot get to the center.

Several special apartments for the disabled are being built in the new suburbs of Belgrade. Plans are also afoot to set up several groups of apartments in such a way that residents can share one or two attendants.

Bibliography

ASIA

THE ACTIVITY OF JAPAN ABILITIES ASSOCIATION. The First Experimental Factory Operated by Laymen. Translation. By H. Itoh. August, 1974.

Homemaking Handbook for Village Workers in Many Countries, Extension Service, United States Department of Agriculture, in cooperation with Agency for International Development, United States Department of State. PA–953. Superintendent of Documents, United States Government Printing Office, Washington, D.C. 20402. March, 1971. $1.75.

Labour Ability of the Paraplegics—Japan Sun Industries. By Y. Nakamura. JOURNAL OF REHABILITATION IN ASIA, Vol. 15, No. 4, pages 7–12, October, 1974.

Working Ability of the Paraplegics. By Y. Nakamura. PARAPLEGIA, Vol. II, No. 2, pages 182–193, August, 1973.

AUSTRALIA

The Development of Rehabilitation Services in Australia. INTERNATIONAL REHABILITATION REVIEW, Vol. 22, pages 4–8. 1971.

DIRECTORY OF SOCIAL WELFARE RESOURCES, SOUTH AUSTRALIA. 1974. Prepared by The Citizens' Advice Bureau (Adelaide).

The Home for Incurables. By J. McLean. PHOENIX NEWS, Vol. 10, pages 14–16, 1971.

THE HOME THAT CARES. Auxiliary to the Home for Incurables. By M. Tuckwell. 1969.

MERMAID ON WHEELS. The Story of Margaret Lester, a paraplegic architect. By June Epstein. Ure Smith Pty Limited, Sydney and London, 1967.

New Commonwealth Rehabilitation Centre at Glen Waverly, Victoria. REHABILITATION IN AUSTRALIA. Vol. 10, No. 1, pages 12–14, January, 1973.

The Paraplegic Association of W.A. By V. Smith. AUSTRALIAN PARAPLEGIC, Vol. 6, pages 10–11, 1970.

THE PARAPLEGIC AND QUADRIPLEGIC ASSOCIATION OF NEW SOUTH WALES TWELFTH ANNUAL REPORT. 1973.

The Phoenix Society Incorporated. PHOENIX NEWS, Vol. 14, pages 26–27, 1974.

THE SEVERELY DISABLED CEREBRAL PALSIED IN INDUSTRY. By Neil McLeod. Published for the 1971 Conference on International Rehabilitation Patterns for the Multi-Handicapped in New York City. Available from The Spastic Centre of New South Wales, Allambie Heights, Sydney 2100

SURVEY REPORT OF PARAPLEGICS AND QUADRIPLEGICS IN NEW SOUTH WALES. Covering a period between 1st May, 1969, and 31st December, 1970. The Paraplegic and Quadriplegic Association of N.S.W.

CZECHOSLOVAKIA

Born Again. By Irena Krausová, CZECHOSLOVAK LIFE, Vol. XXVIII, pages 22–23, 1973.

Solution of the Problem of Housing the Disabled in Czechoslovakia. By Jan Brázdil, draft report, March, 1974.

DENMARK

The Cripples' Building Society. Brochure, 1963.

Samfundet og Hjemmet for Vanføre (The Society and Home for the Disabled). 109-page descriptive booklet in English and Danish, 1974.

The Danish Approach to Residential Care and Community Integration. By F. Frederickson in PERSONAL RELATIONSHIPS, THE HANDICAPPED AND THE COMMUNITY. SOME EUROPEAN THOUGHTS AND SOLUTIONS. Edited by D. Lancaster-Gaye. Routledge & Kegan Paul Ltd., Broadway House, 68–74 Carter Lane, London EC4V 5EL, England, and 9 Park Street, Boston, Massachusetts 02108. Pages 41–51. 1972.

FEDERAL REPUBLIC OF GERMANY

Books

Denk, Horst (editor). *Bundessozialhilfe Gesetz.* Muenchen: Wilhelm Goldmann Verlag, 1974

Kuldschun, Herbert and Erich Rossman. *Planen und Bauen fuer Behinderte.* Stuttgart: Deutsche Verlags-Anstalt, 1974.

Sagi, Alexander. *Das Koerperbehinderte Kind.* Freiburg im Breisgau: Lambertus-Verlag, 1966.

Catalogs of Establishments

Ausbildungseinrichtungen fuer behinderte Jugendliche. Nuernberg: Bundesanstalt fuer Arbeit, 1974.

Berufsfoerderungswerke, Stand 1975/1976. Bonn: Bundesministerium fuer Arbeit und Sozialordung, 1974.

Berufsfoerderungswerke, Stand 1973/1974. same as above.

Katholische Einrichtungen der Heim-und Heilpaedagogik in der Bundesrepublik Deutschland. Freiburg im Breisgau: Verband katholischer Einrichtungen fuer Heim- und Heilpaedagogik, 1973.

Kubale, Siegfried. *Rehabilitations-Einrichtungen fuer Kinder und Jugendendliche.* Berlin—Charlottenburg: Carl Marhold Verlagsbuchhandlung, 1968.

Verzeichnis der Anstalten, Kliniken und Einrichtungen fuer die Eingliederung und Pflege Koerperbehinderter in Deutschland. Heidelberg: Eigenverlag der Deutschen Vereinigung zur Foerderung der Koerperbehindertenfuer—soerge e.V., Orthopaedische Klinik, printed by Beltz Verlag (Weinheim), 1959.

Verzeichnis der dem Diakonischen Werk angeschlossenen Einrichtungen fuer behinderte Menschen. Stuttgart: Das Diakonische Werk (Protestant Church), 1971.

Pamphlets, Periodicals, Similar Publications, (1 Article)

Auf dem Weg zur Umfassenden Rehabilitation. Heidelberg: Verlag der Stiftung Rehabilitation, 1974.

Aufgabenstellung, Organizationsstruktur und Gliederung. Heidelberg: Stiftung, 1975.

Auftrag und Aufgaben. Heidelberg: Stiftung, 1974.

Die Berufstherapie. Heidelberg: Stiftung, 1974.

Die Stiftung. Heidelberg: Stiftung, Januar, 1975.

Fink, (Dr.) "Der bayerische Behindertenplan." *Leben und Weg der Koerperbehinderte,* Krautheim, (February, 1975), page 10.

Fokus-Dokumentation. Hoisbuettel: Fokus Deutschland, 1973. (loose-leaf, large)

Jahrbuch 1973, Josefs-Gesellschaft e.V. Bigge-Olsberg: Josefs-Druckerei, 1974.

Orthopaedische Klinik und Poliklinik der Universitaet Heidelberg. 50 year anniversary publication. Heidelberg, 1972.

Pfennigparade, Muenchen: roughly 10 small pamphlets and leaflets over 5 years.

Sozialpolitische Information. Bonn: Bundesministerium fuer Arbeit und Sozialordnung, Dec., 1973. (bulletin)

Suedwestdeutsches Rehabilitationskrankenhaus. Heidelberg: Stiftung R., 1974.

Zeitgerechte berufliche Bildung fuer Behinderte. Heidelberg: Stiftung, 1974.

FINLAND

Rehabilitation in Finland. By Aulikki Kananoja. Published by the ISRD Finnish Committee, Helsinki, Finland. 1972. Available free from the Finnish Consulate, Washington, D.C.

Social Security in Finland. The National Rehabilitation and Preventive Care Scheme. 1974. Available free from the Finnish Consulate, Washington, D.C.

FRANCE

GUIDE DE LA FRANCE POUR LES HANDICAPÉS PHYSIQUES. Edited by Europe Handicap. Available from Comité National Français de Liaison pour la Réadaptation des Handicapés (Dept. S), 38 Boulevard Raspail, 75007 Paris, France. 52 francs ($8.50 including postage).

GREAT BRITAIN

AN ABC OF SERVICES AND GENERAL INFORMATION FOR DISABLED PEOPLE. Disablement Income Group, Queen's House, 180/182A, Tottenham Court Road, London W1P OBD, England. 10 pence (20¢) or free to disabled.

CHESHIRE SMILE. Quarterly publication of the Cheshire Homes. Order from Greenacres, 39 Vesey Road, Sutton Coldfield, Warwickshire B73 5NR, England. 50 pence/year. (From U.S. send $2.)

Handicapped and Impaired in Great Britain. Part I. By Amelia I. Harris with Elizabeth Cox and Christopher R. W. Smith. Social Survey Division. HMSO. 1971. £3.50. ($7)

Handicapped and Impaired in Great Britain. Part II. Working and Housing of Impaired Persons. By Judith R. Buckle. Social Survey Division. HMSO. 1971. £2.25. ($4.50)

HOUSING FOR PEOPLE WHO ARE PHYSICALLY HANDICAPPED. Department of the Environment and Welsh Office Joint Circular 74/74 and 120/74. London, Her Majesty's Stationery Office, 1974.

INTERNATIONAL PATTERNS OF RESIDENT CARE FOR THE MULTI-HANDICAPPED. By James Loring. Presented at Conference on International Rehabilitation Patterns for the Multi-Handicapped. New York, October, 1971.

A LIFE APART. A Pilot Study of Residential Institutions for the Physically Handicapped and the Young Chronic Sick. By E. J. Miller, G. V. Gwynne. London, Tavistock Publications Ltd., 1972.

RESIDENTIAL ACCOMMODATION FOR DISABLED PEOPLE. By Jean Symons AA Dipl, RIBA. London, Centre on Environment for the Handicapped, 1974.

SPASTIC NEWS. Monthly tabloid. Order from Circulation Clerk, Spastic News, 12 Park Crescent, London W1N 4EQ, England. 5 pence per copy (from U.S. send $2).

SPINAL CORD INJURIES. Comprehensive Management and Research. By Sir Ludwig Guttmann. Oxford, Blackwell Scientific Publications, 1973.

The United Kingdom Approach to Residential Care. By Derek Lancaster–Gaye. In PERSONAL RELATIONSHIPS, THE HANDICAPPED AND THE COMMUNITY. Edited by D. Lancaster–Gaye. London, Routledge & Kegan Paul, pages 11–24, 1972.

THE NETHERLANDS

Het Dorp: A Unique Experiment in Humanity. Brochure by the Het Dorp Foundation.

Is it Right for Everyone? Two Personal Views of Het Dorp. By Rosalie Wilkins and Selwyn Goldsmith. THE CORD, Vol. 24, No. 3, 1972.

"No One at Home" A Brief Review of Housing for Handicapped Persons in Some European Countries. By Deborah Greenstein, Charles Gueli, and Edmond Leonard. REHABILITATION LITERATURE. Pages 2–9. Vol. 37, No. 1, January, 1976.

Operation Matchbox. By David Cohen. SPASTICS NEWS, April, 1972.

Rehabilitation Officer's Report of Visit to Britain and Europe. By Blanche Lindsay. The Paraplegic and Quadriplegic Association of New South Wales, Australia.

NORWAY

BOLIGER FOR ALLE? (FREEDOM FOR ALL?) By Laila Nikolaisen and Marit Skiple. Sosialforlaget A/S. Oslo. 1974.

PROGRAMMERING OG LANLEGGING AV UTBYGGINGSOMRÅDER by Marit Skiple. Norges Vanførelag. 1974.

SPAIN

BOLETIN INFORMATIVO FRATERNIDAD. Monthly bulletin published by Fraternidad Católica de Enfermos, Domicilio Social, Montserrat, 30, Madrid 8, Spain.

SWEDEN

SOU 1970:64 *Bättre socialtjänst för handikappade,* Allmänna Förlaget, Stockholm 1970

SOU 1969:35 *Bättre utbildning för handikappade,* Allmänna Förlaget Stockholm 1969

SOU 1972:30 *Bostadsanpassningsbidrag,* Allmänna Förlaget, Stockholm 1972

Svenska kommunförbundet, *Serviveboende—bostäder för svårt handikappade,* memorandum dated May 7, 1974.

Kungl. Bostadsstyrelsen, *God Bostad i dag och i morgon,* Stockholm 1964.

Satens planverk, *Svensk Byggnorm SBN Kap 691 Handikappbyggnormer* Stockholm 1974.

Bostadsstyrelsen tekniska byrån, *Forslag till bostadsnormer för lägenheter och hus,* Stockholm February 1973.

SWITZERLAND

INSTITUTIONS DE RÉADAPTATION. Zentralsekretariat Pro Infirmis, Feldeggstrasse 71, Postfach 129, CH-8032, Zurich, Switzerland.

YUGOSLAVIA

Travel Notes: Yugoslavia. By Blanche and Lenny Goldwater. REHABILITATION GAZETTE, Vol. XIV, pages 74–77, 1971.

Functional and Physical Obstruction in Living Environment of Disabled Persons. By Bosko M. Zotovic, MD. Joint research project between Social and Rehabilitation Service, Washington, D.C., and Center for Prosthetics, Belgrade, 1975.

Appendices

Appendix A

The International Symbol of Access

The international symbol of access was adopted by Rehabilitation International in 1969 at its 11th World Congress of Rehabilitation of the Disabled. The symbol, indicating that a building or facility intended for public use is accessible to the wheelchaired, is in use throughout the world.

The symbol may not be changed; it should be used in the original design and proportions. It may be reproduced either in black and white or dark blue and white.

Although intended originally to identify accessible facilities, the symbol has also been used on automobile license tags in a number of states to indicate the driver is wheelchaired.

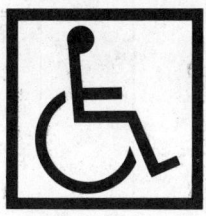

Appendix B

ACCESSIBILITY FOR DISABLED PERSONS—NORMS IN DIFFERENT COUNTRIES

ALL MEASUREMENTS IN METERS. 1 INCH = 0.025. 1 FOOT = 0.33
MEASUREMENTS OF WC-ROOM AND LIFTCAR REFER TO WIDTH × DEPTH

COUNTRY	WIDTH OF WALK (PATH)[1]	WIDTH OF CORRIDOR[1]	FREE WIDTH OF DOORS	MEASUREMENTS OF WC-ROOM	MEASUREMENTS OF LIFTCAR, DOOR-WIDTH OF LIFTCAR	WIDTH OF PARKING AREA	INCLINATION OF RAMP	HEIGHT ABOVE FLOOR OF SWITCHES AND CONTROLS
Belgium	—	2.00	0.86, 0.90	1.80 × 2.10	1.20 × 1.50 0.86, 0.90	3.30, 3.60	1:20	—
Canada	ca 1.65	—	0.81	ca 1.80 × 2.80	—	ca 4.00	1:12	—
Denmark[2]	1.30	1.30 (1.40)	0.83	2.20 × 1.80	1.10 × 1.20 0.83	3.50	1:12	0.90–1.20
Federal Rep. of Germany	1.20	1.40	0.85	1.80 × 2.00 2.20 × 2.00	1.10 × 1.40 0.80, 0.85	3.50	1:10, 1:16	1.05
Finland[2]	1.30 (1.50)	1.30	0.80, 0.90	—	—	3.40	1:12 (1:14)	0.90–1.20
France	1.50	1.20, 1.50, 1.60	0.80	2.10 × 2.17	0.80 × 1.30, 1.20 × 1.50 0.80	3.30	1:20	1.00–1.40
German Democratic Republic	—	1.80	0.83	1.62 × 1.80	—	—	1:12.5	—
Great Britain	—	1.22	0.785	1.37 × 1.75, 1.52 × 1.675	1.345 × 1.125, 1.07 × 1.455, 1.75 × 1.09	—	1:12	0.91, 1.07, 1.37

Country							
Ireland	1.22	1.22	0.785	1.52 × 1.75	1.07 × 1.455 0.835	—	1:12	1.07
Israel	—	1.50	0.80	1.40 × 1.75, 2.40 × 1.30	1.07 × 1.46 0.84	3.00	1:10, 1:12	1.30
Italy	1.50	1.50	0.85, 0.90	1.80 × 1.80	1.70 × 1.50 0.90	3.00	1:12	0.90
Netherlands	1.30	1.10	0.85, 0.90	1.55 × 2.25, 1.90 × 1.90, 2.25 × 2.25	1.10 × 1.40 0.80	3.50, 3.60	1:12, 1.20	1.00
New Zealand	1.22	1.22	0.785	1.52 × 1.75 1.37 × 1.83	1.37 × 1.83	3.05	1:12	1.14
Poland[3]	1.50	—	0.85, 0.90	1.55 × 2.25, 1.90 × 1.90, 2.25 × 2.25	1.10 × 1.50 0.90	3.60	1:8[4]	0.90
Sweden[2]	1.30	1.30	0.75, 0.80	2.10 × 1.40, 1.70 × 1.70, 2.20 × 1.70	1.10 × 1.40 0.80	3.60	1:12	0.90–1.20
Switzerland	—	—	0.80	1.50 × 1.50	1.10 × 1.40 0.80	3.50	1:17	0.90
United States of America[5]	1.22	1.05	0.80	1.65 × 2.00	1.65 × 1.65	3.80	1:12	1.20

[1] Measurements over 1.20 m permit turning a wheelchair and over 1.50 two wheelchairs passing each other.
[2] Columns 1, 2, 7, 8 by a proposal of the Scandinavian Committee for Building Norms.
[3] Columns 3, 4 according to the Netherlands norm.
[4] Assistance required.
[5] Column 2, North Carolina State Building Code. Column 8, the City of South Bend Code.

Reprinted from International Rehabilitation Review, Vol. 1, XXVI, No. 1, 1st Quarter, 1975
Compiled by the International Center on Technical Aids, Housing and Transportation (ICTA), Stockholm, Sweden, 1974.

Appendix C

Michigan State Housing Development Authority Mentally Retarded Housing Program-Guidelines-February, 1974

The Michigan State Housing Development Authority has initiated a housing program for the handicapped providing housing for mentally retarded adults who are capable of relatively independent living in their communities. The housing program will serve retarded persons 18 years of age or older, who are capable of self-care with a reasonable degree of independence, and whose basic needs include the provision of a suitable place of residence in a normal living situation concurrently with employment, placement in a community program or sheltered workshop setting appropriate to their level of functioning.

SPONSOR

A group applying for authority funds must meet the following qualifications:

They must show a reasonable guarantee of their continued existence. While the MSHDA does not expect an absolute commitment of indefinite involvement of all parties, it does need assurance that the people who become involved in this housing endeavor are stable residents of their communities and can be depended upon for their businesslike handling of all matters.

The process involved in planning and construction requires extensive liaison with community groups. A sponsor must have roots in the community which reflect this involvement with interested groups.

They must show a willingness to be intimately involved in the assessment of needed services and delivery of those needed supportive services to the occupants of the house.

The nonprofit housing corporation is the method which is used in the development of this housing. An example of a nonprofit housing corporation might be: four to five parents, three to four members from the public sector such as act 54 boards, interagency coordinating committees, etc. Nonprofit corporations should also include a representative from the local association for retarded children. The nonprofit housing corporation would work in conjunction with the authority housing development officer in charge as well as a development team made up of an architect, builder, etc.

SITE AND ARCHITECTURE

The number of residents thought to be desirable is from 6 to 16. The building should be large enough to comfortably house the number of occupants involved, including adequate space for sleeping, cooking, dining and living; yet small enough to insure a homelike atmosphere:

This housing should be convenient to employment, shopping community services, transportation, etc.

The authority's townhouse development manual will serve as a model and resource in the site designing of this housing.

Several architectural plans already designed and in construction may be used and adapted by sponsors to suit a particular locality.

The FHA minimum property standards for multiple housing will be used as basis for construction standards.

Furnishing and decoration will be appropriate and adequate in quality and quantity to meet the needs of the occupants.

AUTHORITY FINANCING

The authority is now authorized to provide financing for the construction of new low income housing through the following programs:

The authority will finance as mortgagee multiple occupancy housing that is developed and designed for the adult mentally retarded.

This financing will be accomplished with the assistance of federal housing subsidy programs, authority below mortgage interest rates, authority grants, or a combination of these programs. Financing programs will be designed to meet the individual needs of individual projects.

The MSHDA will develop and process these programs by working closely with local community sponsors, as well as state and county agencies that provide supportive services to the adult mentally retarded.

Written agreements concerning the financial commitments of the department of mental health and department of social services will be entered into as is appropriate.

SUPPORTIVE SERVICES

PERSONNEL

Individuals hired to act as managers of these homes must possess attitudes and qualifications suitable to work with the mentally retarded. They must be able to provide the nurturance, guidance, and atmosphere that will be conducive to the occupants' effective use of the home. Persons selected as managers will be required to complete a training program specially designed by and at the expense of the authority. The program will consist of classroom and on-the-job instruction in both property management and work with the mentally retarded.

PROGRAMMING

There will be written agreements to provide for social, therapeutic, and vocational services secured from appropriate public and private agencies in the area, i.e., mental health, Department of Social Services, Public Health, Vocational Rehabilitation, Community Chest Agencies, etc., as evidence that there will be meaningful daytime "work" as well as leisure activity appropriate to the capabilities and needs of the occupants of these homes.

OPERATING BUDGETS

The following expenses are presently projected for a typical 16 person group home which has the benefit of a reduced mortgage amount from an authority grant. A below market interest rate (6%) from the authority, but which is still paying full local real estate taxes:

SHELTER COSTS	TOTAL ANNUAL
Miscellaneous administrative	$ 1,000
Insurance	450
Fuel	1,120
Electricity	528
Water and Sewer	320
Maintenance and Repair	2,080
*Real Estate Taxes	3,000
†Debt Service	11,421
Reserves	1,200
	$21,119

This equals a monthly rental of $110 per person for housing costs ($3.66/day).
*Local tax exemption lowers monthly rental to $101 ($3.38/day).
†Federal housing subsidy lowers monthly rental to $84 ($2.79/day).

NONSHELTER COSTS	TOTAL ANNUAL
House parent/director & substitute	$10,000
Operating/training personnel	4,000
Secretary/bookkeeper (½ time)	4,000
Payroll taxes 15%	2,500
Food and supplies ($1.90 person/day)	10,944
Misc. administrative expense	2,000
Transportation	3,000
	$36,444

This equals a monthly nonshelter cost of $190 per person ($6.36/day).

Total expenses	$57,563
	(Total $10 per person per day)

Income for the group home is to come from a combination of federal (SSI) and state (DSS) sources that will total $10 per person daily. Thus the total annual income for a 16 person group home is

$$\$10 \times 360 \text{ days} \times 16 \text{ persons} = \underline{\$57,600}$$
$$\text{surplus of} = \$37.00$$

DEVELOPMENT COSTS

Total development costs for constructing new group homes are presently running $25–$30 per sq ft depending on varying regional and local costs. Typically a 5500 sq ft group home will have a total mortgage amount of $130,000–$160,000 for all costs, including land, on-site development, landscaping, structures, fees, interest, insurance, and taxes. Land costs vary widely from developed urban areas to the undeveloped countryside. Similarly, on-site development factors, landscaping, and amenity levels in the home may vary considerably, depending on the desires and decisions of the sponsor. Typically the following median costs are presently being experienced for a 5500 sq ft group home.

	TOTAL	PER SQ FT
On-site development	18,000	3.27
Landscaping	3,000	.55
Structures (all construction costs including builder's overhead & profit)	99,000	18.00
Land, fees, interest, insurance & taxes	30,000	5.45
Total development cost	$150,000	$27.27

Since nonprofit sponsors are benefited with a 100% mortgage loan (including provision of a "seed money" loan) by the authority, it is expected that the sponsors will undertake a local fund drive to raise money for the purpose of furnishing the home.

ADDITIONAL SUPPORTIVE SERVICES

In addition to the budgets above it is assumed that residents will be engaged in a meaningful work or activity program in the community during the normal work week. Costs for these services must be secured from other public or private sources such as departments of education, mental health, or vocational rehabilitation, or united fund, etc.

DESIGN

A variety of attractive and reasonable architectural designs have been developed for authority financed homes. Typically the designs include double occupancy bedrooms with attached full bath for the residents, ample living room, dining room, kitchen, activity room, a two-bedroom apartment for the resident manager, and an attached two car garage. Total livable square footage has on the average been 5000 sq ft. (This does *not* include basement space of garage).

Plans and specifications are based on FHA minimum property standards for multifamily housing. Fire safety is based on state standards. (The home is *not* considered a nursing home. It is more comparable to a boarding house). Amenities should typically include carpeting, central air conditioning, drapes, and all modern appliances for kitchen and laundry.

An example of a typical authority-financed group home in Chapter 15.

Groups interested in development of this type of housing should contact and secure application from the Michigan State Housing Development Authority, 900 Commerce Center Building, Lansing, Michigan 48926. (Phone: 517/373-6880). Attention: Harold Mondol, Housing Development Officer.

Appendix D
The Swedish Fokus Society

Though the Swedish Fokus Society was discontinued for lack of funds in 1974, its concepts are of value. The following material was compiled from official publications of the Fokus Society.

The Fokus Society, Västra Hamngatan 24–26, S–411 17, Göteborg, Sweden, was founded in 1964 by Dr. Sven-Olof Brattgård to provide integrated living for severely disabled individuals. Dr. Brattgård has a special understanding of the problems of the disabled, for he became a paraplegic at the age of 27, continued his medical education from a wheelchair, and now occupies the chair of Research for the Handicapped at the University of Göteborg.

The Fokus Society began with a TV program on severely disabled young people who were isolated in their homes or in hospitals. The response was so tremendous that the Swedish Radio and the Swedish Lions arranged a 1-day fund-raising program in April, 1965. The contributions amounted to a total of about 3 million dollars.

With this working capital, the Fokus Society was created to provide the severely disabled with housing and services on a nationwide basis. The Society was organized with a central directorate and local executive committees, whose membership represented the government, organizations of the disabled, the tenants, and local social, medical, and welfare services.

TWO RESEARCH PROJECTS

The Fokus Society determined its course of action with two research projects. The first study was designed to determine the number of severely disabled individuals between the ages of 16 and 40 years of age. A 2-year study, it encompassed all of Sweden, whose population is about 3 million, and uncovered 1000 disabled individuals who were in need of apartments of the Fokus type and another 1000 borderline cases. A preponderance of the disabled were in rural areas, presumably because disability prevented their migration to the cities and towns. Second, a special task force developed new and flexible solutions to the problems of designing housing for the disabled.

The task force consisted of architects, rehabilitation experts, consulting engineers (heating, ventilation, sanitation, and electrical), and disabled persons. They studied the design of dwellings as well as the surrounding environment; they planned common use facilities and worked on details such as an emergency signal system. In 1968 the final manifesto was published in Swedish, German, and English under the title, *Principles of the Fokus Housing Units for the Severely Disabled.*

INTEGRATION

Since integrating the disabled into society was one of the chief purposes of Fokus, all of its apartments are located in regular residential areas near cultural, shopping, and business centers and in communities with relatively good employment opportunities and educational programs.

A fundamental principle of Fokus was that every tenant shall have his own apartment.

Apartments vary from one room with a kitchen and bath for single disabled persons to two and three rooms for disabled individuals who are married or families with disabled persons. The best combination for integration and services was found to be 10–15 apartments at one site. In high-rise buildings these apartments are located near the elevators, with only one or two on each floor to minimize segregation.

FLEXIBLE DESIGNS

The flexible designs of the task force proved adaptable to a wide variety of disabilities. The designers concentrated on communication and the two problem areas, the bathroom and the kitchen.

With electrical controls the tenant can open doors, call for assistance, talk on the house telephone, and turn lights and electrical appliances on and off. These controls are assembled in portable boxes small enough to be carried on a wheelchair. All apartments are connected to the staff room by intercom. Most tenants have their own telephones. Every apartment has a smoke detector. All the elevators have automatic door openers.

The kitchen and bathroom cabinets and fixtures can be located to suit an individual's needs. Their height can be adjusted, and the shower and basin can be changed so that the tenant may transfer to the toilet from the right or the left. The undercounter cabinets in the kitchen are all on rollers so that they may be moved to allow more space for a wheelchair. The water faucets are designed for easy operation by arthritic or paralyzed hands; the sink can be raised or lowered because of its flexible hoses and telescoping drain pipe.

COMMUNAL ROOMS

In each building there are certain rooms that are used by both the disabled and the nondisabled tenants: physical therapy, laundry, sauna, and lounge–lobby–dining rooms. Most of the sites have special parking stalls for the disabled or carports equipped with electrical heaters; some have garages for wheelchairs used outdoors.

The tenant has to furnish his own apartment, though Fokus will help him obtain the capital if he has insufficient money. All tenants must pay for their own food, but they may have dinner service in the common dining room if they wish.

FULL CARE SERVICE

The Fokus system provides a variety of services on a 24-hour basis. Each individual is assessed on the need for services, based on what he can do on his own with special assistive devices and on the time it takes him. Services vary from one locality to another, but the basic anchor is the special staff at each unit which works in 8-hour shifts so that someone is on duty around the clock. Staff members are provided with staff rooms as well as an office or duty room.

The service system is arranged so that every tenant who needs more than occasional assistance will be given his own individual attendant. This attendant will come every day for 1 or more hours to take care of the tenant's personal needs as well as cleaning, cooking, laundry, and shopping. Fokus found it important that the tenant like his attendant and that he have someone who knows his habits, someone who comes in from the outside and brings news as a friend. According to Dr. Brattgård, all service personnel should receive special training so they will be open-minded and not try to act as a nurse in the ordinary way. "The service system is as important as the designing of the flats."

The disabled tenants can call the duty room for any service they need at any hour of the day or night—to be dressed, to be turned over in bed, to be fed. Help with dressing and toileting is needed by 70%; 30% have to be fed; 25% must be turned over in the night. Dr. Brattgård estimates that most of the tenants are disabled by cerebral palsy, muscular dystrophy, or spinal cord injuries. Wheelchairs are used by 80%–90%; half of these are electric wheelchairs, and some of them are operated by sucking and blowing remote controls.

In addition to the services performed by the special staff, county councils and municipalities provide various services such as house cleaning, shopping, washing, or general assistance by "home Samaritans" which are available to the aged, sick, and disabled. The home helpers are usually housewives who have been given special training and who work 3–5 hours/day. They are paid by the local authorities, who in turn charge a small fee, if the person can pay. Experimentally, some young people have done their so-called "civilian military service" by working as service assistants for the disabled for 1 year; they are paid by the government for their services. "All service is given from paid people. Even if the service is given from a wife or a relative they get money for that."

A special transport system has been evolved. Specially equipped buses with trained drivers are available, if arrangements have been made ahead of time, to drive the tenants to work, church, or recreation in their wheelchairs. The prices are the same as those of an ordinary bus. The transport system has greatly increased the independence of the tenants.

MEASURABLE FOKUS BENEFITS

When Fokus was started, more than 90% of the tenants were receiving invalid pensions, that is, they were judged incapable of work. Most of them, 48%, had formerly lived with their parents, while 24% had been in institutions. After being in the Fokus units for only 1 year, 45% of the tenants were employed or pursuing an education. After 2 years, 80% of them were working or attending school. The Fokus dwellings make it possible for more disabled to form families with other disabled or nondisabled persons. After 1 year, "36% of the tenants cohabited or were married." Some of the disabled residents help the nondisabled families with baby sitting or with homework or by receiving mail or packages.

There are a number of fringe benefits in a Fokus apartment. For some, it is the stepping stone to life in an ordinary home. Because it is a nationwide network, tenants may move to another Fokus apartment nearer to friends, relatives, or better job opportunities. Tenants may swap apartments temporarily for vacations. Also, the tenants may provide weekend guest accommodations to other disabled persons who also may receive the special services.

REMAINING PROBLEMS

Despite this good record, many employment and leisure problems remain to be solved. Suitable employment is difficult to find for many who must remain temporarily in sheltered workshops. Some communities are not yet prepared to accept the disabled. Integration has been slow for some who had been overprotected at home or in nursing homes. Inevitably, the Fokus system makes demands on the community as well as on the disabled themselves.

COST COMPARISONS

Dr. Brattgård emphasizes that the only real cost comparison is between an independent life in a Fokus apartment and the corresponding cost of an unproductive life in a nursing home or other institution. The total expense of a Fokus apartment—including rent and service—is approximately half of what the care of a disabled person would be in a long-term clinic and two-thirds of that in a nursing home. "Each time," said Dr. Brattgård, "a disabled person moves from an institution to a Fokus flat he is saving money for society."

The total cost of a Fokus apartment, with service, is approximately $6000/year for each disabled person (1/3 for rent; 2/3 for services). The rental cost per square meter does not appreciably exceed the costs of an ordinary dwelling in the general housing field.

The Society's policy was to get in touch with the builder of a new housing project during the planning stage and rent 10–15 apartments. The government subsidizes the costs of adapting the apartments for the disabled; this includes fire–emergency call, intercom, flexible equipment in kitchen and bathroom, any special technical arrangements, hydraulic lifts for tubs, special laundry and hobby rooms—everything except the rooms for the service staff. The government pays these costs directly, and they are not included in the rent.

Because of the basic flexibility of the entire Fokus concept, it is adaptable for use in other countries. Germany and Holland have built Fokus units, and Canada and several other countries are studying the project.

In August of 1974, just 10 years after founding the Fokus Society, Dr. Brattgård wrote:

We have around 300 disabled tenants in 260 Fokus flats. Above these numbers of tenants there are some nondisabled in the flats. We have today 13 Fokus units in 13 cities. . . . We calculated with a need of around 2000 Fokus flats. From the 1st of July the municipalities in Sweden have taken over the complete responsibility for all Fokus units and for the further development of the idea. They have presented a plan for more units. Some municipalities have already started to build their own units. The experiment made by Fokus Foundation is therefore closed in a great success. The housing and the service for the severely disabled are now looked upon as part of the responsibility of the society.

Bibliography

ACCESSIBLE TOWNS—WORKABLE HOMES. Prepared by National Swedish Research D9. 1972. Order from Svensk Byggtjänst, Box 1403, S–111 84 Stockholm, Sweden. Sw.Kr. 13. (about $3.50 US).

HOUSING AND SERVICE FOR THE HANDICAPPED IN SWEDEN. By Sven-Olof Brattgård, Folke Carlsson, Arne Sandin. 1971. Order from The Fokus Society, Västra Hamngatan 24–26, S–411 17 Göteborg, Sweden.

INFORMATION PAPER 1. SEMINAR—THE FOKUS SOCIETY (DOCUMENT D'INFORMATION 1. SEMINAIRE—LA SOCIÉTÉ FOKUS). September 18, 1972. Order from Architectural and Planning Division, Central Mortgage and Housing Corporation, Ottawa, Ontario KIA OP7.

MODELS OF SERVICE FOR THE MULTI-HANDICAPPED ADULT. Major papers presented at the International Conference on Models of Service for the Multi-handicapped Adult in New York City. October 7–10, 1973. Order from United Cerebral Palsy of New York City, Inc., 122 East 23rd Street, New York, New York 10010.

PRINCIPLES OF THE FOKUS HOUSING UNITS FOR THE SEVERELY DISABLED. Order from Stiftelsen Fokus, Västra Hamngatan 24–26, S–411 17 Göteborg, Sweden. Sw.Kr. 60 (about $14 US).

Appendix E
Rehabilitation Gazette Available Back Issues

In addition to the special features listed below, all the issues contain first person accounts of the experiences of severely disabled individuals in obtaining higher education, training, or employment, reviews of books of special interest, and excerpts from readers around the world seeking pen friends.

1962. Vol. V. Experiences of quads acquiring higher education by telephone, correspondence, and attendance. Reading aids. New approaches to attendants. Voicespondence Club. Self-aspirator.

1963. Vol. VI. Quads and their families at home, marriage, and adoption. Housing around the world. Wheelchair cushions. Australian fibre glass lung. Vacations and camping. English chair/bed.

*1964. Vol. VII. Quads around the world. Foot-typing. Clothing. Mouthsticks. Portable rocking bed. Painting aids. Home study. Contesting. Toileting. Photography. Arm slings. Postal chess. Bowling.

1965. Vol. VIII. Traveling quads. Medical engineering—arm aids, foot-operated aids, multi-controls. Quad driving—foot-controlled steering, ramps, lifts, aids. Adoption. Housing. Narrowers.

1966. Vol. IX. Vocational rehabilitation. Employment experiences of quads. Wheelchairs—self-reclining, respiratory, climbing, foreign. Remote controlled typewriter. Association of Mouth and Foot Painting Artists. Housing. Reading list for quads.

1967. Vol. X. Experiences of 23 disabled college students and 35 employed quads. Citizens band radio. One-hand typing. Wheelchairs—curb-climbing, chin-controlled. Frog breathing. Portable lungs. Sex and the disabled. Alien attendants. Housing summary.

1968. Vol. XI. Tenth anniversary issue. Homemaking experiences of severely disabled individuals. Home-based businesses. Quad driving. Wheelchairs and accessories. Mouth-operated phone. Housing in Mexico and England. Rehabilitation through music. Remote controls.

1969. Vol. XII. The quad in his community. Ramps for home and car. Home care services. Housing complexities. Wheelchairs. Typing aids. Bathroom equipment. Traveling and living in Mexico. Photography.

1970. Vol. XIII. Community service projects. Independent living by quads. Mouthstick typing. Cushions. Bath lifts. Tie-downs. Hydraulic tailgates. One-armed fishing. Chess by mail. Group tours.

*1971. Vol. XIV. Grooming and clothes for men and women. Wheelchaired parents. Legal rights of the disabled. Home-based jobs. Possum. Cut-rate water beds. Veterans. Phone patching. Programming.

1972. Vol. XV. Comprehensive rehabilitation centers. Housing and home services for the disabled in the U.S. Remote controls. Ramps. Amateur radio. Art, music, and religion. Architectural barriers.

1973. Vol. XVI. Social security and Medicare. Annotated bibliography of sex. Vans, lifts, and driving controls. Communications. Curb-jumping. Mouthstick controls. Family reactions to quadness. Yoga, Zen, and Sufism. Periodicals around the world relating to disability. Veterans. Housing and home services for the disabled in the U.S.

1974. Vol. XVII. Travel to Canada, Mexico, and Europe. Travel with respirators. Recreational vehicles for wheelchaired. Rehabilitation Act of 1973. Bills of rights. Coalitions. Education and employment of quads. Volunteer projects. Adjustments to spinal cord injury. Biofeedback. German breathing treatment. Charcot-Marie-Tooth syndrome. New wheelchairs. Vans and lifts. Remote controls.

1975. Vol. XVIII. Compendium of employment experiences of 101 quads. Supplementary Secu-

401

rity Income. Multiple sclerosis. The telephone: a genie of services. IRS regulations on attendants. Quad-adapted camera. Step-vans, lifts, and ramps. New word board. Inexpensive tie-down. Bargain wheelchair narrower. ACCD. Architectural barriers milestones.

*There are so few copies left of the 1964 and 1971 issues that they will be limited to orders for complete sets of the 14 back issues.

Donation per copy: $3 from the disabled
$5 from the non-disabled

Rehabilitation Gazette
*4502 Maryland Avenue
St. Louis, Missouri 63108, U.S.A.
Phone: (314) 361-0475*

Appendix F
Resources for
Architects and Planners

ARCHITECTURAL GUIDELINES

ACCENT ON ACCESS. By Larry Kirk. 45 pages. Illustrated. 8½ × 11. 1975. Available from American Society of Landscape Architects Foundation, 1750 Old Meadow Road, McLean, Virginia 22101. $6.

The author, who is wheelchaired, is staff assistant, Office of Programs for the Elderly and Handicapped, at HUD. He states in his foreword, "In this book I have attempted to bring together the urban planner, the architect, the landscape architect, the engineer, the civil engineer, the industrial engineer, the interior designer, and the transportation expert conceptually in the elimination of design barriers." It is a clear and concise summary of the guidelines to an accessible environment.

ACCESS 76. BLUEPRINT FOR ACTION. By the Easter Seal Society for Crippled Children and Adults of Massachusetts, Inc. and United Community Planning Corporation. 57 pages. Illustrated. 8½ × 11. 1975. Available from the Easter Seal Society, 14 Somerset Street, Boston, Massachusetts 02108. Free.

The combination of the Easter Seal Society and a superb professional team directed by Robert J. Lynch, AIA, who is wheelchaired, produced an artistic and practical publication. Though specifically designed to eliminate or modify barriers for the Bicentennial, the methods of involving the community, the summary of regulations and implementation, conclusions, and recommendations are of universal value.

ARCHITECTURAL FACILITIES FOR THE DISABLED. Nederlandse Vereniging Voor Revalidatie (NVR). The Netherlands' Society for Rehabilitation. The Hague. 32 pages. Illustrated. 8 × 11½. 1973. Order from ICTA Information Centre, FACK S-161 03 Bromma, Sweden. $2.

The booklet of illustrations was compiled from data derived from Dutch and other foreign sources through the cooperation of ICTA, NVR, and Rehabilitation International. Of special interest are the details for planning facilities for people with impaired vision or hearing difficulties. The introduction stresses the words "accessibility and usability" to describe adaptations of buildings.

ARTS AND THE HANDICAPPED. AN ISSUE OF ACCESS. A Report from Educational Facilities Laboratories and the National Endowment for the Arts. 78 pages. Illustrated. 5½ × 11. 1975. Order from EFL, 850 Third Avenue, New York, New York 10022. $4.

This attractive publication is an excellent guide to what has been and what can be done to create accessible museums, theaters, special schools, community service centers, colleges, and nature centers. Information is included relative to all types of permanent and temporary disabilities, including blindness, deafness, age, and pregnancy.

BARRIER FREE DESIGN. Report of a United National Expert Group Meeting held June 3–8, 1974. 35 pages. Illustrated. 8½ × 11. 1975. Order from Rehabilitation International, 122 East 23rd Street, New York, New York 10010. $5.

A flashcard summary of the universality of barrier problems, the report covers public buildings, private housing, legislation, norms in various countries, and includes an international bibliography.

BARRIER FREE DESIGN GRAPHICS. By Robert A. L. Williams, AIA. 23 pages. Loose-leaf. Illustrated. 8½ × 11. 1975. Order from League-Goodwill, Department 1000, 1401 Ash Street, Detroit, Michigan 48208. $2.

This book contains graphic illustrations of the Michigan Construction Commission's "General Rules" to make facilities accessible. The author teaches Barrier Free Design at Lawrence Institute of Technology in Southfield, Michigan.

DESIGNING FOR THE DISABLED. 2nd Edition, Revised and Expanded. By Selwyn Goldsmith, MA (Cantab), ARIBA, Royal Institute of British Architects. 207 pages. Illustrated. 8½ × 12. 1967. Order from Royal Institute of British Architects, 66 Portland Place, London, W1, England £3 10s. ($6.20)

This is the "Bible" of designing for the disabled—the encyclopedic manual. The author feels that the ambulatory and semiambulant should be counted with the average normal population and that only the completely chairbound should be considered as an atypical group in need of special facilities.

While the first edition concentrated on details of domestic housing, the second edition places more emphasis on public buildings. Divided into nine sections, the manual covers general material on the disabled population, measurement data on anthropometrics and circulation spaces, building elements and finishes, service installations, general spaces, detailed recommendations for public buildings, types of public buildings, and domestic housing. Appendices include cost implications, a glossary, selected references, an extensive bibliography, a list of organizations concerned with the planning of facilities for people who are disabled, and a section on siting that covers psychologic needs and social contacts.

Goldsmith concludes this splendid publication with admonitions that disabled people, young or elderly, should not be segregated from the rest of the community and that disabled people do not belong together merely because they are disabled.

The third edition is being written and will be ready in 1976.

HOUSING THE HANDICAPPED. (LOGEMENTS POUR LES HANDICAPÉS). Prepared for Central Mortgage and Housing Corporation. 60 pages in English; 60 pages in French. Illustrated. 8½ × 11. 1974. Order from Central Mortgage and Housing Corporation, Information Services, Ottawa K1A OP7, Ontario, Canada. $3.32.

This handsome book is liberally illustrated with floor plans and elevations. It is of value both to an individual planning a private residence and to architects and builders planning group homes or blocks of apartments.

The publication divides housing needs into three "housing packages:"

1. Minimum criteria to be considered for all new multiple unit buildings: access to the building itself (entrance door, 3 ft) and to all basic facilities including elevators; access to all rooms of the individual units with all doors having a clear passage of 30 in. and all bathrooms slightly larger to allow wheelchair maneuvers and having cantilevered washbasins; all doors, cupboards, drawers, and faucets with lever handles; and window hardware no higher than 4 ft 8 in. from the floor.
2. Residential group homes and apartments for those disabled who want or need the mutual support of a small, close-knit group: maximum size of ten residents plus a director to retain a domestic character. Plans and facilities are included both for homes in residential areas for the exclusive use of disabled and for integrated units in mixed use apartment buildings. The section on elevators, heating, cooling, ventilation, fire systems, and alarm systems is particularly thorough and helpful.
3. Private homes. The basic criteria for the interiors are the same; some suggestions are

included for problems caused by ice and snow: electrically operated garage doors, ceiling-hung trapeze in garage, two-way switch for garage lights, block heaters, heated garages, and underground heating for walks.

The sections on kitchens and bathrooms offer an array of plans and suggestions. In the kitchen, three alternatives are offered: 1) a compromise height of 33-in. counters which would not be ideal for anyone but which would not add any extra cost; 2) limited flexibility by means of a car jack that raises and lowers the range and the base cabinets that are stabilized by a sliding track at the rear; and 3) the Fokus plan of a completely flexible mass-produced system. Six layouts of bathrooms are included, ranging in overall size from 4 ft 7 in. × 8 ft to 7 ft × 9 ft; a compromise height of 33 in. is suggested for the washbasin; also suggested, a standard height installation of 15 in. for the toilet with a separate and removable seat attachment for dwellings where nondisabled persons share the bathroom.

HOUSING FOR THE PHYSICALLY IMPAIRED. A Guide for Planning and Design. By S. L. Tesone, Architectural adviser. U.S. Department of Housing and Urban Development. 49 pages. Illustrated. 8 × 10½ 1967. Published by The Superintendent of Documents, U.S. Government Printing Office.

This guide is out of print but is on file at major libraries. It has been the basic resource for almost every project in the country specially planned for the disabled.

HOUSING FOR SPECIAL NEEDS. Part One. The Physically Handicapped. Prepared for Scottish Local Authorities Special Housing Group. 84 pages. Illustrated. 8 × 12. 1974. Order from P.H. Stringer, Chief Architect, Research Unit, 53 Melville Street, Edinburgh, EH3 7HL, Scotland. £2.50. ($5)

Designed specifically for local Scottish housing authorities, the attractive book correlates the information on technical solutions to the housing problems with legal references and government standards. The emphasis throughout is on "making housing for the physically disabled as close in appearance and form to mainstream housing as is practicable" and on offering a flexibility of arrangements. A special section is devoted to home dialysis with exact details on equipment and home conversions.

Some interesting equipment for the immobile, such as a telephone-controlled electric door lock, is described. For the blind, room thermostats should be removed and sent to the Royal National Institute for the Blind where they will be converted for blind operation, free of charge. For the deaf, there are two methods of hooking up a control box so that lights go on or flash when the doorbell is pushed; an induction loop system that permeates an area with a magnetic field which can be received by a hearing aid fitted with a pickup coil enables the deaf person to listen to TV with the family at normal levels of sound without using headphones.

INTO THE MAINSTREAM: A SYLLABUS FOR A BARRIER-FREE ENVIRONMENT. By Stephen A. Kliment. 44 pages. Illustrated. 8½ × 11. 1975. Single copy free from National Easter Seal Society for Crippled Children and Adults, 2023 West Ogden Avenue, Chicago, Illinois 60612.

This publication is first on the list of required reading "for all those who through concern or legal obligation care about a barrier-free environment and are prepared to do something about it," for all who want "to know what to do and how to start to bring local buildings and sites to a barrier-free level of access."

It was prepared under a grant to the American Institute of Architects (AIA) by the Rehabilitation Services Administration. The AIA considered it so informative that it distributed it to every member of its organization. It includes a history of the development of legislation, codes, and standards, the basic barrier conditions, solutions to the removal of barriers and techniques of organizing action groups, and an annotated list of information sources and concerned agencies, as well as a sample questionnaire for use in evaluating accessibility of buildings.

AN INTRODUCTION TO DOMESTIC DESIGN FOR THE DISABLED. By Felix Walter, FRIBA, FRSA. 32 pages. Illustrated. 8½ × 12. 1968. Order from Disabled Living Activities Group, 346 Kensington High Street, London W14, England. 12s. 6d. ($2)

A clear, untechnical introduction to designing homes for the disabled that functions as a general planning check list. To assist those who are new to the subject, an asterisk indicates the most essential design features; the others may be included only as required. Some of the line drawing pages that are particularly helpful deal with countertop and cupboard adjustability, a combined bath transfer seat and linen container, an extended toilet seat, an adjustable lavatory, a quadrant drawer beneath the bed, and a wall unit with door shelves.

MADE TO MEASURE. Prepared for Domestic Extensions and Adaptions for Handicapped Persons, Cheshire County Council, Department of Architecture. 44 pages. Illustrated. 8¼ × 11. Request from County Architect, County Hall, Chester, Cheshire, England. Free.

In the introduction, the Director of Social Services details the scope of work undertaken by the County Architect in making home adaptations. The thoroughness of the instructions is typified by the directions to the workmen as to making tea, "The contractor should be asked to bring his own tea-making facilities: if a job drags on for 6 months or more it can be quite a burden for a housewife to provide boiling water at least three times a day."

MOBILITY HOUSING. By Selwyn Goldsmith, MA (Cantab), ARIBA. Reprinted from THE ARCHITECTS' JOURNAL, CI/SfB 81 (E3p), pages 43–50, 3 July 1974. Request from Housing Development Directorate, Department of the Environment, 2 Marsham Street, London SW1P 3EB, England. Single copies without charge.

In order to make more housing available to disabled and elderly people as soon as possible, the Department of the Environment (DoE) developed the concept of mobility housing. It involves three requirements: 1) entrances are accessible to those in wheelchairs; 2) interiors allow easy movement by those who use wheelchairs but can stand to transfer; and 3) one bedroom, bathroom, and toilet are at entrance level.

Relating DoE's studies and Great Britain's recent surveys of the disabled population, Goldsmith concludes that 96% of the 1¼ million adult handicapped people and 98% of the 3 million categorized as impaired could use mobility housing. Roughly 2% of the impaired need to be in special wheelchair housing.

Goldsmith points out that "the changeover to metric has given powerful impetus to dimensional coordination, prefabrication, and standarization" and will influence the design of typical housing and its suitability to disabled people. All public housing is now designed to a basic planning grid of 300 mm (11 13/16 in.), within which are increments for components of 100 mm (3 15/16 in.). Standard passages are 900 mm (35 7/16 in.) wide, and doorsets are 900 mm or 800 mm across the frame. To check these measurements, the Institute for Consumer Ergonomics at Loughborough University set up a test simulating a standard 900-mm passage with a 775-mm (30½ in.) door opening and tested the 12 wheelchairs currently available under the National Health Service. All went through the opening except an E & J Powerdrive and an oversized model.

The Institute concluded that it is the characteristics of standard wheelchairs, rather than the characteristics of disabled people which determine whether housing is accessible. Goldsmith suggests that all wheelchairs in the future should be designed so they can be propelled from a 900-mm passage through a 775-mm opening or vice versa.

PRINCIPLES OF THE FOKUS HOUSING UNITS FOR THE SEVERELY DISABLED. 2nd Edition. Prepared by a research group at the request of the Fokus Society. 83 pages. Illustrated. 8 × 11½ 1969. Order from Fokus Society, Västra Hamangatan 24–26, S-411 17, Göteborg, Sweden. Sw. Kr. 60. (About $14 U.S.).

This manual comprises the detailed specifications of the Fokus units, including the surroundings of the buildings as well as the construction elements in the flats and the cabinetry; exact specifications and sources of supply are included on all plumbing and electrical equipment. Further there are analyses of household activities, including the reach areas in terms of work and living space.

Flexibility is an essential part of the Fokus system; over one-half of the units were rearranged within the first 2 weeks of use. Some detailed design notes are: motor drives, costing $400, are available for raising and lowering kitchen and bathroom assemblies; each unit has a smoke detector; balconies, with radiant heat, provide relaxation and change as well as convenient fire escapes; radiant heat in the bathroom floor helps keep the floor dry from the shower splashes; every room has an emergency cord.

REMOVING ARCHITECTURAL BARRIERS. Edited and produced by the Division of Vocational Rehabilitation, New Mexico Department of Education. 83 pages. Illustrated. 8½ × 11. 1975. Available from the DVR, 231 Washington Avenue, P.O. Box 1830, Santa Fe, New Mexico 87503. Free.

This handbook illustrates Chapter 41 of the 1973 New Mexico Uniform Building Code.

SELECTED REHABILITATION FACILITIES IN THE UNITED STATES. An Architect's Analysis. By Thomas K. Fitz Patrick, FAIA. 58 pages. Illustrated. 10 × 8. 1973. Order from Superintendent of Documents, U.S. Government Printing Office, Washington, D.C. 20402. 90¢

An attractive booklet, it covers facilities in urban and regional settings, special facilities for communications disorders, the blind, and mentally retarded, as well as research, hospital and workshop centers.

WHEELCHAIR HOUSING. By Selwyn Goldsmith, MA (Cantab), ARIBA. Reprinted from THE ARCHITECTS' JOURNAL, CI/fSB 81 (E3p), pages 1319–1348, 25 June 1975. Request from Housing Development Directorate, Department of the Environment, 2 Marsham Street, London SW1P 3EB, England. Single copies without charge.

This comprehensive report is intended as a guide to architects who are planning housing for those who are confined to wheelchairs and are unable to use mobility housing. "While the number of people who need wheelchair housing is small, it is also by definition a very variable population, making it impossible for there to be formula solutions which will be universally appropriate." The report includes a summary of a study of housing for 249 disabled people by Janis Morton, a sociologist.

LANDSCAPE

BARRIER-FREE SITE DESIGN. Prepared by American Society of Landscape Architects Foundation and U.S. Department of Housing and Urban Development Office of Policy Development and Research. 82 pages. Illustrated. 11 × 9. 1975. Order Stock Number 023-000-00291-4. HUD-PDR-84 from Superintendent of Documents, U.S. Government Printing Office, Washington, D.C. 20402. $2.30.

Produced under HUD contract by the American Society of Landscape Architects Foundation, the report covers pertinent population data for each of the most frequent disabilities and surveys federal and state guidelines for the design of outdoor areas. It illustrates in drawings and diagrams a number of ways in which such barriers as steps, walkways, curbs, benches, railings, and lighting can be designed or redesigned to permit full use of the outdoor environment by persons with a temporary or permanent disability.

LANDSCAPE DESIGN FOR THE DISABLED. By Jay Jorgensen. 118 pages. Illustrated. 8½ × 11. 1975. Order from Publications Department, American Society of Landscape Architects Foundation, 1750 Old Meadow Road, McLean, Virginia 22101. $5.50.

This publication is an outgrowth of a research report prepared by the Society for HUD. Its purpose is to provide a designer with a guide to making outside spaces and recreational areas accessible.

URBAN PLANNING

ACCESSIBLE TOWNS—WORKABLE HOMES. Planning with Consideration for the Handicapped. Document D9:1972. Prepared by The National Swedish Institute for Building Research. 28 pages. Illustrated. 8¼ × 12. 1972. Order from Svensk Byggtjänst, Box 1403, S-111 84 Stockholm, Sweden. Sw.Kr. 13. (About $3.50 U.S.).

This two-part document by the National Swedish Institute for Building Research recommends that the environment be made accessible to the disabled through personal service, technical aids, and the adaptation of the urban environment and its buildings.

PLANNING FOR DISABLED PEOPLE IN THE URBAN ENVIRONMENT. By Percy Johnson Marshall, The Planning Research Unit, University of Edinburgh. 63 pages. Illustrated. 8¼ × 12. 1969. Order from Central Council for the Disabled, 34 Eccleston Square, London SW1, England. 15s.

An artistic as well as an informative publication, the study covers the range of problems faced by the disabled in urban centers, including private transport, public transport, pedestrian routes, vertical circulation, and individual buildings.

"It has been assumed throughout this study that new buildings can and should be made accessible to disabled people. . . . At least one entrance door, served by an accessible approach, should be not less than 33 in. (835 mm) wide and should give a clear opening width of not less than 31 in. (785 mm)."

BIBLIOGRAPHIES

BARRIER FREE DESIGN: A SELECTED BIBLIOGRAPHY. By Peter L. Lassen, Construction Project Manager, Veterans Administration. 103 pages. 8½ × 11. 1973. Order from Michigan Chapter, Paralyzed Veterans of America, 5646 McMillan Street, Dearborn Heights, Michigan 48127. $6.

This comprehensive collection of national and international references should be in the library of everyone working toward barrier-free design or planning any kind of residence or facility geared to the disabled. It is the most extensive bibliography compiled on the subject.

THE BUILT ENVIRONMENT FOR THE ELDERLY AND THE HANDICAPPED. A Bibliography. Compiled by the Library and Information Division of HUD. 46 pages. 1971. Order Stock Number 2300–1191 from Superintendent of Documents, U.S. Government Printing Office, Washington, D.C. 20402. 75¢.

This publication is particularly useful for its coverage of housing for the elderly.

THE ELIMINATION OF ARCHITECTURAL BARRIERS TO THE DISABLED. A Selected Bibliography and Report on the Literature in the Field. Compiled by Susan Klement. 36

pages. 8½ × 11. 1969. Order from Canadian Rehabilitation Council for the Disabled, 2nd Floor, 242 St. George Street, Toronto, Ontario M5R 2N5, Canada. $1.

In addition to architectural designs and programs to eliminate barriers, the author includes psychologic and sociologic aspects of disability and the anthropometric and work characteristics of the disabled.

LIST OF LITERATURE. Prepared by ICTA Information Centre. 55 pages. 8¼ × 11½. 1971. Order from ICTA Information Centre, FACK, S-161 03 Bromma 3, Sweden. $1.50.

This bibliography includes listings in English, Swedish, French, Dutch, German, and Italian. It covers activities of daily living and rehabilitation in general, clothing, disabled drivers, disabled homemakers, furniture, guides, handicapped children and youth, housing and urban planning, sport and wheelchairs. The listings, mainly covering literature on motor disabilities, are a revision of the list issued by ICTA in 1967.

INFORMATION CENTERS

Central Council for the Disabled, 34 Eccleston Square, London SW1V 1PE, England. The Council functions as the coordinator of information for the disabled on a national and international basis. It publishes a wealth of information on accessibility, covering entire towns, universities, employment, entertainment, and public buildings, as well as journals and bulletins. One of its publications is a compilation of an incredible number of summer accommodations for disabled people in England and all over Europe, *Holidays for the Physically Handicapped 1975* (50 pence ($1) from the Holidays Department). Another is the *Motel Guide for the Disabled,* which covers European highways (25 pence) (50 ¢).

Of particular interest is the Housing Advisory Service which assists individuals with specific problems; questions should be addressed to the Housing Officer. During the summer months, the Council sponsors a traveling exhibition of aids.

Two other briefs of interest, both dated June, 1973: one contains a bibliography on "Access for the Disabled;" the other has notes on design features for university buildings.

Centre on Environment for the Handicapped (CEH) 24 Nutford Place, London W1H 6AN, England. The Centre provides advice on all design phases of facilities for the disabled. Its information services are available to the disabled as well as to architects, builders, universities, doctors, therapists, and housing authorities. In addition to the library, it has a collection of plans, photographs, and slides which can be used at the Centre. Consultation on specific problems and designs with Selwyn Goldsmith, Jean Symons, or Janet Levison is available by appointment. The membership fee of £4.50/year includes the *Newsletter,* which reports projects and research in designing for the disabled and includes book reviews and a forum for discussion of problems in the field of designing. Following are a few of the publications on the extensive list:

Bibliography 1. Introduction to Design for Mentally Handicapped People. Revised 1972. 15 pence. (30¢)

Bibliography 3. Training Centres and Workshops for Mentally Handicapped People. 1972. 10 pence. (20¢)

Bibliography 4. Designing for Old People. 1973. 15 pence. (30¢)

Bibliography 5. Designing for the Physically Handicapped. 1974. 15 pence. (30¢)

Designing for the Handicapped. Edited by Kenneth Bayes and Sandra Francklin. Published by George Godwin, London. 1971. £1.70. ($3.40)

Seven Seminars on Physical Handicap 1973–4. Organized by Selwyn Goldsmith. 30 pence. (60¢)

The CEH Design Guide 2, *Residential Accommodation for Disabled People* (60 pence) is a 36-page booklet by Jean Symons which is especially informative. In order to obtain information on the accommodation needs of disabled persons, the author visited a number of hospitals and various types of residential units. Few of those interviewed wished to live in special communities for the disabled, such as Het Dorp; the chief desire of those living unhappily in institutions was to have or to have had the opportunity to choose their home. In general, they considered residential homes and special workshops symbols of segregation.

As alternatives to segregated accommodation, the author describes two completed schemes in which units for disabled people are mixed with ordinary housing and the disabled residents are provided with supportive services: Haringey and Friendship House.

Points which were considered especially important by wheelchair users and by architects experienced in designing for the wheelchaired are listed in detail. Most of the suggestions, made at a CEH seminar, followed the usual patterns. A few thoughts were quite innovative, however: electric taps should be installed for some severely disabled individuals; baths should be low rather than high; sliding door mechanisms go wrong, concertina doors are unsatisfactory; access or escape are as important as ventilation or drainage.

Disabled Living Foundation (DLF), 346 Kensington High Street, London W14 8NS, England. Under the chairmanship of its redoubtable founder and chairman, Lady Hamilton, this unique organization pioneered the organization of information services for the disabled. In addition to its comprehensive Information Service and Aids Centre with a permanent display of equipment, gadgets, and publications, the Foundation publishes a bimonthly Newsletter on a subscription basis (£7 ($14) overseas). The subscription service publishes up-to-date addresses of manufacturers of every type of aid or equipment and the latest publications and information of concern to both the disabled and elderly, ranging from household equipment to wheelchairs.

The Foundation has created and funded a number of research projects, particularly in the field of clothing for the disabled. Following are some of these published reports as well as relevant publications:

Clothes Sense for Handicapped Adults of All Ages. £1.50. ($3)

Four Architectural Movement Studies for the Wheelchair and Ambulant Disabled. £1.50. ($3)

Sports Centres and Swimming Pools. £1.50. ($3)

Early Days—You and Your New Baby. £1.25. ($2.50)

The Easy Path of Gardening. £1.25. ($2.50)

Two other closely allied aids centers have been patterned after the DLF, one in Scotland and one in Liverpool. The latter, opened by the Liverpool Social Services Department, can be used by disabled persons who wish to make an appointment to try out bathroom aids used with typical local plumbing under the supervision of occupational therapists.

EQUIPMENT FOR THE DISABLED. The National Fund for Research into Crippling Diseases pioneered the publishing of current guides to equipment with a loose-leaf series in 1960 and a revised edition in 1966. In 1971, a series of ten separate booklets was initiated, each dealing with an important aspect of daily living. Between 1971–1974 the following booklets were published: *Wheelchairs and Outdoor Transport, Communication, Clothing and Dressing for Adults, Home Management, Disabled Mother, Personal Care, Leisure and Gardening, Housing and Furniture, Hoists and Walking Aids, Disabled Child.*

In 1974, the Oxford Regional Health Authority, on behalf of the Department of Health and Social Security, assumed responsibility for publishing subsequent editions. Professional inquiries concerning equipment should be addressed to Equipment for the Disabled, Mary Marlborough Lodge, Nuffield Orthopaedic Centre, Headington, Oxford OX3 7LD. Orders for booklets should be sent to Equipment for the Disabled, 2 Foredown Drive, Portslade, Sussex BN4 2BB, England.

All the booklets are superb reference books. They contain commercial sources and approximate prices as well as directions for homemade adaptations. They are all generously illustrated and clearly presented and include selected bibliographies. They average 50–60 pages, with large photographs and drawings and a minimum of text. Price per copy is £1.05 ($2.10); the set of 10 booklets is £10.50 ($21), plus 95 pence ($1.90) for a binder.

ICTA Information Centre, FACK, S-161 03 Bromma 3, Sweden. ICTA collects and disseminates information about technical aids on an international basis. About 20 information sheets are published each year; they are illustrated and have texts in English, French, German, and Spanish. The sheets which give the essential technical data as well as the price and the manufacturer, are available on a subscription basis for $8/year; back issues are available at $15. They are a splendid way of keeping up with equipment developments in the U.S. and Europe.

National Association of Housing and Redevelopment Officials, 2600 Virginia Avenue, N.W., Washington, D.C. 20037. An action and information center that serves local, state, and federal agencies, officials, and civic leaders, NAHRO is concerned with community development and housing action. Free list of publications available.

National Easter Seal Society for Crippled Children and Adults, 2023 West Ogden Avenue, Chicago, Illinois 60612. One of the outstanding services of this voluntary organization is to act as a resource center for published information. A booklet listing all their publications is free.

Following are some of their publications that are particularly relevant:

Sources of Information on Self-Help Devices for the Handicapped. L-6. Free.

A Living Environment for the Physically Disabled. By Dorothy A. Jeffrey, OTR. (A-238). 1973. 10¢.

Avenues of Action for Long-Term Care of the Multiply Handicapped. By Elsie D. Helsel. (D-35). 1965. 25¢.

Designing for the Mentally Handicapped. By Daniel C. Bryant. 1964. 10¢.

Furniture Design for the Elderly. By Barbara Laging. 1966. 25¢.

Home Care Programs. By Cecil G. Sheps and Jack Kasten. 1962. 25¢.

Housing Needs of the Aged With a Guide to Functional Planning For the Elderly and Handicapped. By Alexander Kira. 1960. Free. L-20.

Vehicles for the Severely Disabled. By Peter Bray and Don M. Cunningham. (D-38). 1967. 25¢.

Directory of Resident Camps for Persons With Special Needs. (E-41). 1975. $1.50.

The Wheelabout Garden. By Easter Seal Society of Massachusetts. PR-29. 1975. 10¢.

"No One at Home." A Brief Review of Housing for Handicapped Persons in Some European Countries. By Deborah Greenstein, Charles Gueli, and Edmond Leonard. 1976. L-104.

From Problem to Solution: The New Focus in Fighting Environmental Barriers For the Handicapped. By Rita McGaughey. 1976. L-103.

Current Materials on Architectural Barriers. February 1976 A-200. Free.

Rehabilitation International, 122 East 23rd Street, New York, New York 10010. Founded in 1922, this nongovernmental federation of national and international organizations provides rehabilitation services for the disabled in 61 countries. It promotes the dissemination of information through the International Center on Technical Aids, Housing and Transportation (ICTA) in Stockholm and the newly operating Rehabilitation International Information Service being provided by Stiftung Rehabilitation, Heidelberg, Federal Republic of Germany.

Rehabilitation International, U.S.A., 17 East 45th Street, New York, New York 10017. A recent outgrowth of Rehabilitation International, this voluntary organization is devoting its energies to coordinating the activities of U.S. organizations having an impact on international rehabilitation programs.

AIDS AND ADAPTATIONS FOR THE BLIND

THE BLIND: SPACE NEEDS FOR REHABILITATION. By F. C. Salmon and C. F. Salmon. 82 pages. Illustrated. 1964. $4. Order from Oklahoma State University School of Architecture, Stillwater, Oklahoma 74074.

General information on space requirements and the design of rehabilitation centers is included. A revised edition is being prepared.

INTERNATIONAL CATALOG. Aids and Appliances for Blind and Visually Impaired Persons. Edited by L.L. Clark. 214 pages. 8¼ × 10¼. 1973. Order from American Foundation for the Blind, Inc., 15 West 16th Street, New York, New York 10011. $2.

This comprehensive compilation is a guide to devices and aids that are available for purchase from manufacturers around the world.

THE PHYSICAL ENVIRONMENT AND THE VISUALLY IMPAIRED. By Per-Gunnar Braf. 34 pages. Illustrated. 8¼ × 12. 1974. Order from ICTA Information Centre, FACK, S-161 03, Bromma 3, Sweden. $3.

The author, an architect, carried on extensive research, with the assistance of The Swedish Association of the Blind, on the planning and adaptation of buildings and other forms of physical environment for visually impaired people. The booklet, charmingly illustrated with line drawings, includes definitions and discusses the basic implications of impaired vision as well as making general suggestions for dealing with the total environment. Among the specific suggestions are: design handrails so they give good directional guidance; make lighting and color work in combination with each other; complement optical signals with acoustic signals; design pedestrian circulation routes so that they are easy to follow; and use right-angled solutions.

ELDERLY

COMMUNITY PLANNING FOR THE ELDERLY. By M. Powell Lawton, PhD and Thomas O. Byerts. Prepared for HUD by The Gerontological Society. 66 pages. 8½ × 11. 1974. Order #PB-232 000 from National Technical Information Service, U.S. Department of Commerce, Springfield, Virginia 22151. $3.75.

Intended for the use of community planners, this report suggests alternative types of housing accommodations and community services. Criteria are given for elderly housing site selection and the questions of mixing the elderly by age, income, health, facial and ethnic characteristics are addressed. "A basic premise is that the elderly do not have common characteristics but, if anything, differ among themselves even more than do younger people."

HOUSING FOR THE ELDERLY—FACTORS WHICH SHOULD BE EVALUATED BEFORE DECIDING ON LOW- OR HIGH-RISE CONSTRUCTION. Report to the Congress by the Comptroller General of the United States. 23 pages. 8 × 10½. 1975. Order #RED-75-308. from U.S. General Accounting Office, Distribution Section, P.O. Box 1020, Washington, D.C. 20013. $1.

About 108,500 units, or 49%, of new local housing authority owned (LHA) units for which construction was started during 1970–1973 were for the elderly. Although HUD and LHA officials said more high-rise housing had been built because it was cheaper to construct, operate, and maintain, because of a shortage of land near business districts, and because elderly people preferred to live in high-rise buildings, the General Accounting Office (GAO) found that costs varied so much in different areas that no firm conclusion could be reached as to which should be used more frequently.

Elderly tenants who were questioned did not have a strong preference for either type of building. Most people questioned said they preferred to live in the type of building in which they were currently living.

A NATIONAL DIRECTORY ON HOUSING FOR OLDER PEOPLE. Revised edition. 1969–1970. Including a Guide for Selection. Prepared by the National Council on the Aging. 362 pages. 8½ × 11. 1969. Order from The National Council on the Aging, 315 Park Avenue South, New York, New York 10010. $5.

The directory includes both profit and nonprofit facilities that are designed or adapted for older people. The facilities listed include those for individuals who can maintain their own living quarters and manage their own affairs, either with or without health and social services. Listed are self-contained housekeeping units, residence club or hotel type units, and a combination of housekeeping and nonhousekeeping units, social care, and nursing facilities. Homes for the aged, nursing homes, and public housing units are not included.

The National Council on the Aging has an extensive list of publications which are listed in a free brochure. Among these are FURNITURE REQUIREMENTS FOR OLDER PEOPLE, a 46-page paperback, $2.50, 1974 DIRECTORY OF SENIOR CENTERS AND CLUBS: A NATIONAL RESOURCE, a 558-page directory listing 4900 programs prepared by the National Institute of Senior Citizens, $10, and PLANNING HOUSING ENVIRONMENTS FOR THE ELDERLY by Louis E. Gelwicks, AIA, and Robert J. Newcomer, AIP, a 120-page book, $7.50.

Physiological and Behavioral Characteristics of the Elderly: A Basis for Design Criteria for Interior Space and Furnishings. By Bettyann Raschko. REHABILITATION LITERATURE, Vol.35, No.1, pages 10–13. January, 1974.

The author places particular emphasis on planning for private space which an individual can manage according to his own desires. "Possession of a tangible piece of space seems almost essential for one's identity."

Bedroom units are recommended over studio units; a separate bedroom is a place in which to relax, to store possessions, to work. If a one-room living space is used, an alcove with a window should be screened off for privacy. A living room window for viewing should be located at eye level (the mean eye height of an older person seated on a 17 in. high chair is 3 ft 7-¾ in.). The bathroom should have a nonskid floor; toilet seat height should be 17–18 in. The kitchen should have a pull-out lapboard.

PROCEEDINGS OF HOUSING CONFERENCES

FREEDOM OF CHOICE. REPORT TO THE PRESIDENT AND TO THE CONGRESS ON HOUSING NEEDS OF HANDICAPPED INDIVIDUALS. Vols. I and II. Report of the Architectural and Transportation Barriers Compliance Board Public Hearing on Housing for Handicapped Individuals held in Chicago, Illinois, June 9–10, 1975. Vol. I: 41 pages; Vol. II: 67 pages. 8 × 10½. Available free from Architectural and Transportation Barriers Compliance Board, Washington, D.C. 20201.

The ATBCB invited 130 organizations, groups, and individuals representing the disabled and the housing industry to attend the hearing and submit written testimony. In Volume I testimony is summarized and presented under 19 categories that cover the major areas of concern. Of particular value is the information in the appendices—a comprehensive documentation, prepared by HUD, of existing federal legislation and programs affecting housing for the disabled and a listing of the statistics of people with physical limitations.

Volume II is a transcript of the oral and written testimony presented by the 39 witnesses at the hearing. Both volumes are important sources of information and guidance.

HOUSING ALTERNATIVES FOR HANDICAPPED ADULTS. Proceedings of a conference sponsored by the New York City chapters of the National Rehabilitation Association and the National Association of Social Workers. 78 pages. 8½ × 11. 1975. Request from New York City Chapter National Association of Social Workers, 79 Madison Avenue, New York, New York 10016. Free.

This 1-day conference brought together professional workers and disabled persons to discuss housing alternatives. These included small group residences such as hostels, halfway houses, and congregate living arrangements; large group residences such as nursing homes; and individual and group apartments.

The conference participants recommended that the City of New York establish a central information, referral, and coordinating agency on housing for disabled persons. They also made the following recommendations: strong antidiscrimination provisions, financing for adaptations of existing housing, modification of laws affecting small group residences, and rent subsidies similar to those given to senior citizens.

MODELS OF SERVICE FOR THE MULTI-HANDICAPPED ADULT. Major Papers Presented at the International Conference on Models of Service for the Multi-Handicapped Adult, New York City, October 7–10, 1973. Prepared by United Cerebral Palsy of New York City, Inc. 84 pages. Illustrated. 7 × 9. 1974. Request from United Cerebral Palsy of New York City, Inc., 122 East 23rd Street, New York, New York 10010.

Leslie D. Park, executive director of United Cerebral Palsy of New York City, Inc., has sponsored two conferences which brought together the international leaders of housing and services for the disabled. The 1971 conference, International Rehabilitation Patterns for the Multi-Handicapped, included presentations by Dr. A. Klapwijk the creator of

Holland's Het Dorp, James Loring of the International Cerebral Palsy Society, and Douglas G. Seaton of Canada's Bell woods Park House. At the 1973 biennial conference, Models of Service for the Multi-Handicapped Adult, speakers included Dr. Sven-Olof Brattgård, who established the Fokus Society in Sweden, and Derek Lancaster–Gaye of England; there were representatives from 18 nations, including 9 Latin American countries. The participants discussed the problems of the severely disabled adult in the areas of housing, work and leisure time activities, interrelationships with others, and the inherent rights of the disabled to make decisions for themselves and to be accepted as human beings.

PROCEEDINGS OF NATIONAL CONFERENCE ON HOUSING AND THE HANDICAPPED. Convened by Goodwill Industries of America, Houston, Texas, September 10–12, 1974. 61 pages. Illustrated. 8½ × 11. 1974. Order from Health and Education Resources, Inc., 9650 Rockville Pike, Bethesda, Maryland 20014. $2.

More than 150 representatives of government and volunteer groups participated. Among the speakers were: Edward H. Noakes, AIA, president, National Center for a Barrier-Free Environment; Mercer L. Jackson, minority staff member of the House Banking and Currency Committee and its Housing Subcommittee; Dr. Philip Roos, executive director of the National Association for Retarded Citizens; Jayne Shover, executive director of the National Easter Seal Society for Crippled Children and Adults; Dr. Andrew S. Adams, Commissioner, Rehabilitation Services Administration, HEW; and Dean Phillips, president, Goodwill Industries of America.

Conference recommendations included: form a permanent coalition, develop a data information and referral system, develop a public information program, help educate the disabled toward attaining their civil rights, support research into existing housing, encourage the use of HUD-held unoccupied housing, develop a compliance mechanism, provide technical support services, and endorse national health legislation that includes attendant care for personal needs, prosthetics, and orthopedic equipment.

Index

Abt Associates, 148, 305
Accent on Access [Architectural Guidelines], 403
Access 76. Blueprint for Action, [Architectural Guidelines], 403
Access: Housing, 310, 333
Access, international symbol of, 381, 389
Accessible Towns–Workable Homes, 408
Accessibility
   alternative approaches, 290, 300
   college campuses, 290
   environment, 403–408
   housing, 353
   norms in different countries, 390–391
   public buildings, 10, 289, 291–294, 403, 405
Acoustics, 216
Adaptations and Techniques for the Disabled Homemaker, 11, 29
Adaptive Housing for the Handicapped, 299
Adventure in a Wheelchair, 220, 246
Advertising. *See* Newspaper advertising
Aging. *See* Elderly
Aids for the Severely Handicapped, 23
Aid to Independent Living, 29
Alabama
   information service, 113–114
   Lakeshore Rehabilitation Facility, 145–147
Alarm systems, 19, 20, 23, 56, 179, 220, 222, 225, 231, 233, 376
Alcoholics Anonymous, 87
Alien Attendants, 95, 96
ALPHA, 7
Alpha Place. *See* California
American Association for Retired Persons, 106, 206
American Coalition of Citizens with Disabilities, 8
American Foundation for the Blind, 89
American Institute of Architects, 5, 288, 289, 405
American National Standards Institute (ANSI), 5, 148, 211, 287, 291
   construction standards, 288, 289, 291
American Red Cross, 109
American Society for the Physically Handicapped, 252
Amyotonia congenita, 70, 91

Angus Mitchell House (Australia), 350–351
Annandale Village (Georgia), 271
Apartment living, 162–185, 278–280. *See also* Attendants, California, Independent living, Mexico, Sweden, Transitional facilities
   2100 Bloomington (Minnesota), 182, 184
   without supportive services, 177–184
      accessible housing and environment, 180–182
         Roswell, New Mexico, 180–182
      leased housing, 177–178
         HUD assistance, 177
      private apartments, 177
      subsidized housing (Section 236 program), 178–180
         Elmwood Park Tower (Michigan), 179
         Lakewood Plaza (Virginia), 178
         Ocean Village (New York), 179–180
         Wyandotte Co-op Apartments (Michigan), 179
   with supportive services, 163–177
      Atlantis Community, Inc. (Colorado), 169
         apartment renovation, 169
         attendants, 169
         costs, 169
         HUD financing, 169
      Bird S. Coler Hospital Pilot Study (New York), 171–172
      Creative Handicaps, Inc. (Texas), 166
         attendants, 166
         costs, 166
         transportation, 166
      Free Lives, Inc. (Texas), 166
      Handicapped Adults Association (New York), 172–173
      Independent Life Styles (Texas), 163–165
         admission criteria, 164
         architectural modifications, 163
         attendants, 165
         costs, 164
         legislation, 165
         meals, 165
         services, 164–165
         transportation, 165
      Independent Living for the Handicapped (New York), 170–171

Apartment living, *(continued)*
    Project Independence (Minnesota), 169–170
        apartment renovation, 170
        costs, 170
        services, 170
    Public housing, 173–177
        Massachusetts, 173–176
        Tanya Towers (New York), 176–177
An Apartment Living Plan to Promote Integration and Normalization of Mentally Retarded Adults, 162
Apartment renovation. *See* Architecture
Appliances. *See also* Kitchens
    electrical, 23, 30
    switches, 24–26
Aprons, 46
Architectural barriers, 8, 39, 79, 191, 287, 296, 354
    books about, 407–409
    guidelines, 403–407
    legislation, 288–293
    removal of, 5, 128, 257, 298, 299
    workshops on, 6
Architectural Barriers Board, 294
Architectural Facilities for the Disabled, 403
Architectural and Transportation Barriers Compliance Board, 290, 414
Architecture. *See also* Apartment living, Bathrooms, Barrier free design, Design, Guidelines, Kitchens, Legislation
    apartment renovation, 125, 131, 150, 163, 178
    books about, 281, 310, 370, 381–382, 403–408
    guidelines, 392–395, 403–407
    national design competition, 5
    Planen und Bauen fuer Behinderte, 370
    Selected Rehabilitation Facilities in the United States—An Architect's Analysis, 145, 407
Archives of Physical Medicine and Rehabilitation, 223
Arkansas, Hot Springs Rehabilitation Center, 145
    Our Way, Inc, 202
Arthritis, 12, 30, 31, 89, 132, 164, 173, 192, 213, 225, 232
Arts and the Handicapped. An Issue of Access, 403
Asia, 354–365. *See also* Japan
    books about, 383
    Journal of Rehabilitation in Asia, 356
    uselessness of wheelchairs, 356
Association for Retarded Children, 250, 257, 270
Atlantis Community, Inc. (Colorado), 167–169
Attendants, 84–99
    alien, 95–96
    California programs. *See* California

Attendants *(continued)*
    Danish, 368, 369
    disabled, 88–92
    family members, 369
    Fokus system, 397–398
    foster family, 96–97
    Het Dorp, 373
    hourly, 73–75, 79
    household chores, 64, 65, 67, 71, 91, 94, 123
    how to find, 71, 75, 79, 80, 86–88
    mentally retarded, 89–91, 232
    Mormon missionaries, 92–94
    newspaper advertising for, 75–80, 86–87, 93
    payment of, 65–69, 74, 79, 80, 86, 94, 96, 131, 136–137, 187
    Swedish helpers, 375
    Texas programs, 165
Attitudinal barriers, 5, 8, 296
Auckland Coordinating Council for the Disabled (New Zealand), 352–353
Australia, 342–352
    Angus Mitchell House, 350
    Bedford Industries Vocational Rehabilitation Association, 349
    books about, 383
    Brisbane Spastics Centre, 347
    Cherrywood Village, 346
    Civilian Maimed and Limbless Association, 344–345
    Community Home Care Service, 347
    Deva Hostel, 352
    Glen Waverly Rehabilitation Centre, 351
    Hilltops Holiday House, 351
    home care services, 349–350
    Home for Incurables, 348
    House with No Steps, 342–343
    Meals on Wheels, 349, 350
    Mitchell Park Village, 348
    Paraplegic Association of South Australia, 348–349
    Paraplegic and Quadriplegic Association of New South Wales, 346
    Paraplegic Welfare Association of Queensland, 347
    Phoenix Society, Inc., 347
    Spastic Centre of New South Wales, 345–346
    Western Australia, 352
Automobiles, 40, 67, 83
    VA benefits, 160

Baking, 38, 43, 46
Barrier free design, 5, 6, 10, 128, 158, 182–184, 200, 207, 287, 289, 294, 297–299, 376–380, 397, 399, 403–408
Barrier Free Design, 403, 408
Barrier-Free Design, Accessibility for the Handicapped, 294

Barrier Free Design Graphics, 404
Barrier Free Environment, National Center, 5
Barrier-Free Site Design, 407–408
Barriers, environmental, 6, 10, 128, 200, 220, 237, 287, 300, 406–409. *See also* Architectural barriers, Attitudinal barriers, Legislation, Rehabilitation Act
Bathrooms, 56–63, 220, 230, 241, 293, 368, 405–406
 alarm system, 56
 bath chair, 62
 bathtub, 40, 220
  area, 56
  handrails, 56, 348
  height, 60
  on-the-bed, 60
  slip proofing, 60, 160
  vs. shower, 206, 209, 223, 228, 230, 340
 bedpan, 59
 books about, 12, 29–31, 63, 400, 405–407
 commode chair, 59
 construction standards, 293
 controls, 61, 63
 design, 40, 56–63, 163, 228, 397
 doors, 56, 63, 131, 160, 228, 241, 293
 electric outlets, 33, 56, 160
 floor space, 56, 63, 160, 199, 228, 293, 294
 gadgets, 61
 grab bars, 110, 131, 160, 179, 220, 228, 230, 241, 316, 340, 368
 hydraulic lifts, 40, 61, 131
 lavatory
  faucets, 195, 293, 316, 397
  height, 56, 61, 63, 293, 397, 405
  wall-hung, 294
  wheelchair, 61, 195, 220, 316
 light switch, 63, 160, 163, 293
 medicine cabinets, 56, 196, 293, 397
 mirrors, 56, 184, 293
 mobile homes, 206, 209–210
 remote control cleansing, 57, 58
 shower, 228, 241, 348, 397
  clear space, 56, 293
  controls, 56, 293
  hand-held, 60, 220, 230
  seats, 40, 60, 110, 230, 293, 340
  wheel-in, 157, 163, 184, 199, 230
 toilet, 57–59
  attachments, 57
  chemical, 59
  Clos-o-Mat, 57, 58, 339
  Destroilet, 59
  handrails, 56, 177
  height, 56, 57, 160, 195, 220, 226, 230, 241, 340, 405
  portable, 57–59
  seats, 57, 228

Bathrooms, toilet *(continued)*
  supports, 57, 337, 368
  urinals, 57–59
  wall-hung, 228
Battin-Fielding Memorial Housing (Canada), 322–324
Bedford Industries Vocational Rehabilitation Association (Australia), 349
Bedrooms, 40, 72
 Balkan frame bed, 73
Beitler and Associates, 209–210
Belgium, accessibility norms, 390
 home help services, 101
Bellwoods Park House (Canada), 324–325
Bibliographies, 408–409
Bird S. Coler Hospital, 171, 200
Blind
 aids for, 412
 counseling, 129
 housing, 173, 217, 223–225, 349
 room thermostat, 405
The Blind: Space Needs for Rehabilitation, 412
Books
 architecture, 281, 370, 381–382, 403–408
 barrier free design, 403–408
 bathrooms, 12, 29–31, 63, 400, 405, 406, 407
 blind, 412
 developmentally disabled, 281–285
 elderly and handicapped, 10, 29–31, 403–408, 413
 home health services, 117–118
 housing adaptation, 11, 12, 29–31, 403–407, 414–415
 kitchens, 11, 12, 29, 54–55, 400, 405, 406
 landscape, 407–408
 mental retardation, 281–285
 talking, 115
 urban planning, 408
Boston Center for Independent Living, Inc., 149
Boston Housing Authority, 173–175
Brake, uses for, 71
Brandeis University model home care program, 112
Bread board uses, 33, 35, 40
Brisbane Spastics Centre (Australia) 347
Building codes, 291–294, 299. *See also* Legislation
Building plans, 29–31, 41, 54–55, 110, 135
Built Environment for the Elderly and Handicapped, 408
Burners, 33–35, 51

California Association for the Physically Handicapped, 7

California
  attendant programs, 119–138
    Alpha Place, 130–132
      apartment renovation, 131
      attendants, 131
      expenses, 131
    Center for Independent Living, 8, 119, 139, 140
      client services program, 128
      communications, 128
      community environment, 128
      funding, 130
      student program, 127
      supportive services, 129
    Farm House Motel, 133
    funding to disabled, 119
    Glass Mountain Inn, Inc., 132–133
    Handicapped Independence Proven, 135–137
      attendants, 137
      conversion of existing facilities, 135
      resident costs, 136
      staff salaries, 136
    Homemaker/Chore Service, 119–120, 136
    Medi-Cal, 119–120, 124, 125, 131
    Rancho Los Amigos Hospital Home Care Plan, 120–123
    RSVP at Rippling River, 133–134
    Spastic Children's Foundation, 123–126
      Activity Center, 126
      dependent dorms, 124
      independent apartments, 125
      semidependent housing, 124
      semiindependent housing, 124–125
      Therapy Department, 126
      Transportation Department, 126
  college facilities, 148
  Contempo Care, 203
  housing studies, 294–297
  Pilgrim Tower, 216–217
  solo living, 72
Camphill Village (New York), 263
Canada, 306–333
  accessibility norms, 390
  Action League for Physically Handicapped Advancement (ALPHA), 7
  Cheshire Home Foundation–Canada Inc., 326–331
    Ashby House Group, 330
    Cheshire Homes of York, Inc, 329
    Clarendon House, 329
    Durham Region Home, 330
    Hastings–Prince Edward Home, 329
    McLeod House, 327–328
    Saskatoon Cheshire Home, 331
  group homes, 313
  Handicapped Housing Society of Alberta, 309
    charette, 309–310
    housing master plan, 310–311
    registry and lifestyle research of disabled, 309

Canada (continued)
  home help services, 103, 108
  housing, disabled, 307–311
    low rental, 331–332
  Housing and Urban Development Association of Canada, 314
  information sources, 284–285, 312
  model home, 314–316
  residential facilities, long term, 322–326
    Battin-Fielding Memorial Housing, 322–324
    Bellwoods Park House, 324–325
    Maison Lucie Bruneau, 325–326
    Participation House, 325
  service organization, 311–314
    Canadian Paraplegic Association, 311, 313
    Handicapped Resource Centre, 312–314
    Local Initiatives Program, 311–312
    Social Planning and Review Council of British Columbia, 308
  social security, 306
    Central Mortgage and Housing Corporation, 307, 313–316, 330
    financial assistance for disabled, 306–307
    national registry, 307
    vocational rehabilitation, 307
  Toronto Task Force, 308
  transitional homes, 316–322
    Elves House, 316–317
    Paraplegic Lodge, 316–317
    Point Pleasant Lodge, 322
    Wheelchair Housing Centre, 321–322
Canadian Paraplegic Association, 311, 313, 317–321
Canadian Rehabilitation Council for the Disabled, 307–308
Can openers, 30, 49
Carpeting, 41
Casters, uses for, 19, 44, 50, 337, 356
Catalogs. See Mail catalogs
Center for Independent Living. See California
Center Park Apartments. See HUD housing projects
Cerebral palsy, 76, 88, 113, 133, 141, 155, 173, 175, 192, 206, 253, 254, 326
Chairs, 44, 59, 62
Charette, 309–310
Cherrywood Village (Australia), 346
Cheshire Home Foundation–Canada Inc. See Canada
Cheshire Homes (Great Britain). See Great Britain
Cheshire Homes (New Jersey), 202, 326–311, 335
Christian League for the Handicapped (Wisconsin). See Residential facilities
Christopher Founders, Inc., 248–249

Church-sponsored respite care programs, 109
Civilian Maimed Association (New Zealand), 354
Civilian Maimed and Limbless Association (Australia), 344–345
Civil Rights Act, 8
Civil rights of disabled, 6, 8, 114, 129, 291
Closets, 199, 232, 293
Clothes washing. *See* Laundry
COHOPE (Virginia), 274–275
College living. *See* Transitional facilities
Colorado, apartment facilities, 167–169
 Atlantis Community, Inc., 167–169
Communal living, 71, 77–79, 147–149. *See also* Developmentally disabled, Residential facilities
Community care homes, 115
Community Home Care Service (Australia), 347
Community Living Centers, Inc. (Michigan), 274
Community Planning for the Elderly, 413
Connecticut
 McLean Home, 192–195
 New Horizons Wing, 192, 201
Contempo Care (California), 203
Co-op City (New York), 172
Cooperative Living Concept (Texas), 151–153
Counseling services
 Australia, 342, 345
 California, 122, 129, 134
 New York, 171
Counters. *See* Kitchens
Courage Center (Minnesota), 195
Creative Handicaps, Inc. (Texas), 166
Creative Living. *See* HUD housing projects
Cupboards. *See* Kitchens
Cutting board, 39, 47
Czechoslovakia, 365, 383

Deaf, special housing, 176, 216, 224, 276, 349, 405
Denmark
 accessibility norms, 390
 apartment building for disabled, 4
 Hans Knudsens Plads, 366–369
 home help services, 101–102
Denver Housing Authority, 167–169
Dermatomyositis, 92
Design. *See also* Apartment living, Barrier Free Design, Bathrooms, Guidelines, HUD housing projects, Kitchens, Landscaping
Designing for the Disabled, 404
Deva Hostel (Australia), 352
Developmental Disabilities Acts, 5, 256, 258, 272, 279, 280
Developmentally disabled, 256–285
 books about, 281–285
 foster homes for adults, 262

Developmentally disabled *(continued)*
 group apartments, 278–280
  converted shopping centers (Ohio), 278–279
  Developing Opportunities in Individual Responsibility (Pennsylvania), 279–280
  Young Adult Institute Residence (New York), 278
 group homes, 272–275
  COHOPE (Virginia), 274–275
  Marlborough House (Missouri), 275
  Michigan State Housing Authority Community Centers, 272–274
 Hope Haven Work Training Center (Iowa), 262, 263
 hostel apartments, 275–278
  Elmer Lux Hotel (New York), 277
  Exceptional Persons, Inc. (Iowa), 277–278
  New York State hostels, 275–276
  Tanya Towers (New York), 276–277
 intermediate care facilities, 261–262
  Echoing Hills Residence Center (Ohio), 261
  Phoenix Residence (Minnesota), 261–262
 legislation, 256–257
 nursing homes, 258–261
  Senate report, 260
  suitability for young disabled, 258, 260
  Tender Loving Greed, 260
 state institutions, 258
 villages, 263–271
  Annandale Village (Georgia), 271
  Camphill Village (New York), 263
  Fircrest Halfway Houses (Washington), 263
  Handicap Village (Iowa), 268–269
  Lambs Farm (Illinois), 271
  Mount Olivet Rolling Acres (Minnesota), 269–270
  Opportunity Village (Ohio), 270
  Rainbow Village (Missouri), 270–271
Developing Opportunities in Individual Responsibility (Pennsylvania), 279–280
Developmental disabilities, 256–285
Diabetes, 173
Disabled, civil rights of, 6, 8, 114, 129, 291
 definition of, 286–287
 residential care needs studies, 294–304
Disabled in Action, 7
Disabled Citizens' Society (New Zealand), 353
Disabled Re-Establishment League, Inc. (New Zealand), 353
Dishes. *See* Kitchens.
Doors, 18–19, 406
 accessibility norms, 390–391
 bathroom, 56, 63, 131, 163, 178, 180, 228, 293

Doors *(continued)*
    check, 26
    closet, 199, 216, 232
    garage, 26, 40
    handles, 19, 163, 220, 232
    hinges, 18
    keys, 19
    kitchens, 33, 35-37, 40, 43, 45, 49, 55, 184, 293
    locks, 26, 63, 405
    openers, 25, 26, 397
    oven, 33, 35, 232
    refrigerator, 36, 37
    widening of doorway, 18, 163, 339
Drains, installation of, 33, 39
Dycem, 48
Dystonia, 46

Eastern Paralyzed Veterans Association, 139, 140, 157-159
Echoing Hills Residence Center, 261
Education by telephone, 20
Elderly
    books about, 413-414
    home help services, 102, 109-110, 114
    increasing numbers of, 2, 287
    legislation, 7
    organizations, 6, 7
    public housing, 173-177, 212-245, 276, 299, 332, 336, 342, 349
    vacation program, 115, 116
Electric outlets, 33, 47, 56, 160, 220, 293, 339, 397
Electronic equipment. *See* Alarm systems, Intercom, Remote control systems, Telephones
Elevators, 15-18, 216, 222, 236, 253, 294, 298, 397
Elimination of Architectural Barriers to the Disabled, 408-409
Elmer Lux Hostel (New York), 277
Elmwood Park Towers (Michigan), 179
Elves House (Canada), 316-317
Emphysema, 187
ENCORE, 115
Encyclopedia of Associations, 6
England.
    See Great Britain
Entrances, 12-15, 220, 229
Environmental barriers. *See* Barriers
Environment control system, 21
Epilepsy, 141, 173
Equipment sources
    bathroom, 56
    electrical, 28
        Great Britain, 410-411
    kitchen, 46
        Sweden, 411
    laboratory, 28
    telephone, 27, 28
European home help programs, 100-103

Evergreen Apartments (New York), 177
Exceptional Persons, Inc. (Iowa), 277-278

Farm House Motel (California), 133
Faucets, 30, 45, 47, 61, 72, 195, 220, 231, 397
Federal Housing Authority (FHA), housing project financing, 240, 249
    mobile home financing, 205
    survey of housing needs, 248
Feedback Journal, 132
Filling pans with water, 45, 47
Financing. *See also* Medicare, Medicaid, California, Michigan
    apartments, 169, 179
    European home help programs, 102
    Fokus system, 399
    Hill-Burton, 202, 249
    housing projects, 239-240, 249, 268, 273-275, 279-280
    information centers, 113
    mobile home loan programs, 160, 205
    residential facilities, long term, 202
    self help services programs, 130
    transitional projects, 151, 153, 317, 321
    wheelchair homes (VA), 159-160
Finland, 370, 384
    accessibility norms, 390
    home help services, 101-102
Fircrest Halfway House (Washington), 263
Fishing, 66
Flask holder, 24
Floors, 216
Florida
    Goodwill Industries-Suncoast, Inc., 199
    Key Palm Villa, 203
    Rambling Pelican Garden Villa Condominium, 203
Foam rubber, 41, 48, 59
Food preparation, 33, 44, 46-50, 53, 54.
    See also Independent living, Kitchens
Fokus Society. *See* Sweden
Ford Foundation, 248
Foster family attendants, 96-97
Foster homes, 262
France, 371-373
    accessibility norms, 390
    home help services, 101-102
    travel guide for disabled, 371, 385
Free Lives, Inc. (Texas), 166
Freedom Gardens for the Handicapped (New York), 186-187
Friedreich's ataxia, 155, 326

Gadgets
    bathroom, 61
    books about, 29-31
    kitchen, 30, 46

Garage, 12, 40, 220, 232, 340, 397, 405
Garage door openers, 26, 28
Georgia, Annandale Village, 271
  Georgia Rehabilitation Center, 145
Germany, 369-370
  accessibility norms, 390
  Fokus housing, 399
  health insurance, 369
  home help services, 101-102
  publications, 384
  residential facilities, 370
  Stiftung Rehabilitation, 369
Glass Mountain Inn, Inc. (California), 132-133
Glen Waverly Rehabilitation Centre (Australia), 351
Goodwill Industries of America, 5, 166, 233-237, 278. *See also* Residential facilities, long term
Grab bars, 110, 131, 160, 179, 220, 226, 316, 340
Great Britain.
  accessibility norms, 390
  disabled and elderly, care of, 7, 303-304
  disabled, statistics, 385, 406
  Disabled Living Foundation, 11, 21, 54
  disablement income group (DIG), 7
  home help services, 101-103
  hospital training, 141
  housing
    mobility, 406
    prefabricated, 339-340
    public, 406
    self-contained, 336-339
      Habinteg, 337-338
      Inskip St. Giles Housing Association, 338
      John Groom's Association for the Disabled, 339
      Thistle Foundation, 339
      Wheelchair, 407
  legislation
    Chronically Sick and Disabled Persons Act, 103, 117, 341
    Department of Environment circular, 341
    Working Party on Housing for Disabled People, 341
  publications, 385
  remote control systems, 21
  residential facilities, 334-336
    Charities digest, 336
    Cheshire Homes, 335, 354
      adaptations, 335
      costs, 335
      management, 335
      residents, 335
    Marie Foster Home, 336
    Royal Hospital and Home for Incurables, 336
    Spastics Society, 335, 338
  spinal cord injuries facilities, 340
  younger chronic sick units, 340

Group homes, Canada, 313
Group Homes: One Alternative, 272
Guardrails, 13
Guide de la France pour les Handicapés Physiques, 371, 385
Guidelines
  architectural, 403-407
  housing programs, 392
  mentally retarded, 395

Habinteg (Great Britain), 337-338
Handbook for Housing the Handicapped in Public Housing Facilities, 176
Handicap Village (Iowa), 268-269
Handicapped Adults Association, 172-173
Handicapped Independence Proven, 135-137
Handicapped Services Center, 175-176
Handi-Ramp, 13, 14
Handles, door, 19, 163, 220, 232
Handrails, 13, 56, 177, 216, 293, 339
Health insurance, 8, 104, 369. *See also* Medicaid, Medicare, Social security
Hearing impairment, 141
  telephone services, 19
Heat, radiate, 407
Helping All the Handicapped, 298
Het Dorp: A Unique Experiment in Humanity, 373, 385
HEW, 5, 148-151, 261
  approval of state social services, 107
  funding, electronic control systems, 22
    New Jersey Statewide Computerized Referral Information Program (SCRIP), 113
    Texas Institute for Rehabilitation and Research, 151
  housing studies, 252, 300-301
  report on Medicare, 105
  study of facilities for college students, 148
  vacation program, 115-116
  Vocational Rehabilitation Administration, 262
Highland Heights Apartments (Massachusetts), 224-227
Hill-Burton Act, 202, 249
Hilltops Holiday Home (Australia), 351
Hinges
  card table, 33
  door, 18
  oven, 37
Holland. *See* Netherlands
Home economists, 110
Home health care agencies
  church-sponsored respite care program, 109
  home economists' programs, 110
  information centers, 113-114

Home health care agencies *(continued)*
  occupational therapy programs, 109–110
  Oklahoma program, 110–112
  Personal Care Organization, 112–113
  Red Cross aides training course, 109
  Visiting Nurse Association, 108–109
  voluntary organizations, 114
Home Health in Chinatown, 115
Home help services, 100–118
  Canadian programs, 103
  European programs, 100–103
    Denmark, 368–369
    financing, 102
    Fokus system, 397–398
    services, 102, 398
    Sweden, 375
    training, 101
  United States programs, 103–114
    health care agencies, 108–114
    Medicaid, 105–106
    Medicare, 104–105
    National Council for Homemaker-Health Aide Services, 107–108
    Social Services Amendments, 106–107
Home for Incurables (Australia), 348
Homemaker, disabled. *See also* Home help services, Information centers
  books about, 11, 12, 29–31, 54, 55
  model home, 314–316
  traveling demonstration, 116
Homemaker/Chore Service, 119–120, 136, 166
Hope Haven Work Training Center (Iowa), 262
Hospitality Home (California), 250
Hostels, 275–278
House, ownership, 64, 77
  rental, 71, 80
House With No Steps (Australia), 342–343
Household chores, 65, 67, 71, 80, 91, 123.
  See also Kitchens
Housing
  adaptation, 11–28
  basic library, 11, 12
  conference proceedings, 414–415
  failures, 247–255
  group, 271–275
  HUD-assisted, 212–245
  in 1950s and early 1960s, 2–4
  in late 1960s and early 1970s, 4–6
  prototype, 5
  public, 173–177, 406
    Boston Housing Authority program, 173–176
    Great Britain, 406
    Handicapped Services Center, 175–176, 212
    Tanya Towers, 176–177
  studies of, 294–304
Housing Alternatives for Handicapped Adults (1974 conference), 158

Housing Authorities
  Boston, 297
  Denver, 167–169
  Fall River, 224
  Federal (FHA), 205, 240, 248, 249
  Madison, 153–154
  Michigan State, 272–274, 392–395
  Philadelphia, 301
  Seattle, 219–221
  Toledo, 213
Housing and Community Development Act.
  See Legislation
Housing for the Elderly, 413
Housing the Handicapped, 404–405
Housing Needs of the Handicapped, 297–298
Housing the Physically Impaired, 405
Housing project failures, 247–255
  Christopher Founders, Inc. (Michigan), 248
  Hospitality Home, Inc. (California), 250–251
  Iron Lung Polios and Multiplegics, Inc. (Ohio), 247–248
  Motel, 66 (California), 255
  New Horizons, Inc. (Connecticut), 251–252
  Overbrook Hall (Pennsylvania), 253–254
  Rochester complex (New York), 249–250
Housing for Special Needs, 405
Housing and Urban Development (HUD), 149, 177, 248, 272–273
  definition of disabled, 286
  financing of housing for disabled, 134, 153, 169, 173, 273
  housing projects, 212–245
    Center Park Apartments (Washington), 219–223
      alarm systems, 222
      elevators, 222
      garage doors, 220
      kitchens and bathrooms, 220
      public transportation, 223
      residents, 222
      services, 222
    Creative Living (Ohio), 237–245
      architectural features, 240–241
      community involvement and fund raising, 239–240
      costs, 242–243
      federal assistance, 240
      meals, 244
      residents, 241–242
      staff, 243
      transportation, 245
    Highland Heights Apartments (Massachusetts), 224–227
      architectural features, 226
      costs, 227
      research report, 226–227
      services, 225–226
    Independence Hall (Texas), 233–237

Housing and Urban, projects *(continued)*
    architectural features, 236–237
    costs, 237
    services, 236
  New Horizon Manor (North Dakota), 228–233
    architectural features, 228–232
    residents, 232–233
    transportation, 233
  Pilgrim Tower (California), 216–217
    communication system, 217
  Vistula Manor (Ohio), 213–216
    architectural features, 215–216
    services, 216
  Walter B. Roberts Manor (Nebraska), 223–224
  Interim Report on ANSI standards, 287, 291
  legislation and regulations
    FHA Section 236, 166, 178, 179, 183, 233, 237, 273, 279
    Section 8, 154, 177, 184, 279
    Section 202, 153, 177
    Section 815, 212
  mobile home design, 210–211
  mobile home loan program, 204–205
  national design competition for adaptable housing, 5
Housing and Urban Development Association of Canada (HUDAC), 314–316
HUD Challenge, 116, 211
Hydraulic lifts, 12, 18, 40, 60–62, 68, 261

Illinois
  Chicago building code, 294
  Lambs Farm, 271
  Winning Wheels, Inc., 201–202
Income tax
  information, 115
  rehabilitation expense, 18
  renovation costs, 292–293
Independence Hall (Texas), 200, 233–237
Independent Life Styles. *See* Apartment living
Independent living. *See also* Attendants, California, Mexico, Transportation
  cooking, 65, 72, 94
  employment, 64, 67, 70, 72, 73, 74, 77–79, 83, 97
  expenses, 65, 67, 69, 71, 74, 75, 78–80, 92, 94, 96, 97
  home care routine, 65, 67, 68, 71, 73, 75, 78, 94, 96, 97
  housing, 64, 67, 69, 71, 72, 77, 79, 80
  income, 64, 67, 69, 71, 74, 75, 77
  laundry, 67, 94
  marriage, 68–70, 79, 80, 91–94
  personnel management, 65, 67, 69, 71, 74, 75, 76, 79, 83
  shopping, 65, 69, 71

Independent living *(continued)*
  social life and entertainment, 66–73
  travel, 67, 73, 77
Independent Living for the Elderly, 109
Independent Living for the Handicapped, 170–171
Indiana, Pleasant View Nursing Home, 210
Information centers, 113–114, 409–412
  Alabama, videotape and newsletter, 113, 114
  California Center for Independent Living, 119, 126–130
  Central Council for the Disabled, 409
  Disabled Living Foundation, 410
  Equipment for the Disabled, 410–411
  ICTA Information Centre, 411
  National Association of Housing and Redevelopment Officials, 411
  National Easter Seal Society for Crippled Children and Adults, 411–412
  New Jersey Statewide Computerized Referral Information Program, 113
  New York City Mayor's Office of the Handicapped, 114
  Philadelphia Mayor's Office of the Handicapped, 114
  Rehabilitation International, 412
  Rehabilitation International USA, 412
Information sources, Developmentally Disabled
  Canada, 284
  Great Britain, 285
  United States, 282–284
Inglis House (Pennsylvania), 198
Inskip St. Giles Housing Association (Great Britain), 338
Institute of Rehabilitation Medicine, 141, 215
Institutions de Réadaption, 382
Intercom systems, 20, 40, 163, 166, 240, 241, 397
INTERFACE, 6
International Commission on Technical Aids (ICTA), 11, 411
Into the Mainstream: A Syllabus for a Barrier-Free Environment, 405–406
Introduction to Domestic Design for the Disabled, 406
Iowa
  building conformance study, 289
  Exceptional Persons, Inc., 277–278
  Goodwill Industries of Des Moines, 199
  Handicap Village, 268–269
  Hope Haven Work Training Center, 262–263
  Wall Street Mission Goodwill Industries, 200
Ireland, accessibility norms, 391
Iron lung polios, 2, 247–248
Iron Lung Polios and Multiplegics, Inc., 247–248

Ironing, 33, 43, 44, 52
Israel, accessibility norms, 391
Italy, accessibility norms, 391

Japan, 356-365
  Abilities Data Service, 363, 365
  Japan Abilities, Inc., 363-364
  Japan Sun Industries, 356-360
  medical rehabilitation, 360
  model home Tetra-Ace, 356-360
John Groom's Association for the Disabled (Great Britain), 339
Journal of Rehabilitation in Asia, 356

Kennedy-Mills bill, 106
Keys, door, 19
Kitchens, 32-55, 220, 231, 241, 293, 367, 376-380, 397, 405, 407
  baking, 38, 43, 46
  books about, 11, 12, 29, 54-55, 400, 405, 406
  bread board uses, 33, 35, 40
  built-in appliances, 30, 33, 35, 40, 54, 55
  burners, 33-35, 51, 228
  cabinet toe space, 40, 54, 184, 231, 293, 348
  can openers, 30, 49, 51, 72
  carpeting, 41
  construction standards, 293
  counters, 30, 33, 40, 184, 216, 220, 226, 337, 376-380, 397
    adjustable heights, 184, 220, 232, 376, 379, 405
  countertops, 33, 38, 41, 54, 220, 228, 231, 293
  cupboards, 33, 43, 220, 226, 230-231, 339, 348
  cutting boards, 39, 47
  design, 33-46
  dishes, 38, 39, 41, 43, 51, 52
  dishwasher, 30, 38-41, 43, 54
  doors, 40, 293
    oven, 29, 33, 35, 43, 184, 348
    refrigerator, 36, 37, 43, 45, 49
    sink, 43
  drains, 33, 39, 397
  drawers, 35, 37, 39, 40, 43, 40, 220
  Dycem, 48
  electric outlets, 33, 47, 55
  faucets, 29, 30, 45, 47, 72, 220, 231, 321, 397
  filling pans with liquids, 33, 45-48
  foam rubber, 41
  iron, 33, 44
  lapboard, 29, 43, 44, 48, 414
  lazy Susan, 30, 38-40, 43, 55
  light switches, 33, 39, 40, 231
  lighting, 33, 39, 40, 231
  magnets, 49, 50

Kitchens *(continued)*
  mixers, 38, 48, 51
  mobile home, 210
  oven, 33, 35, 37, 38, 40, 41, 46, 184, 226, 232, 348
  pantry, 37, 38, 40
  pegboard, 33, 43, 51, 54
  plastic bowl, 33, 48
  potholders, 48
  pots and pans, 33-35, 51
  push button controls, 35, 45
  range, 40, 45, 54, 199, 220, 293, 321
  refrigerator-freezer, 36-38, 41, 43-45, 72, 293, 339
  removing food from cooking liquid, 50
  serving carts, 50, 54
  shelves, 37, 40, 41, 43, 45, 50, 54, 220, 231, 293
  sinks, 29, 30, 33, 39, 40, 43, 47, 52, 53, 54, 72, 184, 199, 220, 293, 339, 348, 376, 397
  storage space, 33, 40, 50, 54, 199, 220, 293
  stove, 33, 51
  tongs, 49, 50
  utensils, 33, 35, 38, 43, 49-51, 72
  windows, 39
  work board, 45
  work space, 33, 45, 231, 293
Knives, 30, 47

Lakeshore Rehabilitation Center. *See* Transitional facilities
Lakewood Plaza (Virginia), 178
Lambs Farm (Illinois), 271
Landscape Design for the Disabled, 408
Landscaping, 348, 403, 407-408
Lapboard, 29, 43, 44, 48, 414
Laundry, 43, 50, 52, 67, 71
Lavatory. *See* Bathrooms
Lazy Susan. *See* Kitchens
Legal aid, 10
Legislation
  architectural barriers, 288-291
  Architectural Barriers Act (1968), 288-289
  building codes, 291-294, 307
    California, 128
    Canada, 307
    Chicago, 294
    Massachusetts, 294
    national, 291-292
    New Mexico, 407
    New York City, 294
    North Carolina, 292-294
  Civil Rights Act (1964), 8
  Developmental Disabilities Acts, 5, 256, 258, 272, 279, 280
  future, 165
  Housing and Community Development Act (1974), 5, 257

Index   427

Legislation, Housing *(continued)*
  construction loans, 290
  mortgage insurance programs, 290
  Massachusetts barrier-free housing, 297–298
  Mental Retardation and Community Health Centers Construction Act (1963), 258
  Minnesota barrier-free legislation, 289
  National Commission on Architectural Barriers, 288
  North Carolina barrier-free legislation, 289
  Older Americans Act, 7, 106
  Rehabilitation Act (1973), Amendments (1974), 5, 257, 286, 290
    Architectural and Transportation Barriers Compliance Board, 290, 414
    barrier-free work areas, 290
    definition of disabled, 286
    nondiscrimination under federal grants, 290
  Social Services Amendments (1974), 5, 106–107, 257
Liberation movements
  disabled, 7–8, 374–375
  elderly, 6–7
Lights. *See also* Switches
  kitchen, 33, 39, 40, 231
  remote control, 23
  signals, 217
Lifts
  hydraulic, 12, 61–62, 68, 261
  bathtub, 40, 60
  Hoyer, 61, 67, 94
  stair, 78
  wheelchair, 16–18

Made to Measure, 406
Madison Housing Authority, 153–154
Magnets, 48–50
Mail catalogs
  bathroom, 57, 60, 61
  Japan, 364–365
  kitchen gadgets, 46
  self-help, 31, 57
Maine, Abilities and Goodwill, Inc. 199
Maison Lucie Bruneau (Canada), 325–326
March of Dimes, 2, 3, 249
Marie Foster Home (Great Britain), 336
Marlborough House (Missouri), 275
Maryland
  community care homes, 115
  Rehabilitation Center, 145
Massachusetts
  building code, 294
  college student facilities, 149
  Highland Heights Apartments, 224–227
  information for disabled, 115
  public housing, 173–176, 297–300
Massachusetts Association of Paraplegics, 297–298

Mayor's Office of the Handicapped, New York City, 114
  Philadelphia, 114
McLean Home (Connecticut), 192–195
Meals on Wheels, 114, 349, 350
Mealtime Manual for the Aged and Handicapped, 12, 29
Measurements. *See also* Bathrooms, Kitchens, Accessibility (norms in different countries), Ramps
Medicaid, 105–106, 108–110, 114, 117, 140, 149, 192, 249
Medi-Cal. *See* California
Medicare, 104–106, 108–109, 117, 140, 149, 192
Medicine cabinets, 56
Mental retardation, 89–91, 141, 256
  books about, 162, 281–285
  housing, 162, 199, 263, 268, 269, 272, 274, 344, 392, 395
Mentally retarded attendants, 89–91, 112
Metric, 406
Mexico
  architectural barriers, 156
  Guadalajara residences, 156–157
  independent living for disabled, 154–157
  transportation, 156
Michigan
  Elmwood Park Tower, 179
  Housing Authority Community Centers, 272–274
  State Housing Authority Mentally Retarded Housing Program guidelines, 392–395
  Wyandotte Co-op Apartments, 179
Microwave oven, 38
Minnesota
  barrier-free apartments, 182–184
  barrier-free legislation, 289
  Commission for the Handicapped, 6
  Courage Center, 195
  Mount Olivet Rolling Acres, 269–270
  Phoenix Residence, 261–262
  Project Independence, 169–170
Mirrors, 51, 56, 184, 216
Missouri
  Marlborough House, 275
  Paraquad, Inc., 202
  Rainbow Village, 270–271
Mitchell Park Village (Australia), 348
Mixers, 38, 48, 51
Mobile homes, 160, 204–211
  advantages, 205
  disadvantages, 204
  factory adaptations, 206–209
  financing, 205
  floor plan, 206
  HUD studies, 210–211
  parks, 205–206
  Tips on Buying a Mobile Home, 204
Mobility for Handicapped Students, 149
Mobility Housing, 406

Model homes
  Canada, 314–316
  Japan, 356–360
Mormon attendants, 92–94
Moss, Senator Frank E., 106
Motel 66 (California), 255
Motion impairment, remote control systems, 21
  telephone services, 20
Mount Olivet Rolling Acres (Minnesota), 269
Mouthstick, 66–68, 81
Multiple sclerosis, 46, 68, 173, 192, 225, 232, 326
Multiple Sclerosis Society, 89, 167, 239, 250, 322, 323
Muscle atrophy, 46
Muscular dystrophy, 46, 164, 173, 187, 225, 326
Muscular Dystrophy Associations of America, 89, 167

National Aeronautics and Space Administration (NASA), 21
National Association of Physically Handicapped, 201
  NAPH Farm-Home, Inc. (New York), 201
National Center for Barrier Free Environment, 287
National Center for Voluntary Action, 114
National Council for Homemakers–Home Health Aide Services, 107–108
National Easter Seal Society for Crippled Children and Adults, 89, 178, 210, 403, 411
National Institute of Senior Centers, 115
National Paraplegia Association, 210
National Retired Teachers Association, 106
Nebraska
  traveling demonstrations for disabled, 116
  Walter B. Roberts Manor, 223–224
Netherlands, 373
  accessibility norms, 391
  Fokus housing, 399
  home help services, 101–102
  publications, 385
New Horizon Manor (North Dakota), 228–233
New Horizons, Inc. (Connecticut), 201, 251
New Horizons Wing (Connecticut), 192
New Jersey
  Cheshire Home, 202
  information centers, 113
New Mexico, accessible housing, 180–182
New York City
  Bird S. Coler Hospital Pilot Study, 171–172
  building code, 294
  Handicapped Adults Association, 172–173
  Housing Authority, 158

New York City *(continued)*
  Independent Living for the Handicapped, Inc., 170–171
  Mayor's Office of the Handicapped, 114
  Roosevelt Island, 200
  Tanya Towers, 176–177, 276–277
New York State
  Camphill Village, 263
  Elmer Lux Hostel, 277
  Freedom Gardens for the Handicapped, 186–187
  hostel program for developmentally disabled, 275–276
  housing studies, 302–303
  NAPH Farm-Home, Inc., 201
  Ocean Village, 179–180
New Zealand
  accessibility norms, 391
  Auckland Coordinating Council for the Disabled, 352–353
  Civilian Maimed Association, 354
  Disabled Citizens' Society, 353
  Disabled Re-Establishment League, Inc., 353
  home services, 354
  Laura Fergusson Trust for Disabled Persons, Inc., 353
Newspaper advertising for attendants, 75–80, 86, 87
North Carolina
  barrier-free legislation, 289, 292–293
  building codes, 292–294
  income tax deductions, 292–293
North Dakota, New Horizon Manor, 228–233
Norway, home help services, 101–102
  publications of architectural details, 381–382, 385
Nursing Home Care in the United States: Failure in Public Policy, 260, 281
Nursing homes, 70, 136, 167, 187, 193, 210, 258–261, 281–282, 299, 368. *See also* Developmentally disabled

Occupational therapy
  home service programs, 109–110, 117
  in-hospital training, 141
  Medicare, 104
Ocean Village (New York), 179
Ohio
  Christ Mission Goodwill Industries, 199
  Creative Living, 237–245
  Echoing Hills Residence Center, 261
  Iron Lung Polios and Multiplegics, Inc., 247–248
  Opportunity Village, 270
  Vistula Manor, 213–216
Oklahoma home care program, 110–112
Older Americans Act, 7, 106, 109

Ombudsman, 129
One hander's book, 30
Opportunity Village (Ohio), 270
Oregon, Portland Housing Authority, 178
Osteogenesis imperfecta, 132
Our Way, Inc. (Arkansas), 202
Outdoor adaptations, 12-15
Ovens. *See* Kitchens
Overbrook Hall (Pennsylvania), 253-254

Pantry. *See* Kitchens
Paper towels, 47
Paralyzed Veterans of America, 8, 54, 154, 203, 297-298
Paraplegia, 43, 115, 134, 139, 141, 164, 175, 239
Paraplegic Association of South Australia, 348-349
Paraplegic Lodge (Canada), 139, 317-321
Paraplegic and Quadriplegic Association of New South Wales (Australia), 346
Paraplegic Welfare Association of Queensland (Australia), 347
Paraquad, Inc. (Missouri), 202
Participation House (Canada), 325
Partitions, use of, 258-259
Pegboard, 33, 43, 51, 54
Pennsylvania
  Goodwill Industries of North Central Pennsylvania, 199
  information centers, 114
  Inglis House, 198
  Overbrook Hall, 253-254
  Pennsylvania Rehabilitation Center, 145
  Philadelphia housing studies, 300-301
  Philadelphia Mayor's Office of the Handicapped, 114
Personal Care Organization, 112, 113, 117
Phoenix Residence (Minnesota), 261
Phoenix Society (Australia), 347
Physical Environment and the Visually Impaired, 412
Physically Disabled Students Program, 72
Physically Impaired Association of Michigan, 7
Pilgrim Tower (California), 216-217
Planen und Bauen fuer Behinderte, 370
Planning for Disabled People in the Urban Environment, 408
Planning Kitchens for the Handicapped Homemakers, 54
Pleasant View Nursing Home (Indiana), 210
Plumbing. *See* Bathroom and Kitchens
Pneumobelt, 68
Point Pleasant Lodge (Canada), 322
Poland, accessibility norms, 391
Poliomyelitis, 2-4, 23, 41, 44, 68, 80, 130, 139, 187
  Fourth International Conference, 3

Porch lift, 16, 17
Possum Selector Unit. *See* Switches, Remote controls
President's Committee on Employment of the Handicapped, 8
Principles of the Fokus Housing Units for the Severely Disabled, 407
Project Independence, 169-170
The Promethean, 153
Prostheses, 8
Public housing. *See* Accessibility, Housing

Quadriplegia, 4, 23, 32, 41, 46, 64, 72, 77, 79, 80, 86, 94, 97, 134, 135, 139, 144, 151, 155, 159, 164, 166, 239, 248, 360, 361

Radio
  remote control, 23, 397
  switches, 24
Rainbow Village (Missouri), 270
Rambling Pelican Garden Villa Condominium (Florida), 203
Ramps
  automobile, 77, 80
  entrance, 131, 142, 160, 178
  folding, 13-15
  guardrails, 13
  handrails, 13
  indoor, 184
  motorcycle, 15
  portable, 13-15
  rehabilitation expense, 18
  standards, 13, 160, 294, 390-391
  street, 128
  surface, 13, 15, 160
Rancho Los Amigos Hospital Home Care Plan, 120-123
Range. *See* Kitchens
Refrigerator-freezer. *See* Kitchens
Rehabilitation Act (1973), Amendments (1974). *See* Legislation
Rehabilitation centers. *See* March of Dimes, Transitional facilities
Rehabilitation Digest, 307
Rehabilitation Gazette, 11, 46, 83, 192, 209, 248
  back issues, 401-402
Rehabilitation Record, 89, 174
Remote controls, 21-23, 57, 58, 219
Removing Architectural Barriers, 407
REPORT, 5
Residential care needs. *See* Surveys
Residential facilities
  building codes, 291-294
  long-term, 186-203. *See also* Canada, Great Britain
    Cheshire Home (New Jersey), 202

Residential facilities, long-term *(continued)*
  Christian League for the Handicapped (Wisconsin), 189–191
    costs, 190
    Intermediate Care Facility, 190
    spiritual emphasis, 190–191
    transportation, 190
    vocational training, 190
  Contempo Care (California), 203
  Courage Center (Minnesota), 195
  Freedom Gardens for the Handicapped (New York), 186–187
  Goodwill Industries of America, 198–200
    Abilities and Goodwill (Maine), 199
    Christ Mission Goodwill Industries (Ohio), 199
    Goodwill Industries of Des Moines (Iowa), 199
    Goodwill Industries of North Central Pennsylvania, 199
    Goodwill Industries–Suncoast (Florida), 199
    Goodwill Industries of Western Connecticut, 200
    Goodwill Terrace Apartments (New York), 199
    Independence Hall (Texas), 200
    Wall Street Mission (Iowa), 200
  Inglis House (Pennsylvania), 198
  Key Palm Villa (Florida), 203
  McLean Home (Connecticut), 192–195
    independent living, 193
    Nursing Home, 193
    Rest Home, 193
  NAPH—Farm-Home, Inc. (New York), 201
  New Horizons, Inc. (Connecticut), 201
  New Horizons Wing (Connecticut), 192
  Our Way, Inc. (Arkansas), 202
  Paraquad, Inc. (Missouri), 202
  Rambling Pelican Garden Villa Condominium (Florida), 203
  Roosevelt Island (New York), 200
  Virginia Home (Virginia), 191–192
Resource Guide for the Disabled of Massachusetts, 115
Respiratory centers, 3, 4
Rocking bed, 67, 68, 88
Roosevelt Island (New York), 200
Royal Hospital and Home for Incurables (Great Britain), 336
RSVP at Rippling River. *See* California

Safety-Walk, 13
St. Louis
  American Red Cross, 109
  Association for Retarded Children, 109
  Hearing and Speech Center, 116
San Francisco Home Health Service, 115
Scissors, 47, 71
Scotland
  Scottish Housing Authorities, 405
  Thistle Foundation, 231
Seattle Handicapped Club, 219–220
Seattle Housing Authority, 219–222
Selected Rehabilitation Facilities in the United States, 145, 407
Self-help aids, books about, 12, 29
Self-Help Manual for Arthritis Patients, 12, 30, 31
Self-help programs, 126–130
Services for Special Needs, 19
Serving carts, 50, 54
Showers. *See* Bathrooms
Sight switches, 21, 22
Signals for help, 26, 83, 396
Sinks. *See* Bathrooms, Kitchens
Smoke Detectors, 222, 241, 397
Social Security Act, 97, 106, 119, 136, 164, 257
  definition of disabled, 286
Social services agencies, 87
Social Services Amendments (1974), 5, 106–107, 118
Solo living, 72, 73
Sound switches, 23
Spain, 382
Spastic Centre of New South Wales (Australia), 345–346
Spastic Children's Foundation. *See* California
Spastics Society (Great Britains), 335
Specialty Homes, Inc. (Illinois), 209
Speech defects, 19, 20, 141
Spina bifida, 141, 164, 326
Spinal cord injury, 4, 141, 147, 151, 157, 225, 288, 326, 340
Spoons, 30, 47, 50
Stairway lifts, 17, 18
Standards. *See also* Legislation
  ANSI, 211
  building construction, 289, 293–294
  Great Britain, 406
  mobile homes, 210–211
  ramps, 13
  VA housing, 160, 288
State reports. *See* Individual states
Statistics
  disabled, 287–288
  elderly, 287
  Great Britain disabled, 385, 406
  United States Disabled, 287–288
Stiftung Rehabilitation, 369
Storage space. *See* Kitchens
Stoves. *See* Kitchens
Student attendants. *See* Attendants
Student Organization for Every Disability United for Progress (SO FED UP), 7
Supplemental Security Income (SSI), 71, 105, 114, 124, 125, 131, 134, 136, 140, 166

Surveys and Studies, 294–304
  residential care needs
    California, 294–297
    Great Britain, 303–304
    Massachusetts, 297–300
    New York State, 302–303
    Philadelphia, 300–301
Sweden
  accessibility norms, 391
  Fokus Society, 376, 381, 396–399, 407
    background, 396
    benefits, 398
    cost comparisons, 399
    design, 397
    home helpers, 398
    integration, 396–397
    research projects, 396
    services, 397–398
  home help services, 101–102, 116, 375
  housing for handicapped, 374, 376
  organizations for handicapped, 374–375
  Service Houses, 380–381
  transitional facilities, 139
Switches
  accessibility norms, 390–391
  head operated, 361–362
  light, 24, 33, 63, 150, 160, 231, 241, 321, 339
  Possum, 21, 357, 360
  sight, 21, 22
  sound, 23
  toggle, 24
  wall, 24
  whistle, 23
Switzerland, 382
  accessibility norms, 391
  home help services, 101–102

Talking books, 115
Tanya Towers (New York), 176–177, 276–277
Telephones, 27–28
  buying of, 27
  dialing, 27, 81–83, 93
  education by, 20
  equipment, 19–20, 27, 28
  remote control, 23
  special services, 19, 114
  support, 24
Telephone Services for the Handicapped, 20
Television
  remote control, 22, 23
  switches, 24, 25
Test tube holders, 28
Tetra-Ace model home, 356–360
Texas
  Creative Handicaps, 166
  Free Lives, Inc., 166
  Independence Hall, 233–237
  Independent Life Styles, 163–165

Texas Institute for Rehabilitation and Research, 139, 140, 149–153, 163, 165
Texas Rehabilitation Commission, 164–166
Thermostats, 241
  Thistle Foundation (Scotland), 339
Title XIX, 110, 249, 261
Title XX. *See* Social Services Amendments
Toggle switches, 24, 27, 28
Toilets. *See* Bathrooms
Toledo Metropolitan Housing Authority, 213
Toothbrushes, 61
Totally Disabled Helpers Association, 122
Transfer board, 19
Transitional facilities, 139–161. *See also* Canada
  college arrangements, 147–149
    Boston University, 149
    California, 148
    St. Andrews Presbyterian College, 148
    Southern Illinois University, 147–148
    University of Illinois, 147
    Wellington Hall, 149
  in-hospital training, 141
  Madison Housing Authority, 153–154
  Mexican projects, 154–157
  residential rehabilitation centers, 141–147
    Lakeshore Rehabilitation Facility, hospital unit, 146
      recreation, 147
      transitional unit, 146
      transportation, 146
      vocational training, 146
    Maryland Rehabilitation Center, model apartment, 145
      vocational training, 145
    Woodrow Wilson Rehabilitation Center, 141–145
      driver training, 144
      personal care training, 144
      vocational training, 144
  Texas Institute for Rehabilitation and Research, 149–153, 163
    background, 150
    Cooperative Living Concept, 151–153
    funding, 150–151
    HEW study grant, 151
  Veterans Administration, 157–160
    apartment housing plan, 157–159
    benefits, 159–160
    hospital-based home care, 157
Transmitter, 26
Transverse myelitis, 32
Transportation
  barriers, 296, 414
  communal, 110, 122, 125, 126, 131, 132, 146, 152, 165, 166, 170, 190, 233, 245, 261, 398
  information about, 114, 305
  legislation, 290
  in Mexico, 156

Transportation *(continued)*
 private, 67, 68, 71, 72, 75, 77, 80
 public, 128, 129, 223, 289, 290
Travel guide for disabled (Paris), 371
Traveling demonstrations, 116, 304
Typewriter
 remote control, 23
 use of toes, 82–83

Union of the Physically Disabled against Segregation (UPIAS), 7, 9
United Cerebral Palsy Associations, Inc., 89, 109, 170, 257, 263, 284
 Denver, 167
 Franklin County, Ohio, 278
 New York City, 276–277, 414
 Oregon, 178
 Philadelphia, 253–254
 Pittsburgh, 279–280
 Rochester, 250
 St. Louis, 275
 Western New York, 277
United Handicap Federation, 182–184
United States, accessibility norms, 391
United Way, 109, 169, 311
Urban America, 248
Urban planning, 408
Urinals, 57–59
Utensils. *See* Kitchens

Vacation residential exchange, 115–116
Velcro, 29, 59, 61, 62
Veterans Administration (VA), 4, 21, 167, 204–205
 automobiles, 160
 benefits, 159–160
 construction standards, 288, 291
 environment control system, 21, 22
 mobile home loan program, 204–205
 transitional living, 157–159
 wheelchair or 702 homes, 159–160
Villages. *See* Developmentally disabled
Virginia
 COHOPE, 274–275
 Lakewood Plaza, 178–179
 Virginia Home, 191–192
Vision impairment, telephone services, 20
Visiting Nurse Association, 108–109, 225
Vistula Manor (Ohio), 213–216
Vocational training, 144–146, 190, 195, 232, 243, 342–343, 349
Voluntary organizations, 9, 114

Wall switch, 24
Walks, outdoor, 12
Walter B. Roberts Manor (Nebraska), 223–224
Washington
 Center Park Apartments, 219–223
 Fircrest Halfway Houses, 263
West Germany. *See* Germany
West Virginia Rehabilitation Center, 145
Wheelchair. *See also* Accessibility, Bathroom, Kitchens
 battery-powered, 358
 dancing, 40
 dimensions, 31, 55, 406
 elevators for, 15–18
 garages for, 12, 40, 220, 232, 340
 lavatory, 61, 316
 mobile home adaptations, 206–210
 model home, 314–316, 356–360
 narrowing, 18, 55
 outdoor walks for, 12
 ramps, 13–15, 128
 remote control, 22, 23
 repair, 129, 148
 uselessness in Asia, 356
 VA housing, 159–160
Wheelchair Housing, 407
Wheelchair Housing Centre (Canada), 321–322
Wheelchair Interiors, 31
The Wheelchair in the Kitchen, 55
Whistle switch, 23
White House Conference on Aging, 6
White House Conference on Handicapped Individuals, 5
Windows, 39, 199, 293, 404, 414
Winning Wheels (Illinois), 201–202
Wisconsin
 Christian League for the Handicapped, 189–191
 Madison Housing Authority transitional facility, 153–154
Woodrow Wilson Rehabilitation Center. *See* Transitional facilities
Work board, 45
World Association to Remove Prejudice Against the Handicapped (WARPATH), 7
Wyandotte Co-op Apartments (Michigan), 179

Young Adult Institute Residence (New York), 278
Yugoslavia, 382